MEDICAL RADIOLOGY

Diagnostic Imaging

Editors:
A. L. Baert, Leuven
M. Knauth, Göttingen
K. Sartor, Heidelberg

M. Oudkerk · M. F. Reiser (Eds.)

Coronary Radiology

2nd Revised Edition

With Contributions by

S. Achenbach · M. Ackerman · H. Alkadhi · C. R. Becker · T. Boskamp · A. Broekema
N. Bruining · P. Buszman · P. J. de Feyter · G. J. de Jonge · W. F. A. den Dunnen · S. de Winter
R. Dikkers · R. R. Edelman · R. Erbel · T. G. Flohr · B. Goedhart · M. J. W. Greuter
J. M. Groen · P. Guyon · S. S. Halliburton · R. Hamers · A. Hennemuth · C. Herzog
U. Hoffman · J. P. Janssen · W. A. Kalender · M. T. Keadey · G. Koning · W. Kristanto
C. Kuehnel · A. Lansky · D. Li · G. Ligabue · J. Ligthart · M. J. Lipton · R. Marano
C. H. McCollough · S. Möhlenkamp · B. Ohnesorge · M. Oudkerk · G. L. Raff · P. Raggi
A. Rareş · G. P. Reddy · M. R. Rees · J. H. C. Reiber · G. D. Rubin · J. R. T. C. Roelandt
J.-L. Sablayrolles · A. Schmermund · U. J. Schoepf · L. J. Shaw · V. E. Sinitsyn · W. Stanford
A. E. Stillman · A. J. H. Suurmeijer · G. Tarulli · A. J. Taylor · J. C. Tuinenburg
E. J. R. van Beek · P. M. A. van Ooijen · R. Vliegenthart Proença · L. Wexler · C. S. White
J. C. M. Witteman · F. Zijlstra

Foreword by

A. L. Baert

With 267 Figures in 405 Separate Illustrations, 170 in Color and 37 Tables

Springer

Matthijs Oudkerk, MD, PhD
Professor of Radiology
University Medical Center Groningen
University of Groningen
Hanzeplain 1
P. O. Box 30.001
9700 RB Groningen
The Netherlands

Maximilian F. Reiser, MD
Professor and Chairman
Department of Clinical Radiology
University Hospitals – Grosshadern and Innenstadt
Ludwig-Maximilians-University of Munich
Marchioninistrasse 15
81377 Munich
Germany

Medical Radiology · Diagnostic Imaging and Radiation Oncology
Series Editors:
A. L. Baert · L. W. Brady · H.-P. Heilmann · M. Knauth · M. Molls · C. Nieder · K. Sartor

Continuation of Handbuch der medizinischen Radiologie
Encyclopedia of Medical Radiology

ISBN 978-3-642-06954-3 e-ISBN 978-3-540-32984-8

DOI 10.1007 / 978-3-540-32984-8

Medical Radiology · Diagnostic Imaging and Radiation Oncology ISSN 0942-5373

Softcover reprint of the hardcover 2nd edition 2009

Cover-Design and Layout: PublishingServices Teichmann, 69256 Mauer, Germany

Printed on acid-free paper – 21/3180xq
9 8 7 6 5 4 3 2 1 0

springer.com

Foreword

It is a great privilege to introduce this second, completely revised and updated edition of the first monograph dealing with both invasive and non-invasive coronary imaging.

This volume offers a comprehensive overview of the latest technological advances in coronary imaging and of the actual clinical role of this technique.

As in the first edition, the illustrations are numerous, of outstanding technical quality and selected appropriately to underscore facts and statements.

I am very much indebted to the editors, M. Oudkerk and M. F. Reiser, for their outstanding engagement and meticulous editing task in order to prepare this second volume in a record brief period of time, enabling us to include the latest developments in coronary radiology. They have been supported by a superb group of leading experts in the field for individual chapters.

This splendid volume should be on the shelves of all radiologists involved in cardiac radiology. Radiologists in training will find all relevant basic information to help them better understand and conduct coronary imaging, while the book is equally recommended to cardiologists and cardiac surgeons as a support in their daily clinical management of patients.

I am convinced that this second edition will meet with the same great success among readers as the first.

Leuven

Albert L. Baert

Preface

The coronary circulation was first described by Ibn al Nafis (1213–1288) in the thirteenth century. He published *Kitab Mujiz - The concise book* (1250) in Damascus (Syria) in which he writes the following: *"the nourishment of the heart is from the blood that goes through the vessels that permeate the body of the heart"*. After the first anatomical opening of the human body by Mundinus (1270–1326) in Bologna in 1305, it took almost 250 years before Vesalius (1514–1564) published the first anatomical drawing of the coronary arteries from observations of the post mortem human body in his famous *De Humani Corporis Fabrica* (1543), although Leonardo da Vinci (1452–1519) visualized the coronaries of animals earlier in his famous anatomical sketches. Visualization of the coronaries in the living human body had to wait for the development of radiology. In 1907, an X-ray atlas of the coronary arteries composed of analysis of human cadavers by Jamin and Merkel was published. In 1933, Rousthoi experimentally performed the first left ventriculography and coronary visualization. Radner, of Sweden, performed the first in vivo coronary angiogram by direct sternal puncture of the ascending aorta in the year 1945. The first selective cine frame coronary arteriogram was recorded by Mason and Sones, Jr., on October 30, 1958.

Diagnostic coronary angiography was developed through the 1960s and 1970s with diminishing procedure-related complication and mortality rates. Gruentzig performed the first percutaneous transluminal coronary angioplasty on September 16, 1977, in Zurich (Switzerland). In 1972, the first computerized tomographic images of the living human brain were made by Hounsfield and Cormack. Data acquisition took up to almost 5 min per rotation. In 1988, the first clinical continuously rotating CT systems were installed, enabling one-second and subsecond scanning. With the introduction of the multidetector systems from 2000 onwards, rotation times reached levels beyond 350 ms, permitting image time resolution down to 150 ms, which almost equals the time resolution of the non-mechanical electron beam computed tomography which was introduced in 1983. Since the coronaries move over a 3- to 5-cm distance per second and only rest in diastole for no longer than 100 ms, this high performance technology is absolutely mandatory for non-invasive imaging of the coronary arteries.

With this new CT technology, routine non-invasive examination of the coronary vessel wall becomes feasible and will provide information that could only be gathered previously with intra-vascular ultrasound. Initial studies on 4D coronary imaging, virtual coronary angioscopy and thrombus detection within the coronary arteries have been published, proving the feasibility of a wide range of new diagnostic applications in the coronaries. Also, new developments in magnetic resonance imaging open up non-invasive coronary vessel wall examination, in particular with recently released MR contrast agents.

This book covers the full scope of radiological modalities to examine the coronary arteries and the coronary vessel wall. Today, a complete new era has emerged in cardiac and coronary imaging in which everyone can be informed about the condition of his or her coronary arteries non-invasively and in one simple, short examination. Since every radiologist will visualize many coronaries daily during routine CT examinations, including those in asymptomatic patients, it is of the utmost importance not to neglect this information but to learn how to interpret and communicate it within the medical community and to the patient.

Since the release of the first edition, the field of coronary radiology has developed with turbulent speed. As breaking news is presented in the leading international media, non-invasive coronary imaging is requested by the patients themselves before any invasive procedure can be performed. With all these incentives, the major manufacturers of the radiological equipment involved are engaging in a real competition for the best image quality within the limitations of acceptable radiation exposure. Researchers from all over the world are publishing a vast body of evidence that non-invasive imaging of the coronaries is indeed a method from which almost every cardiovascular patient can profit.

It is foreseeable within the near future that not only the coronaries but a full cardiac examination, including cardiac function, can be assessed within acceptable radiation dose limits in one study. Furthermore, non-invasive coronary imaging will be mandatory for optimal planning of revascularization procedures.

This second edition of *Coronary Radiology* covers the latest developments. Not only new acquisition technologies, but also the substantial improvements made by postprocessing software developers, new fields of indication for coronary imaging and the latest guidelines on acute chest pain and coronary calcification assessment are discussed. All authors contributing to this edition are key international authorities in the field endorsed by both the European Society of Cardiac Radiology as well as the North American Society of Cardiac Imaging.

Together, they are moving non-invasive coronary imaging in a direction in which adequate detailed information on the condition of the coronaries will be available for every patient, not only in the Western world, but worldwide to a very high degree of standardization and quality.

Groningen
Munich

Matthijs Oudkerk
Maximilian F. Reiser

Contents

Coronary Anatomy

1

Gonda J. de Jonge, Peter M. A. van Ooijen, Jean-Louis Sablayrolles, Guido Ligabue, and Felix Zijlstra

CONTENTS

G. J. de Jonge, MD; P. M. A. van Ooijen, PhD
Department of Radiology, University Medical Center Groningen, University of Groningen, Hanzeplein 1, P.O. Box 30.001, 9700 RB Groningen, The Netherlands
J.-L. Sablayrolles, MD
Centre Cardiologique du Nord, 32–36 Rue de Moulins Gémeaux, 93200 Saint Denis, France
G. Ligabue, MD
Cattedra e Servizio di Radiologia, Policlinico di Modena, Via del Pozzo 71, 41100 Modena, Italy
F. Zijlstra, MD, PhD
Professor, Thorax-Center, Department of Cardiology, University Hospital Groningen, P.O. Box 30.001, 9700 RB Groningen, The Netherlands

1.1 Introduction

Knowledge of the physiology, normal and variant anatomy and anomalies of coronary circulation is essential for the assessment of coronary disease. Coronary disease accounts for a high morbidity and mortality, therefore, proper evaluation is necessary.

Traditionally, the coronary arteries were evaluated using conventional catheter coronary angiography. This technique, however, has some major disadvantages: The exact course of the coronary arteries may be difficult to assess, because of their complex three-dimensional anatomy which is displayed in two dimensions. This is a major problem, especially in the diagnosis of coronary artery anomalies. A misdiagnosis of the course of an anomalous coronary artery is reported to occur in up to 50% of cases (Schmid et al. 2006). Furthermore, catheter coronary angiography only provides information on the coronary artery lumen and not on the vessel wall, and it is an invasive procedure with a morbidity and mortality of 1.7% and 0.1%, respectively (Dikkers et al. 2006). Therefore, a non-invasive alternative was greatly desired.

In 1998, multi-detector computed tomography (MDCT) was introduced and since then, cardiac CT has played a major role in the evaluation of the coronary arteries. Before the introduction of this new technique, electron beam computed tomography (EBCT) had already been used to evaluate the heart, but because of the inferior spatial resolution compared with MDCT and the fact that it is not widely available, EBCT does not play a major role in cardiac imaging today (Wintersperger and Nikolau 2005).

With the advent of newer generations of CT scanners, the 64-slice MDCT, and more recently, the dual-source CT (DSCT), temporal and spatial resolution have improved dramatically, due to a higher gantry rotation speed. Consequently, image quality has improved and the number of motion artefacts have substantially decreased compared to earlier scanner generations (Achenbach et al. 2006). As a result of these developments, evaluation of the coronary artery tree is increasingly performed with CT.

In MDCT, the coronary anatomy is shown in axial slices, as in all other radiological studies. But besides these axial slices, coronary anatomy can also be evaluated using a three-dimensional visualization derived from these axial slices. With current software, oblique multiplanar reconstructions, curved multiplanar reconstructions, three- and four-dimensional volume rendering can be achieved without extensive manual manipulation necessary.

In this chapter, the physiology of the heart will be discussed, including the normal and aberrant anatomy of the coronary arteries using both two- and three-dimensional images.

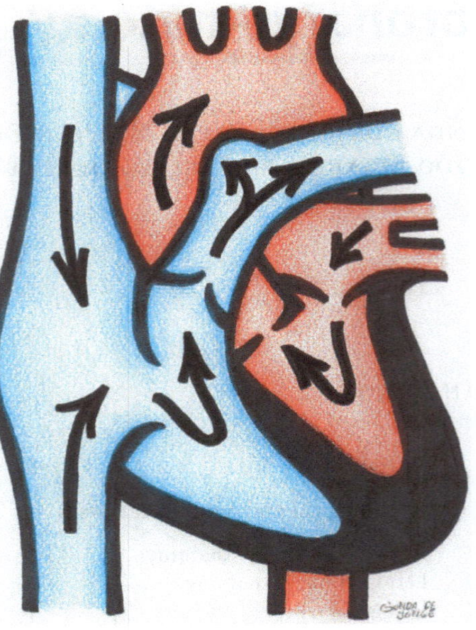

Fig. 1.1. The double pump-function of the heart

1.2 Physiological and Anatomical Bases

The heart can be considered as a regular ovoid lodged in the thorax between the lungs. This ovoid can be divided into four chambers: the two atria and the two ventricles with the aorta originating from the left ventricle and the pulmonary artery from the right ventricle. Each chamber has its own muscular wall, and the pericardial sac surrounds the whole structure. Due to the oblique position of the heart in the thorax, the chambers are positioned as follows:

- The left atrium is the most posterior of the chambers.
- The right atrium and the left ventricle are in a median position.
- The right ventricle is the most anterior of the chambers.

The pulmonary artery is situated anterior to the ascending aorta, which is slightly further to the left than the aorta.

The heart is made up of two parts: the right side of the heart, which pumps blood with low oxygen saturation into the lungs for oxygenation and the left side of the heart, which receives the oxygenated blood from the lungs and pumps it into the ascending aorta, from where it flows into the systemic circulation (Fig. 1.1) (Moore and Dalley 1999). The right side as well as the left side of the heart consist of a two-chamber pump, with both an atrium and a ventricle. With an atrial contraction, the blood is emptied into the ventricle, and the ventricle in turn supplies the main force that pushes the blood into the pulmonary trunk (right ventricle) or the systemic circulation (left ventricle) (Guyton and Hall 1996). The cardiac cycle consists of a period of ventricular relaxation (diastole) and a period of ventricular contraction (systole).

The heart has a fast, specialized nervous system which causes a smooth rhythmical contraction of the myocardium. The sinus node (also called the sinoatrial node or SA-node) generates an electrical impulse which causes atrial contraction. It is located in the wall of the right atrium at the junction of the right atrium and the superior vena cava. The impulse travels through the atria via the internodal pathways to the atrioventricular node (the AV-node) where the impulse is delayed before passing into the ventricle. This allows some time for the atria to fill the ventricle before ventricular contraction. The posterior septal wall of the right atrium immediately behind the tricuspid valve and adjacent to the opening of the coronary sinus is where the AV-node is located. The AV-node conducts the impulse further into the ventricles, through the Bundle of His and the Purkinje fibers (Guyton and Hall 1996).

The coronary arteries supply the myocardium with well oxygenated blood directly from the ascending aorta. They are the first branches of the aorta and originate from the left and right aortic sinus, just above the aortic valve. The distributional pattern of the coronary artery defines its name rather than its origin.

The walls of the left ventricle can be divided into three main segments (basal, medial and apical) (Fig. 1.2) with a further division into 16 sub-segments. The apical segment is divided into four sub-segments (Fig. 1.3), the medial segment (Fig. 1.4) and basal segment (Fig. 1.5) are both subdivided into six identical sub-segments. Each coronary artery provides a specific part of the myocardium with blood (Figs. 1.6–1.9). Depending on which coronary main branch is dominant, distribution may vary.

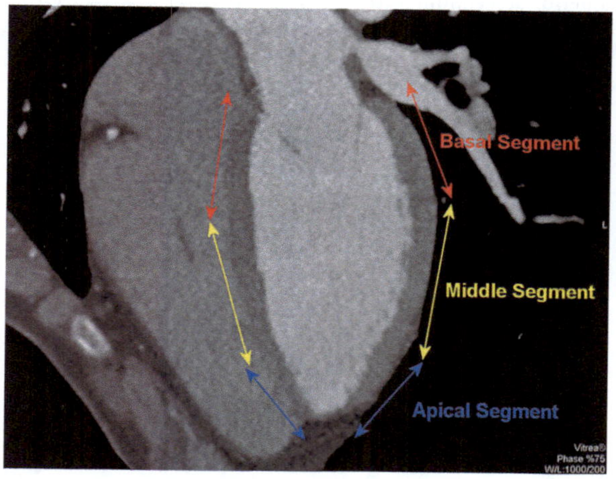

Fig. 1.2. Four-chamber view of the heart, subdivision of the left ventricle into three segments

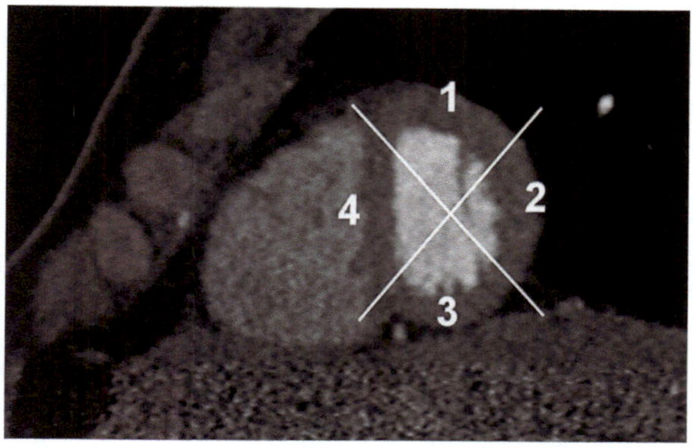

Fig. 1.3. Cross-section of the heart (*short axis*) through the apical segment, which can be divided into four sub-segments

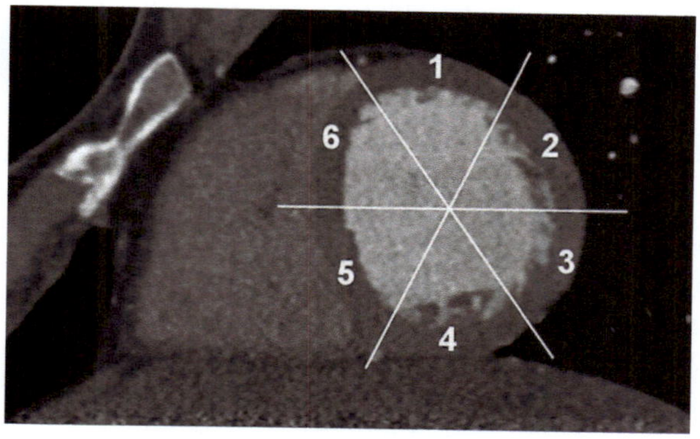

Fig. 1.4. Cross-section of the heart (*short axis*) through the middle segment, which can be divided into six sub-segments

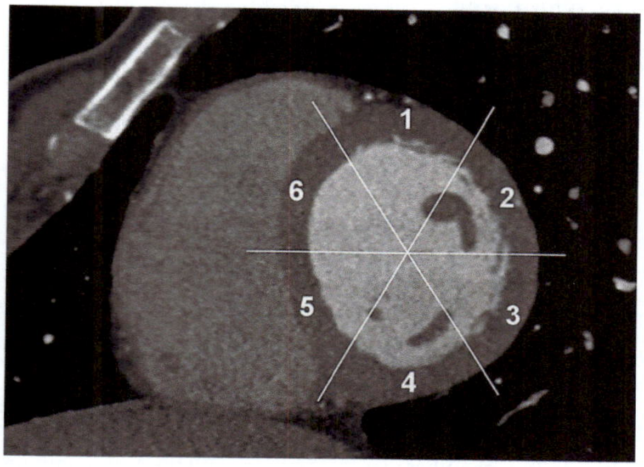

Fig. 1.5. Cross-section of the heart (*short axis*) through the basal segment, which can be divided into six segments

The heart is mobile around its axis, with rotation during systole and a varying volume between systole and diastole. The heart's volume is also affected by displacement of the diaphragm.

In systole, the opening of the aortic valve and the ventricular ejection jet creates a "vacuum pump" effect at the aortic coronary sinuses which hampers the movement of blood through the ostia of the coronary arteries. During contraction of the ventricular myocardium the subendocardial coronary vessels are compressed due to high intraventricular pressure. However, the epicardial coronary vessels remain patent. Because of this, blood flow in the subendocardium stops. As a result, most myocardial perfusion occurs during heart relaxation when the subendocardial vessels are patent and under low pressure. Cardiac diastole represents the moment of muscular and vascular silence: the heart is immobile, positions are fixed (apart from movements of the diaphragm controlled by breath-hold) and there is easier and thus better filling of the coronary arteries during the full diastolic phase.

On the ECG the periods of cardiac immobility or diastole begins slightly later than the R-wave and lasts until the Q-wave (on the ECG the centre of diastole is situated at about 70% of an RR-complex) (Fig. 1.10).

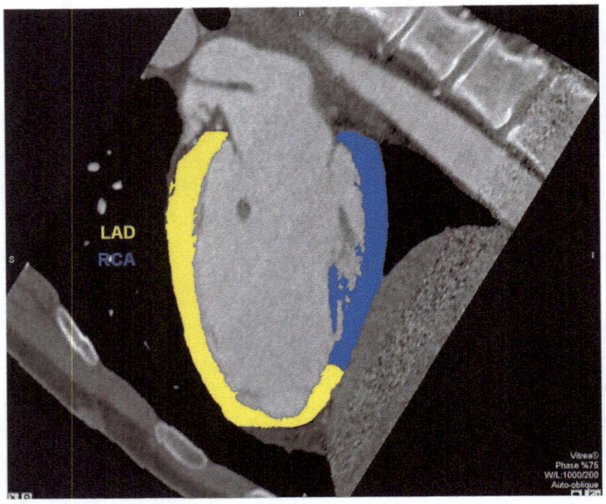

Fig. 1.6. Two-chamber view of the heart with the most common distribution of the left anterior descending artery (*LAD*) and right coronary artery (*RCA*) (anterior wall/posterior wall)

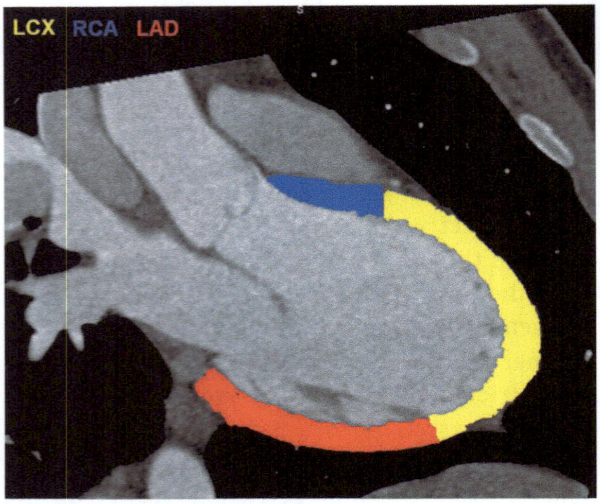

Fig. 1.7. Three-chamber view of the heart with the most common distributional pattern of the left circumflex (*LCX*), left anterior descending (*LAD*) and right coronary arteries (*RCA*)

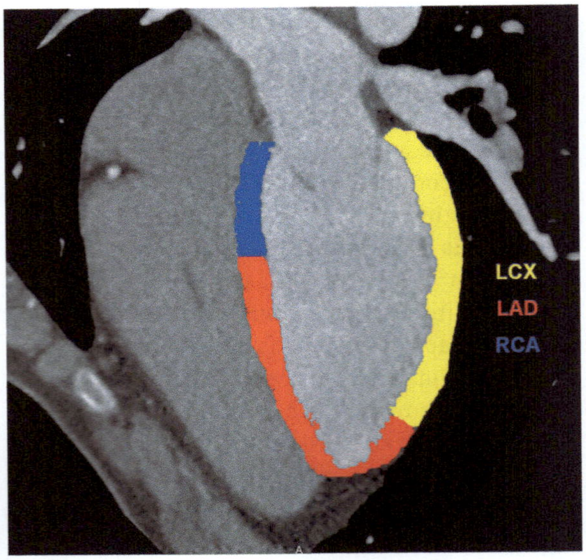

Fig. 1.8. Four-chamber view of the heart with the most common distributional pattern of the left circumflex (*LCX*), left anterior descending (*LAD*) and right coronary arteries (*RCA*)

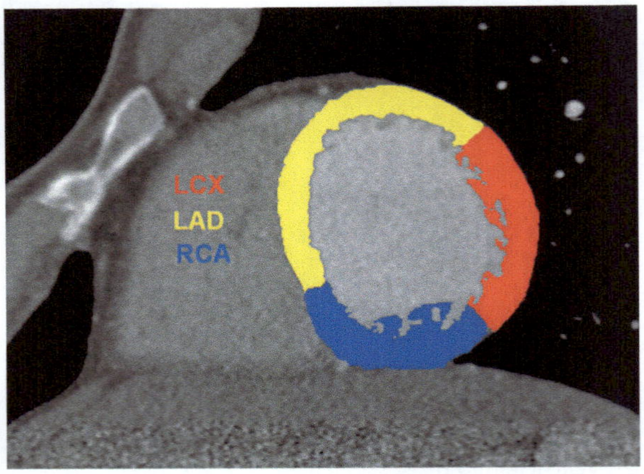

Fig. 1.9. Short-axis view of the heart with the most common distributional pattern of the left circumflex (*LCX*, lateral wall), left anterior descending (*LAD*, anterior wall and septal wall) and right coronary arteries (*RCA*, inferior wall)

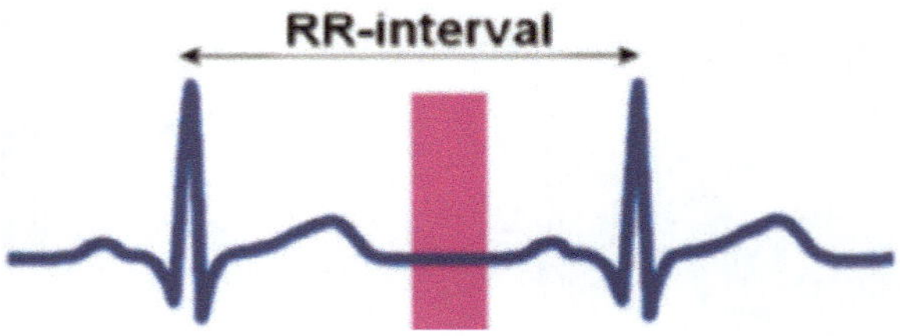

Fig. 1.10. Electrocardiogram with the scan reconstruction interval (*pink box*) set at approximately 60% of the RR-interval

1.3 Normal Coronary Anatomy

The coronary arteries normally arise perpendicular from the aorta below the sinotubular ridge (the transition between the tubular aorta and the sinuses of Valsalva). Usually, two coronary ostia exist; one of the right coronary artery (RCA) which originates from the right aortic sinus, usually but not always in its central portion, and one of the left coronary artery (LCA) which originates from the left aortic sinus, nearly always from its central portion (Fig. 1.11). The LCA is subdivided into a left main coronary artery (LM), a left anterior descending artery (LAD) and a left circumflex artery (LCX) (Figs. 1.12, 1.13).

Furthermore, a posterior or non-coronary cusp exists in a normal three leaflet aortic valve. Coronary ostia are typically equal to, or larger than, the vessel which they supply.

The four main coronaries can be schematically seen as a "circle and half-loop".

Because of the high variability in the anatomy and distribution of the coronary arteries, a general, prevailing anatomy will be described first.

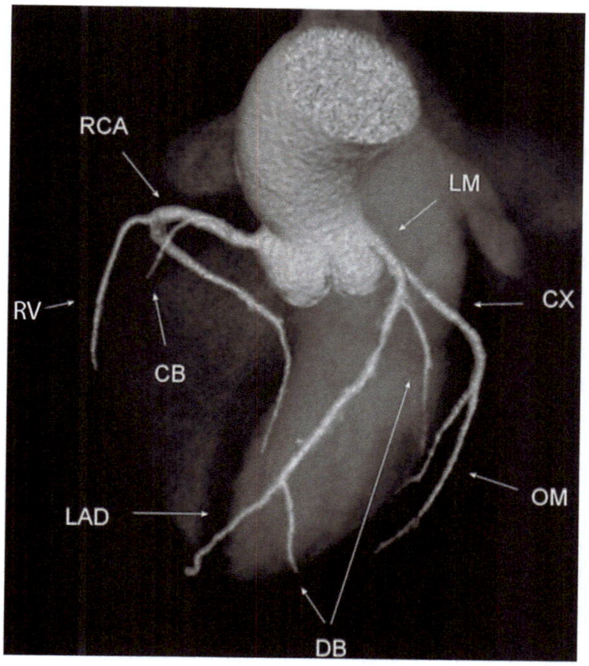

Fig. 1.12. Three-dimensional CT image of the ascending aorta and the coronary artery tree, with transparent other cardiac structures. *RCA*, right coronary artery; *LM*, left main coronary artery; *CX*, circumflex artery; *OM*, obtuse marginal branch; *DB*, diagonal branches; *LAD*, left anterior descending artery; *CB*, conus branch ; *RV*, right ventricular branch

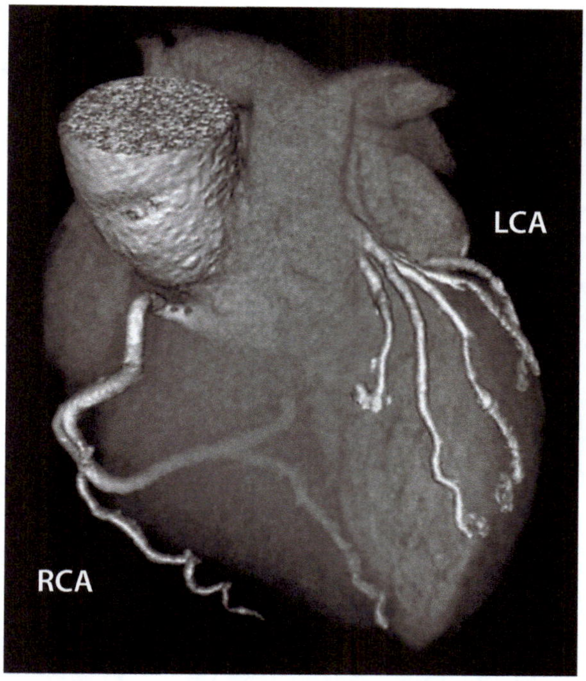

Fig. 1.11. Three-dimensional CT image of the heart with the right coronary artery (*RCA*) and the left coronary artery (*LCA*)

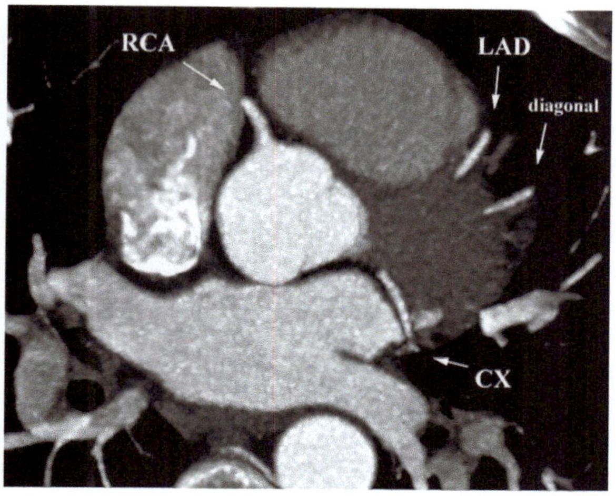

Fig. 1.13. Maximum intensity projection (MIP) of the heart showing the right coronary artery (*RCA*), left anterior descending artery (*LAD*), a diagonal of the LAD and the circumflex artery (*CX*)

1.3.1 Left Coronary Anatomy

1.3.1.1 Left Main Coronary Artery

The LM arises just above the left sinus of Valsalva and courses behind the pulmonary trunk [right ventricular outflow tract (RVOT)]. The diameter of the LM ranges from 3 to 6 mm and its length is also variable, usually 10–30 mm. Quantitative analysis has shown that the diameter of the LM varies with the existence and location of coronary artery disease. LM artery diameter is 4.5 mm in patients with entirely normal coronary arteries, 4.0 mm in patients with distal LCA disease and 3.8 in patients with disease in the adjacent segment of the LCA. The LM bifurcates into the LAD and the LCX. It may give rise to a ramus intermedius branch (approximately 37% of cases) which arises between the LAD and the LCX creating a trifurcation. This branch supplies the myocardium between diagonal and marginal territories. The LM may be absent; the LAD and LCX then have separate origins.

1.3.1.2 Left Anterior Descending Coronary Artery

The LAD passes behind the pulmonary trunk and then moves forward between the pulmonary trunk and the left atrial appendage to the anterior interventricular sulcus. It gives rise to diagonal branches and septal perforating branches. The first branch is the left conal branch, which supplies the infundibulum. The septal branches originate from the LAD at approximately 90° angles, so when seen on axial images these vessels are in cross-section. They pass into the interventricular septum with a wide variation in number, size and distribution. A first distribution comprises a large, vertically orientated, first septal branch dividing up into a number of secondary branches which ramify throughout the septum. Another possible distribution involves a large, more horizontally orientated first septal branch, with a trajectory parallel to and below the LAD. A third distribution shows a number of septal arteries with roughly comparable sizes. By interconnection of the septal branches originating from the LAD with similar septal branches originating from the posterior descending branch of the RCA a network of potential collateral channels is created. As the first branch irrigates the interventricular septum, which is the most vascularized area of the heart, it is the most important potential collateral channel. All septal branches from the LAD supply the anterior 2/3 of the interventricular septum.

The diagonal branches are muscular branches extending from the LAD supplying the anterolateral free wall of the left ventricle and the anterolateral papillary muscle. A wide variation in number and size of diagonal branches exists which all originate from the LAD and pass over the anterolateral aspect of the heart. In over 90% of the human population one to three diagonal branches originate from the LAD and less than 1% has no diagonal at all. This indicates that when diagonal branches are not visualized, acquired atherosclerotic occlusion of the diagonal branches is highly probable especially in patients with unexplained contraction abnormalities of the anterolateral left ventricle. The LAD courses beyond the left ventricular apex and terminates along the diaphragmatic aspect of the left ventricle in 78% of patients (Fig. 1.14). In the remaining 22%, the distal segment of the LAD is smaller and shorter than usual, terminates at or before the cardiac apex and does not reach the diaphragmatic surface. In this latter case a "superdominant" RCA will exist with a posterior descending branch which is larger and longer than usual and supplies the cardiac apex. In these cases, early attenuation and a distal narrow segment of the distal LAD does not necessarily indicate LAD

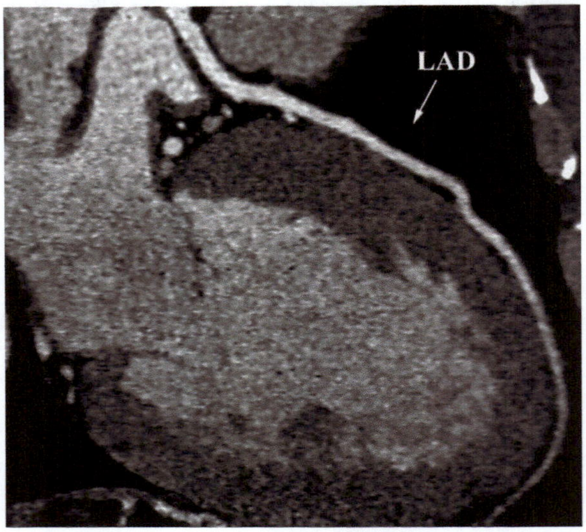

Fig. 1.14. Left anterior descending artery (*LAD*) coursing from the anterior wall of the left ventricle to the apex. Left circumflex artery

disease when some or all of the cardiac apex is supplied by the posterior descending artery.

1.3.1.3
The Circumflex Artery

The LCX angles posteriorly from the bifurcation (or trifurcation) to pass below the left atrial appendage and enters the left atrioventricular groove along the obtuse margin of the heart (Fig. 1.15). It gives rise to obtuse marginal branches and left atrial branches (Fig. 1.16). In general, three obtuse marginal branches originate from the LCX: the anterolateral branch (AL), the obtuse marginal branch (OM) and the posterolateral branch (PL), of which the second is generally the largest. They originate from the LCX supplying the posterolateral wall of the left ventricle. Usually, non-invasive techniques only visualize this second OM branch. Beyond the origins of the OM branches, the distal LCX tends to be small. The LCX also gives rise to one or two left atrial circumflex branches. These branches supply the lateral and posterior aspects of the left atrium. A wide variation in circumflex anatomy is seen and it is the non-dominant vessel in 85% of the population.

In 10% of the population the LCX gives off the posterior descending artery (PDA) and the AV nodal arterial branch. Such patients are termed left-dominant. In 40% of cases the LCX supplies the SA node branch.

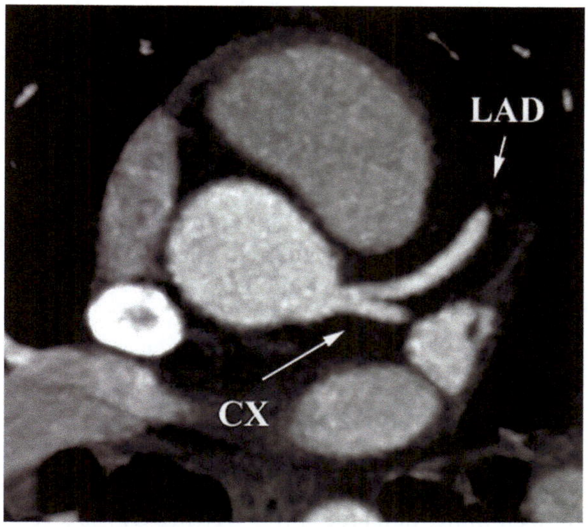

Fig. 1.15. Axial CT slide showing the bifurcation of the left anterior descending artery (*LAD*) and the circumflex artery (*CX*)

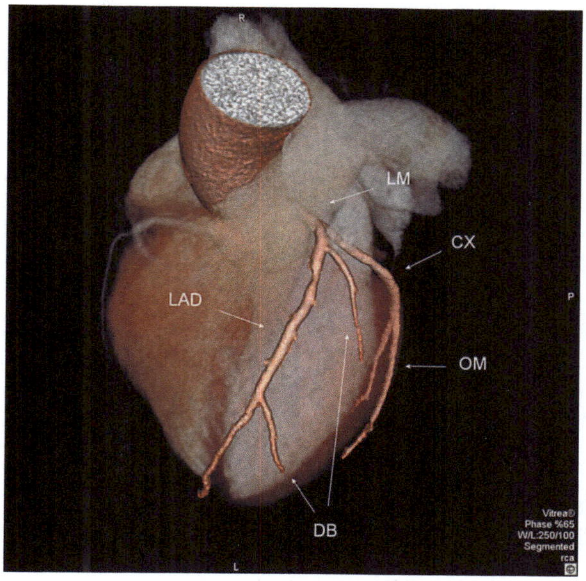

Fig. 1.16. Left coronary artery system. *LM*, left main coronary artery; *CX*, circumflex artery; *OM*, obtuse marginal branch; *DB*, diagonal branches; *LAD*, left anterior descending artery

1.3.2
Right Coronary Anatomy

1.3.2.1
Right Coronary Artery

The RCA arises above the right sinus of Valsalva, slightly lower than the origin of the left main coronary artery, and follows its trajectory between the right ventricular outflow tract (RVOT) and the right atrial appendage and courses into the right atrioventricular groove (Fig. 1.17). Proximal branches of the RCA are the conus branch (CB), the right ventricular branches (RV) and the acute marginal branch (AM). The first branch is often the conus branch, which supplies the infundibulum. In half of the population, the conus branch arises at the right coronary ostium or within the first few millimetres of the RCA. The conus branch travels anteriorly and upward over the RVOT toward the LAD (Fig. 1.18). It may serve as a source of collateral circulation in patients with LAD occlusion. In the other half of the population, the conus branch arises from a separate ostium in the right aortic sinus just above the right coronary ostium. The RCA also provides the right atrial branches and in 60% of cases it provides the SA node branch. The AM branches branch off the RCA and arise at an acute angle and extend anteriorly

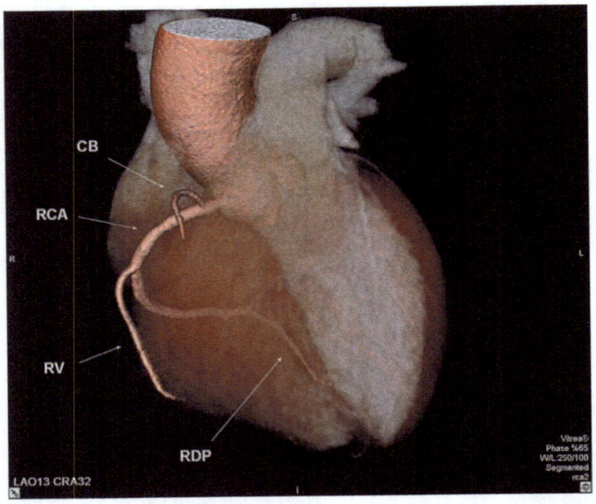

Fig. 1.17. Right coronary artery system. *CB*, conus branch; *RCA*, right coronary artery; *RV*, right ventricular branch; *RDP*, right descending posterior branch

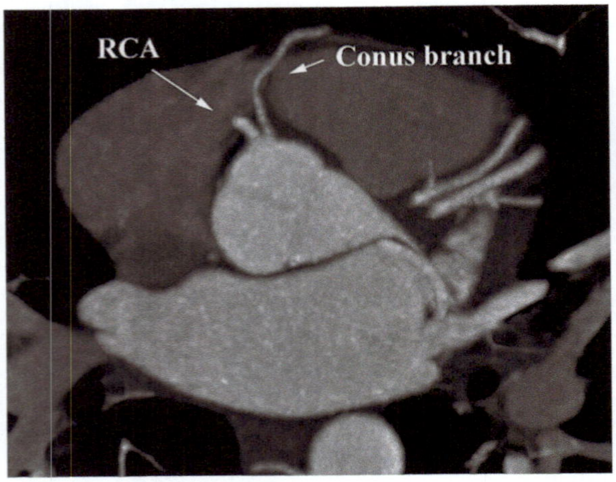

Fig. 1.18. Maximum intensity projection (MIP) of a cardiac CT showing the separate origin of the right coronary artery (*RCA*) and conus branch

over the right ventricle, where they supply the anterior free wall. Despite their relative unimportance they may serve as sources of collateral circulation in patients with LAD occlusion.

The distal RCA starts just after the AM branch and passes horizontally along the diaphragmatic surface of the heart, giving rise to the posterior descending artery (PDA) in 85% of individuals. This is called right-dominance. The PDA adjoins the middle cardiac vein and runs anteriorly in the posterior interventricular sulcus. It supplies the posterior third of the ventricular septum with septal perforators. After giving rise to the PDA, a dominant RCA continuous beyond the crux (joining point of the left and right atrioventricular and posterior interventricular sulci on the diaphragmatic surface of the heart) in the left atrioventricular sulcus in which it terminates into the PL. This branch supplies the posterior aspect of the left ventricle. In cases in which the RCA supplies the AV nodal branch, this branches off the RCA at the crux and courses towards the AV node.

1.3.2.2 Determination of Dominance

The artery which crosses the crux of the heart and gives rise to the PDA, AV nodal branch and the posterolateral artery (PLA) is considered to be the dominant coronary artery.

If the RCA gives off the PDA and the LCX gives off the PLA then the heart is so-called co-dominant. In a general population, 70% is right-dominant, 20% is co-dominant and 10% is left-dominant.

1.4 Visualization of the Normal Coronary Artery Tree

1.4.1 Anatomy on Catheter Coronary Angiography

Standard projection angles have been determined for catheter coronary angiography. An optimal angiographic projection has been appointed for each of the segments of the coronary artery tree. Figures 1.19–1.33 show the different standard projection angles.

Each figure consists of three elements, first the positioning of the X-ray tube and image intensifier are shown, next the corresponding catheter coronary angiogram is shown, and finally a schematic drawing describing the branches.

1.4.2 Anatomy on Multi-detector CT

Multiple studies demonstrate that contrast-enhanced multi-detector spiral CT (MDCT) is a reliable non-invasive technique to provide a good anatomical overview of the coronary anatomy. Most of the shortcomings of catheter angiography have been overcome with contrast-enhanced MDCT. First, immediate visualization of the anomalous coronary artery is possible due to systematically administered contrast agent and secondly, complete cardiac CT data sets provide a good inside into the relation of the coronary artery to other cardiac structures such as the pulmonary artery and the aorta (Schmitt et al. 2005; Van Ooijen et al. 2004).

Although MDCT has proven to provide an accurate depiction of origin and course of coronary arteries, the small dimensions and fast movement of the coronary arteries make their visualization difficult. The occurrence of motion artefacts has been an important limiting factor for cardiac CT, especially in patients with high heart rates. Earlier generations of CT scanners were limited because of the insufficient spatial and temporal resolution and needed drug induced heart rate control to obtain images with good quality (Achenbach et al. 2006). Small coronary side branches, such as the diagonal branches of the LAD, were often impossible to evaluate. These limitations of coronary CT angiography seem to have been overcome by dual-source CT (DSCT) (Johnson et al. 2006). Dual-source CT is a new concept of CT. The system combines two arrays of an X-ray tube plus detector (64 slices) mounted on a single gantry at an angle of 90°, allowing a higher temporal resolution. Heart rate independent temporal resolution allows visualization of the coronary artery tree without motion artefacts in a larger number of patients as compared to earlier scanner generations. An advantage of DSCT is the capability to provide reconstructions of diagnostic quality throughout the cardiac cycle (Achenbach et al. 2005).

Axial images are useful to display the coronary arteries and for the recognition of coronary vessels; a combination of axial images with other visualization techniques such as oblique and curved multiplanar reconstruction and three-dimensional volume rendering can also be useful in the recognition of coronary artery segments. Using current commercially available visualization software, a clear visualization is possible without the need for extensive manual manipulation.

The origin of the left coronary artery from the left sinus of Valsalva is visible in the upper axial transverse image. At this level, the short common stem (left main artery or LMA) of the left coronary artery which commonly presents a horizontal course is displayed. This segment is 0.5–2.5 cm long, then it bifurcates into the LAD and the LCX; the most proximal segment of the LAD present a course which is slightly oblique cranial-caudally so it can be seen in the same axial image as the left main artery.

The other part of the LAD passes between the left atrial appendage and the pulmonary artery. Then it courses downwards into the interventricular sulcus, largely surrounded by epicardial fat, rounds the acute margin of the heart just to the right of the apex: those segments of the LAD are displayed with round or oval shape and lie just interior to the interventricular septum. Diagonal branches, usually two, are also very frequently seen on axial images: they arise from the left side of the LAD and run on the obtuse margin of the heart in a perpendicular course.

The LCX arises from the bifurcation of the LMA and passes under the left auricula, then runs into the atrioventricular sulcus perpendicular to the scanning plane giving off to the lateral left ventricular wall and atrium; the largest collateral vessels of the circumflex artery are the marginal branches which can be readily identified on the obtuse surface of the left ventricle; usually the circumflex artery terminates at the obtuse margin of the heart, but in some cases it reaches the crux.

The RCA arises from the anterior surface of the right sinus of Valsalva at a slightly caudal level of the left coronary artery. The first segment is usually parallel to the scan plane; in some cases it describes a curve with upper convexity so it is possible to have this tract displayed two times in the same image. This segment gives off the conus branch artery and the artery supplying the sinus node. The second segment of the RCA runs along the right atrioventricular sulcus embedded in fat; it may be difficult to evaluate this part of the RCA due to the presence of high concentration of contrast media in the right atrium and due to the greater movement of the right cardiac chambers than the left ones during diastole. The third portion of the RCA runs horizontally in the right atrioventricular groove and, in subjects with right dominance, gives rise to the right descending posterior (RDP) and to other branches for the diaphragmatic surface of the heart and to the PL that supply the posterolateral side of the left ventricle; those vessels are almost always easily identified.

For some of the previously shown catheter coronary angiograms, the corresponding multislice CT angiograms are shown in Figures 1.34–1.44.

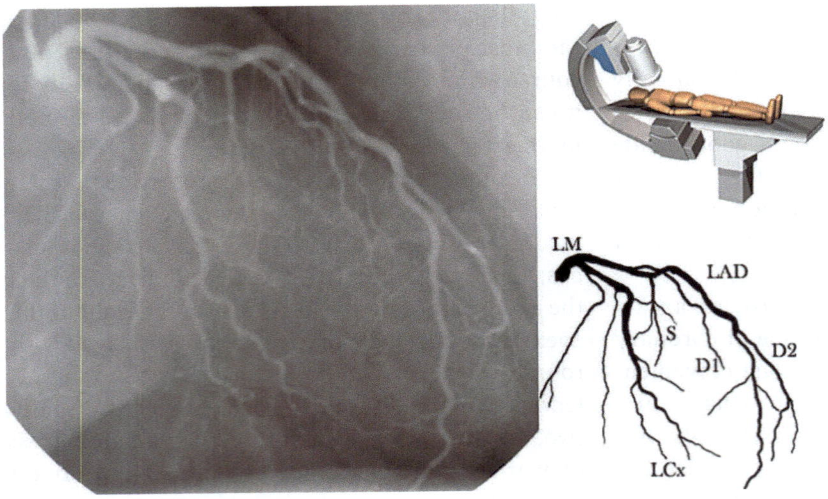

Fig. 1.19. Left coronary artery – RAO (30°) straight. The *left image* shows a coronary angiogram with a schematic drawing of the same angiogram at the *bottom right*. The *top right* shows the positioning of the C-arm to obtain this coronary angiogram. *LM*, left main; *LAD*, left anterior descending; *S*, septal branch; *D1*, first diagonal branch; *D2*, second diagonal branch; *LCx*, left circumflex artery

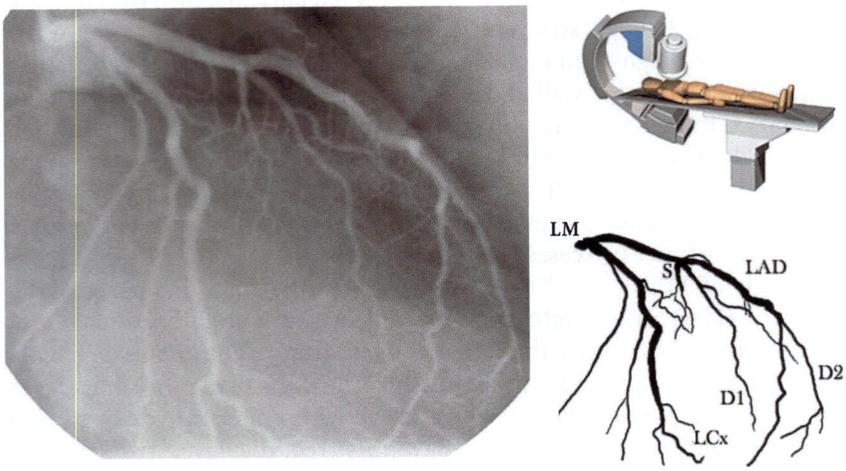

Fig. 1.20. Left coronary artery – RAO (29°) caudal (30°). The *left image* shows a coronary angiogram with a schematic drawing of the same angiogram at the *bottom right*. The *top right* shows the positioning of the C-arm to obtain this coronary angiogram. *LM*, left main; *LAD*, left anterior descending; *S*, septal branch; *D1*, first diagonal branch; *D2*, second diagonal branch; *LCx*, left circumflex artery

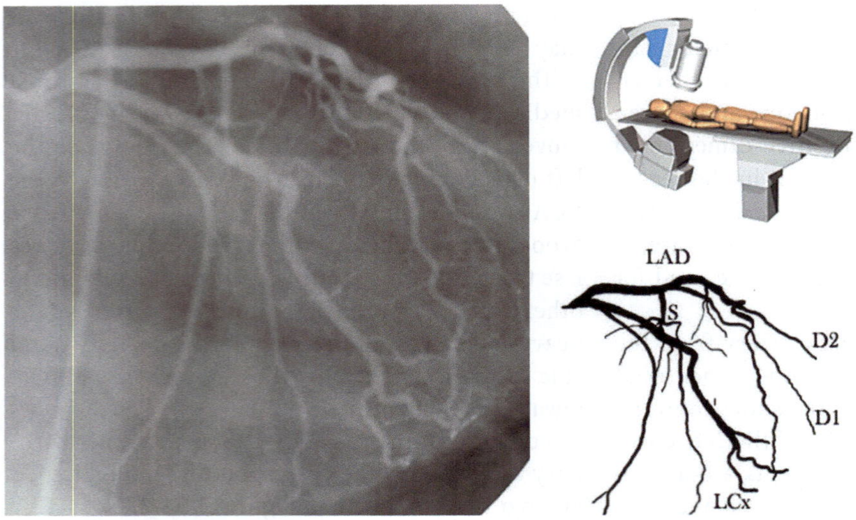

Fig. 1.21. Left coronary artery – AP caudal (28°). The *left image* shows a coronary angiogram with a schematic drawing of the same angiogram at the *bottom right*. The *top right* shows the positioning of the C-arm to obtain this coronary angiogram. *LAD*, left anterior descending; *S*, septal branch; *D1*, first diagonal branch; *D2*, second diagonal branch; *LCx*, left circumflex artery.

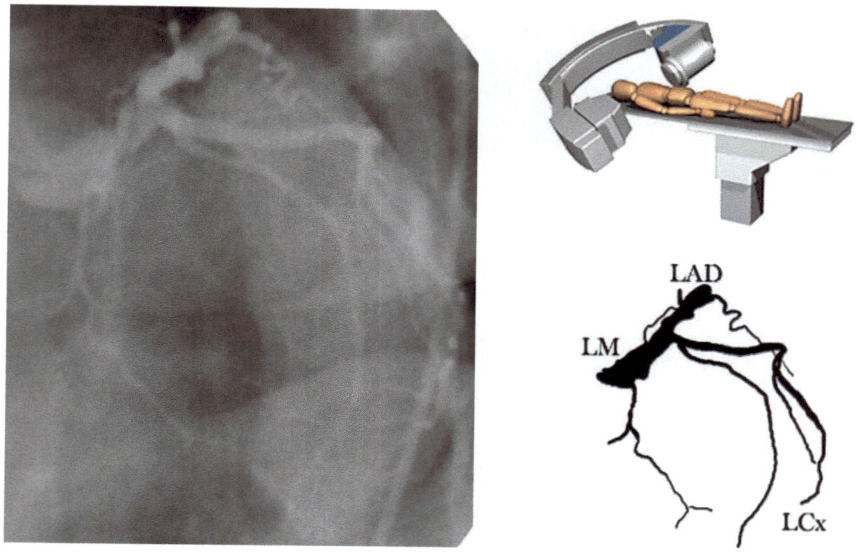

Fig. 1.22. Left coronary artery – LAO (51°) caudal (30°) (spider view). The *left image* shows a coronary angiogram with a schematic drawing of the same angiogram at the *bottom right*. The *top right* shows the positioning of the C-arm to obtain this coronary angiogram. *LM*, left main; *LAD*, left anterior descending; *LCx*, left circumflex artery

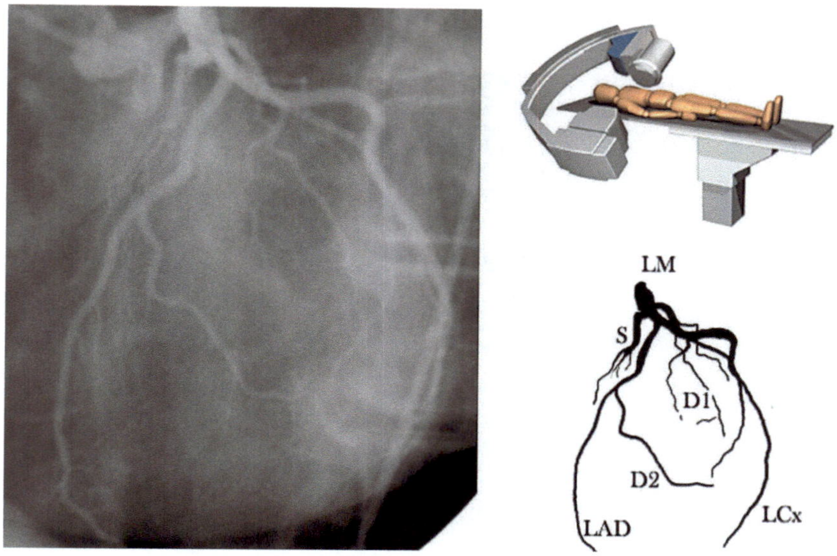

Fig. 1.23. Left coronary artery – LAO (60°) straight. The *left image* shows a coronary angiogram with a schematic drawing of the same angiogram at the *bottom right*. The *top right* shows the positioning of the C-arm to obtain this coronary angiogram. *LM*, left main; *LAD*, left anterior descending; *S*, septal branch; *D1*, first diagonal branch; *D2*, second diagonal branch; *LCx*, left circumflex artery

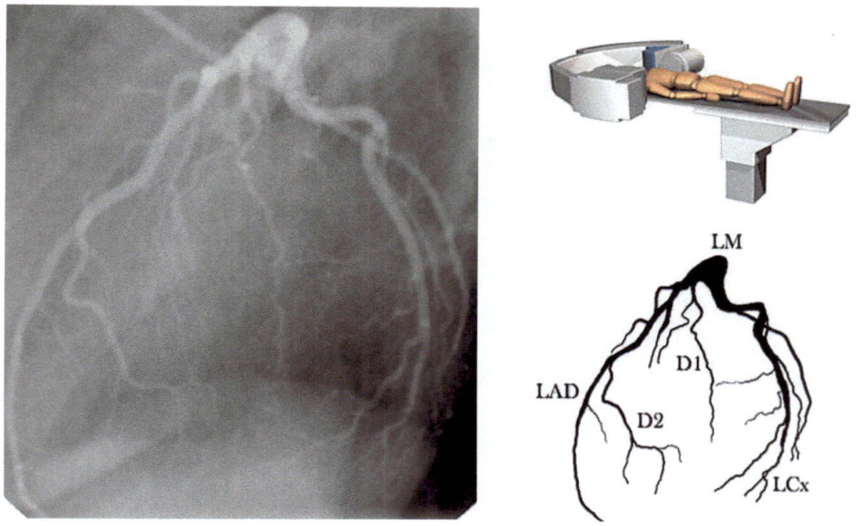

Fig. 1.24. Left coronary artery – LAO (89°) straight (lateral). The *left image* shows a coronary angiogram with a schematic drawing of the same angiogram at the *bottom right*. The *top right* shows the positioning of the C-arm to obtain this coronary angiogram. *LM*, left main; *LAD*, = left anterior descending; *D1*, first diagonal branch; *D2*, second diagonal branch; *LCx*, left circumflex artery.

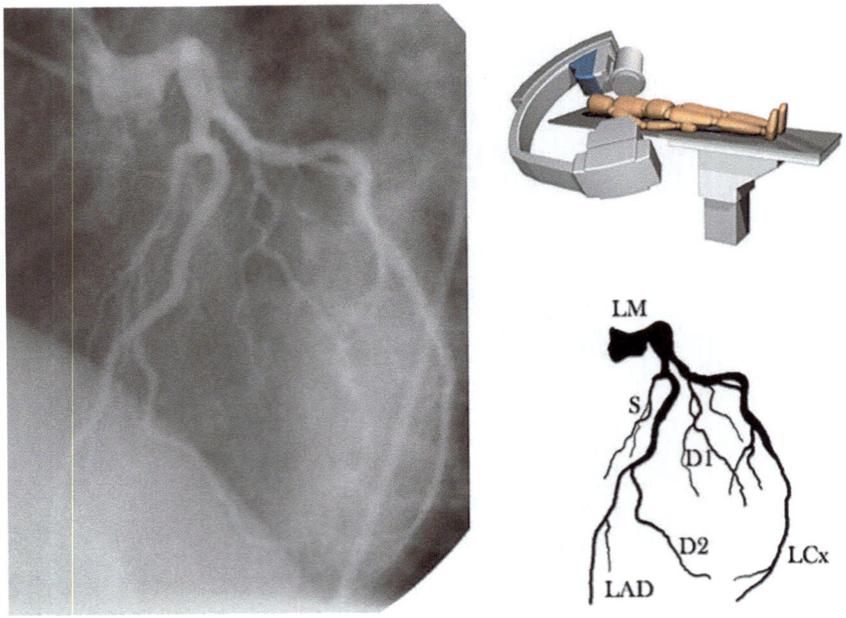

Fig. 1.25. Left coronary artery – LAO (60°) cranial (16°) – normally LAO (45°) cranial (30°) but this was not optimal for this patient. The *left image* shows a coronary angiogram with a schematic drawing of the same angiogram at the *bottom right*. The *top right* shows the positioning of the C-arm to obtain this coronary angiogram. *LM*, left main; *LAD*, left anterior descending; *S*, septal branch; *D1*, first diagonal branch; *D2*, second diagonal branch; *LCx*, left circumflex artery

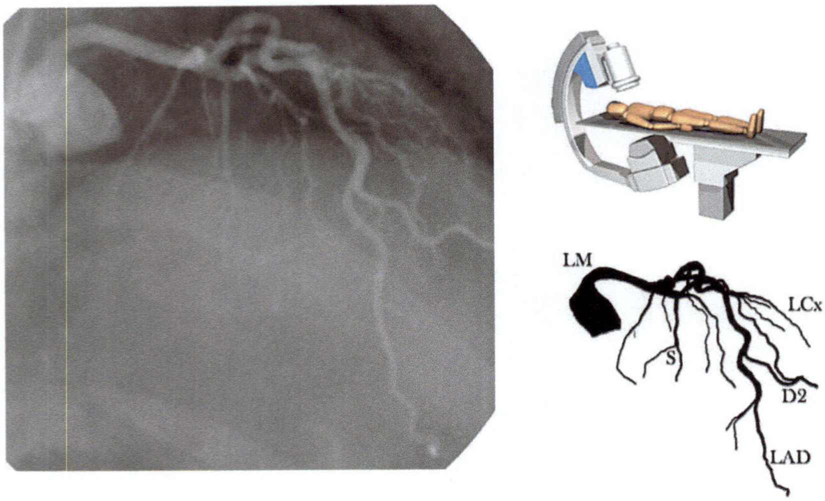

Fig. 1.26. Left coronary artery – AP cranial (30°). The *left image* shows a coronary angiogram with a schematic drawing of the same angiogram at the *bottom right*. The *top right* shows the positioning of the C-arm to obtain this coronary angiogram. *LM*, left main; *LAD*, left anterior descending; *S*, septal branch; *D2*, second diagonal branch; *LCx*, left circumflex artery

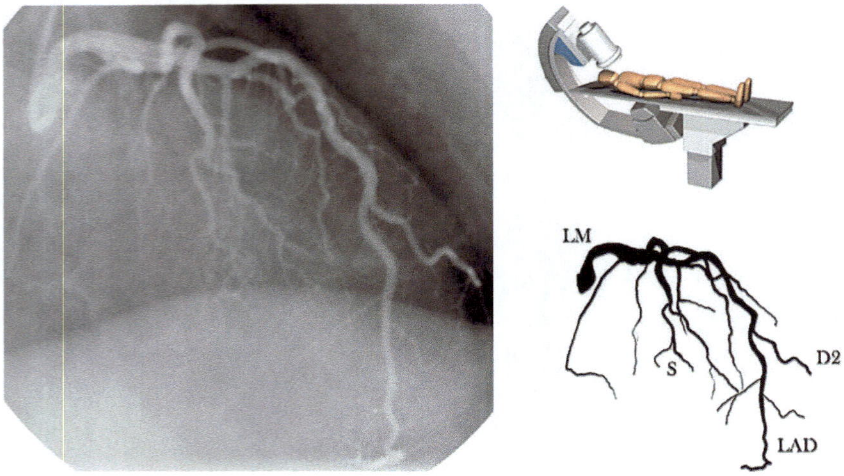

Fig. 1.27. Left coronary artery – RAO (28°) cranial (30°). The *left image* shows a coronary angiogram with a schematic drawing of the same angiogram at the *bottom right*. The *top right* shows the positioning of the C-arm to obtain this coronary angiogram. *LM*, left main; *LAD*, left anterior descending; *S*, septal branch; *D2*, second diagonal branch

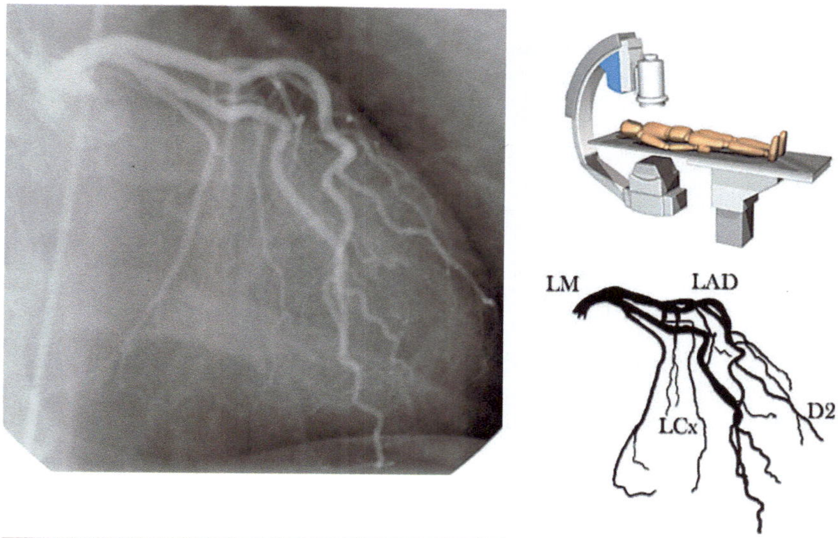

Fig. 1.28. Left coronary artery – AP straight. The *left image* shows a coronary angiogram with a schematic drawing of the same angiogram at the *bottom right*. The *top right* shows the positioning of the C-arm to obtain this coronary angiogram. *LM*, left main; *LAD*, left anterior descending; *D2*, second diagonal branch; *LCx*, left circumflex artery

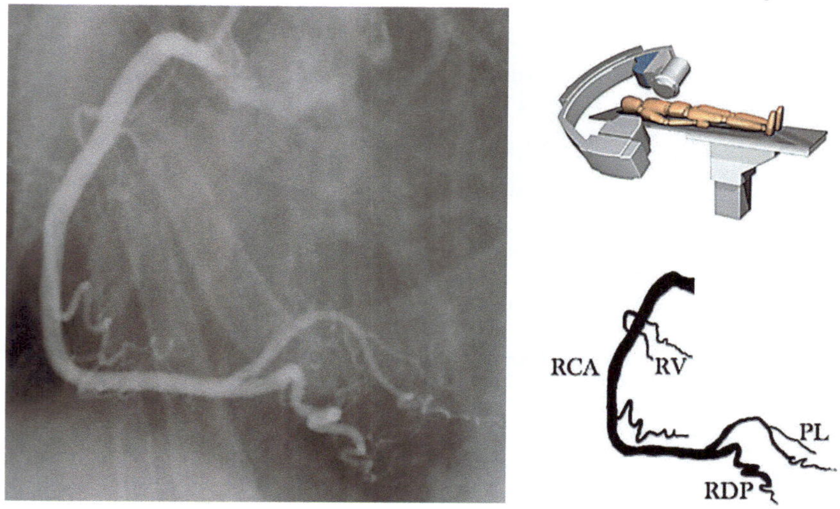

Fig. 1.29. Right coronary artery – LAO (45°) straight. The *left image* shows a coronary angiogram with a schematic drawing of the same angiogram at the *bottom right*. The *top right* shows the positioning of the C-arm to obtain this coronary angiogram. *RCA*, right coronary artery; *RV*, right ventricular branch; *PL*, posterior left ventricular branch; *RDP*, right descending posterior

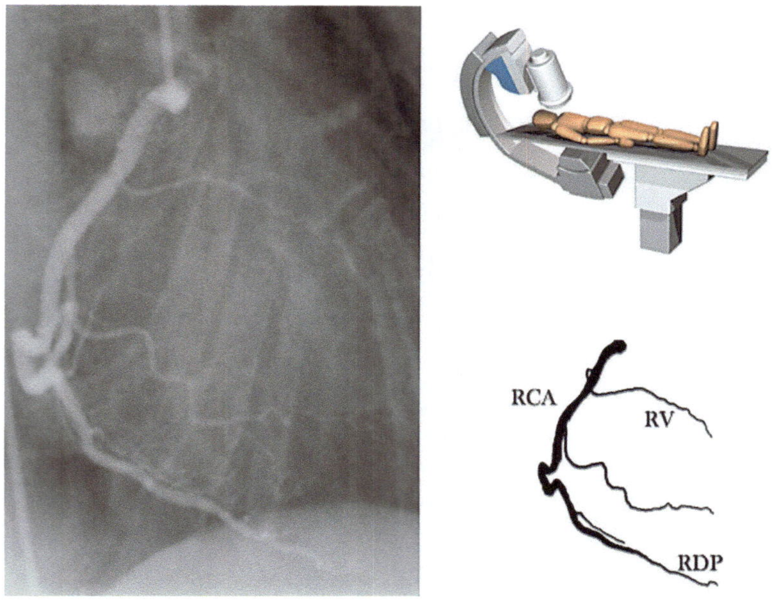

Fig. 1.30. Right coronary artery – RAO (30°) straight. The *left image* shows a coronary angiogram with a schematic drawing of the same angiogram at the *bottom right*. The *top right* shows the positioning of the C-arm to obtain this coronary angiogram. *RCA*, right coronary artery; *RV*, right ventricular branch; *RDP*, right descending posterior

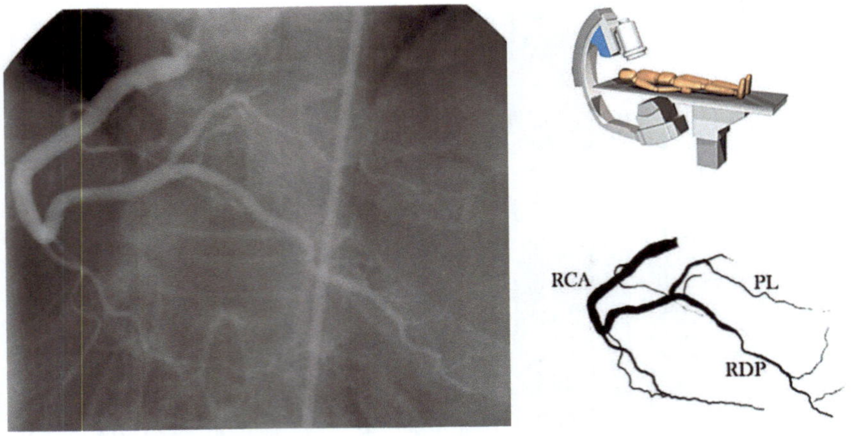

Fig. 1.31. Right coronary artery – AP cranial (30°). The *left image* shows a coronary angiogram with a schematic drawing of the same angiogram at the *bottom right*. The *top right* shows the positioning of the C-arm to obtain this coronary angiogram. *RCA*, right coronary artery; *PL*, posterior left ventricular branch; *RDP*, right descending posterior

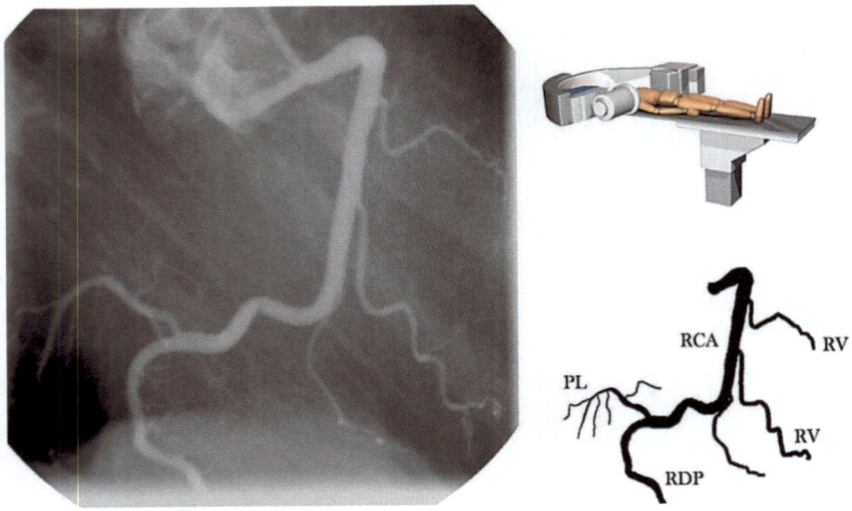

Fig. 1.32. Right coronary artery – RAO (90°) straight. The *left image* shows a coronary angiogram with a schematic drawing of the same angiogram at the *bottom right*. The *top right* shows the positioning of the C-arm to obtain this coronary angiogram. *RCA*, right coronary artery; *RV*, right ventricular branch; *PL*, posterior left ventricular branch; *RDP*, right descending posterior

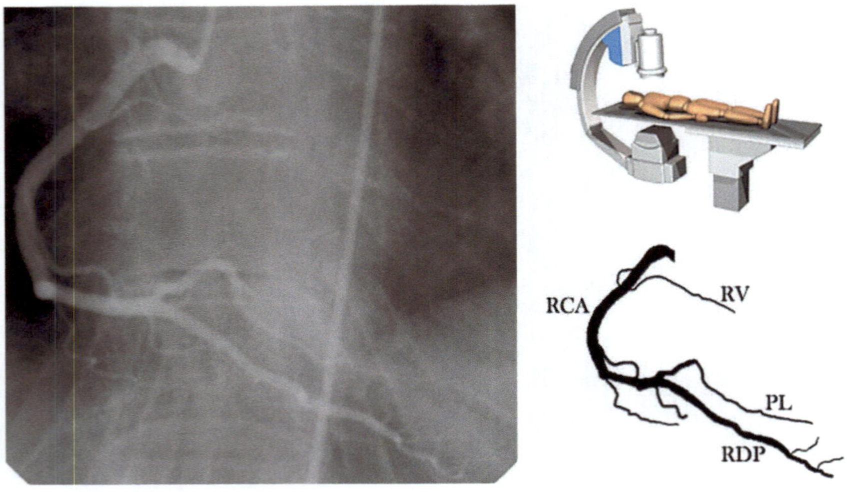

Fig. 1.33. Right coronary artery – AP straight. The *left image* shows a coronary angiogram with a schematic drawing of the same angiogram at the *bottom right*. The *top right* shows the positioning of the C-arm to obtain this coronary angiogram. *RCA*, right coronary artery; *RV*, right ventricular branch; *PL*, posterior left ventricular branch; *RDP*, right descending posterior

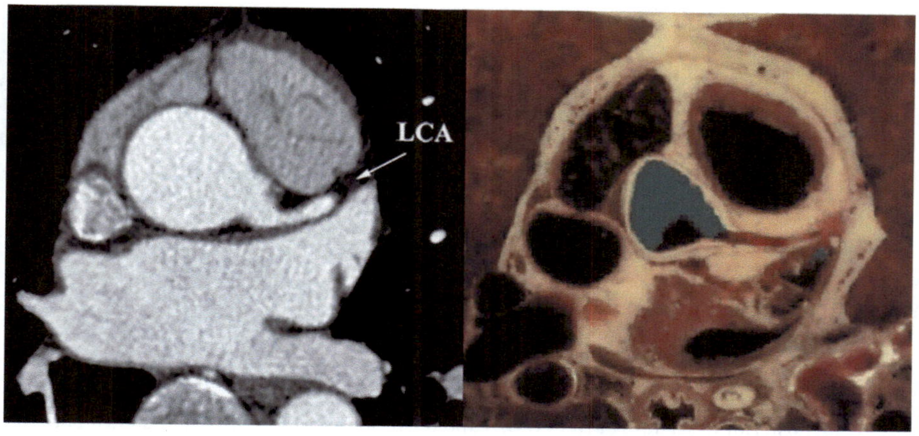

Fig. 1.34a,b. Left coronary artery (*LCA*) both in axial CT slice (**a**) and real anatomy (**b**)

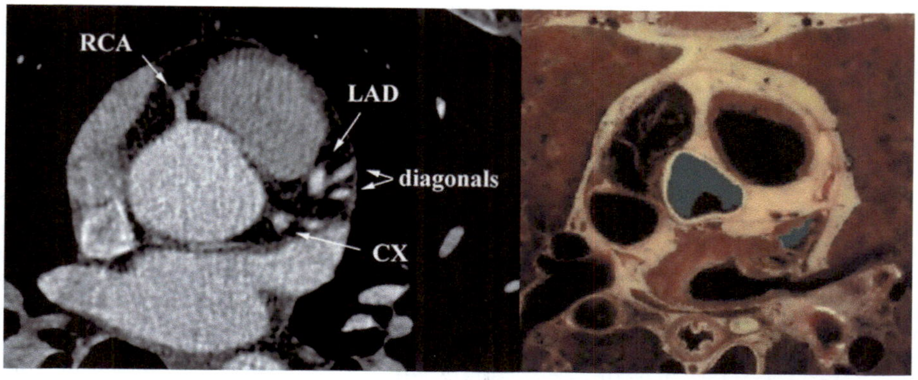

Fig. 1.35a,b. Left anterior descending artery (*LAD*), circumflex artery (*CX*) and diagonals of the LAD in axial CT slice (**a**) and real anatomy (**b**)

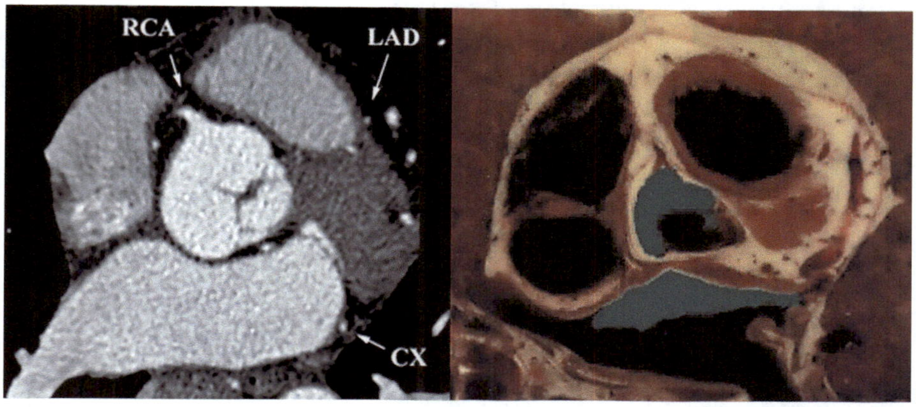

Fig. 1.36a,b. Origin of the right coronary artery (*RCA*), left anterior descending artery (*LAD*) and circumflex artery (*CX*) in axial CT slice (**a**) and real anatomy (**b**)

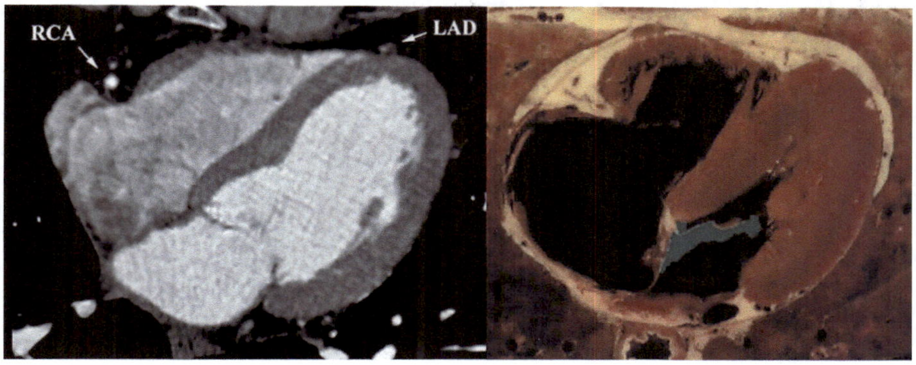

Fig. 1.37a,b. Mid right coronary artery (*RCA*) and distal left anterior descending artery (*LAD*) shown both in axial CT slice (**a**) and real anatomy (**b**)

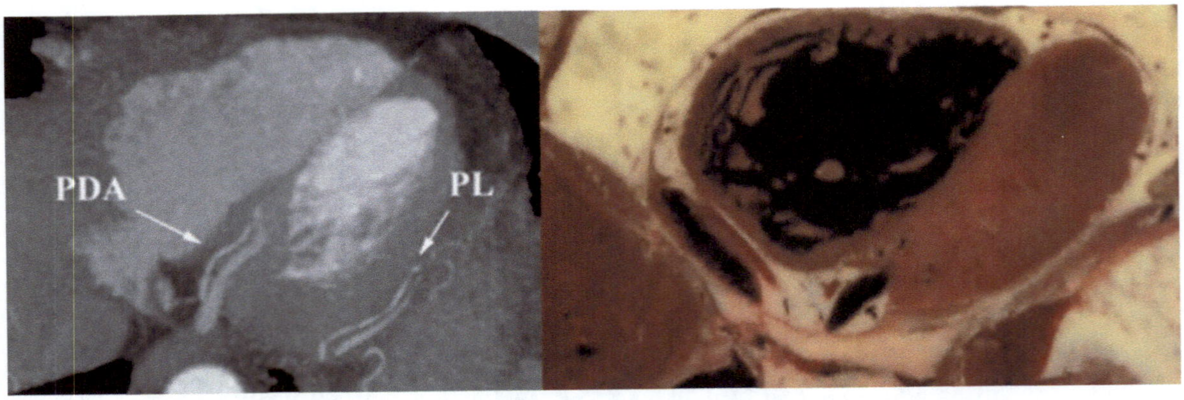

Fig. 1.38. Posterior descending artery (*PDA*) and posterior left (*PL*) ventricular shown both in CT slice (**a**) and real anatomy (**b**)

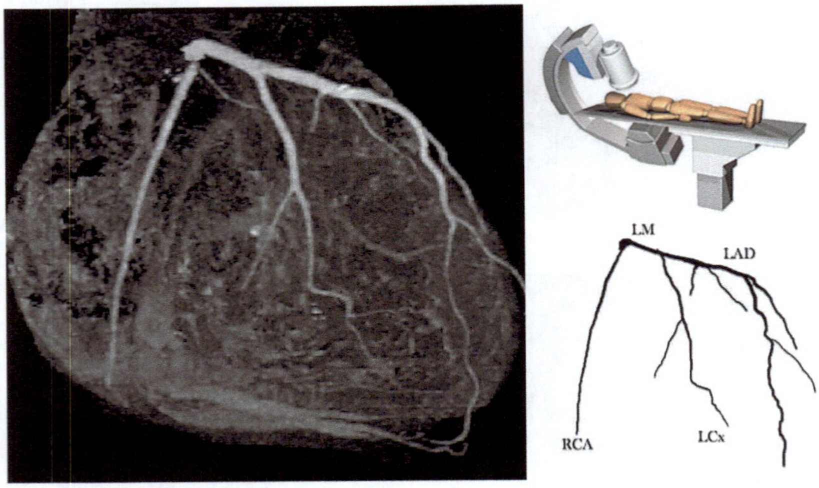

Fig. 1.39. RAO (30°) straight. The *left image* shows a segmented maximum intensity projection of a multi-detector computed tomography angiogram with a schematic drawing of the same angiogram at the *bottom right*. The *top right* shows the positioning of the C-arm that would be used to acquire the correspoding catheter coronary angiogram (Figs. 1.19 and 1.30). *LM*, left main; *LAD*, left anterior descending; *LCx*, left circumflex artery; *RCA*, right coronary artery

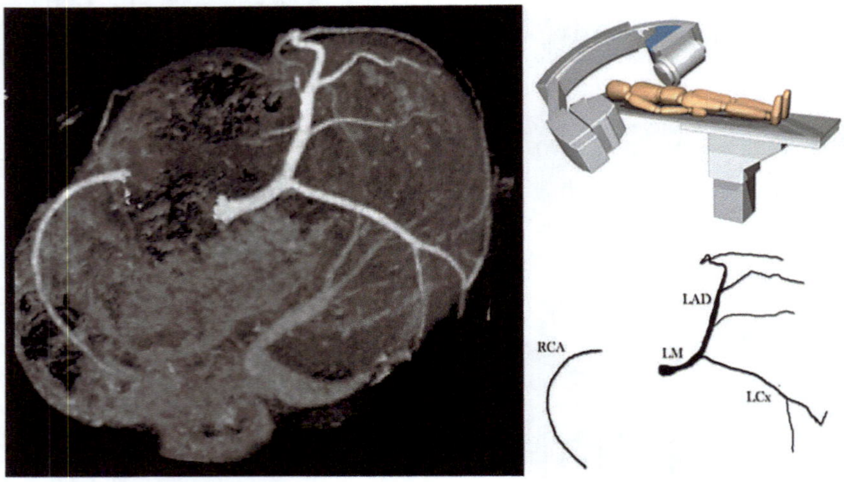

Fig. 1.40. LAO (51°) caudal (30°) (spider view). The *left image* shows a segmented maximum intensity projection of a multi-detector computed tomography angiogram with a schematic drawing of the same angiogram at the *bottom right*. The *top right* shows the positioning of the C-arm that would be used to acquire the correspoding catheter coronary angiogram (Fig. 1.22). *LM*, left main; *LAD*, left anterior descending; *LCx*, left circumflex artery; *RCA*, right coronary artery

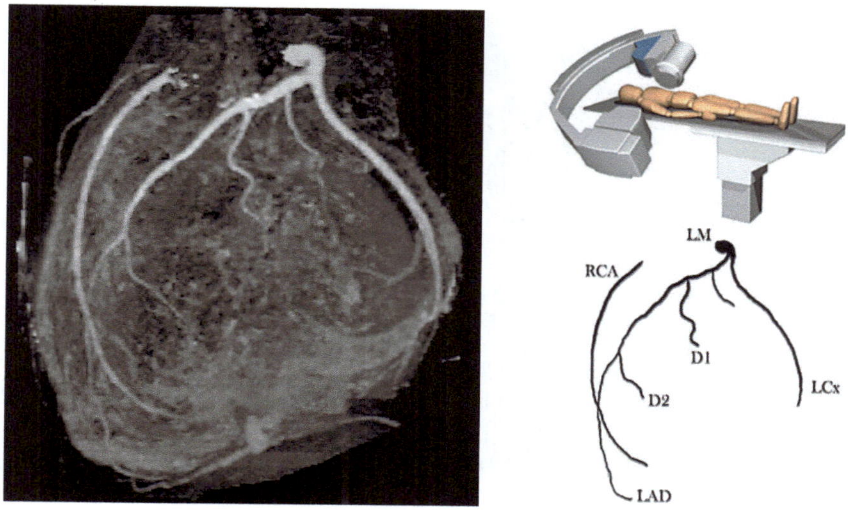

Fig. 1.41. LAO (60°) straight. The *left image* shows a segmented maximum intensity projection of a multi-detector computed tomography angiogram with a schematic drawing of the same angiogram at the *bottom right*. The *top right* shows the positioning of the C-arm that would be used to acquire the correspoding catheter coronary angiogram (Fig. 1.23). *LM*, left main; *LAD*, left anterior descending; *D1*, first diagonal branch; *D2*, second diagonal branch; *LCx*, left circumflex artery; *RCA*, right coronary artery

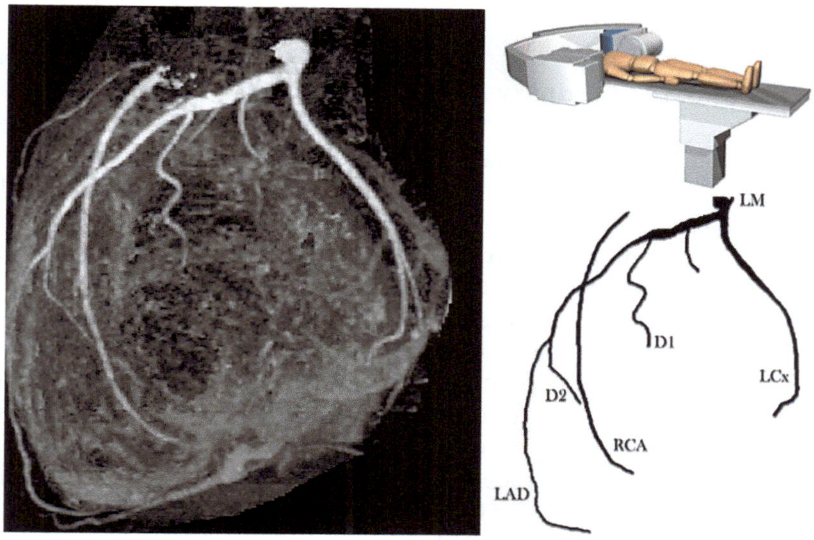

Fig. 1.42. LAO (89°) straight (lateral). The *left image* shows a segmented maximum intensity projection of a multi-detector computed tomography angiogram with a schematic drawing of the same angiogram at the *bottom right*. The *top right* shows the positioning of the C-arm that would be used to acquire the correspoding catheter coronary angiogram (Fig. 1.24). *LM*, left main; *LAD*, left anterior descending; *D1*, first diagonal branch; *D2*, second diagonal branch; *LCx*, left circumflex artery; *RCA*, right coronary artery

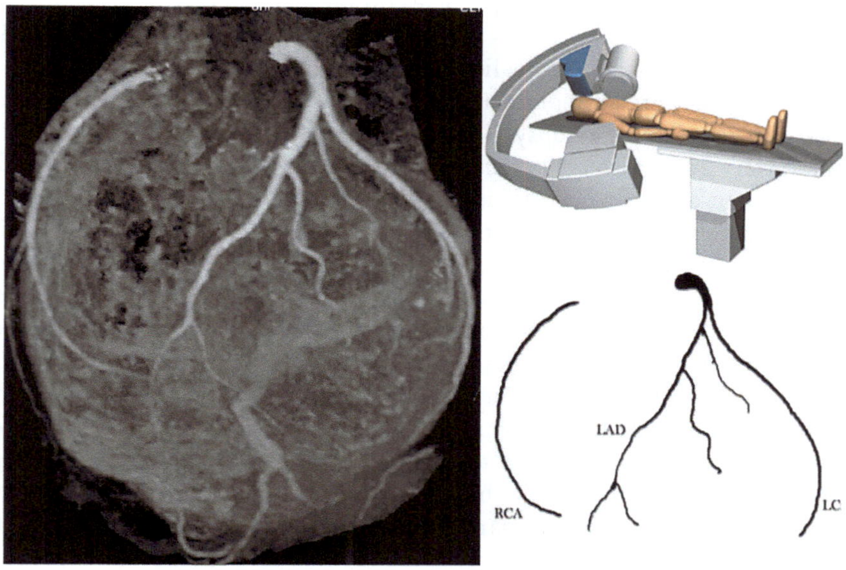

Fig. 1.43. LAO (45°) cranial (30°). The *left image* shows a segmented maximum intensity projection of a multi-detector computed tomography angiogram with a schematic drawing of the same angiogram at the *bottom right*. The *top right* shows the positioning of the C-arm that would be used to acquire the correspoding catheter coronary angiogram (Fig. 1.25). *LAD*, left anterior descending; *LCx*, left circumflex artery; *RCA*, right coronary artery

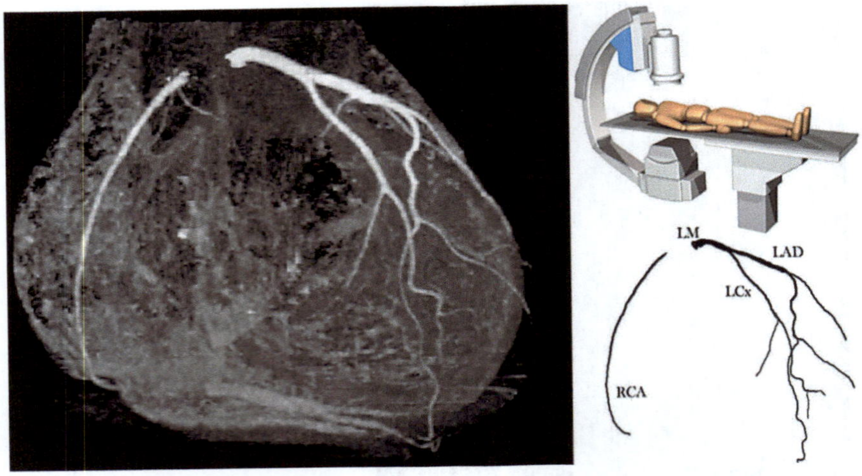

Fig. 1.44. AP straight. The *left image* shows a segmented maximum intensity projection of a multi-detector computed tomography angiogram with a schematic drawing of the same angiogram at the *bottom right*. The *top right* shows the positioning of the C-arm that would be used to acquire the correspoding catheter coronary angiogram (Figs. 1.28 and 1.33). *LM*, left main; *LAD*, left anterior descending; *LCx*, left circumflex artery; *RCA*, right coronary artery

1.5 Anomalies of the Coronary Artery Tree

Congenital abnormalities are rare, although enormous variations in coronary anatomy exist in number, position and both origin and distribution of arteries. They occur in approximately 1% of the general population. They are often associated with congenital heart disease, such as transposition of the great arteries or tetralogy of Fallot, but they also occur in isolated events (Schmitt et al. 2005). A higher incidence of coronary artery anomalies is observed in young athletes, who die of sudden death more frequently than the general population (13% vs 1%). After hypertrophic cardiomyopathy, coronary artery anomalies are the second most common cause of sudden death in young athletes (Maron et al. 2003).

Most coronary artery anomalies are not clinically important; they are asymptomatic and accidentally discovered on CAG or autopsy. However, some coronary artery anomalies are potentially life-threatening and can cause myocardial ischemia or sudden death. Therefore, precise evaluation of the coronary arteries is very important (Datta et al. 2005).

Coronary artery anomalies can be classified according to anatomical morphology, but some studies propose that it would be more effective to classify them on the basis of their correlation and association with myocardial ischemia or sudden death (Rigatelli et al. 2005).

Coronary artery anomalies which can cause myocardial ischemia include coronary artery fistula, an anomalous origin of a coronary artery from the pulmonary trunk, and myocardial bridging. Vessels originating from the contralateral side with an interarterial course, between the aorta and the pulmonary artery, also pose a risk for myocardial ischemia: ectopic origins of the RCA from the left sinus of Valsalva of the LCA, and ectopic origins of the LCA from the right sinus of Valsalva or the proximal RCA (Schmitt et al. 2005). When the contralateral vessel follows another pathway, anterior to the right ventricular outflow tract, posterior to the aortic root or within the interventricular septum, there is no risk for myocardial ischemia and these anomalies can be seen as benign. Other benign anomalies are a LCX originating from the right sinus of Valsalva or the RCA, a separate origin of the LCX and LAD (absent LMCA) and a high takeoff.

1.5.1.1 Coronary Artery Fistula

Congenital arteriovenous coronary artery fistula are a rare condition of a direct communication between a coronary artery and one of the cardiac chambers, the coronary sinus, the superior vena cava or the pulmonary artery (Fig. 1.45). Most fistula are accidentally found during CAG, with a prevalence of about 0.1%–0.2% of all patients who undergo CAG. The most frequent sites of origin are the right coronary artery (60%) and the left coronary artery (40%). Very rarely, fistulas originate from both coronary arteries. The major termination sites are the right ventricle (45%), the right atrium (25%), and the pulmonary artery (15%). The fistulas less frequently drain into the left atrium or left ventricle (10%). When there is a termination to the systemic right

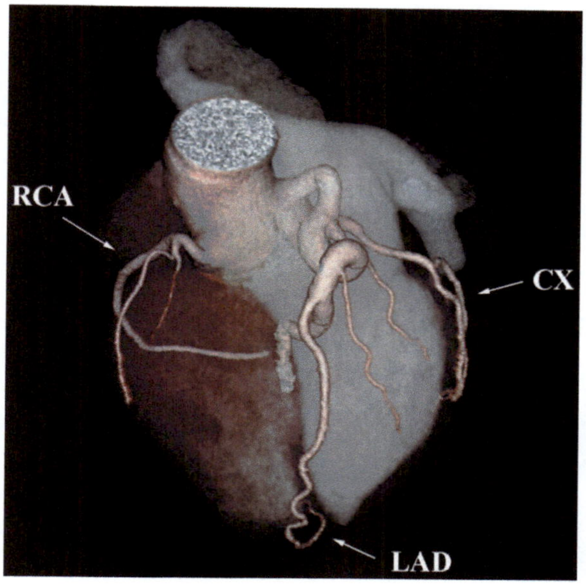

Fig. 1.45. Three-dimensional image of the heart with opaque ascending aorta and coronary arteries, as well as transparent other cardiac structures. The image shows a fistula arising from the first septal branch of the left anterior descending artery (*LAD*). The proximal LAD is tortuous and dilated with a maximum diameter of approximately 8 mm. The dilatation continues distally, until the first septal branch, ending into the right ventricle. After the first septal branch, the LAD has a normal calibre. The proximal part of the circumflex artery is also dilated, with no other abnormalities seen in other parts of the coronary artery system. *RCA*, right coronary artery; *CX*, circumflex artery

side, this is called a left-to-right shunt. When the termination is in a left-sided cardiac chamber, this is referred to as a left-sided volume overloading. The part of the myocardium supplied by the abnormally connecting artery can have decreased blood flow. Without treatment this can result in myocardial ischemia (Kim et al. 2006).

1.5.1.2 Anomalous Origin of a Coronary Artery from the Pulmonary Trunk

An anomalous origin of a coronary artery from the pulmonary artery (ACAPA) is a rare congenital defect (Figs. 1.46–1.48). These anomalies are often haemodynamically significant and can cause myocardial ischemia and sudden cardiac death. The part of the myocardium which is supplied by the abnormally arising coronary artery receives less well oxygenated blood.

An anomalous origin of the LCA from the pulmonary trunk is known as Bland-White-Garland syndrome and most children with this syndrome die in their first year of life (80%–85%). LCA arising from the PA is treated surgically, with ligation and reimplantation of the LCA to the aorta (Nicholson et al. 2004).

An anomalous origin of the left coronary artery from the pulmonary artery (ALCAPA) has a higher incidence than an anomalous origin of the right cor-

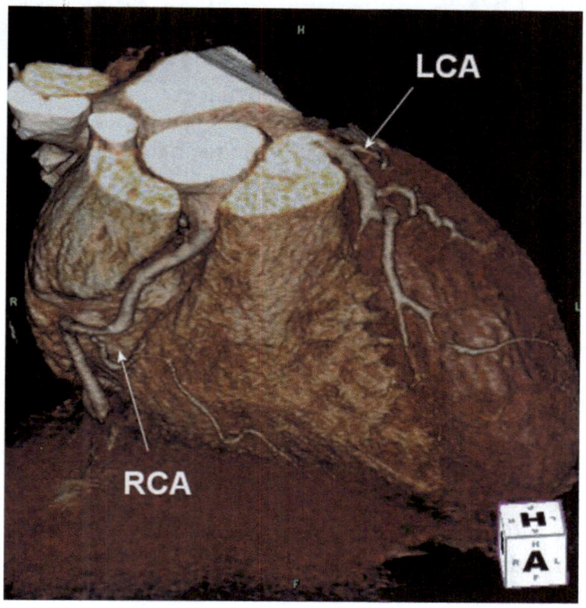

Fig. 1.46. Left coronary artery (*LCA*) coming from the pulmonary trunk, with a normal origin of the right coronary artery (*RCA*) from the aorta

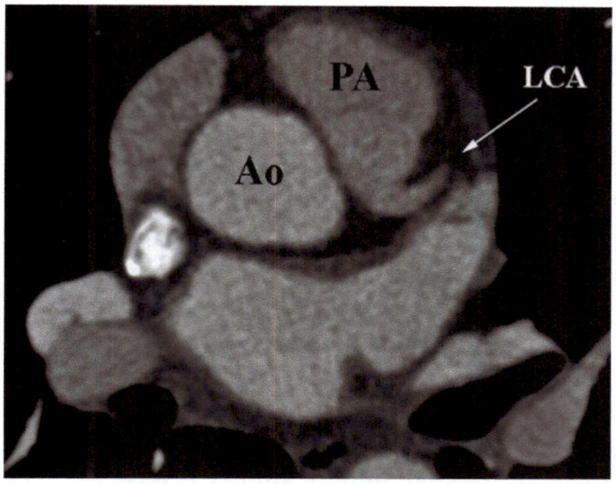

Fig. 1.47. Axial CT slide showing a left coronary artery (*LCA*) originating from the pulmonary artery (*PA*). *Ao*, aorta

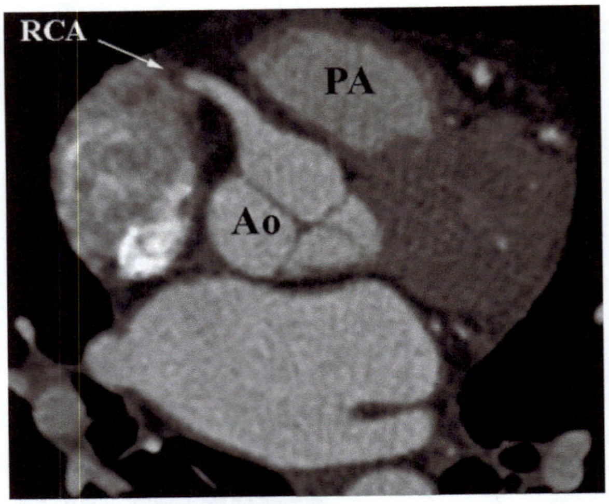

Fig. 1.48. Axial CT slide showing the right coronary artery (*RCA*) having a normal origin from the right sinus of Valsalva. *PA*, pulmonary artery; *Ao*, aorta

onary artery from the pulmonary artery (ARCAPA). The incidences are estimated at 0.008% and 0.002%, respectively. The higher incidence of ALCAPA compared to ARCAPA is explained by the proximity of the left coronary bud to the pulmonary artery sinus during embryological development. The age of presentation is usually earlier in ALCAPA than ARCAPA (<1 year vs >2 years).

ARCAPA less often leads to myocardial ischemia or sudden cardiac death. The possible reason for this is the lower oxygen demand of the right ventricle compared to the left ventricle and the RCA supplies a smaller part of myocardium compared to the LCA (Williams et al. 2006).

1.5.1.3
Myocardial Bridging

Myocardial bridging, an inborn coronary anomaly, is an intramyocardial segment of a coronary artery which is normally located on the surface of the heart. This anomaly results in a wide range of possible clinical manifestations, and its clinical relevance is debated. Myocardial bridging is usually asymptomatic, but has also been associated with angina, myocardial infarction and sudden death. During systole the tunnelled coronary artery is compressed (Alegria et al. 2005). The incidence varies between conventional coronary angiogram studies (0.5%–2.5%) and autopsy studies (15%–85%). The part immediately proximal to the tunnelled artery seems most prone to atherosclerotic plaques because of haemodynamic disturbances. Some articles state that the tunnelled segment is spared from atheromatous changes (Zeina et al. 2007). Myocardial bridging most frequently affects the mid LAD.

Although this malformation is present at birth, symptoms usually do not develop before the third decade (Alegria et al. 2005).

1.5.2
Vessels Originating from the Contralateral Side, With an Interarterial Course

1.5.2.1
Right-Sided Left Coronary Artery

The four most common pathways a right-sided left coronary artery can take are an interarterial (between the aorta and the pulmonary artery), retroaortic, prepulmonic or septal pathway (Fig. 1.49). The course which the anomalous coronary artery has taken is of great significance, because an interarterial course can cause myocardial ischemia or even sudden death, but the other pathways seem to have no clinical significance. The incidence of a left coronary artery from the RSV or RCA in patients receiving conventional catheter coronary angiography is assessed to be 0.09%–0.11%. In three quarters of these patients the anomalous LCA has an interarterial pathway, and thus they are at risk of sudden death (Kim et al. 2006). The mechanism of the cause of the ischemia may be either kinking or compression of the interarterial running coronary artery because of the increased blood flow through the aorta and the pulmonary artery (Figs. 1.50–53).

1.5.2.2
Left-Sided Right Coronary Artery

The incidence of an RCA coming from the LSV or LCA in patients undergoing CAG is estimated to be 0.03%–0.17%. Just as a right-sided LCA, the most common course of the anomalous coronary artery is an interarterial pathway (Figs. 1.54, 1.55). In a left-sided RCA this can also cause myocardial ischemia and sudden death (Kim et al. 2006). However, an RCA running between the aorta and the pulmonary artery has a somewhat lower risk of ischemia than an anomalous LCA. When symptoms of ischemia occur, this can be explained by the same mechanism as described with right-sided LCA.

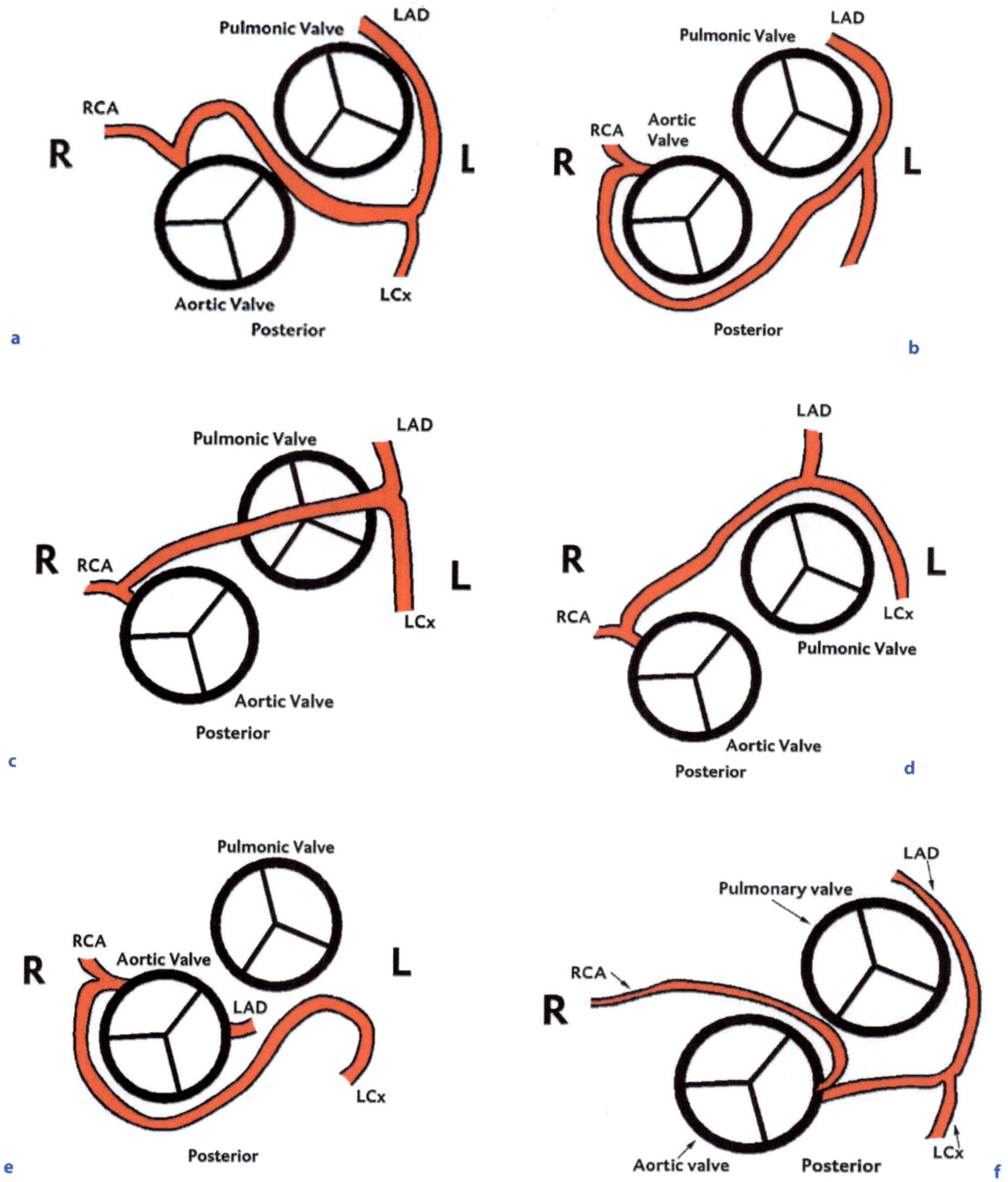

Fig. 1.49a–f. Schematic overview of four different courses of a left coronary artery coming from the right sinus of Valsalva (**a–d**), the most common course of a circumflex artery coming from the right (**e**) and the right coronary artery (*RCA*) coming from the left (**f**). *LAD*, left anterior descending artery; *LCx*, left circumflex artery

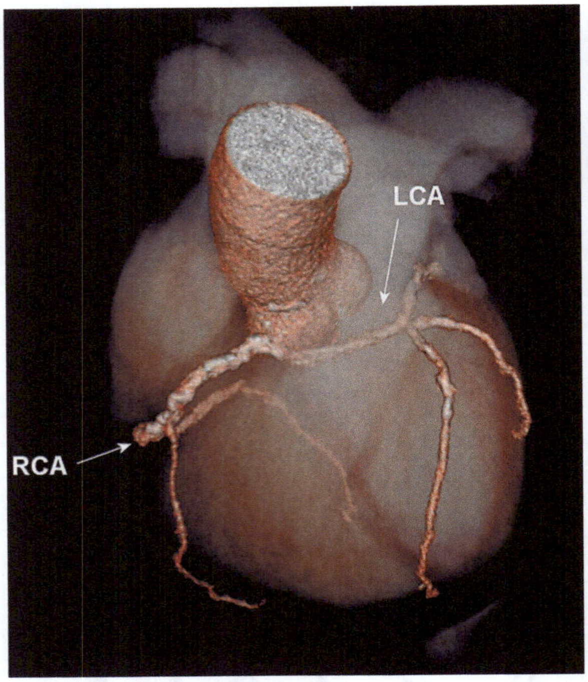

Fig. 1.50. Left coronary artery (*LCA*) originating from the right, sharing the same ostium with the right coronary artery (*RCA*). The LCA crosses over to its normal distributional area between the aorta and pulmonary artery

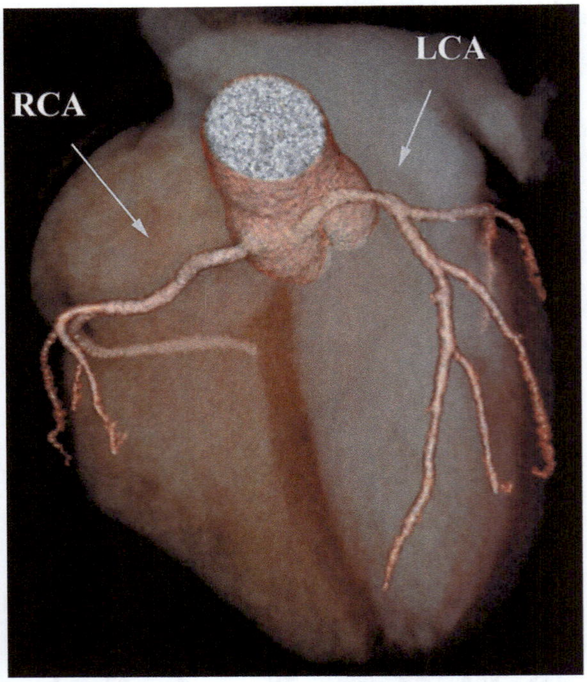

Fig. 1.51. Left coronary artery (*LCA*) coming from the right sinus of Valsalva. *RCA*, right coronary artery

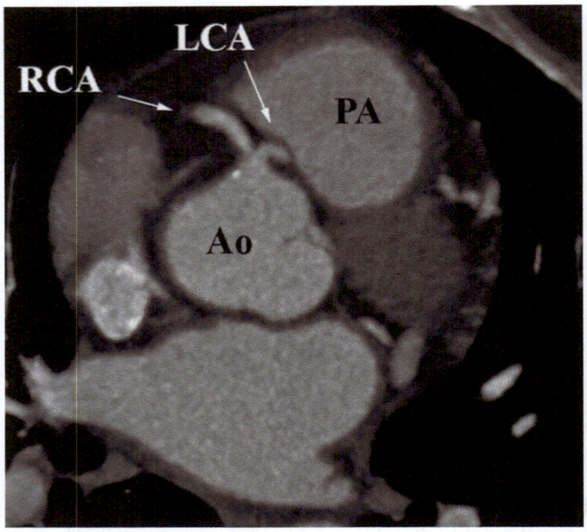

Fig. 1.52. Right coronary artery (*RCA*) and left coronary artery (*LCA*) sharing the same ostium from the right sinus of Valsalva. *PA*, pulmonary artery; *Ao*, aorta

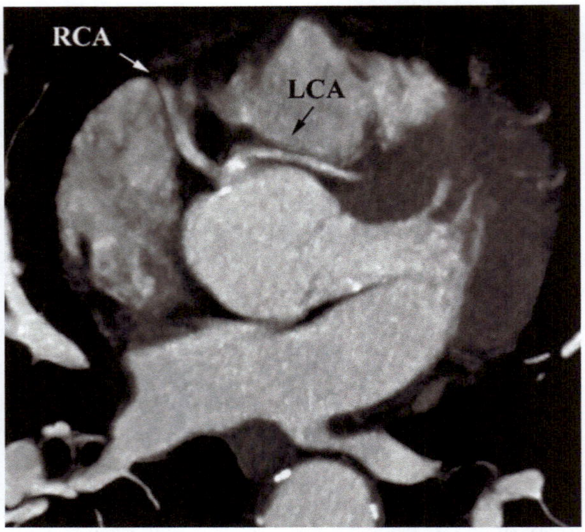

Fig. 1.53. Left coronary artery (*LCA*) sharing the ostium with the right coronary artery (*RCA*) originating from the right sinus of Valsalva. The LCA courses between the aorta and pulmonary artery to its normal distributional area

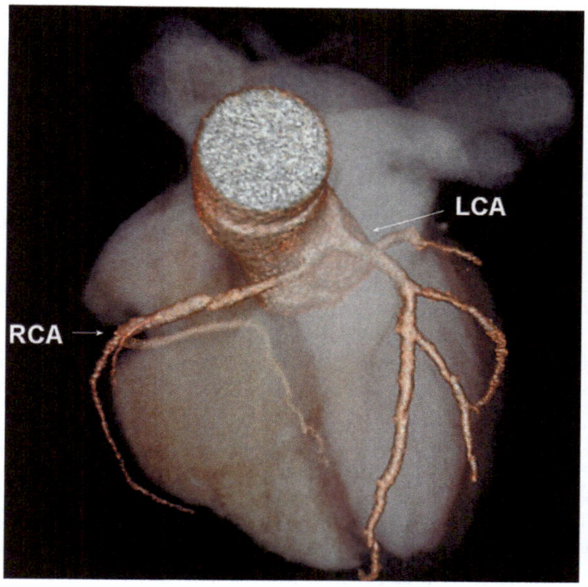

Fig. 1.54. Right coronary artery (*RCA*) coming from the left sinus of Valsalva, sharing the ostium with the left coronary artery (*LCA*). The RCA has an interarterial pathway

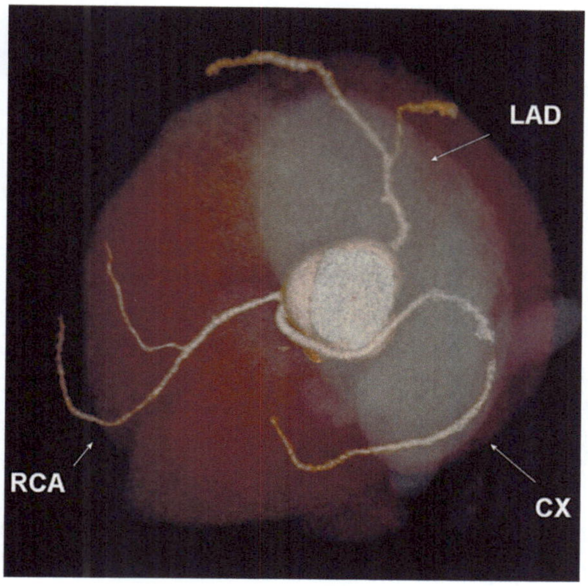

Fig. 1.56. Circumflex artery (*CX*) coming from the right coronary cusp, with the origin just next to the origin of the right coronary artery (*RCA*). *CX*, circumflex artery

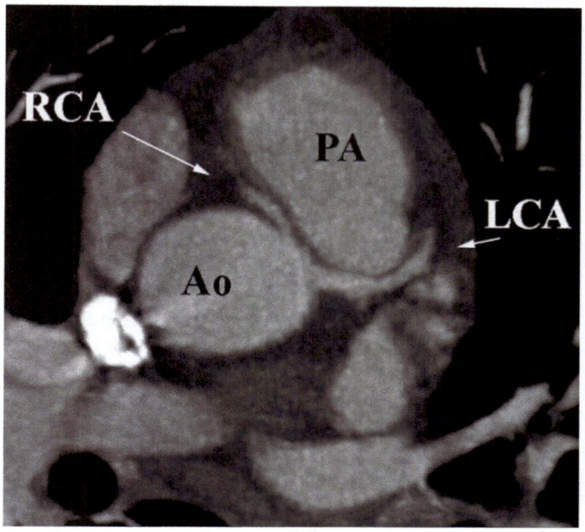

Fig. 1.55. Right coronary artery (*RCA*) coming from the left sinus of Valsalva, coursing between the pulmonary artery (*PA*) and aorta (*Ao*). *LCA*, left coronary artery

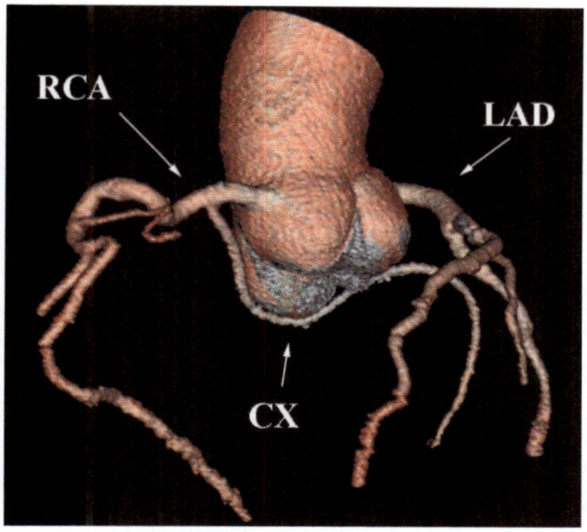

Fig. 1.57. Circumflex artery (*CX*) coming from the right coronary artery (*RCA*) with retroaortic course. *LAD*, left anterior descending artery

1.5.2.3 Congenital Coronary Anomalies Not Causing Myocardial Ischemia

Most coronary artery anomalies are not clinically relevant and are often discovered as an accidental finding in asymptomatic patients. Myocardial blood flow in these patients is not decreased. These anomalies occur in approximately 0.5%–1.0% of adult patients who undergo CAG. The problem with these anomalies is hooking up the origin when performing CAG, because the entrance of the coronary artery is at an unusual position.

An anomalous origin of the CX from the right aortic sinus or as proximal branch of the RCA is frequently encountered (Figs. 1.56, 1.57). In almost every case, the anomalous CX courses behind the aortic root to its normal distributional area, without the risk of interarterial compression, and thus, without risk of myocardial ischemia or sudden death.

A frequently seen anomaly is a high origin of the RCA or LCA. A high takeoff is defined by an origin above the junctional zone between the sinus of Valsalva and the tubular part of the ascending aorta. There is usually no risk of impaired myocardial blood flow.

Another coronary artery anomaly without risk of myocardial ischemia is an absent left main coronary artery. In this case, the LAD and CX arise separately from the aorta. It occurs in approximately 0.41% of individuals with otherwise normal coronary anatomy. Although multiple ostia represent a technical difficulty for the angiographer, they may also allow alternate collateral sources in patients with proximal coronary artery disease (Kim et al. 2006).

References

Achenbach S, Ropers D, Kuettner A, Flohr T, Ohnesorge B, Bruder H, Theessen H, Karakaya M, Daniel WG, Bautz W, Kalender W, Anders K (2006) Contrast-enhanced coronary artery visualization by dual-source computed tomography – initial experience. Eur J Radiol 57:331–335

Alegria JR, Herrmann J, Holmes Jr DR, Lerman A, Rihal CS (2005) Myocardial bridging. Eur Heart J 26:1159–1168

Datta JD, White CS, Gilkeson RC, Meyer CA, Kansal S, Jani ML, Arildsen RC, Read K (2005) Anomalous coronary arteries in adults: depiction at multi-detector row CT angiography. Radiology 235:812–818

Dikkers R, De Jonge GJ, Willems TP, Van Ooijen PMA, Piers LH, Tio RA, Oudkerk M (2006) Clinical implementation of dual-source computed tomography for diagnostic cardiovascular angiography: initial experience. Imaging Decisions, 2

Guyton AC, Hall JE (1996) Textbook of medical physiology, 9th edn. W.B. Saunders, Philadelphia

Johnson TRC, Nikolau K, Wintersperger BJ, Leber AW, Von Ziegler F, Rist C, Buhmann S, Knez A, Reiser MF, Becker CR (2006) Dual-source CT cardiac imaging: initial experience. Eur Radiol 16:1409–1415

Kim SY, Seo JB, Do KH, Heo JN, Lee JS, Song JW, Choe YH, Kim TH, Yong HS, Choi SI, Song KS, Lim TH (2006) Coronary artery anomalies: classification and ECG-gated multi-detector row CT findings with angiographic correlation. RadioGraphics 26:317–334

Maron BJ, Carney KP, Lever HM, Lewis JF, Barac I, Casey SA, Sherrid MV (2003) Relationship of race to sudden cardiac death in competitive athletes with hypertrophic cardiomyopathy. JACC; 41:974–980

Moore KL, Dalley AF (1999) Clinically orientated anatomy, 4th edn. Lippincott Williams & Wilkins, Baltimore

Nicholson WJ, Schuler B, Lerakis S, Helmy T (2004) Anomalous origin of the coronary arteries from the pulmonary trunk in two separate patients with a review of the clinical implications and current treatment recommendations. Am J Med Sciences 328:112–115

Rigatelli G, Docali G, Rossi P, Bandello A, Rigatelli G (2005) Validation of a clinical-significance-based classification of coronary artery anomalies. Angiology 56:25–34

Schmid M, Achenbach S, Ludwig J, Baum U, Anders K, Pohle K, Daniel WG, Ropers D (2006) Visualization of coronary artery anomalies by contrast-enhanced multidetector row spiral computed tomography. Int J Cardiol 111:430–435

Schmitt R, Froehner S, Brunn J, Wagner M, Brunner H, Cherevatyy O, Gietzen F, Christopoulos G, Kerber S, Fellner F (2005) Congenital anomalies of the coronary arteries: imaging with contrast-enhanced, multidetector computed tomography. Eur Radiol 15:1110–1121

Van Ooijen PMA, Dorgelo J, Zijlstra F, Oudkerk M (2004) Detection, visualization and evaluation of anomalous coronary anatomy on 16-slice multidetector-row CT. Eur Radiol 14:2163–2171

Williams IA, Gersony WM, Hellenbrand WE (2006) Anomalous right coronary artery arising from the pulmonary artery: a report of 7 cases and a review of the literature. Am Heart J 152:5

Wintersperger BJ, Nikolau K (2005) Basics of cardiac MDCT: techniques and contrast application. Eur Radiol 15[Suppl 2]:B2–B9

Zeina AR, Odeh M, Blinder J, Rosenschein U, Barmeir E (2007) Myocardial bridge: evaluation on MDCT. AJR Am J Roentgenol 188:1069–1073

Invasive Coronary Imaging

2

2.1 Conventional Catheterisation

Michael R. Rees and Felix Zijlstra

CONTENTS

M. R. Rees, MD, PhD
Professor, Bangor University, Bangor, Gwynedd, LL57 2DG, UK
F. Zijlstra, MD, PhD
Professor, Thorax Center, Department of Cardiology, University Hospital Groningen, P.O. Box 30.001, 9700 RB Groningen, The Netherlands

2.1.1 The Development of Cardiac Catheterisation

The study of the circulation by cardiac catheterisation started in 1844 when Claude Bernard performed retrograde left and right heart catheterisation, from the jugular vein and carotid artery, in a horse. Application of these principles and techniques in patients was made possible by the discovery of X-rays by William Conrad Roentgen (1845–1923) on November 8, 1895, at the University of Wurzburg. He received the Nobel Prize for his discovery in 1901. Roentgen's discovery enabled Werner Forssmann to perform the first cardiac catheterisation on himself under fluoroscopic guidance in 1929 in a small hospital in Eberswald in Germany. He passed a urethral catheter from an arm vein into his right heart. To do this he needed the co-operation of a surgical nurse whom he persuaded to help against the orders of his hospital chief. Forssmann wrote of his findings in 1929 (Forssman 1929); however, the medical establishment failed to recognise his findings. He gave up his work and continued training as a urological surgeon. In 1930, O. Klein described right heart catheterisation and the use of the Fick principle to study cardiac output (Klein 1930).

There was also early research into contrast media in 1929. This was first used by Dos Santos to demonstrate the aorta by direct injection into the lumbar aorta (Dos Santos et al. 1929). In the late 1930s, Robb and Steinberg (1938) demonstrated that the heart and central circulation could be opacified by an intravenous injection of contrast medium.

Others, notably Andre F. Cournand and Dickinson W. Richards, read Forssmann's work. Cournand and Richards performed their first cardiac catheterisation procedure on a patient in 1941 (Cournand and Ranges 1944). Their work led to a greater understanding of the physiology of cardiac circulation and in particular the body's response to shock. These three scientists were jointly awarded the Nobel Prize for their work in cardiac catheterisation in 1956. The use of cardiac catheterisation to study the functional consequences of congenital disease was described in 1944 by Brannon, Weens and Warren at Emory University in Atlanta in a patient with atrial septal defect (Brannon et al. 1945). The development of radiological contrast media had established right heart catheterisation and angiography as well recognised procedures. The study of the left side of the heart was more difficult; the first documented retrograde left heart procedure was performed in 1947 and described by Dr. Henry Zimmerman (Zimmerman et al. 1950).

Angiography was advanced by the development of percutaneous needle puncture techniques by Seldinger, a Swedish radiologist, in 1953 (Seldinger 1953).

In 1958, Dr. Mason Sones observed that a catheter which was intended to be placed in the aorta prolapsed into the right coronary artery. Approximately 30 cc of Hypaque were injected by accident into the artery opacifying it. This caused asystole from which the patient recovered by coughing with no ill effects. Dr. Sones was the first to demonstrate that coronary angiography was possible and went on to demonstrate that much smaller doses of contrast could be injected into the coronary arteries safely and effectively. He started the modern practice of coronary angiography via the brachial cut down approach using his own catheter (Sones et al. 1959). In 1959, Ross developed transseptal puncture whereby a catheter is placed in the left atrium by puncturing the intra-atrial septum from the right atrium (Ross 1959). A percutaneous coronary angiography technique was developed in 1963 and described in 1967 by Dr. Kurt Amplatz (Wilson et al. 1967). Dr. Sven Paulin, a radiologist who developed a technique for coronary arteriography by placing a spiral catheter in the aortic root, also promoted work on coronary arteriography. He published his thesis on coronary arteriography in 1965 and published his findings a year later (Paulin 1966).

In 1967, Dr. Melvin Judkins, working in Charles Dotter's department, developed the preshaped catheters for coronary angiography that are the most common method of coronary arteriography today. His concept was to provide a catheter that was consistent and safe with positive rotational control. His original catheter was 8 F with a tip thinned to 1.8 mm in diameter and 18 mm in length, with a catheter body that was 100 cm in length (Judkins 1967). Right heart catheterisation was further advanced by the development of flow directed catheters by Dr. Jeremy Swan and combined with the work of Dr. William Ganz on the thermodilution method of measuring cardiac output (Swan et al. 1970).

2.1.1.1 Cardiac and Coronary Catheters

Early cardiac catheterisation was carried out using ureteric catheters, which were measured traditionally in French gauge. This method of measurement has persisted with modern cardiac catheterisation and coronary angiography. French gauge is converted into millimetres by dividing by three.

Selective coronary catheters replaced early loop or spiral catheters, which injected contrast into the aortic root as suggested by Bellman et al. (1960) and later by Paulin et al. (1987). The original Sones catheters were made in 7- or 8-F sizes and tapered towards the tip to a 5-F diameter with two holes placed by the tip. They were inserted by a brachial arteriotomy. Originally the catheters were straight but the last few centimetres were often fixed into a curve by forming the tip in heat by an autoclave or steam from a kettle.

Judkins catheters are still the most commonly used catheters. The left Judkins catheter is designed to be inserted directly into the left coronary ostium by placing the secondary curve on the aortic wall and the primary curve directs the catheter into the coronary ostium. The catheters are manufactured in a variety of curve sizes (commonly 3–6 cm). The curve size denotes the distance between the primary and secondary curve in centimetres to accommodate different sized aortic roots. The larger curve sizes are used to cannulate a larger aortic root. The right coronary catheter has to be manipulated into the right coronary artery by clockwise and anterior rotation. Originally Melvin Judkins designed the catheter to be rotated above the coronary ostium so that it would rotate down into the anterior right coronary ostium (Judkins and Judkins 1985). Most angiographers, however, are now taught to place the catheter above the aortic valve and withdraw and rotate the catheter. The right coronary catheter also has a range of curve sizes, which are measured from the primary curve to the midpoint of the secondary curve.

Amplatz catheters are designed such that the secondary curve of the catheter lies across the aortic root and the primary curve points downwards into the coronary artery. This type of catheter is less frequently used and requires a different technique from Judkins catheterisation. Great care should be taken in withdrawing the catheter from the left coronary ostium as when the catheter is withdrawn the tip may plunge deeper into the coronary ostium and cause dissection. For that reason it is recommended by some angiographers that the catheter be withdrawn by advancing the catheter so that the tip prolapses upwards out of the ostium.

Since the introduction of these basic catheters in the 1960s there have been a number of modifications to catheter shape to account for different permutations of coronary anatomy. Catheter design has also had to take account of a number of issues including torsion strength, radio-opacity, thrombogenicity and size. In the latter case there has been a gradual reduction in French size for coronary angiography. Most coronary angiograms are now undertaken with smaller French size catheters (usually 5- or 6-F), but catheters as small as 3-F have been used. The smaller size of catheters has resulted in further modifications of design resulting in proportionately larger lumen sizes to the overall catheter diameter.

2.1.1.2 Cardiac Catheterisation Laboratories

There has been a rapid development of cardiac catheterisation radiological equipment. The resolution of a standard coronary image intensifier should be > 3 line pairs. And acceptable signal-to-noise of 20–25 microR/frame (Moore 1990). The standard catheterisation laboratory consists of angiographic equipment, which is now usually digital with quantification packages for measurement of coronary artery diameter together with modern sophisticated physiological measuring equipment. Other types of imaging and measuring devices are used including intravascular ultrasound (IVUS) (Yock et al. 1988) and pressure wires (Pijls et al. 1995). It is estimated that there are more than 2000 cardiac catheterisation laboratories in the USA, many of which provide on site cardiac surgery. The ACC/SCA&I expert consensus document published in 2001 states that: In the hospital without cardiac surgery capability many patients can undergo cardiac procedures safely. Exclusions for cardiac catheterisation in this setting include patients with acute coronary syndromes, severe congestive heart failure, pulmonary oedema due to acute ischaemia, a high likelihood of severe multi-vessel or left main stem disease based on non-invasive testing, severe left ventricular dysfunction associated with valvular disease and patients with vascular disease. Patients with these problems are at a higher risk of developing adverse complications (Lasky et al. 1993).

With the introduction of digital radiology some had hoped that coronary imaging could be carried out by intravenous injection. This has now been discarded for adult cardiac disease in favour of continuing intra-arterial angiography and pressure measurements. Although some information, particularly on left ventricular contraction and function, can be obtained by intravenous injection (Mancini 1988), adequate visualisation of the coronary arteries, with a view to performing a revascularisation procedure, still requires intracoronary contrast injection. Intravenous injection has a role in the assessment of congenital heart disease (Bogren and Bursch 1984). Digital imaging does in fact have a lower resolution than standard cine film especially in a 512 matrix, an average resolution being 0.2–0.3 mm. Newer digital systems with larger matrix sizes and improved TV chains gain resolution by noise reduction and optimisation of the imaging pathway. This has resulted in a resolution in the range of 0.1–0.15 mm. Digital imaging has allowed for a reduction in radiation dose and reduction in contrast usage compared to film cine angiography.

There has also been progress in the introduction of the DICOM (digital imaging and communication in medicine) format and media for the exchange of cardiac catheterisation information between laboratories and centres (Tuinenburg et al. 2000), but there is still no uniformity of storage methods. Many manufacturers are using a web-based format for transmission and storage of information, but there are significant problems with the transferral of non-DICOM image data into DICOM format images. Despite this non-uniformity there has been a steady growth in the use of telemedicine approaches to the transmission of data.

2.1.1.3 Radiation Safety and Exposure

Coronary angiography and coronary intervention result in significant radiation doses to the operators and the rest of the staff in the catheter laboratory and this must be considered as one of the main health and safety issues in this type of diagnostic and therapeutic procedure. It is also a significant factor in career choice for physician's (Limacher et al. 1998).

Interventional cardiac procedures result in 0.004–0.016 rem/case to the operator. Background radiation exposure is approximately 0.1 rem/year. The recommended maximum radiation exposure is 5 rems/year. Given that there is a general international consensus emerging that doctors should undertake a minimum of 75 cases for intervention a year a cardiac interventionist will be exposed to a significant degree of radiation in order to treat patients and remain within general bounds of accepted practice. Figures for a minimum number of cardiac catheterisations have not been established but range between 75 and 150 per year. The radiation exposure of a diagnostic cardiac case is generally lower than an interventional case on digital equipment, but might be higher on cine angiography.

The increased risk to the operator in terms of development of fatal cancer is generally accepted as 0.04% × total cumulative rem exposure.

The measured exposure for doctors working in cardiac catheter laboratories is from 0.2–6 rems/year with an average exposure of 3 rems/year. Those doctors working in cardiac intervention as well as diagnosis have a higher exposure and the collar level exposure for these physicians is 4–16 mrem/case (Zorzetto et al. 1997; Huiskens and Hummel 1995). Since radiation exposure may also increase the risk of cataract formation, the maximum recommended exposure for the eye lens is 15 rems/year.

Different views alter the radiation dose to the operator; the left anterior oblique view results in a six-fold increase in radiation dose compared to the right anterior oblique view.

Although the radiation dose is higher during cine exposure, fluoroscopy accounts for a higher operator dose because of its prolonged use in interventional procedures.

2.1.1.4
Coronary Contrast Injection

Contrast injection is predominantly carried out manually for coronary artery opacification. Usually 6–9 ml are injected manually into the left coronary artery per coronary 'run' and 3–6 ml for the right coronary artery per 'run'. The rate and force of the injection can then be adjusted to the coronary anatomy being visualised and to account for the clinical condition.

Some authors have advocated pump injections for coronary visualisation as well as for left ventriculography. This approach has the disadvantage of loss of control by the operator but has the advantage of a known injection rate and amount for quantification purposes. Newer pumps have been designed to account for the loss of operator control and are currently being introduced to clinical practice. Pump injection has been advocated as a means of reducing catheter size to 4-F (Arora et al. 2002).

2.1.1.5
Views for Coronary Angiography

Since the branching of the coronary arteries forms a complex three-dimensional pattern, the coronary arteries have to be visualised in a number of different views to obtain a complete picture of coronary anatomy. These views are named after the position of the X-ray image intensifier in relation to the patient and not as in normal radiological nomenclature to the position of the passage of the beam through the patient. Therefore, a right anterior oblique view relates to the position of the image intensifier in the right anterior oblique position to the patient and is located by the degree of displacement from the vertical position. The tube is usually angulated in two planes right and left oblique and in caudal or cranial tilt, again denoting the position of the image intensifier from the vertical in relation to the patients head (cranial) or feet (caudal). It is usual to perform a series of six or more views of the left coronary and three views of the right coronary arteries to obtain all the necessary information (Grover et al. 1984). Multiple views may be required to fully appreciate the nature of disease in some patients. Knowledge of the normal and abnormal anatomy of the coronary tree in these different views is required for full clinical interpretation.

2.1.1.6
Quantification of Coronary Angiography

All modern cardiac catheterisation laboratories contain X-ray equipment, which is equipped with measurement packages for two-dimensional (2D) quantification of the coronary arteries. These measurements can be extrapolated to three-dimensional (3D) measurements. In this way the equipment can measure coronary stenoses and therefore help the operator make predictions about the optimal balloon and stent sizes for coronary angioplasty (Reiber et al. 1993). Digital imaging and quantification packages combined with injection pumps have been used to make measurements of coronary flow and myocardial perfusion. Most of these measurements have been supplanted by other methodologies, in the case of coronary flow-by-flow wires and in the case of dynamic measurement of stenoses by pressure wires or intravascular ultrasound. In the case of myocardial perfusion this is most commonly measured by perfusion scintigraphy, stress echocardiography, perfusion magnetic resonance imaging or by perfusion computed tomography.

2.1.2 Normal Coronary Anatomy

The normal human coronary arterial circulation has two main coronary arteries. The left coronary artery arises from the left posterior aortic sinus (left coronary sinus), after a short distance the artery divides beneath the left atrial appendage into two main branches: the circumflex artery and the left anterior descending artery. The left anterior descending artery runs down the anterior intraventricular groove to the apex and the circumflex artery runs posteriorly in its initial course and then down the posterior atrioventricular groove. The left anterior descending artery gives off septal branches which supply the intraventricular septum and diagonal arteries which supply the anterolateral wall. The right main coronary artery is a single vessel which arises from the anterior coronary sinus (right coronary sinus) and which runs anteriorly down the anterior atrioventricular groove to the crux where the grooves of the heart meet. In most people the right coronary artery then continues anteriorly in the posterior intraventricular groove to supply the inferior surface of the heart and the inferior septum via the septal arteries. From the crux the right coronary artery also usually gives off the artery which supplies the atrioventricular node and arteries which supply the posterior aspect of the left ventricle. The right coronary gives off proximal branches to the conus, sinoatrial node (in 55% of subjects) and right ventricle. The conus artery may have a separate origin or multiple origins. Both the left and right coronary arteries supply vessels to the atria via atrial circumflex arteries. The distribution of the coronary arteries describe a loop around the intraventricular grooves (left anterior descending and posterior descending) and a circle around the atrioventricular grooves (circumflex and right coronary arteries). This loop and circle model can help in the interpretation of coronary artery anatomy in oblique views of the arteries (Franch et al. 1982).

2.1.3 Arterial Dominance

The proportion of the left ventricle supplied by the left and right coronary arteries is variable. By convention the artery that supplies the posterior descending artery determines arterial dominance. If the posterior descending artery arises from the right coronary artery the circumflex artery is small; correspondingly, if the posterior descending artery arises from the circumflex coronary artery the right coronary artery is small and may not contribute any branches to the left ventricle. Approximately 80% of the population have right dominance, 10% have left dominance and 10% are balanced.

2.1.3.1 Normal Variants

In approximately 1% of coronary angiograms the left main stem coronary artery is missing and the left anterior descending and circumflex arteries have separate origins from the left coronary sinus. There are minor variations in location of the ostia within the coronary sinus which are of no clinical importance but which may necessitate the use of specialist catheters for cannulation (Vlodaver et al. 1972).

2.1.3.2 Muscle Bridge

This is a specific coronary variant where part of the coronary artery runs sub-epicardially or within the myocardium. This has been shown to occur in 1% of individuals. A recent study of 3200 angiograms revealed 21 cases (0.6%). The artery usually affected is the left anterior descending artery (Harikrishnan et al. 1999). The prognosis for this condition is good. Occasionally this condition gives rise to symptoms of angina. The usual treatment in these cases is beta-blockers, placement of a coronary stent or bypass surgery.

2.1.3.3 Coronary Artery Anomalies Presenting in the Adult

Coronary artery anomalies account for approximately 1% of all adult cases undergoing coronary angiography; however, some of these cases are missed on initial angiography. Estimates of up to 40% failure to complete visualisation of the whole coronary tree at initial angiography have been made (Yacoub and Ross 1983).

In the USA coronary anomalies are found in 1% of routine autopsy examinations; however, this rises to 4%–15% of patients who suffered sudden death. Despite this the majority of coronary anomalies are clinically silent, although there are specific coronary abnormalities associated with mortality. These include: (a) Origin of the left main coronary artery from the pulmonary trunk; (b) anomalous shape of the ostium; (c) aberrant course of the coronary arteries between the origin of the great vessels; (d) origin of the coronary arteries from the wrong coronary sinus; (e) large coronary fistulae (Angelini 1989).

Other coronary abnormalities may have a lesser, but still significant, risk of sudden cardiac death. These include abnormally high take-off of the coronary arteries, generally defined as being higher than 1 cm above the sinotubular ridge.

The most common anomaly is the origin of the circumflex coronary artery from the right coronary sinus; this has been reported to occur on between 0.37% and 0.67% of coronary angiograms and is generally thought to be benign, although the proximal segment of the circumflex artery often develops coronary artery disease and at least one case of sudden death with this anomaly has been reported (Donaldson et al. 1982). Less commonly the left anterior descending artery arises from the right coronary sinus (0.04% of patients). The clinical significance of this anomaly depends on the subsequent course of the vessel; if it passes between the origins of the great vessels the risk of sudden death is increased. This abnormality has a high degree of association with tetralogy of Fallot. Even rarer (0.02%) and of much greater clinical significance is the origin of the left main stem from the right coronary sinus, with a course of the left main stem between aorta and pulmonary trunk which increases the risk of sudden death. The right coronary artery originating from the left coronary sinus is the rarest of the left/right sinus coronary artery anomalies and is again also associated with sudden death (Basso et al. 2000). This abnormality may be difficult to demonstrate angiographically and may be missed more frequently than is realised. Finally, a single coronary artery is a very rare abnormality and accounts for 0.02% of the catheterised population. This anomaly has a number of variants and its clinical significance depends on the type of orifice and course.

2.1.4 Coronary Abnormalities Presenting in Infancy and Childhood

Any of the above abnormalities may present in the young, the most common abnormality presenting in childhood being the origin of the left coronary artery from the pulmonary artery. Usually, the right coronary artery arises from the normal right coronary sinus and if this is a large and dominant artery this abnormality may not present early. The majority of infants with this abnormality die in the first 3 months of life as the postpartum pressure in the pulmonary artery is not sufficient to supply flow to the myocardium (Mintz et al. 1983). Some infants survive a period of heart failure and improve due to the development of collateral circulation and may present later in life or be asymptomatic.

Patients with congenital heart disease (TGA, pulmonary trunk, Fallot) may also have coronary artery anomalies and careful assessment of the coronary circulation in congenital heart disease is an important part of the assessment of these patients.

2.1.4.1 Coronary Fistulae

A coronary fistula is formed from an abnormal connection between a coronary artery or branch to another structure such as the pulmonary artery, coronary sinus, right atrium or right ventricle. This condition is more common in patients with congenital heart disease and accounts for 0.2%–0.4% of congenital cardiac disease. It is one of the most common congenital coronary abnormalities accounting for approximately 50% of the total of coronary anomalies. In the original studies in the Cleveland Clinic 15 cases were reported in 6000 angiograms (Effer et al. 1967).

Most fistulae arise from the right coronary artery (60%) and terminate in the right heart.

Most fistulae are benign and asymptomatic, they tend to enlarge with time and symptoms occur later in life. Patients may develop angina and heart failure in later life, and presentation in childhood is usually associated with fatigue and dyspnea.

There are rare causes of acquired coronary fistulae, which include trauma, post-surgery including by-pass grafting to a coronary vein and myocardial infarction.

2.1.5 Risks of Coronary Angiography

Although coronary angiography is generally regarded as a safe procedure, it is an invasive procedure. One of the first studies on the complications of coronary angiography by Adams et al. (1973) demonstrated a mortality rate of coronary angiography of 0.44% in a study of 55,640 cases. However, by the time a second study had been carried out by the same authors a much lower mortality rate of 0.17% was observed in 35,500 patients (Abrams and Adams 1975). In the USA, the registry of the Society for Cardiac Angiography participating centres showed that between 1978 and 1981 the risk to life of coronary angiography was 0.125% (Kennedy 1981). In the Society for Cardiac Angiography registry the risk of myocardial infarction was 0.09%, stroke 0.07% and vascular complications 0.5% (Kennedy 1983). In the Bristol General Hospital prospective data were collected over a 7-year period on patients undergoing repair of iatrogenic vascular injury following arterial cannulation. From 9375 procedures (7790 coronary angiograms, 835 coronary angioplasties, 445 other cardiac catheterisations, 155 femoral angiograms, 150 peripheral angioplasties) surgical repair was required in 26 patients. The overall incidence of significant injury was 0.28% and higher in therapeutic than diagnostic procedures (Waller et al. 1993).

Surveys have shown that the risk of angiography rises with the severity of disease and is also inversely proportional to the number of cases carried out in the centre. The highest mortality risk occurred with patients with left main stem disease, which was identified as having a mortality rate of 0.86% in the Society of Cardiac Angiography data (Kennedy 1981, 1983).

Specific risks are associated with patients with systemic disease. Adequate hydration is important in patients with renal disease. Diabetic patients on Metformin have been reported to develop lactic acidosis, therefore the drug should be withheld on the day of procedure and not restarted for 48 h. There are also reports of rare but significant complications of coronary angiography which include air embolism (Hung et al. 2002), coronary perforation (Timurkaynak et al. 2001), radiation injury (Vano et al. 2001), peripheral embolism (Katus et al. 2001), cortical blindness (Kwok and Lim 2000), and spinal cord infarction (Aramburu et al. 2000). The current rate of complications for diagnostic coronary angiography should be less than 1%.

2.1.5.1 Selection of Patients for Coronary Angiography

Over 1 million coronary angiograms were performed in the USA in 1993, representing a figure of 4000 per million of the population. This is projected to rise to 3 million procedures in 2010 (Scanlon and Faxon 1999).

The ACC expert consensus document suggests that, with proper screening and baseline decision-making prior to catheterisation, the number of normal coronary angiograms performed should be in the range of 20%–27%. There is relatively little information available on the documentation of unnecessary coronary angiograms, which is not the same as the number of normal coronary angiograms. Studies have reported figures of between 2% and 58% of unnecessary procedures performed.

It is well established that the risk of coronary angiography rises with age and the degree of severity of the coronary and cardiac disease present.

It is important that patients should be properly investigated prior to coronary angiography in order to reduce these risks and to reduce the number of events. In recent years the role of screening and risk stratification of patients with coronary disease have been investigated.

Despite the fact that coronary angiography is one of the world's most common medical procedures the strategies offered for selection of patients varies considerably. Chest pain is a common symptom and experience with open access chest pain clinics in the UK has demonstrated that approximately only 10% of patients who present with chest pain to an open access chest pain clinic have coronary disease requiring re-vascularisation

2.1.5.2 Development of Coronary Revascularisation

The treatment of coronary disease was advanced by the development of an effective surgical method of bypassing the stenotic or occluded segment of a coronary artery by using a vein graft sown from the aorta into the distal coronary vessel. This operation was first performed by Dr Rene Favarolo in Cleveland, USA, in 1967 (Roncroni et al. 1973).

2.1.6 Percutaneous Coronary Intervention

Interventional cardiology, defined as the application of catheter-based techniques to treat cardiac disease, was developed as a culmination of the use of catheters as instruments for the diagnosis of cardiac disease (Douglas and King 2001). The earliest described procedure was the Raskind balloon septostomy to create interatrial defects in patients with transposition of the great vessels (Douglas and King 2001).

Dotter and Judkins were the first to treat vascular stenosis in peripheral atherosclerotic disease by means of an angioplasty procedure. Although this method of multiple catheters to dilate stenotic arteries failed to gain widespread acceptance because of frequent complications, the modern era of intervention started as an outgrowth of these ideas (Dotter and Judkins 1964; Gruntzig and Hopff 1974). In September 1977 in Zurich Andreas Gruntzig performed the first percutaneous transluminal coronary angioplasty and dilated with success a high grade narrowing in the proximal left anterior descending coronary artery of a 37-year-old man (Gruntzig 1978). The follow-up angiographies after 1 month, 1 year, 10 years and even 20 years in this first patient have shown sustained resolution of this coronary stenosis (Meier et al. 2003).

Since this initial application of balloon angioplasty, this field of interventional cardiology has grown explosively and current indications for this procedure have expanded to include unstable angina and acute myocardial infarction, elderly patients and those with depressed left ventricular function, multivessel coronary artery disease and stenosis with complex characteristics (Smith et al. 2001). Examples are shown in Figure 2.1.1–2.1.7. After the development of balloon angioplasty a variety of additional new devices for intracoronary intervention or intracoronary diagnosis were developed (Simpson et al. 1982; Cumberland et al. 1986; Richens et al. 1987; Hansen et al. 1988; Stack et al. 1989; Simpson et al. 1988; Sigwart et al. 1987; Michalis et al. 1999; Boehrer et al. 1995). Diagnostic techniques, including intravascular ultrasound, pressure measurements and flow assessments have provided a wealth of diagnostic and physiologic information, complementary to data derived from conventional angiography. Many technically very advanced therapeutic alternatives to balloon angioplasty, such as lasers, atherectomies, etc., have been developed, but none of these have gained widespread acceptance (Douglas and King 2001), with the exception of the introduction in to clinical practice of coronary stenting. This procedure is now used in a large majority of percutaneous coronary interventions. These stents are scaffolding devices that prevent elastic recoil and can be used to treat flow-limiting dissections.

In the last 10 years the number of percutaneous revascularisation procedures have outgrown the number of coronary artery bypass surgeries as a consequence of the extended technical possibilities of the percutaneous procedures. This has been made possible by substantial improvements in the quality of radiographic imaging in the cardiac catheterisation laboratory, with the development of high-resolution fluoroscopy, digital image reconstruction and online computerised quantitative analysis. Technical improvements with regard to the catheterisation material, such as guiding catheters, guidewires, low-profile balloon catheters (that can take pressures as high as 26 atm) and a wide range of designs of coronary stents (Carter et al. 1998), make a large majority of stenotic lesions in coronary arteries amenable to percutaneous treatment.

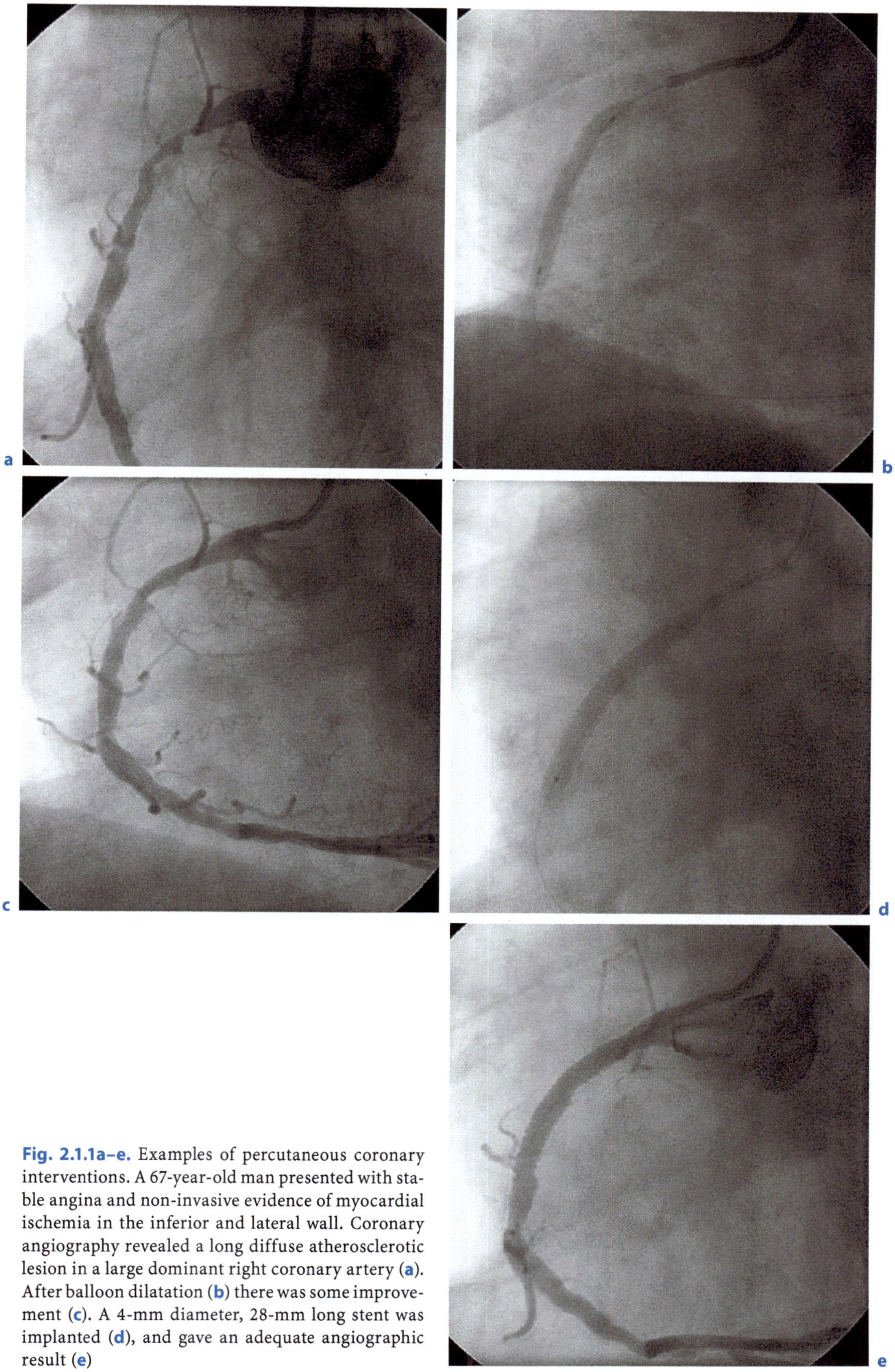

Fig. 2.1.1a–e. Examples of percutaneous coronary interventions. A 67-year-old man presented with stable angina and non-invasive evidence of myocardial ischemia in the inferior and lateral wall. Coronary angiography revealed a long diffuse atherosclerotic lesion in a large dominant right coronary artery (a). After balloon dilatation (b) there was some improvement (c). A 4-mm diameter, 28-mm long stent was implanted (d), and gave an adequate angiographic result (e)

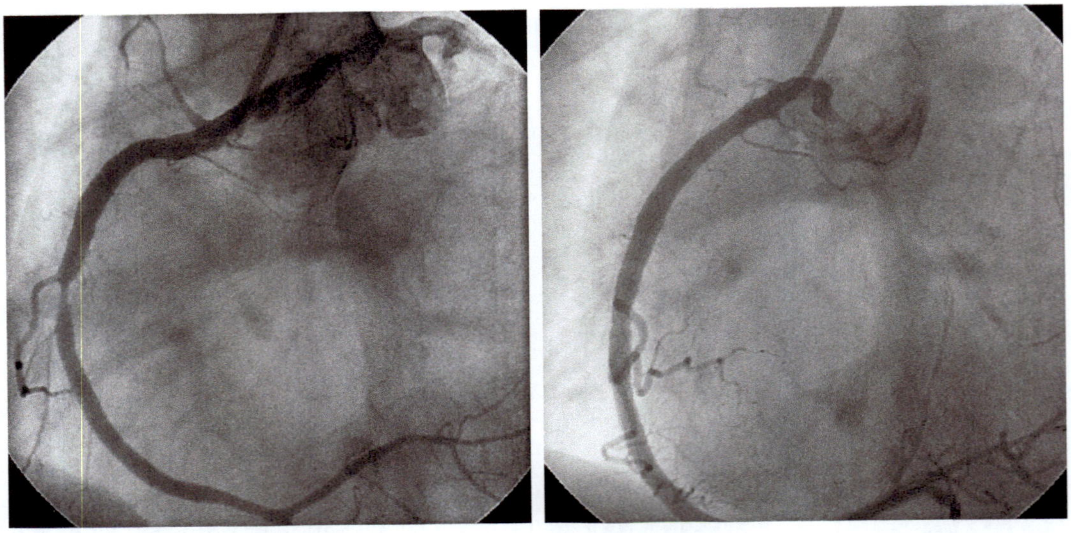

a b

Fig. 2.1.2a,b. A 62-year-old man presented with recent onset angina and ST-T segment changes in the inferior electrocardiographic leads. Coronary angiography showed a short stenosis in a dominant right coronary artery (**a**) that responded well to primary stenting (**b**)

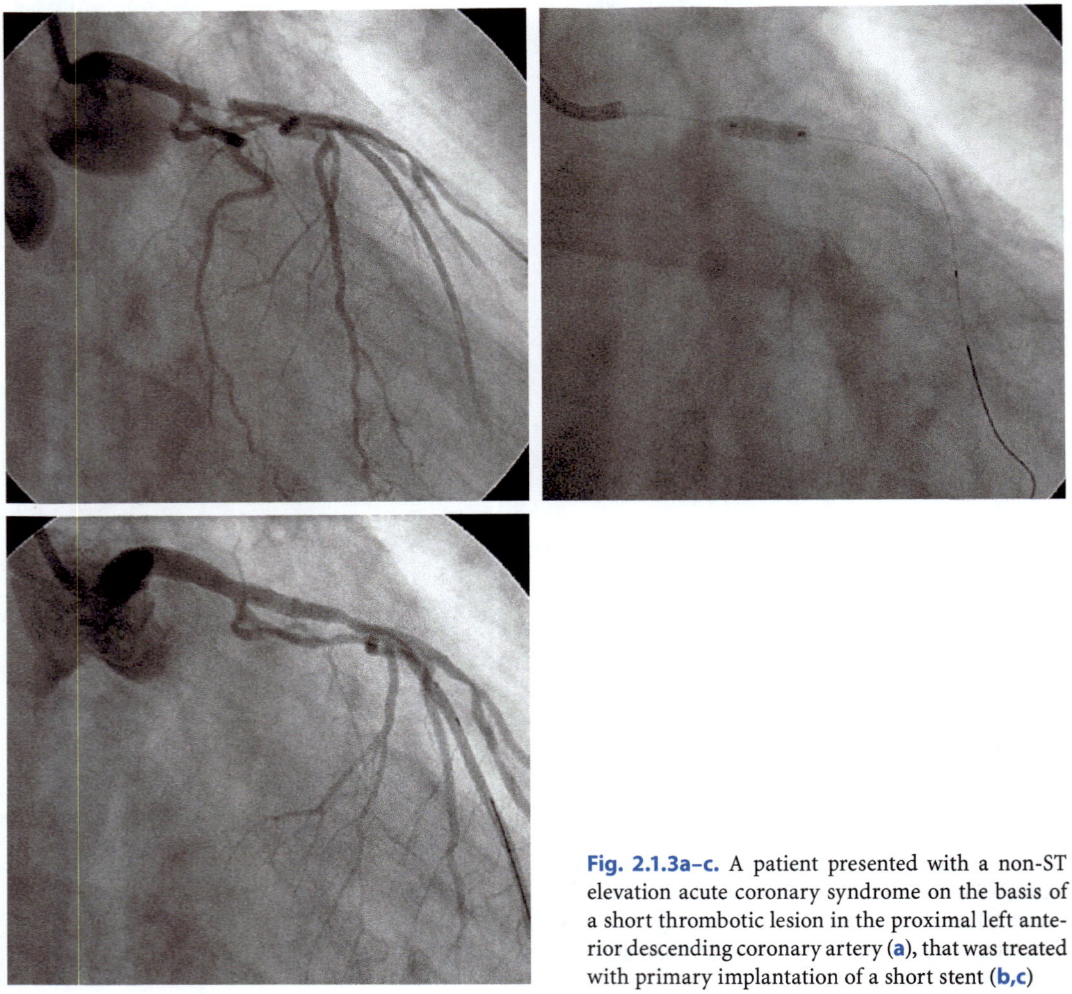

a b c

Fig. 2.1.3a–c. A patient presented with a non-ST elevation acute coronary syndrome on the basis of a short thrombotic lesion in the proximal left anterior descending coronary artery (**a**), that was treated with primary implantation of a short stent (**b,c**)

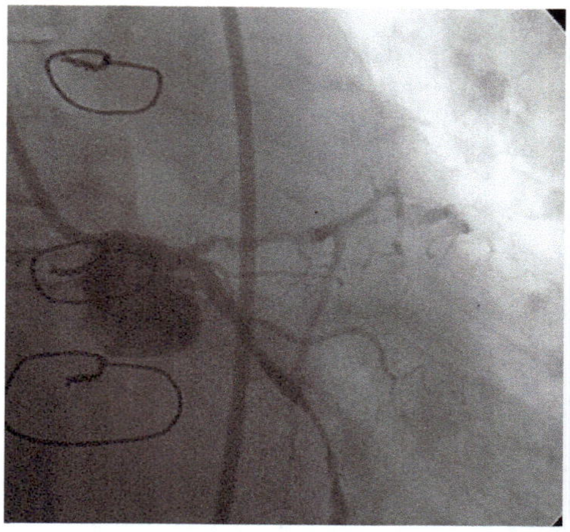
a

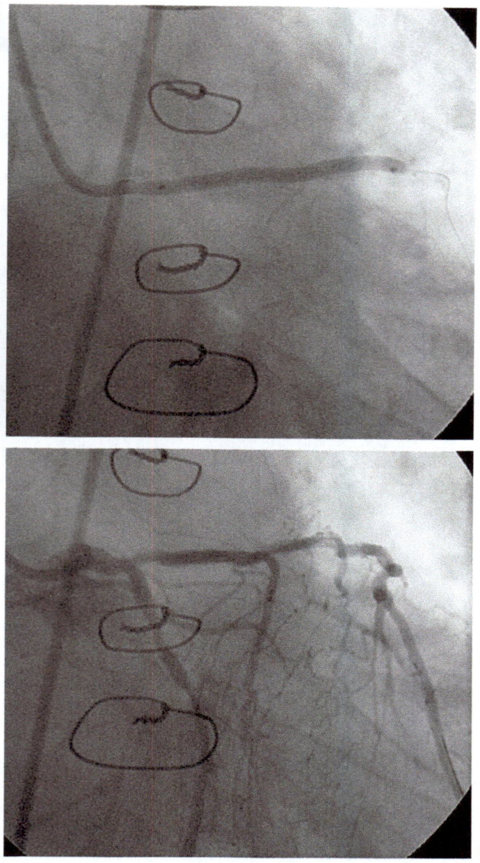
b

c

Fig. 2.1.4a–c. A 76-year-old man presented with angina and heart failure 11 years after triple vessel coronary bypass grafting. Coronary angiography showed triple vessel native disease as well as graft failure towards the anterior wall. There was poor antegrade flow towards the left anterior descending artery due to diffuse disease (**a**). Following multiple inflations with a 3-mm diameter, 40-mm long balloon (**b**), prompt antegrade flow to the left anterior descending artery and its sidebranches was established (**c**)

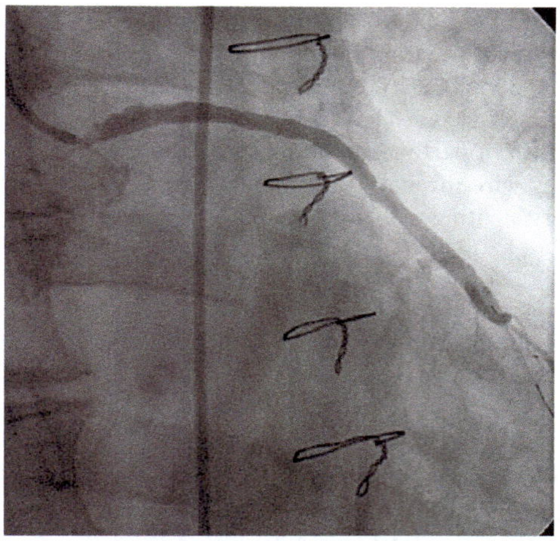
a

Fig. 2.1.5a–c. A 72-year-old man, 18 years after triple vessel coronary bypass grafting presented with unstable angina. Two venous jump grafts showed severe proximal lesions, one of which is shown in (**a**). Direct stenting (**b**) resulted in good angiographic recanalization (**c**) and the patient had a good clinical outcome

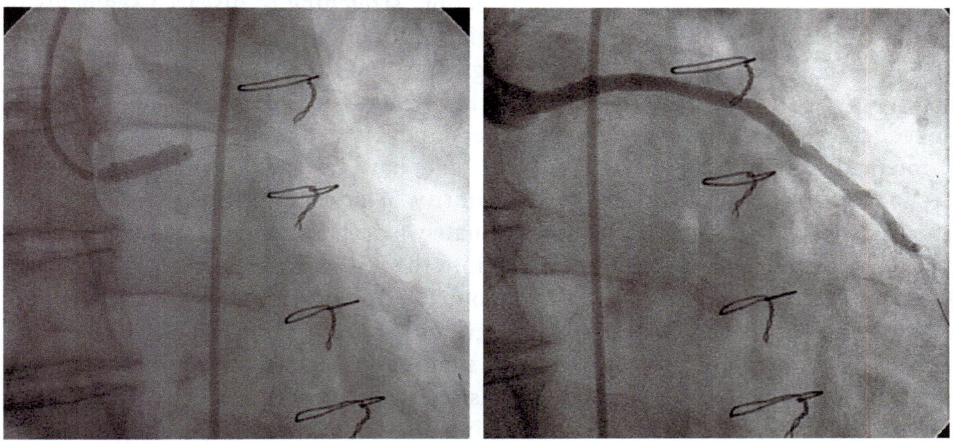
b

c

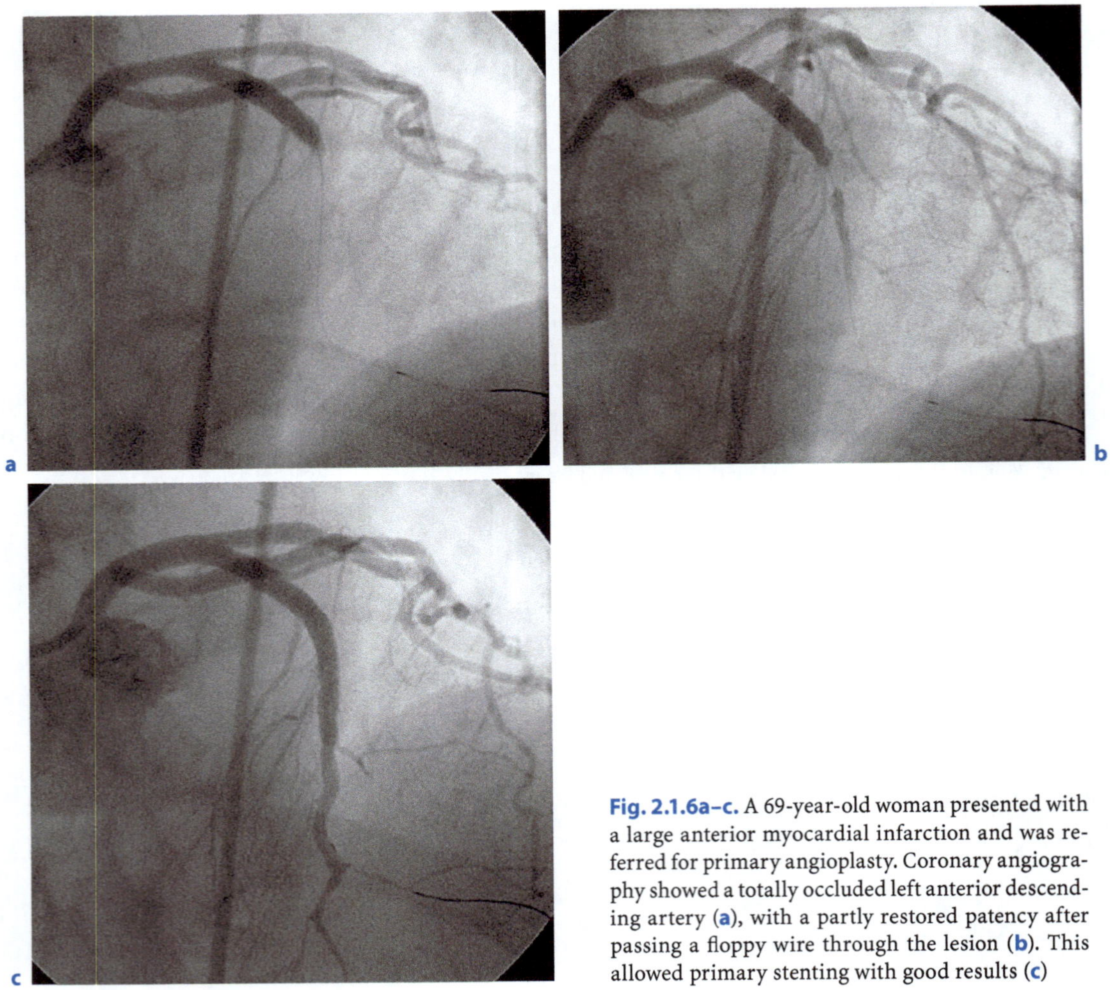

Fig. 2.1.6a–c. A 69-year-old woman presented with a large anterior myocardial infarction and was referred for primary angioplasty. Coronary angiography showed a totally occluded left anterior descending artery (a), with a partly restored patency after passing a floppy wire through the lesion (b). This allowed primary stenting with good results (c)

2.1.6.1 Concomitant Pharmacological Therapy

Antiplatelet therapy with aspirin and clopidogrel starting preferably at least 1 day before the procedure, anti-ischemic therapy with beta-blockers and nitrates, peri-procedural heparinisation and selective use of glycoprotein 2B, 3A inhibitors have put complication rates for large series of patients at below 5% (Douglas and King 2001; Smith et al. 2001; EPIC Investigators 1994; EPISTENT Investigators 1997), and a large majority of complications can nowadays be managed in the catheterisation laboratory. Acute cardiac surgical intervention for angioplasty complications has become rare. Pathological studies have shown that angioplasty is effective by five different mechanisms: plaque compression, plaque fracture, media dissection, stretching of diseased segments of the arterial wall and stretching of plaque-free arterial segments (Douglas and King 2001). Given these rather crude modes of action of angioplasty, it is understandable that scaffolding devices in the form of stents have become an essential part of a large majority of procedures. Provided that they are adequately placed and that all metal is well impressed into the wall, stenting results in improved clinical outcome. Stent thrombosis, a catastrophic complication that occurred frequently in the early years of stenting, has now become rare, although the occasional patient with a stent thrombosis is still the interventional cardiologist's nightmare.

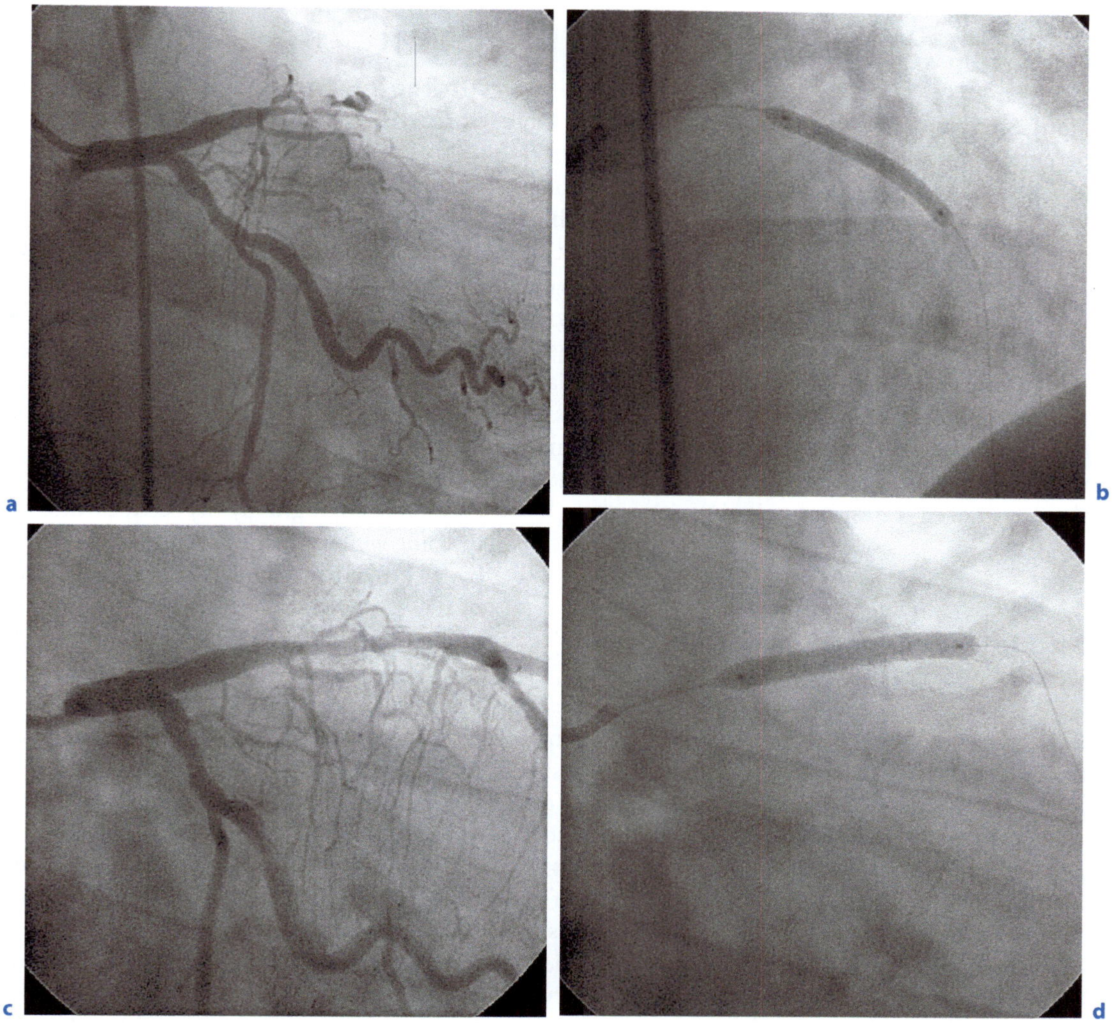

Fig. 2.1.7a–d. A 52-year-old man was referred for primary angioplasty for a large anterior myocardial infarction complicated by cardiogenic shock. Coronary angiography demonstrated a very large left anterior descending coronary artery with acute occlusion (**a**). A wire was passed to the distal vessel and following balloon inflation (**b**) flow was re-established (**c**). Following stent implantation (**d**) a widely patent artery was obtained and the patient made an uneventful recovery

2.1.6.2 Long-Term Outcome

Among patients who have undergone successful coronary angioplasty, the incidence of death or non-fatal infarction in the years after the procedure is low. The most frequently occurring problem is the development of reoccurrence of stenosis at the treated site. Elastic recoil, negative remodelling and ingrowth of tissue induce this re-stenotic process. The first two mechanisms are effectively controlled by stenting; however, most types of stent induce an exaggerated tissue growth response, making the problem of in-stent restenosis a frequent clinical issue that, in particular in long stented segments, is associated with impaired clinical outcome. Recent attempts with drugs loaded on the stents show promising results with regard to a reduction in tissue ingrowth. However, some types of drug eluting stents have been associated with serious hazards such as late stent thrombosis, and late malapposition of stents. Therefore, although they induce a reduced rate of restenosis, an improved clinical outcome is not always the final result. Nevertheless, theoretically these developments will resolve the important clinical issue of restenosis over the coming years.

2.1.6.3
Comparison with Bypass Surgery

Many randomised trials have compared current day percutaneous coronary intervention with coronary artery bypass surgery (Douglas and King 2001). With regard to major clinical endpoints, such as death and myocardial infarction, most of these studies do not show a difference. Most studies show a difference with regard to more morbidity in the surgical group around the surgical procedure and a higher rate of repeat procedures for recurrent ischemia in the percutaneous coronary intervention groups. In daily practice, patient and physician preferences usually determine the mode of revascularisation therapy chosen for an individual patient.

2.1.6.4
Percutaneous Coronary Intervention Versus Conservative Therapy

Randomised studies of patients with stable coronary artery disease have confirmed that angioplasty results in less ischemia and a somewhat better clinical outcome compared to medical therapy alone in selected patients with proven myocardial ischemia (Douglas and King 2001; Smith et al. 2001). In this type of patient with stable coronary artery disease, there is no proof that angioplasty lowers mortality. In patients admitted to hospital with an unstable coronary syndrome, randomised trials in recent years have confirmed that in patients with unstable angina or non-ST elevation myocardial ischemia, and objective evidence of ischemia, for instance ECG changes and/or positive troponins, intervention with a percutaneous coronary procedure results in a lower incidence of the combination of death and non-fatal myocardial infarction.

Finally, many studies have confirmed the important benefits of percutaneous coronary intervention in the setting of acute myocardial infarction in comparison with thrombolytic therapy (Keeley et al. 2003). Percutaneous intervention results in a higher rate of successful reperfusion of the epicardial coronary artery, consequently resulting in a smaller infarct size, better clinical outcome and improved short- as well as long-term mortality. The acute coronary syndromes are therefore the main indications for angioplasty. Today, careful attention to the concomitant pharmacological therapy in these patients is of utmost importance and in most countries the majority of angioplasties are performed for these indications (Smith et al. 2001).

2.1.7
Alternative Strategies to the First Line Use of Coronary Angiography

Ideally, only patients with coronary disease who require treatment dependent on the angiographic appearances of the coronary tree should undergo this procedure. This would reduce the requirement for coronary angiography and reduce the general population risk. It would also be desirable to have advanced knowledge of conditions that increase risk in coronary angiography, particularly left main stem disease. Significant valve abnormalities and poor left ventricular function can be diagnosed prior to coronary angiography by echocardiography. Significant ventricular arrhythmias can be diagnosed by electrocardiography. Prior to the introduction of new cross-sectional imaging techniques by MRI and spiral and electron beam CT it was difficult to diagnose coronary disease and the main method of investigation was exercise testing. This is an imprecise method and is poorly sensitive in some groups of patients. Results from chest pain centres in the USA have shown a range of sensitivity from 29% to 73% and a specificity of 50%–99% (Gibbons et al. 2002).

It has been demonstrated that the appropriate use of imaging in a chest pain clinic may improve the sensitivity and specificity of patient selection for angiography (Rees and Cripps 2002). The use of new imaging techniques has been demonstrated to score the probability of coronary disease (Agatston et al. 1991), while even newer technologies such as multislice CT and faster MRI may be able to select out patients who are at high risk from adverse complications at coronary angiography.

References

Abrams HL, Adams DF (1975) The complications of coronary angiography. Circulation 52[Suppl 2]:27

Adams DF, Fraser DB, Abrams HL (1973) The complications of coronary angiography. Circulation 48:609

Agatston AS, Janowitz WR, Nobuyuki A, Gasso J, Hildner F, Viamonte M (1991) Quantification of coronary calcium reflects the angiographic extent of coronary disease. Circulation 84:II-159

Angelini P (1989) Normal and anomalous coronary arteries definitions and classification. Am Heart J 117:418–434

Aramburu O, Mesa C, Arias JL, Izquierdo G, Perez-Cano R (2000) Spinal cord infarctions as a complication of coronary angiography. Rev Neurol 30:651–654

Arora P, Naik N, Bahl VK, Mishra S, Yadav R, Sharma S, Manchanda SC (2002) Coronary angiography using 4 French catheters with power injection: a randomized comparison with 6 French catheters. Indian Heart J 54:184–188

Basso C, Maron BJ, Corrado D (2000) Clinical profile of congenital coronary artery anomalies with origin from the wrong aortic sinus leading to sudden death in young competitive athletes. J Am Coll Cardiol 35:1493–1501

Bellman S, Frank HA, Lambert PB, Littman D, Williams JA (1960) Coronary arteriography: differential opacification of aortic stream catheters of special design. Experimental development. N Engl J Med 262:325

Boehrer JD, Ellis SG, Pieper K, Holmes DR, Keeler GP, Debowey D, Chapekis AT, Leya F, Mooney MR, Gotleib RS et al. (1995) Directional atherectomy versus balloon angioplasty for coronary ostial and nonostial left anterior descending coronary artery lesions: results from a randomized multicentre trial. The CAVEAT-I investigators. Coronary Angioplasty Versus Excisional Aatherectomy Trial. JACC 25:1380–1386

Bogren HG, Bursch JH (1984) Digital angiography in the diagnosis of congenital heart disease. Cardiovasc Intervent Radiol 7:180–191

Brannon ES, Weens HS, Warren JW (1945) Atrial septal defect: study of hemodynamics by the technique of right heart catheterisation. Am J Med Sci 210:480

Carter AJ, Scott D, Bailey I (1998) Stent design: in the end it matters. Circulation 961:402

Cournand A, Ranges HA (1944) Catheterization of the right auricle in man. Proc Soc Exp Biol Med 55:34

Cumberland DC, Sanborn TA, Taylor DI, Moore DJ (1986) Percutaneous laser thermal angioplasty: initial clinical results with a laser probe in total peripheral artery occlusions. Lancet 1:1457–1459

Donaldson RM, Raphael M Radley-Smith R, Patterson FK (1982) Sudden death in a young adult with anomalous origin of the posterior circumflex artery. South Med J 75:748

Dos Santos R, Lamas AC, Perierira-Caldas J (1929) Arteriographia da aorta e dose vasos abdominalis. Med Contemp 47

Dotter CT, Judkins MD (1964) Transluminal treatment of arteriosclerotic obstruction: description of a new technique and a preliminary report of its application. Circulation 30:654

Douglas JS, King SB (2001) Percutaneous coronary intervention. In: Fuster V, Alexander RW, O'Rourke RA (eds) Hurst's The Heart, 10th edn. McGraw-Hill, New York, pp 1440–1442

Effer DB, Sheldon WC, Turner JJ, Groves LK (1967) Coronary arteriovenous fistulas: diagnosis and surgical management. Report of 15 cases. Surgery 61:41

EPIC Investigators (1994) Use of monoclonal antibody directed against the platelet glycoprotein IIb/IIIa receptor in high risk coronary angioplasty. N Eng J Med 330:956–961

EPISTENT Investigators (1997) Randomised placebo controlled and balloon angioplasty controlled trial to assess safety of coronary stenting with the use of platelet glycoprotein-IIb/IIIa Blockade. Lancet 349:1429–1435

Forssman W (1929) The catheterisation of the right side of the heart. Klin Wochenschr 8:2085

Franch RH, King SB, Douglas JS (1982) Techniques of cardiac catheterisation including coronary arteriography. In: Hurst JW (ed) The heart, 5th edn. McGraw-Hill, New York, p 1866

Gibbons RJ, Balady GJ, Timothy Bricker J, Chaitman BR, Fletcher GF, Froelicher VF, Mark DB, McCallister BD, Mooss AN, O'Reilly MG, Winters WL, Gibbons RJ, Antman EM, Alpert JS, Faxon DP, Fuster V, Gregoratos G, Hiratzka LF, Jacobs AK, Russell RO, Smith SC; American College of Cardiology/American Heart Association Task Force on Practice Guidelines. Committee to Update the 1997 Exercise Testing Guidelines (2002) ACC/AHA 2002 guideline update for exercise testing: summary article. A report of the American College of Cardiology/American Heart Association Task Force on Practice Guidelines (Committee to Update the 1997 Exercise Testing Guidelines). J Am Coll Cardiol 40:1531–1540

Grover M, Slutsky R, Higgins C, Atwood JE (1984) Terminology and anatomy of angulated coronary arteriography. Clin Cardiol 7:37

Grüntzig AR (1978) Transluminal dilatation of coronary artery stenosis. Lancet 1:263

Grüntzig A, Hopff H (1974) Percutaneous recanalization after chronic arterial occlusion with a new dilator-catheter (modification of the Dotter technique). Dtsch Med Wochenschr 99:2502–10, 2511

Hansen DD, Auth DC, Vrocko R, Richie JL (1988) Rotational atherectomy in atherosclerotic rabbit iliac arteries. Am Heart J 115:160–165

Harikrishnan S, Sunder KR, Tharakan J, Titus T, Bhat A, Sivasankaran S, Bimal F (1999) Clinical and angiographic profile and follow-up of myocardial bridges: a study of 21 cases. Indian Heart J 51:503–507

Huiskens CJ, Hummel WA (1995) Data analysis on radiation exposures in cardiac angiography. Radiat Protect Dosim 57:475–480

Hung MJ, Kuo LT, Wang CH, Cherng WJ (2002) Irreversible myocardial damage after coronary air embolism. Angiology. 53:213–216

Judkins MP (1967) Selective coronary arteriography: a percutaneous transfemoral technique. Radiology 89:815

Judkins MP, Judkins E (1985) Coronary arteriography and left ventriculography: Judkins technique. In: King S, Douglas JS (eds) Coronary arteriography and coronary angioplasty. McGraw-Hill, New York, pp 182–238

Katus HA, Richardt G.A, Jain D, Kurz T (2001) Unique complication during coronary angiography: peripheral embolism by selective right coronary engagement. Angiology 52:493–499

Keeley EC, Boura JA, Grines CL (2003) Primary angioplasty versus intravenous thrombolytic therapy for acute myocardial infarction: a quantitative review of 23 randomised trials. Lancet 361:13–20

Kennedy JW (1981) Complications associated with cardiac catheterisation and angiography. Report of the registry committee of the society of cardiac angiography. Coronary disease today. Proceedings of an international symposium, Utrecht, 25–27 May

Kennedy JW (1983) Report of the registry committee, Society for Cardiac Angiography, Annual meeting, Scottsdale Arizona May

Klein O (1930) Zur Bestimmung des Zerkulatorischen Minutens Volumen nach dem Fickschen Princip. Munch Med Wochenschr 77:1311

Kwok BW, Lim TT (2000) Cortical blindness following coronary angiography. Singapore Med J 41:604–605

Lasky W, Boyle J, Johnson LW (1993) Multivariable model for prediction of risk of significant complication during diagnostic cardiac catheterisation. The registry committee of the Society for Cardiac angiography and interventions. Cathet Cardiovasc Diagn 30:185–190

Limacher MC, Douglas PS, Germano G, Laskey WK, Lindsay BD et al. (1998) ACC expert consensus document. Radiation safety in the practice of cardiology. American College of Cardiology. J Am Coll Cardiol 31:892–913

Mancini GBJ (1988) Clinical applications of cardiac digital angiography. Raven, New York

Meier B, Bachmann D, Lüscher TF (2003) 25 Years of coronary angioplasty: almost a fairy tale. Lancet 361:527

Michalis LK, Rees MR, Davis JAS, Pappa EC, Naka KKM, Rokkas S, Agrios N, Loukas S, Goudevenos J, Sideris DA (1999) Use of vibrational angioplasty for the treatment of chronic total coronary occlusions: preliminary results. Cathet Cardiovasc Interv 46:98–104

Mintz GS, Iskandrian AS, Benis CE et al. (1983) Myocardial ischaemia in anomalous origin of the right coronary artery from the pulmonary trunk. Am J Cardiol 51:610

Moore RJ (1990) Imaging principles of cardiac angiography. Aspen, Rockville Ogden JA (1970) Congenital anomalies of the coronary arteries. J Cardiol 25:474

Paulin S (1966) Coronary arteriography. Postgrad Med. 40: A53–59; and 100:232–240 (1997)

Paulin S, von Schulthness GK, Fossel E, Krayenbuehl HP (1987) MR imaging of the aortic root and proximal coronary arteries. AJR Am J Roentgenol 148:665–670

Pijls NH, Van Gelder B, Van der Voort P, Peels K, Bracke FA, Bonnier HJ, el Gamal MI (1995) Fractional fl ow reserve. A useful index to evaluate the influence of an epicardial coronary stenosis on myocardial blood fl ow. Circulation 92:3183–3193

Rees MR, Cripps T (2002) The use of imaging in chest pain. CARS Proceedings 2002, Springer, Berlin Heidelberg New York, p890–894

Reiber JH, van der Zwet PM, Koning G et al. (1993) Accuracy and precision of quantitative digital coronary arteriography: observer, short and medium term variables. Cathet Cardiovasc Diagn 28:187–198

Richens D, Rees MR, Watson D (1987) Laser coronary angioplasty under direct vision. Lancet ii:183

Robb RG, Steinberg I (1938) A practical method of visualisation of the chambers of the heart, the pulmonary circulation and the great blood vessels in man. J Clin Invest 17:507

Roncoroni A, Weischelbaum E, Vedoya RC, Kaplan MV, Navia JA, Favarolo JJ, Favarolo RG (1973) Surgical treatment of coronary disease. Angiologia 25:183–189

Ross J Jr (1959) Transseptal left heart catheterisation: a new method of left atrial puncture. Ann Surg 149:395

Scanlon PJ, Faxon DP (1999) ACC/AHA Guidelines for coronary angiography. J Am Coll Cardiol 33:1756–1824

Seldinger SI (1953) Catheter replacement of the needle in percutaneous arteriography. Acta Radiol 39:368–376

Sigwart U, Puel J, Mirkovitch V, Joffre F, Kappenburger L (1987) Intravascular stents to prevent occlusion and restenosis after transluminal angioplasty N Eng J Med 316:701–706

Simpson JB, Baim DS, Robert EW, Harrison DC (1982) A new catheter system for coronary angioplasty. Am J Cardiol 49:216–222

Simpson JB, Robertson GC, Selmon R (1988) Percutaneous coronary atherectomy. J Am Coll cardiol 11:110A

Smith SC, Dove JT, Jacobs AK, Kennedy JW, Kereiakes D, Kern MJ, Kuntz RE, Popma JJ, Schaff HV et al. (2001) ACC/AHA guidelines for percutaneous coronary intervention (revision of the 1993 PTCA guidelines) – executive summary: a report of the American College of Cardiology/American Heart Association Task Force on practice guidelines (Committee to revise the 1993 guidelines for percutaneous transluminal coronary angioplasty) endorsed by the Society for Cardiac Angiography and Interventions. J Am Coll Cardiol 37:2215–2239

Sones FM Jr., Shirey EK, Proudfi t WL, Wescott RN (1959) Cine coronary arteriography. Circulation 20:773

Stack RS, Perez JA, Newman GE, McCann RL, Wholey MH, Cummins FE, Galichia JT, Hoffman PU, Tcheng JE, Sketch MH, Lee MM, Phillips HR (1989) Treatment of peripheral vascular disease with the transluminal extraction catheter: results of a multicentre study. J Am Coll Cardiol 13:227A

Swan HJC, Ganz W, Forrester J, Marcus H, Diamond G, Chonette D (1970) Catheterisation of the heart in man with use of a fl ow directed balloon tipped catheter. N Eng J Med 283:447

Timurkaynak T, Ciftci H, Cemri M (2001) Coronary artery perforation: a rare complication of coronary angiography. Source Acta Cardiologica 56:323–325

Tuinenburg JC, Koning G, Hekking E, Zwinderman AH, Becker T, Simon R, Reiber JH (2000) American College of Cardiology/European Society of Cardiology International Study of Angiographic Data Compression Phase II: the effects of varying JPEG data compression levels on the quantitative assessment of the degree of stenosis in digital coronary angiography. Joint Photographic Experts Group. J Am Coll Cardiol 35:1380–1387

Vano E, Goicolea J, Galvan C, Gonzalez L, Meiggs L, Ten JI, Macaya C (2001) Institution skin radiation injuries in patients following repeated coronary angioplasty procedures. Br J Radiol 74:1023–31

Vlodaver Z, Neufeld HN, Edwards JE (1972) Pathology of coronary disease. Semin Roentgenol 7:376–394

Waller DA, Sivananthan UM, Diament RH, Kester RC, Rees MR (1993) Iatrogenic vascular injury following arterial cannulation: the importance of early surgery. Cardiovasc Surg 1:251–253

Wilson WJ, Lee GB, Amplatz K (1967) Biplane selective coronary arteriography via a percutaneous transfemoral approach. Am J Roentgenol Radium Ther Nucl Med 100:318–321

Yacoub MH, Ross DN (1983) Angiographic identification of primary coronary anomalies causing impaired myocardial perfusion. Cathet Cardiovasc Diagn 9:237

Yock P, Linker D, Saether O et al. (1988) Intravascular two dimensional catheter ultrasound: initial clinical studies. Circulation 78[suppl II]:II–21

Zimmerman HA, Scott RW, Becker NO (1950) Catheterisation of the left side of the heart in man Circulation 1:357

Zorzetto M, Bernardi G, MoraccuttiG, Fontanelli A (1997) Radiation exposure to patients and operators during diagnostic catheterisation and coronary angioplasty. Cathet Cardiovasc Diagn 40:348–351

Invasive Coronary Imaging

2

2.2 Quantitative Coronary Arteriography

Johan H. C. Reiber, Joan C. Tuinenburg, Gerhard Koning, Johannes P. Janssen, Andrei Rareş, Alexandra J. Lansky, and Bob Goedhart

CONTENTS

2.2.1 Introduction

The dynamics of coronary atherosclerosis, that is to say the progression and regression of coronary atherosclerotic lesions, the healing of lesions, and the development of new ones, have intrigued cardiologists since the time that this process could be followed by repeated coronary arteriographic X-ray examinations (Bruschke et al. 1981; Jukema et al. 1996).

A complicating factor in the evaluation of severity and extent of the degree of coronary atherosclerosis is the occurrence of compensatory mechanisms, which is nowadays denoted by the term coronary artery remodeling. Glagov et al. (1987) were the first to describe that compensatory enlargement of the human atherosclerotic coronary arteries occurs during the early stages of plaque formation, followed by Stiel et al. (1989). This compensatory enlargement results in the preservation of a nearly normal lumen cross-sectional area so that an atherosclerotic plaque will have less haemodynamic effects. This "outward" growth process stops at a certain point in time as it reaches the maximal stretching capacities of the vessel, followed by subsequent further "in-

J. H. C. Reiber, PhD
J. C. Tuinenburg, MSc
G. Koning, MSc
J. P. Janssen, MSc
A. Rareş, PhD
Division of Image Processing (LKEB), Department of Radiology, Leiden University Medical Center, Albinusdreef 2, 2300 RC Leiden, The Netherlands
A. J. Lansky, MD
Cardiovascular Research Foundation, New York-Presbyterian Hospital, Columbia University, 161 Fort Washington Avenue 5th FL, New York, NY 10032, USA
B. Goedhart, PhD
Medis Medical Imaging Systems B.V., Schuttersveld 9, 2316 XG Leiden, The Netherlands

ward" growth of the plaque. Once the lumen of the vessel becomes impaired, it becomes visible by X-ray arteriography, which is a two-dimensional projection technique, allowing only the visualization of the contrast-filled lumen. For this reason, the X-ray arteriogram is often also called a "luminogram".

Usually, atherosclerosis is present as a focal narrowing over a limited length, superimposed on a diffuse atherosclerotic process within the entire artery. Because X-ray arteriography only depicts the remaining opening of an artery, it underestimates the presence of diffuse atherosclerosis and is unable to detect the early stages of coronary atherosclerosis. Until recently, cross-sectional imaging of the individual coronary arteries and the assessment of the arterial wall was the exclusive domain of intravascular ultrasound (IVUS). IVUS is able to provide real-time high-resolution (pixel size about 0.1 mm) tomographic images of sections of the arterial wall and to demonstrate the presence or absence of compensatory arterial enlargement. Recent developments with IVUS include the assessment of the stiffness of the vessel wall using palpography (Schaar et al. 2004, 2006), and the composition of the plaque derived from the original high frequency signal content (virtual histology) (Nasu et al. 2006). Intravascular ultrasound has proved to be very important for the development and validation of new coronary interventional devices (in particular stents) and is used as a gold standard for the validation of new non-invasive coronary visualization techniques [multi-slice computed tomography (MSCT) and magnetic resonance imaging (MRI)]. Another recently developed intravascular approach with even higher resolution but less vessel wall penetration is optical coherent tomography (OCT) (Pinto and Waksman 2006), although in practical terms it is still limited by the fact that the vessel needs to be flushed with saline to obtain acceptable image quality.

With the extremely rapid developments in MSCT over the last several years, there has been enormous interest in the non-invasive three-dimensional (3D) visualization and quantitation of the coronary arteries plus the plaque burden and the presence of calcium. The great advantage of MSCT is of course the 3D visualization of the entire heart and its surroundings (Leber et al. 2006). Although the resolution is far behind that of invasive arteriography, the technique is rapidly improving with 256-slice MSCT becoming available in 2007. Also, MRI is a powerful and harmless technique to visualize the cardiovascular system and in particular the vessels by magnetic resonance angiography (MRA), certainly in combination with vessel wall imaging (VWI), which has the highest potential to accurately describe the composition of the vessel wall and to assess changes in the wall as a result of therapies (Adame et al. 2006).

In general, the purely visual interpretation of images is subjective and therefore associated with significant inter- and intra-observer variations (Reiber and Serruys 1991). There has been continuing interest in developing robust and automated segmentation techniques to obtain objective and reproducible data for all imaging modalities. In fact, X-ray left ventriculography was one of the very first arising cardiovascular imaging fields, which led to significant activities in the quantification of the regional left ventricular function and the automated segmentation of the left ventricular contours in the 1960s and 1970s (Heintzen 1971; Reiber et al. 1986). Despite these early efforts, very few, if any, of the quantitative approaches developed have proved to be ideal: each technique requires a certain amount of user interaction, as well as corrections to the detected contours in a significant percentage of the cases. Recently, we developed an entirely new approach based on statistical models of the left ventricle (so-called active appearance models, or AAMs), that has proved to be quite robust and requires minimal user interaction. A semi-automated version with manual model initialization showed a success rate of 100% for end-diastolic frames and of 99% for end-systolic frames in a study based on image data of 70 patients, while a fully-automated version gave success rates of 91% and 83%, respectively (Oost et al. 2006).

In the late 1970s, quantitative coronary arteriography (QCA) was developed to quantify vessel motion and the effects of pharmacological agents on the regression and progression of coronary artery disease (Brown et al. 1977). So far, QCA has been the only technique that allows the accurate and reliable assessment of arterial dimensions within the entire coronary vasculature over time (regression/progression studies), despite its known limitations (de Feyter et al. 1993). For the main coronary segments, quantitative coronary ultrasound (QCU) has also been used with analytical software packages based on automated detection of lumen, vessel and stent contours (Tardif and Lee 1998; Dijkstra et al. 1999).

In interventional cardiology, QCA has been used for on-line vessel sizing for the selection of interventional devices and the assessment of the efficacy of the individual procedures; for the on-line selection of patients to be included or excluded in clinical trials based on quantitative parameters (e.g. small vessel disease); and for training purposes. But, in particular, it has been applied worldwide in core laboratories and clinical research sites to study the efficacy of these procedures and devices in smaller and larger patient populations.

The goal of this chapter, therefore, is to provide an overview of the basic principles of QCA, including the latest applications in both coronary and peripheral vessels; drug eluting stent and brachytherapy (straight) analyses; ostial and bifurcation analyses; and finally, to present some of the results from validation studies.

2.2.2 Analog or Digital Image Acquisition and Analysis

In the current era, previously widely used cinefilm-based X-ray systems have been largely replaced by complete digital systems. For that reason we will not describe the cinefilm-based approaches anymore. If needed, the reader is referred to one of our previous publications in this field (Reiber et al. 1994a).

In the digital approach, the output image of the image intensifier is projected onto the input target of a video camera. The analog video output signal is modified electronically in the so-called white compression unit, resulting in greater contrast differences in the parts with high X-ray absorption (e.g. vertebrae and contrast filled arteries or the ventricle) and lower contrast differences in the areas with low X-ray absorption (e.g. lung area). This markedly improves the image quality of the images. Next, the resulting video signal is digitized at a resolution of 512 × 512 pixels × 8 bits on most X-ray systems or up to 1024 × 1024 pixels × 12 bits on some other X-ray systems and stored on the high-speed disks (RAID system) of the digital imaging system for subsequent review and possibly quantitative analysis. An entire patient study can be stored in DICOM format on CD-R after the procedure or stored in a picture archiving and communication system (PACS) by means of the DICOM messaging protocol for the exchange of image data over a network.

New developments in the technology of digital X-ray imaging systems have resulted in the replacement of the conventional vacuum-tube image intensifier [in combination with a CCD (charge-couple device)-based camera, an A/D (analog-to-digital) converter, etc.] by a completely digital flat-panel detector. The main advantages of these flat-panel detectors, among others, are the ability to preserve significantly more of the original signal, e.g. due to the large reduction of veiling glare (the scattering process within the image intensifier) and the absolute absence of spatial distortions, e.g. the magnetic field distortion and pincushion distortion (the latter being due to the curvature of the input screen of the image intensifier) (van der Zwet et al. 1995; Holmes et al. 2004), providing better image quality and enabling further image enhancement. In clinical practice, this means improved visibility of vessels, lesions, and guide-wires, even at reduced X-ray dose levels (Geijer 2002; Tsapaki et al. 2004). Typical matrix sizes for the flat panel systems nowadays are 1024 × 1024 pixels at 12.5–30 frames/s, or 512 × 512 at 60 frames/s with 8-, 10- or 12-bit depth for cardiac acquisitions.

From the user's point of view, the evidently better image characteristics of the flat-panel-based images [e.g. they are distortion free, have an excellent contrast resolution, a large dynamic range, a high sensitivity to X-rays, a spatial resolution that is determined by the actual size of the detector elements, etc. (Holmes et al. 2004; Spahn et al. 2003)] do not have any significant influence on the results of QCA and QVA analyses. In fact, we have demonstrated that the data obtained from both image intensifier-based and flat-panel-based X-ray systems can be used collectively in (multi-center) clinical trials (Tuinenburg et al. 2006).

2.2.3 Brief History of Quantitative Coronary Arteriography

Since the first papers on QCA were published in 1977 and 1978, this field has grown substantially (Brown et al. 1977; Reiber et al. 1978). First-generation QCA systems, developed in the 1980s, were based on 35-mm cinefilm analysis. Second-generation systems (1990–1994) were characterized by further improvements in the quality of the edge detection, often applied to digital images, and included corrections for the overestimation of the vessel sizes below approximately 1.2 mm (Reiber et al. 1994a). It should be noted that the edge-detection algorithm for the cinefilm analysis could not simply be applied to digital images, which have other image characteristics [e.g. well-defined and constant nonlinear functions (white compression), the absence of film grain noise, a dark structure on a bright background, and the possibility of edge enhancement]. Therefore, digital images required further tuning of these algorithms. Third-generation (1995–1998) QCA systems provided solutions for the quantitative analysis of complex lesion morphology using, for example, the gradient field transform (GFT®) (van der Zwet and Reiber 1994) and improved diameter function calculations (Reiber et al. 1996a). With the establishment of DICOM for digital image exchange and HL7 for administrative data, the need for integration of QCA systems into the complex environment of the hospital was recognized. Finally, with the greatly enhanced capabilities of modern workstations, fourth-generation QCA systems have been available since 1999. These systems are characterized by simplified portability to digital DICOM viewers, network connectivity, improved reporting and database storage functions, and options for specialized QCA functions, such as brachytherapy analysis (Lansky et al. 2002). Although most modern QCA packages are based on the linear programming approach, i.e. minimum cost algorithm (MCA), for contour detection, there are still differences in the quality of these packages, which need to be documented by extensive validation reports (Reiber et al. 1994b). Finally, the fifth generation systems became available in around 2005, characterized by further extensions towards ostial and bifurcation analyses, an option for drug eluting stents (DES), the applicability towards both coronary and peripheral vessels all in one and in the same analytical software package, the development of a new robust pathline technique, as well as further improved diameter function calculations, and finally the quantification of both obstructive and aneurysmal lesions. These developments will be described in more detail in the following paragraphs.

2.2.4 Basic Principles of Quantitative Coronary Arteriography

2.2.4.1 Basic Principles of Automated Contour Detection

The general principles and characteristics of a modern QCA software package are best illustrated by the QAngio® XA (Medis medical imaging systems bv, Leiden, the Netherlands) algorithms developed in our laboratory (Reiber et al. 1985, 1993, 2001).

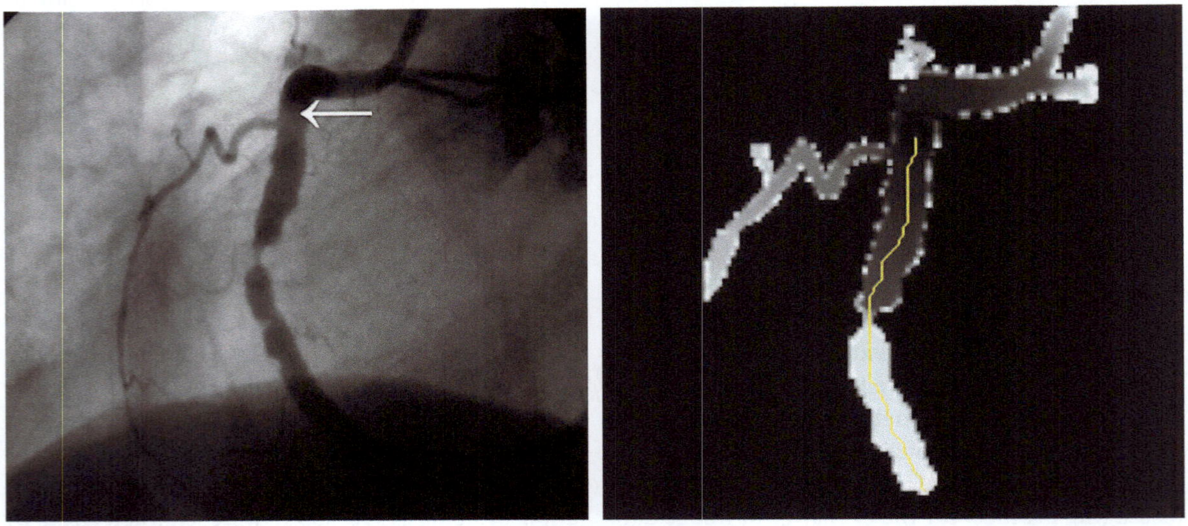

a b

Fig. 2.2.1a,b. The wavefront pathline detection. **a** The *arrow* indicates the proximal point of the segment. **b** The local arrival times of the wavefront (traveling faster through darker regions and slower through brighter regions) and the pathline representing the fastest route

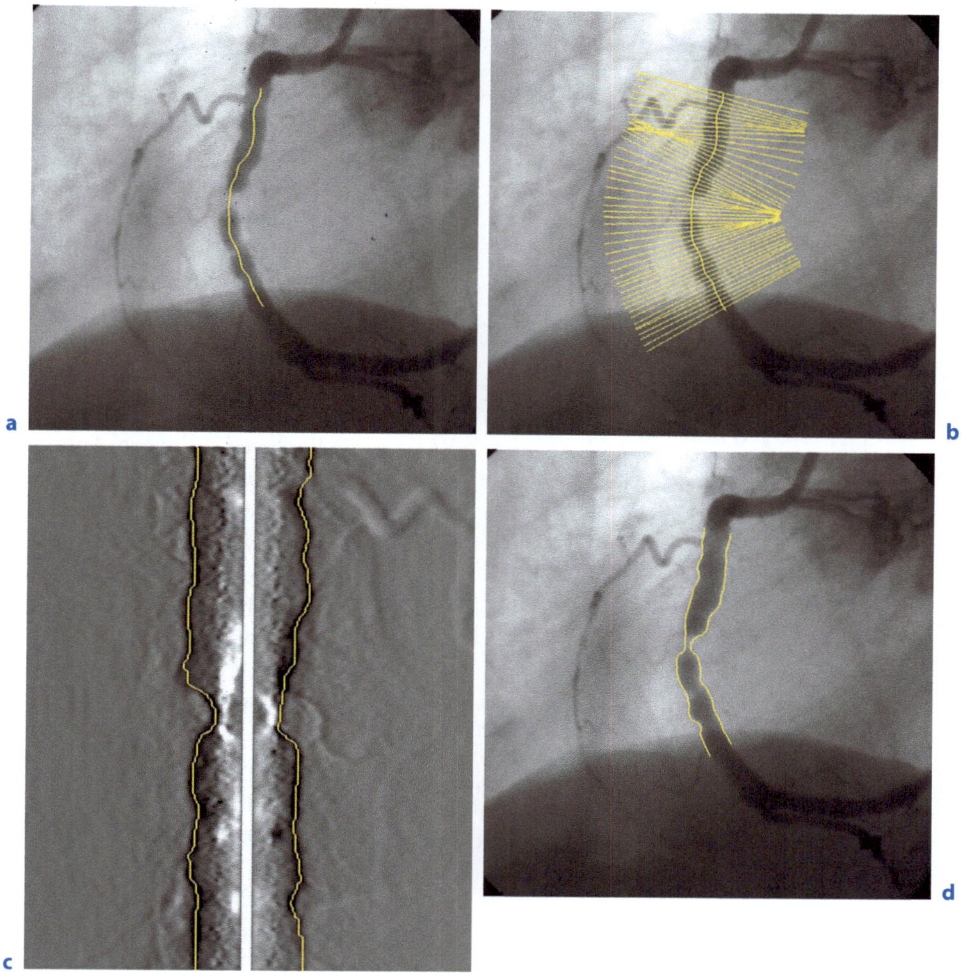

Fig. 2.2.2a–d. Basic principles of the minimum cost contour-detection algorithm (of Fig. 2.2.1). **a** Initial segment with pathline. **b** Scanlines defined. **c** Straightened for analysis; contours calculated. **d** Contours returned to initial image; diameter measurements performed

The QCA operator selects the coronary segment to be analyzed by using the computer mouse to define the start and end points of that segment. Next, an arterial pathline through the segment of interest is computed based on the wavefront propagation principle ('the wavepath approach'). The algorithm is initiated in the proximal point (Fig. 2.2.1a) and expands through the image (like a wavefront), traveling faster through darker regions and slower through brighter regions, and therefore following the vessel structures, until the distal point is reached. This results in an image that represents the local arrival time of the wavefront (Fig. 2.2.1b). Subsequently, a traceback is performed on this arrival time image, starting at the distal point taking the fastest route to the point with the lowest arrival time: the proximal point. This results in the pathline, representing this fastest route (Fig. 2.2.1b) (Janssen et al. 2002, 2004).

The contour-detection procedure is carried out in two iterations relative to a model. In the first iteration, the detected pathline is the model (Fig. 2.2.2a). To detect the contours, scanlines are defined perpendicular to the model (Fig. 2.2.2b). For each point or pixel along such a scanline, the corresponding edge-strength value (local change in brightness level) is computed as the weighted sum of the corresponding values of the first- and second-derivative functions applied to the brightness values along these scanlines (Fig. 2.2.3). The resulting edge-strength values are input to the so-called minimum cost contour-detection algorithm (MCA), which searches for an optimal contour path along the entire segment (Fig. 2.2.2c). The individual left and right vessel contours detected in the first iteration now serve as models in the second iteration, in which the MCA contour-detection procedure is repeated relative to the new models. At the end this results in initially detected arterial contours (Fig. 2.2.2d).

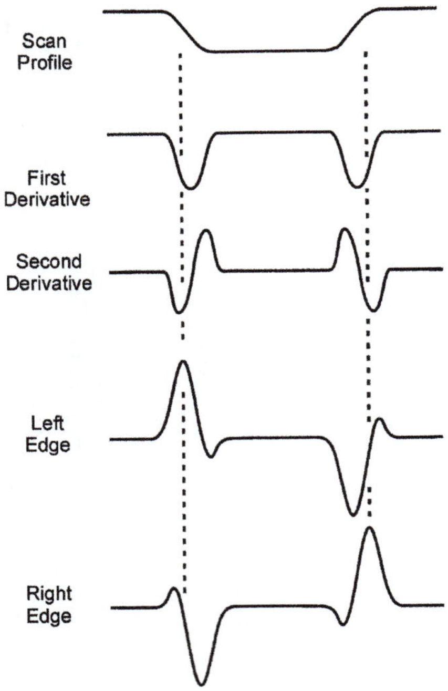

Fig. 2.2.3. The edge strength values along a scanline. Schematic representation of the brightness profile of an arterial vessel assessed along a scanline perpendicular to the local pathline direction and the computed 1st derivative, 2nd derivative, and the combinations of these 1st and 2nd derivative functions; the maximal values of the last functions determine the edge positions

To correct for the limited resolution of the entire X-ray system, the MCA algorithm is modified in the second iteration based on an analysis of the quality of the imaging chain in terms of its resolution, which is of particular importance for the accurate measurement of small diameters, as in coronary obstructions. If such a correction was not applied, significant overestimations of vessel sizes below approximately 1.2 mm would occur. In the literature, other approaches have also been described (Kirkeeide et al. 1982; Sonka et al. 1997).

If the QCA operator does not agree with one or more parts of the initially detected contours, they can be edited in various ways. However, each manual editing is followed by a local MCA iteration, so that the newly detected contours are truly based on the local brightness information. In other words, the operator indicates roughly where the contour should be detected, and the MCA algorithm searches for the final contour based on the available image information. The MCA approach has been demonstrated to be very robust.

2.2.4.2 Calibration Procedure

Calibration of the image data is performed on a non-tapering portion of a contrast-filled catheter using an MCA edge-detection procedure similar to that applied to the arterial segment. In this case, however, additional information is used in the edge-detection process because this part of the catheter is known to be characterized by parallel boundaries. It should also be recognized that the catheter calibration procedure is the weakest link in the analysis chain because of the variable image quality of the displayed catheters. Another potential problem with calibration is the out-of-plane magnification, which occurs when the catheter and the coronary segment of analysis are positioned at different distances from the image intensifier. Biplane calibration could overcome this problem (Reiber et al. 2001; Büchi et al. 1990; Wahle et al. 1995), but is rarely applied in routine QCA. A number of recommendations for catheter calibration are reviewed in Sect. 2.2.5.1.

2.2.4.3 Coronary Segment Analysis

From the left- and right-hand contours of the arterial segment, a diameter function is determined (Fig. 2.2.4a), which is not a trivial task, certainly not in a situation of complex anatomy or strongly curved vessels (Reiber et al. 1996a). To calculate the diameter function (the width of a vessel segment along its trajectory from proximal to distal), the exact centerline of the vessel is derived from the arterial contours, followed subsequently by the assessment of the width values at every pixel distance along the centerline and measured perpendicular to this centerline. This represents the diameter function.

In conventional X-ray imaging, pincushion distortion caused by the convex input screen of the image intensifier may be present, which may influence the diameter calculations. Correction for this distortion should not be applied in routine single-plane QCA, as this may introduce more artifacts rather than resolve problems (van der Zwet et al. 1995). It should also be noted that the pincushion distortion is minimal in modern image intensifiers, and certainly absent in the latest solid-state flat-panel detectors.

The most widely used parameter to describe the severity of a coronary obstruction is the percentage a 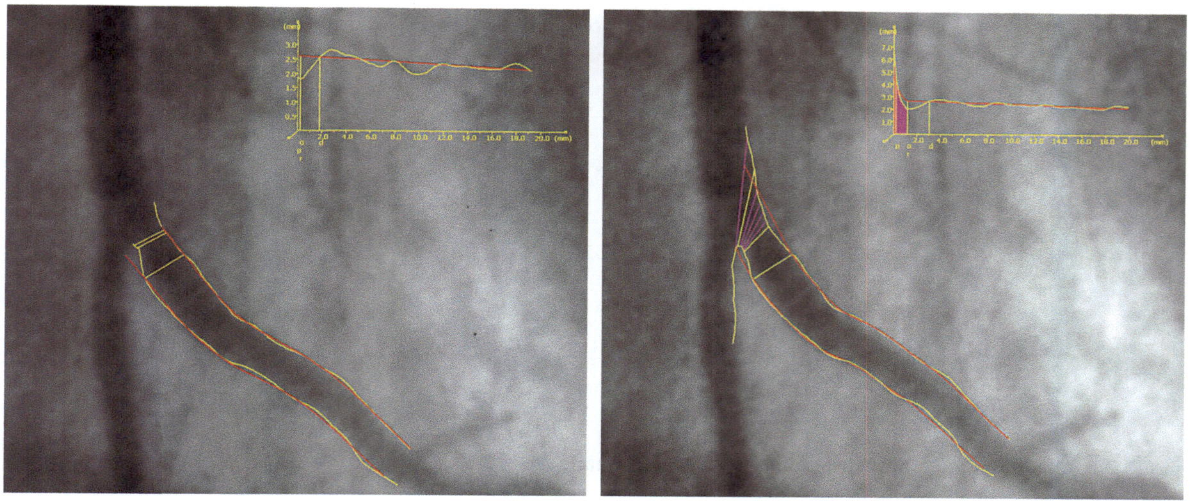 b

Fig. 2.2.4a,b. The diameter function. **a** The contours and the diameter function of a straight analysis. **b** The contours and the diameter function of an ostial analysis

of diameter stenosis. Calculation of this parameter requires that a reference diameter value is computed, for which two options are available: (1) a user-defined reference diameter as positioned by the user at a so-called normal portion of the vessel, and (2) the automated or interpolated reference diameter value. In practice, this last approach is preferred because it requires no user interaction and takes care of any tapering of the vessel. For that purpose, a reference diameter function is calculated by an iterative regression technique and displayed in the diameter function as a straight line. The iterative approach has been used to exclude the influence of any obstructive or ectatic areas (Fig. 2.2.5a,b) as much as possible, so that it represents a best approximation of the vessel size before the occurrence of the focal narrowing or aneurysm. Moreover, this approach works also if both obstructive and ecstatic areas are present in one and the same vessel segment.

Now that the reference diameter function is known, reference contours can be reconstructed around the actual vessel segment, representing the original size and shape of the vessel before the focal disease occurred. However, the possible presence of any diffuse atherosclerosis along the vessel segment cannot be corrected for as it is not visible by X-ray imaging. Finally, the difference in area between the detected lumen contours and the reference contours is a measure for the atherosclerotic plaque in this particular angiographic view and is shaded in Figure 2.2.5a.

The actual reference diameter value corresponding to a selected obstruction is now taken as the value of the reference diameter function at the site of the obstruction, so that neither overestimation nor underestimation occurs. From the reference diameter value and the obstruction diameter, the percent diameter stenosis is calculated. This automated approach has been found to be very reproducible.

A few years ago, we introduced and validated a new quantitative parameter, the diffuse index (DI), which allows us to differentiate objectively whether in-stent restenosis is focal or diffuse in nature. It was demonstrated that the DI correlates very well with the plaque area in the stent, regardless of the type of stent implanted. This parameter combines two angiographic factors: the longitudinal morphology of the stenosis and the plaque area in the stent. In addition, the combination of the DI and percentage plaque area was found to have a strong correlation with subsequent major adverse cardiac events (MACE), including target lesion revascularization (TLR), myocardial infarction, and death. Therefore, the DI is an objective parameter that works complementary to the percentage diameter stenosis, especially in cases of TLR, to indicate whether additional therapies are necessary or not (Ishii et al. 2001).

2.2.4.4 The Flagging Procedure

In the vast majority of QCA analyses, the calculation of the reference diameter function and the reconstruction of the reference contours provide a reliable representation of the vessel segment. However, over-

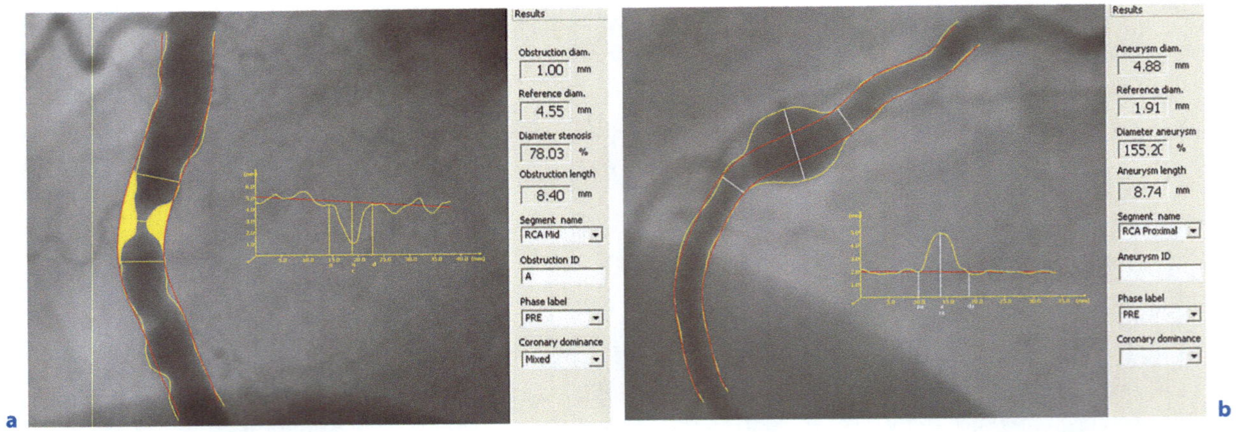

Fig. 2.2.5a,b. Lesion types. **a** Obstruction type. **b** Aneurysmatic type

dilated stents, vessels with extremely ectatic areas, overlap of vessel segments, and so forth, negatively influence the calculation of the reference diameter function. This is illustrated in Figure 2.2.6a: The ectatic area distal of the obstruction results in a significant tapering of the reference diameter function, such that the normal vessel size would not be measured correctly. In this case, a stenosis of 41% would be measured (obstruction diameter of 2.27 mm, reference diameter of 3.84 mm); this is a very undesirable situation. Therefore, another option called the "flagging" procedure has been implemented. The user can "flag" the portion of the vessel segment (in Fig. 2.2.6b, the ectatic area), and the corresponding diameter values are excluded from the subsequent calculation of the reference diameter function. The correctly calculated reference diameter function and reconstructed reference contours are presented in Figure 2.2.6b, which is more in line with what one would expect. For this case, a narrowing of 34% (obstruction diameter of 2.27 mm, and reference diameter of 3.43 mm) is measured.

From the calculated diameter function, many parameters are derived automatically, including the site of maximal percentage of stenosis, the obstruction diameter, the corresponding automatically determined reference diameter, and the extent of the obstruction (Reiber et al. 1993). Additionally, other derived parameters include obstruction symmetry, inflow and outflow angles, the area of the atherosclerotic plaque, and functional information, such as the stenotic flow reserve (SFR) (Fig. 2.2.7). The

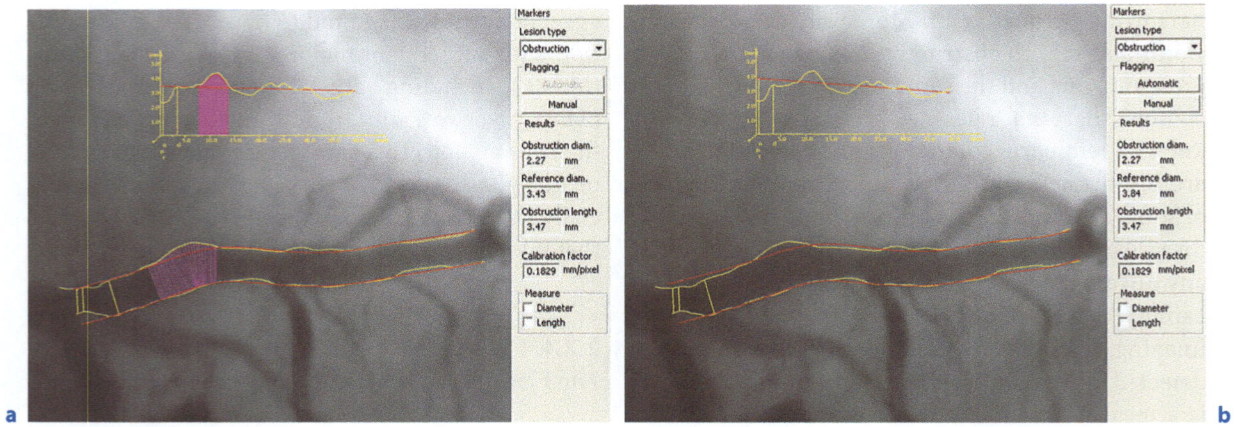

Fig. 2.2.6a,b. Example of a vessel with an ectatic area. **a** The initial (interpolated) reference diameter function would lead to arbitrary, erroneous results, in this case in significant tapering of the reference diameter function. **b** By "flagging" the ectatic area, a proper tapering of the reference diameter function is obtained. The reference diameter changed from 3.84 mm before flagging to 3.43 mm after flagging

Patient Name [ID]	QCA0003 [01]
Phase Label	FU
Calibration Method	CATHETER
Calibration Factor	**0.1829 mm/pixel**
Calibration Device Size	2.00 mm(6.0 French)
Frame (Original Fra...	1 of 1 (34)
Flagging Used	Manual
GFT Used	No
Reference Marker	Automatic

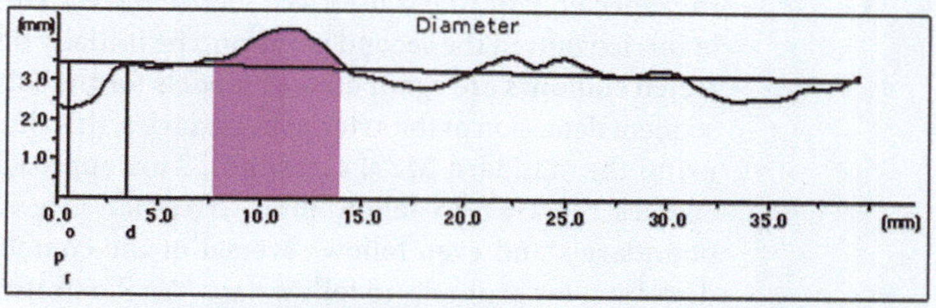

	Diameter (mm)	Area (mm²)	Length (mm)
Obstruction	2.27	4.06	3.47
Reference	3.43	9.23	
%Stenosis	33.72	56.07	

	Diameter (mm)	Area (mm²)
Mean	3.22	8.31
Minimum	2.27	4.06
Maximum	4.32	14.69
Std. dev.	0.47	2.45

	Mean Diameter (mm)	Vessel Area (mm²)	Vessel Length (mm)
Proximal		0.00	0.00
Lesion	2.68	9.63	3.47
Distal	3.27	118.05	36.01
Segment	3.22	127.68	39.49

	Symmetry	Area (mm²)
Plaque	0.47	2.60

a

Patient Name [ID]	QCA0003 [01]
Phase Label	FU

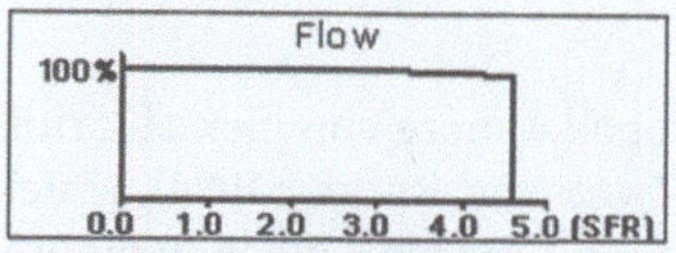

Stenotic Flow Reserve	4.64
Poisseuille Resistance	0.07
Turbulent Resistance	0.38
Normal Flow	0.88 ml/s
Inflow Angle	9 °
OutflowAngle	21 °

b

Fig. 2.2.7a,b. The obstruction and flow parameters (of Fig. 2.2.6).

SFR describes, on the basis of a mathematical/physiological model, how much the flow can potentially increase under maximal hyperemic conditions in that particular coronary segment due to that single obstruction. It can also be described as a wind tunnel test of that stenosis under standardized conditions (Kirkeeide 1991). In a disease-free segment, the SFR equals 4–5, a value that decreases as the severity of the obstruction increases.

2.2.4.5 Complex Vessel Morphology

As explained earlier, modern contour detection approaches are based on the MCA algorithm, which has been demonstrated to be fast and robust for images that may vary significantly in image quality. This approach has been shown to work very well as long as the vessel outlines are relatively smooth in shape. However, complex vessel morphology may occur after coronary intervention (e.g. when a dissection occurs).

In its design, the MCA technique is hampered when tracing very irregular and complex boundaries. First, the algorithm can select only one point per scanline. However, when the coronary artery has irregular boundaries, for example, at a complex lesion, this condition may not be satisfactory (see Fig. 2.2.8; light blue contour). Second, the edge strength or derivative values are calculated only along the direction of the scanlines, whereas the highest edge strength values may occur in other directions. Third, the results are therefore highly dependent on the actual directions of these scanlines; a slight change in direction may result in other contour points. To circumvent these problems and limitations, and as a result be able to adequately analyze such very irregular stenoses, we

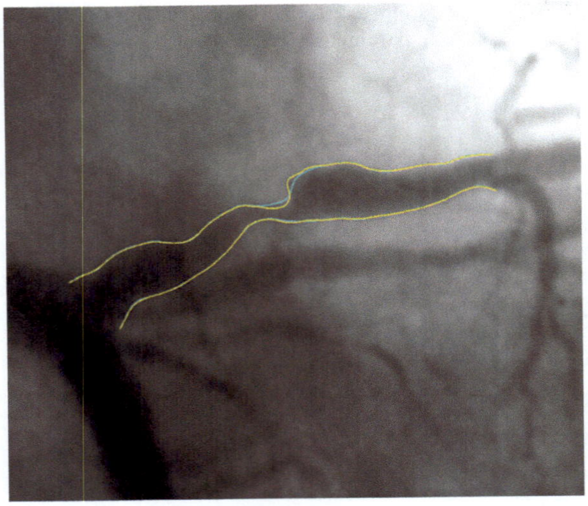

Fig. 2.2.8. Example of outcome of gradient field transform (GFT) analysis on a vessel segment with very severe complex stenosis. Conventional approaches with the minimum cost algorithm (MCA) are not able to follow automatically the abrupt changes in morphology. The *light blue contour* is MCA, and the *yellow contour* is GFT

developed a more complex algorithm, the GFT (van der Zwet and Reiber 1994), which is illustrated by the graphic example given in Figure 2.2.9.

Scanlines are defined perpendicular to the pathline as in standard MCA. The closed circles in Figure 2.2.9 represent pixels along the scanlines. Pixel A is a contour point under consideration. When searching for the next point of the arterial boundary, the MCA algorithm would only consider points C7, C8, and C1. In contrast, the GFT algorithm takes all of its eight neighboring points (C1–C8) into account. Each branch from a particular scan point to a neighboring scan point is assigned a different cost value (a mathematical technique), which is a function of its edge

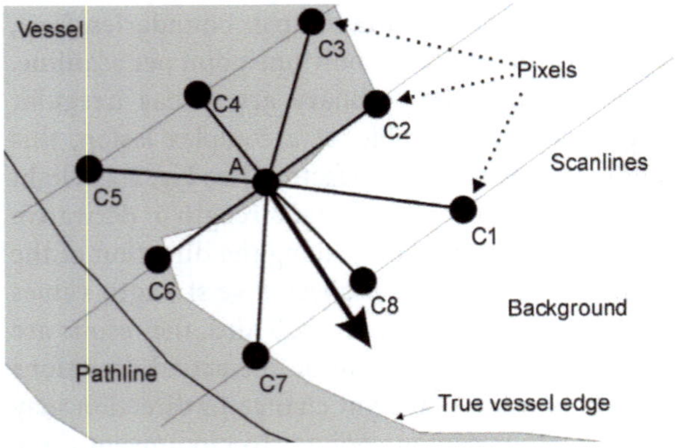

Fig. 2.2.9. Schematic representation of a vessel with its pathline, the scanlines, and the search directions for the GFT algorithm

strength and the angle between the direction of the edge and the direction of the branch. The goal of the algorithm now is to find an optimal path between one node on the first scanline of the vessel segment and one node on the last scanline of this segment.

In practice, the entire contour detection procedure is applied twice to a coronary segment: the first time the detected pathline is used as a model and the GFT is carried out. In the second iteration, the initially detected contours are again used as models for the subsequent detection of the arterial boundaries, this time using the standard MCA algorithm. This approach enables the GFT to follow more irregular arterial boundaries and even follow reversal of the contour direction, for example, to follow flaps. An illustrative example of the GFT is given in Figure 2.2.8.

The obstruction diameters of complex lesions assessed by GFT analysis are, on average, 0.25 mm smaller than those detected by the MCA algorithm (van der Zwet and Reiber 1994). The detected contours are a little more irregular because the algorithm is more sensitive to noise in all possible spatial directions. However, we believe that these data represent a correct reflection of the vessel's morphology. These irregularities may also provide prognostic information (Kalbfleisch et al. 1990). This is a subject that needs to be investigated in future studies.

Our experiences with GFT analyses indicate that this approach is recommended for the analysis of complex lesions and radiopaque stents. For the latter, GFT analysis is able to follow the outer boundaries of the stent struts and the contrast lumen in between the stent struts.

2.2.4.6 Densitometry

Because the X-ray arteriogram is a two-dimensional projection image of a three-dimensional structure, measured vessel sizes may be of limited value in vessels with very irregular cross sections. For many years, great efforts have been devoted in trying to derive information about the path lengths of the X-rays through these vessels from the brightness levels within the coronary arteries (Reiber and Serruys 1991). If such a relationship could be established, one would obtain the information required to compute the cross-sectional areas from a single angiographic view. This approach is called the densitometric measurement technique.

Theoretically, densitometry would seem the ultimate solution for the computation of the vessel's cross-sectional area from a single angiographic view. However, so far, densitometry has not provided reliable results to the extent that it can be used in clinical trials and research. Too many problems remain to make this an acceptable technique, i.e. the nonlinear transfer functions of the X-ray system, the difficulties in correcting for the variable background beyond the vessel of interest in these morphologically complex images, etc. (Reiber 1991).

2.2.4.7 Standardized QCA Methodology for Assessing Brachytherapy Trials

Although brachytherapy is hardly used anymore in interventional cardiology, its requirements a number of years ago led to the design of a new way of analyzing sequential images, which at a later point in time became useful in an adapted format for DES. For that reason, a short paragraph is devoted to this subject, followed by a more generous explanation for the DES application.

The angiographic evaluation of brachytherapy trials became challenging due to the extent of the segment receiving therapy (up to 60 mm in length) and the multiple associated landmarks (lesion, balloon injury, stent, and radiation delivery). Conventional QCA analysis was limited in this regard due to the extensive editing and reanalyses that would be required to execute these multiple segmental analyses.

Based on a consensus of experts (Ravello, Italy, March 2000), new terminology was defined for vascular brachytherapy (VBT) studies, based on markers or physical landmarks obtained during the vascular intervention, in an attempt to achieve global consistency in the angiographic analysis and reporting of VBT trial results. Under the guidance of world-renowned brachytherapy experts, this new terminology was incorporated in the VBT analysis of the QAngio XA. It features comprehensive subsegment analyses required for a thorough evaluation of the interventional brachytherapy (Lansky et al. 2002). The main advantage of this VBT analysis is the reduced interface required by the QCA analyst in obtaining all segmental results. From a practical standpoint, all parameters can be derived from the same diameter function, which results in higher consistency, while simplifying and minimizing the user interface.

2.2.4.8 Standardized QCA Methodology for Drug-Eluting Stent Analyses

In the last few years, the use of DES has demonstrated a dramatic expansion worldwide. It already became clear at the beginning of the first DES trials that the angiographic evaluation of DES trials required new parameters and that multiple associated landmarks (lesion, balloon injury and stent) had to be dealt with, which is not possible with the conventional QCA analysis (only the lesion). As a result, the previously used extensive editing for bare metal stent analyses was not acceptable for DES analyses anymore.

Building upon the previously established terminology for VBT (Lansky et al. 2002), a new terminology for DES has been defined, based on markers or physical landmarks obtained during the vascular intervention, in an attempt to achieve global consistency in the angiographic analysis and reporting of DES trial results. Under the guidance of world-renowned DES experts, this new terminology has been incorporated in the DES analysis of the QAngio XA. It features comprehensive subsegment analyses required for a thorough evaluation of the interventional drug-coated stent therapy.

The main advantage of this DES analysis module is the reduced interface required by the QCA analyst in obtaining all segmental results. Guided by a detailed drawing demonstrating the precise location of each one of the landmarks, the QCA analyst will perform a single DES analysis (at baseline, post-intervention or at follow-up) of the entire coronary segment of analysis, while indicating with pairs of markers the positions of the procedural landmarks in the vessel or corresponding diameter function. From a practical standpoint, all parameters can be derived from this same diameter function, which results in higher consistency, while simplifying and minimizing the user interface. To properly understand all the features of the DES analysis of the QAngio XA, the new nomenclature needs to be explained in detail.

2.2.4.8.1 Definition and Assessment of the Segments Based on Markers or Physical Landmarks

The *coronary segment of analysis* is the part of the target vessel that is used for QCA analysis. In practice, the start- and end-points of the contours define this segment (in other words, the total segment). Within a coronary segment of analysis, there are three different segments that can be identified based on markers or physical landmarks (Fig. 2.2.10).

1. The *obstructed* segment is the part of the coronary segment of analysis showing the lesion intended for treatment (i.e. the only segment part used in a conventional QCA analysis).
2. The *stented* segment is the part of the coronary segment of analysis extending from the most proximal to the most distal stent edge/marker, when one or more drug-eluting stents have been deployed or already exist as for in-stent restenosis. The unique pathophysiology of intimal hyperplasia within stented segments is the rational for distinguishing this segment from adjacent non-stented vessel segments, where combined hyperplasia and negative remodeling contribute to late lumen loss. The effect of the pharmacologic agent within stented versus non-stented arterial segments can thereby be differentiated.
3. The *injured* segment is the part of the coronary segment of analysis that extends from the most proximal to the most distal marker or landmark of any physical vessel injury caused by one or multiple balloon inflations during PTCA, stent placement, a drug delivery balloon, by the use of atherectomy devices, etc. Analysis of the zones of injury may provide insight into the interaction between vessel injury and some of the pharmacologic agent solely, with the caveat that this parameter is entirely dependent on the operator's compulsive recording of all components of the intervention. In practice, this aspect is no routine, with the result that the injured segment is quite often omitted from a study set-up. Nevertheless, the most important (drug-eluting) stent related parameters are still obtained within a relatively short analysis time.

In the ideal situation each segment described is included in, or is equal to, its successor, i.e. the obstructed segment is included in the stented segment, which is included in the injured segment, which in turn is included in the coronary segment of analysis (see Fig. 2.2.10). However, in practice, this may not be the case and segment shifts (i.e. where an obstruction segment is not included in its successor(s) and/or its boundaries do not coincide) may occur (see Fig. 2.2.11).

2.2.4.8.2 Definition and Assessment of the Segments Based on Biologically Relevant Landmarks

Within a coronary segment of analysis, there are two biologically relevant segments (being proximal and distal of the stent) that can be derived from the stented segment, and one segment that is derived from these segments. All these segments are defined by the extent of drug elution (see Fig. 2.2.12):

1. The *DES edge* segments are segments positioned adjacent to the proximal and distal boundaries of the stented segment. The length of the proximal and distal DES edges depends on the study design. Usually, the proximal and distal DES edge segments will be set by default at 5 mm, immediately adjacent to the outer side of the stented boundaries, both proximally and distally.
2. The *analyzed* segment is the injured segment, including the proximal and distal DES edge segments. In practice, this means that the two outer-most

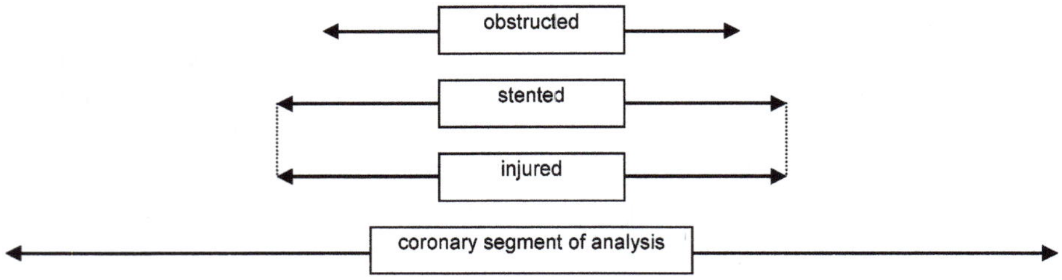

Fig. 2.2.10. DES analysis segment definitions based on markers or physical landmarks (ideal case)

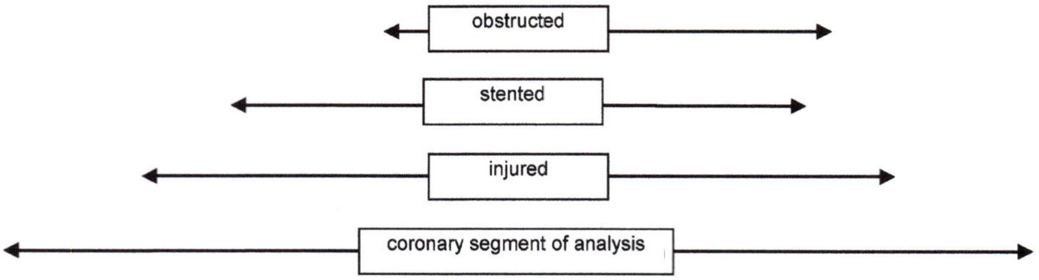

Fig. 2.2.11. DES analysis segment definitions based on markers or physical landmarks (shifted case)

boundaries of any of the segments used (except the obstructed segment) define the analyzed segment.

In a theoretically "ideal" situation, each segment described is included in, or is equal to, its successor (see Fig. 2.2.12). However, in practice, this may not be the case and segment shifts may occur. In that case, the analyzed segment will extend from the most proximal boundary (e.g. of the proximal DES edge) to the most distal boundary (e.g. of the injured segment) (see Fig. 2.2.13).

2.2.4.8.3 Definition and Assessment of the "Normal" Segment

- The *proximal and distal normal reference* segments are segments of 5 mm length (default), both proximal and distal to the analyzed segment (default), which represents the most normal reference vessel segment. These normal segments represent the normal "non-diseased" vessel (i.e. showing normal progression/regression of the vessel), which have not been touched at all by any of the devices (see Fig. 2.2.14).

The position and length of the normal segments will be user-defined and can be set independently from each other, based on the appearance of the coronary artery. The average of the mean diameters of the proximal and distal normal segments (i.e. averaged mean normals) or the interpolated diameter of the proximal and distal normal segments (i.e. interpolation on normals) can be used for comparison purposes. Because the first approach does not take any vessel tapering into account, theoretically its value is only correct for the center position along the vessel. On the other hand, the automatic interpolated reference diameter approach, which provides a reference diameter value for each position along the vessel, thereby corrected for any possible vessel tapering at each individual position, is the first choice for the correct percent diameter stenosis measurements.

2.2.4.8.4 Definition and Assessment of the Related Parts

The *Injured-not stented (I-nS)* segment is the part of the coronary segment of analysis that has been subjected to injury, but that has not been stented. In practice, this means that the boundary of the injured segment and the corresponding boundary of the stented segment define the I-nS segment (see Fig. 2.2.15).

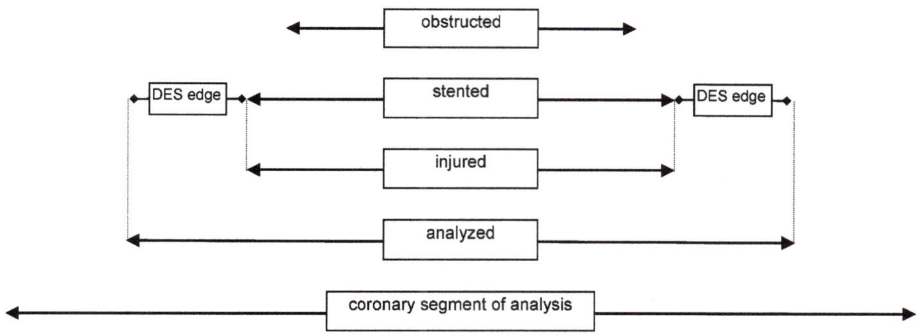

Fig. 2.2.12. DES analysis segment definitions based on biologically relevant landmarks (ideal case)

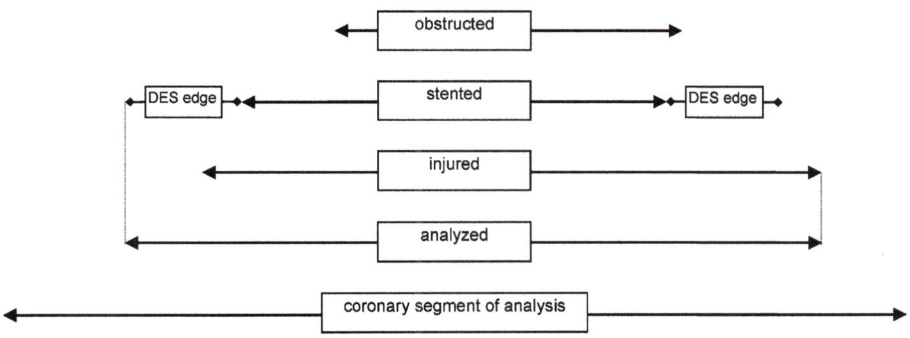

Fig. 2.2.13. DES analysis segment definitions based on biologically relevant landmarks (shifted case)

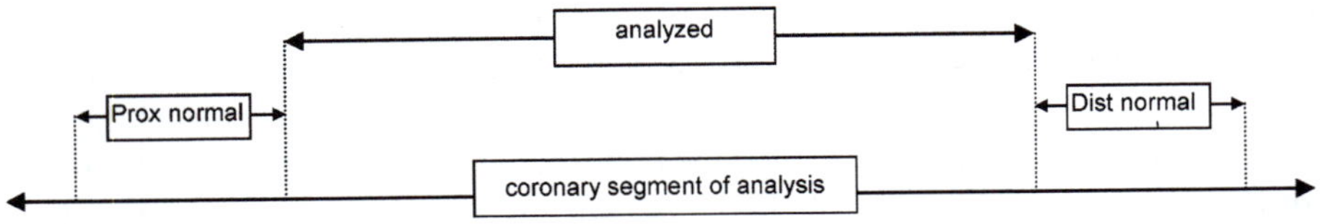

Fig. 2.2.14. The normal segments definition

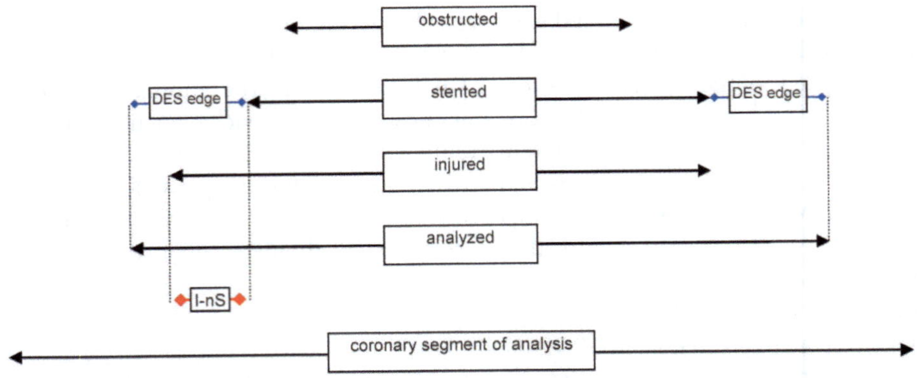

Fig. 2.2.15. Definition of the injured-not stented (I-nS) segment

2.2.4.8.5 Data Collection and Reporting for Drug-Eluting Stent Trials

For each of the defined segments (11 in total), the following 10 parameters are reported:

(1) the minimal lumen diameter (MLD), (2) the position of the MLD relative to the start position of the coronary segment of analysis, (3) the obstruction length of the MLD, (4) the mean diameter, (5) the reference diameter corresponding to a particular MLD (i.e. the reference diameter measurements will be based on a user-defined reference diameter or, preferably, on an interpolated reference diameter, including the use of flagging), (6) the percent diameter stenosis derived from the MLD and its corresponding reference diameter at the site of MLD, (7) the individual segment length, (8) the position of the proximal boundary of an individual segment relative to the start position of the coronary segment of analysis, (9) the plaque area (in the projected plane), and (10) the percentage area stenosis (in the transversal plane).

For the proximal and distal DES edge segments one additional parameter will be calculated: The distance (L) between the MLD of these edge segments and the accompanying boundary of the stented segment (see Fig. 2.2.16).

For the total segment one additional parameter will be calculated: The DI (see Sect. 2.2.4.3).

All these data will be reported automatically during a DES analysis. See Figure 2.2.17 for an example of an actual DES analysis.

2.2.4.9 Ostial Analysis

For the quantitation of a true ostial lesion, whether in a coronary or peripheral vessel, the ostial analysis option was developed. The particular advantage of this option is that the contours of the arterial seg-

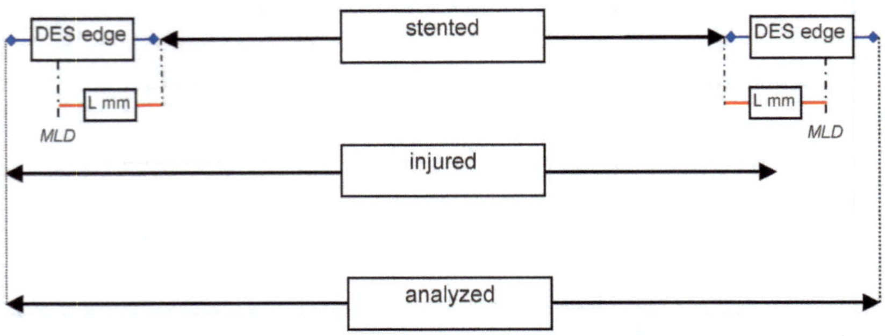

Fig. 2.2.16. Definition of the distance L (in millimeters) between the minimal lumen diameter (MLD) within the drug eluting stent (*DES*) edge and the stented segment boundary

Fig. 2.2.17a–c. Example of a drug eluting stent (DES) analysis on coronary artery

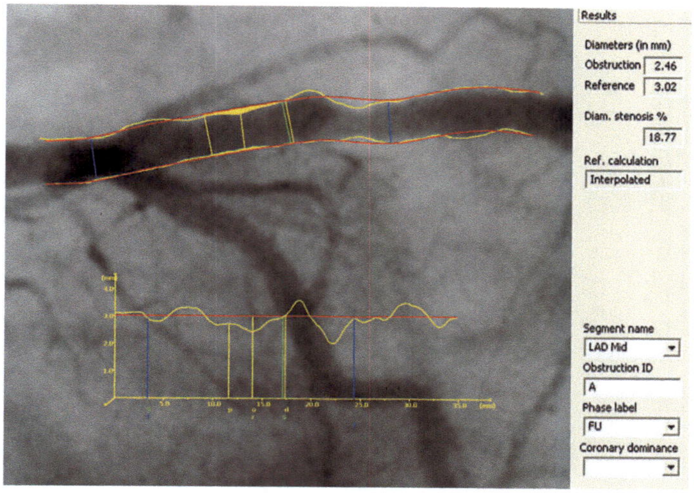

a

Patient Name [ID]	
Phase Label	FU
Calibration Method	CATHETER
Calibration Factor	**0.2419 mm/pixel**
Calibration Device Size	2.00 mm(6.0 French)
Frame (Original Fra...	1 of 2 (27)
Flagging Used	No
GFT Used	No
Reference Marker	Automatic
Reference Method	Interpolated
MLD Calculation	Relative

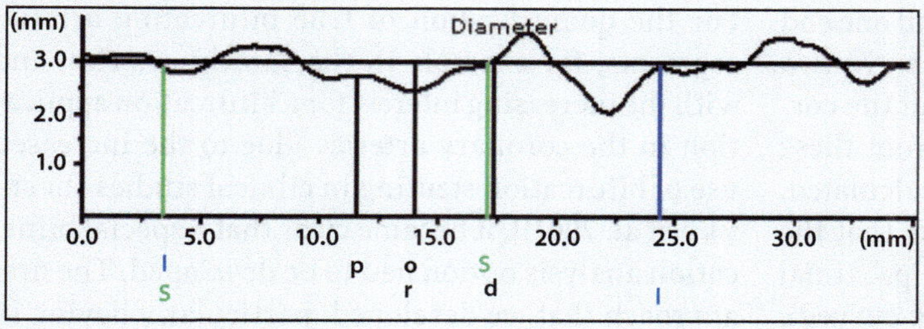

	Diameter (mm)	Area (mm²)	Length (mm)
Obstruction	**2.46**		**5.79**
Reference	**3.02**		
%Stenosis	**18.77**	34.02	

	Distance MLD-stent (mm)	Minimal Diameter (mm)
DES Prox	**0.00**	2.90
DES Dist	**5.07**	2.03

	Mean Diameter (mm)	Segment Length (mm)
Obstruction	2.72	5.79
Stented	2.88	13.76
Injured	2.86	21.00
Total Segment	2.94	34.76

	Area (mm²)
Plaque	1.78
Diffuse Index	0.11

b

Patient Name [ID]
Phase Label FU

	Minimal Diameter (mm)	Position MLD (mm)	Obstructi... Length (mm)	Reference Diameter (mm)	Diameter Stenosis (%)	Area Stenosis (%)	Mean Diameter (mm)	Segment Start (mm)	Segment Length (mm)	Plaque Area (mm²)
Obstruction	2.46	14.00	5.79	3.02	18.77	34.02	2.72	11.59	5.79	1.78
Stented	2.46	14.00	5.55	3.02	18.77	34.02	2.88	3.38	13.76	1.78
Injured	2.03	22.21	4.59	3.03	32.96	55.06	2.86	3.38	21.00	2.35
Total Segment	**2.03**	**22.21**	**4.59**	**3.03**	**32.96**	**55.06**	**2.94**	**0.00**	**34.76**	**2.35**
DES Prox	2.90	3.38	0.48	3.02	3.93	7.70	3.11	0.00	3.38	0.02
DES Dist	2.03	22.21	2.41	3.03	32.96	55.06	2.94	17.14	5.07	1.25
Analyzed	2.03	22.21	4.59	3.03	32.96	55.06	2.89	0.00	24.38	2.35
Prox. Normal										
Dist. Normal										
InS Prox										
InS Dist	**2.03**	**22.21**	**4.59**	**3.03**	**32.96**	**55.06**	**2.81**	**17.14**	**7.24**	**2.35**

c

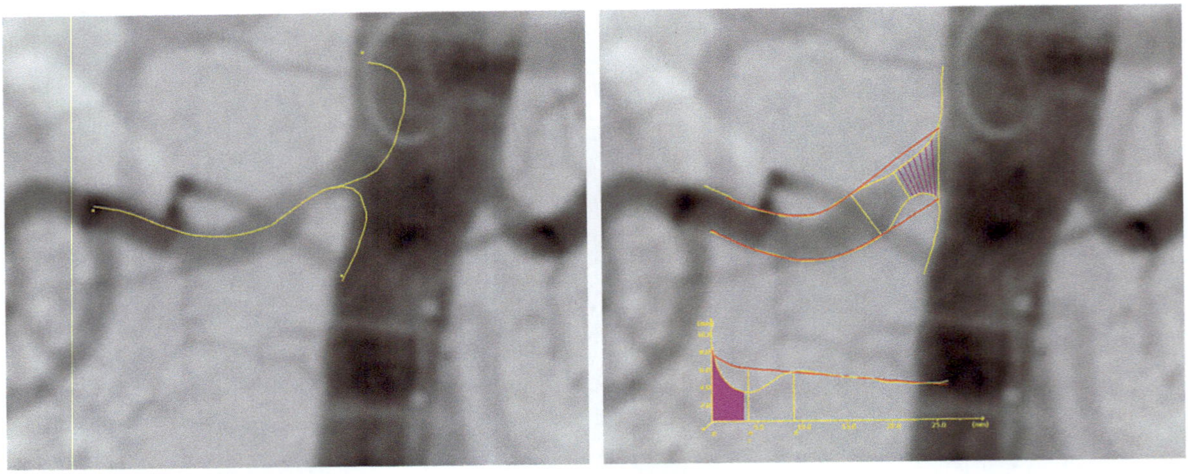

a b

Fig. 2.2.18a,b. Example of an ostial analysis on a renal artery. **a** Pathlines of the ostial analysis. **b** The contours and diameter function of an ostial analysis

ment are properly detected at the ostium, which is not possible with the conventional straight analysis approach (see Fig. 2.2.4a,b).

An example of an ostial analysis on a renal artery is given in Figure 2.2.18. In this ostial analysis, the user is requested to provide three points to define the arterial segment: two start points in the mother segment at either side of the side branch, and one end point distally in the side branch. Subsequently, two pathlines are determined (Fig. 2.2.18a) and the corresponding arterial contours detected. From these contours, the ostial diameter function is calculated. In such an ostial case, we must make sure that the arterial diameter function includes the proximal part at the ostium (which can be strongly curved). Therefore, firstly the exact location where the vessel separates from the main vessel and the direction of the vessel at that location are determined. Secondly, the position where a straight analysis would start in this case is calculated. This information is then used to interpolate the diameter values near the ostium (pink lines), which results in a complete arterial diameter function (Fig. 2.2.18b). However, a straight tapering reference diameter function (red line) would not be the best approximation in such cases. At the position near the ostium, the direction of the reference diameters changes in order to match the direction of the main vessel. Therefore, the reference diameter function is adjusted according to a model that takes into account the angle between the side branch and the main vessel. Because of the increasing arterial diameter function at the ostium, this part is flagged by default (pink lines) in order to obtain a suitable reference diameter function, leading to a proper assessment of the percentage narrowing (Fig. 2.2.18b).

2.2.4.10 Bifurcation Analysis

For the quantification of true bifurcating arterial segments, for example in the carotid arteries, and with the increasing interest for a bifurcation application in the coronary arteries [due to the increased use of bifurcation stenting in clinical studies (Lefevre et al. 2001)], it became clear that a special bifurcation analysis option had to be developed. The first approach that we developed, particularly having in mind the clinical research on (coronary) bifurcation stenting, is the so-called three-section analysis model. The particular advantage of this model is that it combines the proximal and two distal artery segments (fragments) with the central fragment of the bifurcation, resulting in three separate analyses (sections) each with its own set of parameters, all derived in one analysis procedure.

An example of a bifurcation analysis on a coronary artery is given in Figure 2.2.19. In this bifurcation analysis, the user is requested to provide three points to define the arterial bifurcation segment: one start point in the proximal segment and an end point in each of the two distal segments. Subsequently, two pathlines are detected (see Fig. 2.2.19a) and the corresponding arterial contours determined. Next, the central fragment of the bifurcation is defined by three automatically determined delimiters: one distally in the proximal segment and two proximally in each distal segment (see Fig. 2.2.19b). The other three fragments combined with this central fragment form the three sections of the bifurcation analysis.

From the section contours, three arterial and reference diameter functions are calculated. As in our conventional QCA approach, the reference diameter function is calculated by an iterative regression technique, which excludes any obstructive area as much as possible. In our three-section bifurcation analysis the reference diameter function should only be based upon the arterial diameters outside the central fragment, since the normally increasing arterial diameters in the central fragment are not representative for the fragments outside the central fragment. Therefore, the central fragment arterial diameters are all flagged by default in the analyses of all three sections (see Fig. 2.2.19c).

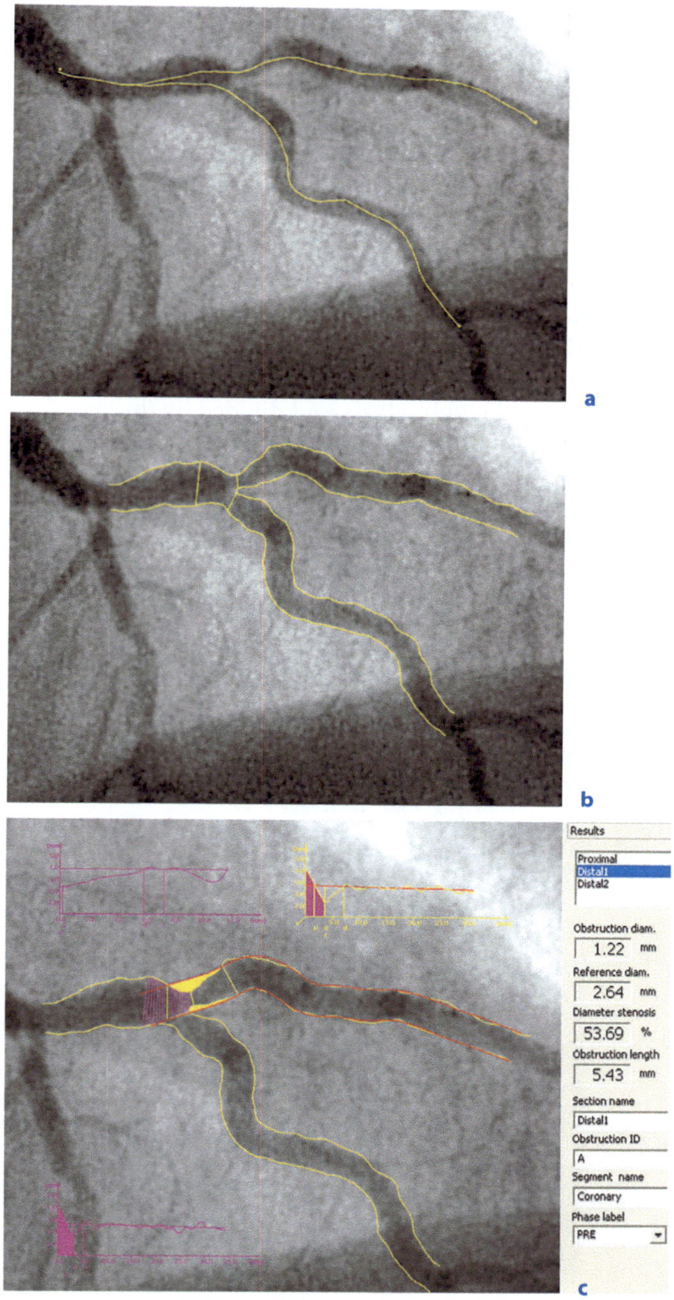

Fig. 2.2.19a–c. Example of a bifurcation analysis on coronary artery. **a** The pathlines of the bifurcation analysis. **b** The delimiters of the bifurcation analysis. **c** The three diameter functions for each section. In this case the distal 1 section is selected

2.2.5 Guidelines

2.2.5.1 Guidelines for Catheter Calibration

The calibration procedure is one of the most important procedures in any QCA or QVA analysis procedure. The goal of the calibration procedure is to assess the size of each picture element or pixel in the image as expressed in millimeters per pixel based on the calibration device with known dimensions. Therefore, any error in the calibration will directly translate into an error in the absolute measures of the arterial segment. For that reason, extra attention to the quality of the outcome of the calibration is really mandatory. The most widely used objects for calibration are the coronary catheters for coronary applications, and either one of the following for peripheral applications: marker catheter or guidewire, cm-grid or ruler, or sphere or coin of known size.

For the coronary applications, a frame is chosen in which the contrast filled catheter is in a "stable" position, i.e. minimal motion with respect to neighboring frames to prevent motion blur. Following these rules will result in an image in which the image contrast of the catheter and the sharpness of the edges are maximal. Other restrictions have been formulated as to the size and type of the catheters, resulting in so-called QCA-approved catheters (Lespérance et al. 1998).

Our recommendations for coronary applications include the following: (1) only catheters of size 6-F or bigger should be used to prevent large unknown variations in the calibration factors, (2) if only smaller catheters (5-F) are available, a test to verify the suitability of these catheters should be carried out, and (3) the variability in repeated calibration measurements (minimal three times) in digital images should be less than 0.01 mm/pixel.

For peripheral applications other devices might be used for calibration as well. The advantage of each of these devices is that the distance over which the calibration is carried out is larger than in the diameter measurements in the coronary applications, leading to more accurate calibration factors. An example of a calibration on a marker catheter is illustrated in Figure 2.2.20a. Here, the average distance between the automatically detected markers is calculated in pixels and divided by the true distance in millimeters, leading to the calibration factor in millimeters per pixel. The advantage of the marker catheter is that it is inside and very close to the arterial segment of interest, thereby avoiding any out-of-plane errors. One disadvantage is the use of a more expensive marker catheter. Examples of using the centimeter ruler and the sphere for calibration purposes are given in Figure 2.2.20b,c, respectively.

2.2.5.2 Guidelines for QCA Acquisition Procedures

The primary objective of QCA measurements in clinical trials is to allow more precise and reliable analyses of the real changes after interventions, namely, acute lumen gain, late lumen loss, and net lumen gain expressed in millimeters. This is best achieved when exactly the same setting is applied during the procedure at baseline and at the follow-up studies, that is, replication of same angiographic X-ray views, same doses of intra-coronary nitroglycerin,

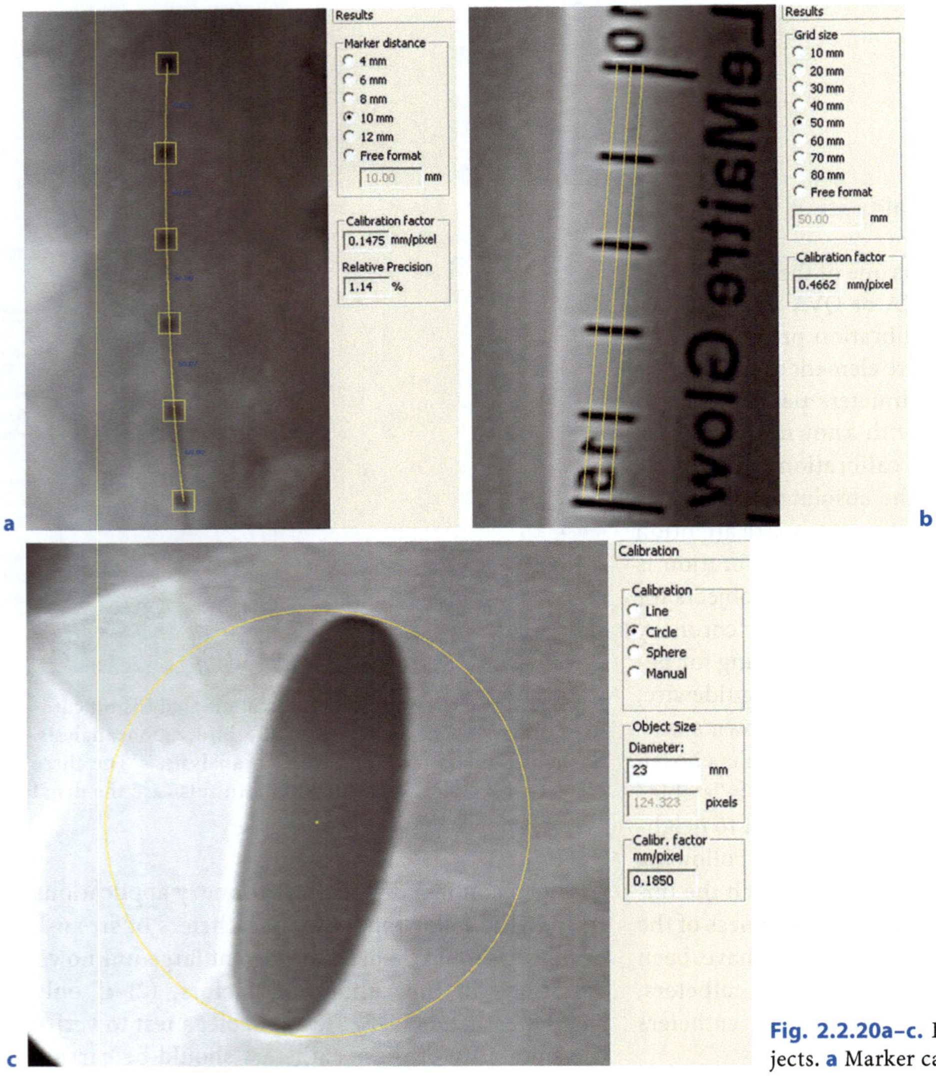

Fig. 2.2.20a–c. Examples of calibration objects. **a** Marker catheter. **b** cm-ruler. **c** Coin

same contrast agent, same catheter type or material, and, if feasible, same catheterization room (Reiber et al. 1996b).

2.2.6 QCA Validation

Whichever QCA analytical software package is being used, it will always produce numbers describing the morphology of the coronary segment analyzed. However, validation studies must demonstrate the true strengths and weaknesses, as well as the clinical validity of such analytical package.

It has been well accepted that the results from validation studies on clinical materials are to be described in terms of the systematic error or accuracy, defined as the average signed difference between repeated measurements (i.e. measurement 1 minus measurement 2), and the random error or precision, is defined as the standard deviation of these signed differences. For objects with known dimensions, such as phantoms, the systematic error is defined by the average signed difference between the measurement and the true phantom tube size, and the random error is defined by the pooled standard deviation of these measurements. For a QCA technique to be acceptable, guidelines for systematic and random error values of absolute vessel dimensions have been established. These guidelines are shown in Table 2.2.1 (Reiber et al. 1993, 1994a,b; Tuinenburg et al. 2002). The systematic error values for the Plexiglass phantom apply to each of the individual measurements. Over the many years that we have developed QCA analytical software, extensive calibration procedures have always been carried out and described in publications (Lespérance et al. 1998; Reiber et al. 1993, 1994a). We will describe in the following paragraphs some of the results of validation studies.

2.2.6.1 Plexiglass Phantom Studies

The QAngio XA analytical package was validated using a coronary Plexiglass phantom with tube sizes in the range of 0.80–5.00 mm. The tubes were filled with 100% contrast medium and positioned horizontally and vertically in the image. The data was obtained at 60, 75, and 90 kV, using both 5″ and 7″ image intensifier sizes. Analyses were carried out on three different image types: (1) digitized 35 mm cinefilm images, (2) digital 512^2 images, and (3) digital 1024^2 images. The results are presented in Table 2.2.2.

The data from Table 2.2.2 can be summarized as follows: Both systematic and random errors were within the guidelines for all three acquisition modes. Variability or random errors increased with increasing kilovolt level due to the decreasing image contrast levels. The lowest variability was obtained with the digital 512^2 images, although the differences are small. The overall variability was found to be slightly higher when the phantom was positioned on a patient's chest compared with an off-patient situation (data not presented here) (Reiber et al. 1994a).

Table 2.2.1. Guidelines for systematic and random errors of a state-of-the-art quantitative coronary arteriography system

	Systematic error (mm)	Random error (mm)		
Type of study		Guidelines	Result ranges	
Plexiglass phantom, off patient	<0.10	0.10–0.13	0.06–0.12	
Plexiglass phantom, on patient	<0.10	0.10–0.13	0.10–0.11	
		Guidelines	Dobs	Dref
Intra-observer variabilities		0.10–0.15	0.10	0.13
Inter-observer variabilities		0.10–0.15	0.11	0.13
Short-term variabilities		0.15–0.25	0.19	0.22
Medium-term variabilities		0.20–0.30	0.18	0.34
Inter-core lab variability			0.14	0.15

Table 2.2.2. QCA results for a Plexiglass phantom acquired on a homogeneous background

		Digital 512	Digital 1024	Cine film
II-Size	kV-Level	S.E.±R.E.	S.E.±R.E.	S.E.±R.E.
5"	60 kV	0.00 ± 0.04	0.00 ± 0.04	0.04 ± 0.04
	75 kV	0.00 ± 0.07	0.00 ± 0.09	-0.01 ± 0.07
	90 kV	-0.03 ± 0.11	-0.02 ± 0.12	-0.04 ± 0.10
7"	60 kV	0.02 ± 0.04	0.03 ± 0.04	0.05 ± 0.04
	75 kV	0.01 ± 0.07	0.01 ± 0.08	0.00 ± 0.08
	90 kV	0.00 ± 0.11	0.00 ± 0.12	-0.04 ± 0.11

S.E., systematic error; R.E., random error.

2.2.6.2 In Vivo Plexiglass Plugs

The ultimate test for a QCA system is the analysis of clinical images of obstructions with known dimensions. For this purpose, small Plexiglass plugs (outer diameters: of 2.5–3.5 mm, inner diameters of 0.5–1.57 mm, length of approximately 7.5 mm) were introduced with a catheter into the coronary arteries of dogs. Images were acquired on cinefilm, as well as in digital format. From the obstructive region, the mean diameter and the standard deviation of the diameter measurements were assessed. The mean diameter was compared with the known true inner diameter of the plug. Systematic and random errors were of the same magnitude as the results from the coronary Plexiglass phantom on a homogenous background and on patient anatomy (Reiber et al. 1994a).

2.2.6.3 Inter- and Intra-observer and Short- and Medium-term Variabilities

Extensive data on inter- and intra-observer and on short- and medium-term variabilities are available (Reiber et al. 1993). The inter- and intra-observer variability studies on a set of routinely obtained digital coronary arteriograms demonstrated that the systematic errors were approximately zero; in other words, no systematic differences were found. The random errors for the obstruction diameter were less than 0.11 mm, and for the interpolated reference diameter these were less than 0.13 mm. Larger variabilities were observed when the study was extended to so-called "short-term" investigations with repeated angiographic acquisition after 5 min, and "medium-term" investigations, with repeated acquisitions at the end of the catheterization procedure under standardized circumstances. These larger variabilities can be explained mainly from variations in the repeated calibration procedures based on the catheter.

2.2.6.4 Inter-laboratory Variability

With the widespread use of QCA in different laboratories, the question came up of how well the results from these QCA laboratories correlate. This is of particular relevance for core laboratories, which at a certain point in time may wish to combine their QCA data from similar trials for meta-analysis purposes or otherwise want to compare data, for example, from angiographic procedures, carried out in different countries. Systematic differences most likely exist in the absolute dimensions between the two laboratories. Hopefully, the two laboratories show the same trends between baseline and follow-up studies. However, these assumptions cannot be taken for granted. Validation studies need to be carried out to demonstrate the differences in an objective manner.

If two laboratories use the same equipment, differences will exist in the image quality of the coronary arteriograms, in the way the angiograms are analyzed in terms of the frame selection, frame digitization (for cinefilm), and the definition of the coronary segments, and in the experience of the technicians in the actual analysis of the images. Studies have clearly demonstrated that significant analysis differences may occur between different angiographic core laboratories, particularly when different QCA systems are used (Beauman et al. 1994).

Two core laboratories, Heart Core B.V. (now Bio-Imaging Technologies) in Leiden, the Netherlands, and the Montreal Heart Institute in Montreal, Canada, standardized their entire QCA procedure through the implementation of common standard operating procedures (SOPs) and the subsequent validation (Tuinenburg et al. 2002). The errors between the two sites for the most important QCA parameters are given in Table 2.2.3. These data indicate that the systematic errors between the two sites are very small and that the random errors are within ranges similar to earlier reported inter-observer variabilities

Table 2.2.3. Inter-laboratory systematic and random errors in the individual measurements for two highly standardized and collaborating core labs

n = 63	Systematic error	Random error
Obstruction diameter (mm)	−0.06	0.14
Reference diameter (mm)	−0.02	0.15
Percentage diameter stenosis (%)	1.83	4.96
Mean segment diameter (mm)	0.00	0.10

(Reiber et al. 1993). It should be noted that an additional potential error source was the different video systems on the cinefilm digitizers (PAL and NTSC) used by the two sites. Nowadays, with digital data, this error source has disappeared. From this study, it can be concluded that inter-laboratory variabilities between highly organized and standardized QCA core labs can be in the same range as the reported inter- and intra-observer variabilities (Reiber et al. 1993; Tuinenburg et al. 2002). Furthermore, it is clear that regular testing of the entire analysis procedure is necessary to remain within the standards that have been set. In practical terms this means that the two sites can function as a single "global" core lab.

2.2.7 Applications of QCA: Off-Line and On-Line

QCA is clearly used in different ways, which we will refer to for reasons of simplification by the notations "off-line QCA" and "on-line QCA".

By off-line QCA, we mean one or more QCA workstations that are not directly connected to the image-generating X-ray system in the catheterization laboratories. Furthermore, it is possible that multiple QCA workstations are connected to an internal network to exchange image data with a file server for central storage purposes. The coronary arteriograms are thus analyzed after the catheterization procedure, and the QCA results have no effect anymore on the actual (interventional) procedure.

Typical applications for such off-line workstations include core laboratory activities and smaller, single-center clinical research studies in a particular cardiology department. Also, the quantitative data can be used for quality assurance purposes in the catheterization laboratory, as well as used as supportive data in cases of questionable lesions. A schematic diagram of such a set-up is shown in Figure 2.2.21. A QCA workstation should be able to accept all available forms of image media.

In recent years we have seen increased use of QCA in the review stations used by the PACS. The availability of patient studies is no longer a problem, since these are stored in the (cardio-) PACS by default nowadays. Thus, patient studies can be retrieved anywhere within the hospital, a QCA analyses can be applied and the results can also be stored in the PACS. DICOM offers several possibilities for this purpose: as a DICOM structured report (SR), a DICOM secondary capture (SC) image or simply as a DICOM encapsulated PDF report. In this way, the results are available for every other user of the PACS and beyond (referring physician).

By on-line QCA, we mean a situation in which the QCA workstation is directly connected to the image-generating X-ray system in the catheterization labo-

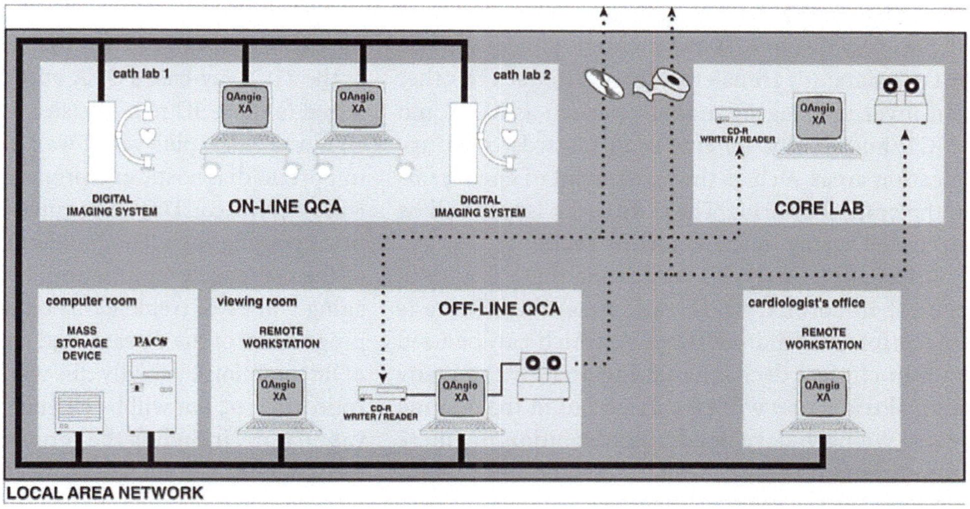

Fig. 2.2.21. Off- and on-line applications of QAngio XA workstations

ratory. This connection can be realized in different ways, from a simple analog video connection to the output of the X-ray system, which requires a selected frame to be digitized [analog-to-digital conversion (A/D)] by the QCA workstation, to a preferred digital connection to the imaging system using DICOM exchange protocols. A schematic diagram of a networked on-line set-up is also given in Figure 2.2.21.

Typical applications of on-line QCA include support of clinical decision-making during the procedure, (e.g. vessel sizing and length measurement of stenosis for the optimal selection of an interventional device), an immediate assessment of the efficacy of the intervention, in- or exclusion of patients for clinical trials based on vessel size (e.g. small vessel disease) or percentage diameter stenosis, and training purposes of fellows. New developments may lead to integration of functional indices with the morphologic information.

It is evident that the great advantage of having the same brand of workstation for on- and off-line applications is that the same software package is being used. As a result, the outcomes of these analyses are directly compatible and comparable.

2.2.8 Future QCA Directions

For the next several years, developments in the following directions can be expected: (a) further optimization of the bifurcation analyses both for coronary and peripheral applications; (b) 3D reconstruction of the coronary vessels from biplane views or rotational angiography with subsequent derivation of optimal angiographic views; (c) from a research point of view, the fusion of X-ray angiographic and IVUS or OCT data; (d) transfer of the techniques to other non-invasive imaging modalities such as MRA and MSCT; and finally, (e) extension towards other application areas such as the assessment of aneurysms in the cranial arteries. These different issues will be discussed briefly in the following sections.

Bifurcation analyses: Worldwide there is a lot of interest in coronary bifurcation stenting. There is a need for quantitative support, which can be used both in clinical decision making and for the many clinical trials that will be carried out in the coming years. We have developed a first solution for these applications; however, given the complex morphologies of these possible cases, further refinements/extensions will be developed and validated extensively in the coming few years so that these are applicable in a robust manner for all clinical and research applications with minimal user interactions.

3D reconstruction: Solutions have been provided for the 3D reconstruction of coronary segments based on biplane acquisitions or rotational angiography. The goal of such analysis is the assessment of the optimal views, particularly for bifurcating vessels, where overlap and foreshortening limit the possibilities of the 2D approach. Although visualization of the vessels is attractive, the true diagnostic value and accuracy of QCA analyses are still to be determined. For the calculation of the optimal views, it would be sufficient to have the centerlines only.

Fusion of X-ray and intravascular data: Certainly for research purposes, there is a need for fusion of the 3D ultrasound data with the reconstructed X-ray angiographic data from biplane angiography or rotational angiography. Typical applications include: computational haemodynamics to calculate wall shear stress, analyses to determine the correlation between vessel curvature and circumferential plaque distribution and simulation of intravascular procedures. Furthermore, from the 3D description of the coronary system, other interesting data can be derived, such as wall shear stress based on computational fluid dynamics, stress and strain on the vessels in relation to the sites of the development of local atherosclerosis, etc. (Chen and Carroll 2000).

Transfer of the techniques to non-invasive imaging: Over the last few years there has been tremendous interest in attempting to visualize the coronary arteries by MSCT (CTA) and by MRA, being 3D acquisition techniques. The additional advantages of these techniques are the potential to visualize the arterial wall and possibly the composition of the plaque at the site of the stenosis. It will be clear that many basic principles of the 2D X-ray-based QCA approaches can be transferred to these 3D non-invasive techniques (3D QCA). CTA and MRA plus vessel wall imaging may provide important diagnostic and prognostic information, but will not replace 2D QCA for interventional cardiology in the coming years. On the other hand, the assessment of the composition of the wall by MR vessel wall imaging will be of tremendous interest for studying the progression of the disease, and particularly the effects of interventions. Initially this will be applied to the carotid arteries, but will be extended towards the entire vasculature, including the coronary arteries, although the spatial resolution will be the limiting factor here.

Other applications: In addition to applying QCA in peripheral vessels, there is also a growing interest in developing approaches for tracking cranial blood vessels and quantifying size, shape and volume of aneurysms, such that the interventional procedure can be optimally prepared. Such approaches can be applied to the rotational angiographic data or to the MSCT data that is often available prior to treatment of such patients.

2.2.9 In Conclusion

Semi-automated segmentation techniques are able to trace the luminal boundaries of coronary arteries from two-dimensional digital X-ray arteriograms after minimal user interaction. QCA allows the derivation of such luminal dimensions and derived indices with small systematic and random errors as demonstrated by a range of validation studies. QCA can be used in an off-line mode for clinical research studies and in an on-line mode during the interventional procedure to support the clinical decision-making process. New options have become available for more extensive analyses in both coronary and peripheral vessels, such as the brachytherapy and DES analyses, the ostial and bifurcation analyses, and the quantification of both obstructive and/or aneurysmal lesions.

Over the last few years, QCA tools such as QAngio XA have become a commodity of PACS review and reporting workstations. This enables the possibility of using (off-line) QCA from every workstation in the hospital, at any given time. Reports of the QCA analysis can be restored back into the PACS/patient record, enabling other users to review the results.

New applications will include integration with QCU or OCT, 3D reconstruction and analysis of coronary segments, allowing the determination of optimal angiographic views, wall shear stress in the vessels, and better guidance of the interventional procedure, but also transfer of the basic principles to non-invasive MSCT and MR applications, resulting in 3D QCA, plus the additional advantage of assessing vessel wall characteristics, which will be of tremendous research interest. Overflow to other areas are also foreseen, such as cranial interventional approaches.

References

Adame IM, Koning PJH de, Lelieveldt BPF, Wasserman BA, Reiber JHC, Geest RJ van der (2006) An integrated automated analysis method for quantifying vessel stenosis and plaque burden from carotid MR images: combined post-processing of MRA and vessel wall MR. Stroke 37:2162–2164. [Epub 2006 Jun 29]

Beauman G, Reiber JHC, Koning G, van Houdt R, Vogel R (1994) Angiographic core laboratories analyses of arterial phantom images: comparative evaluations of accuracy and precision. In: Reiber JHC, Serruys PW (eds) Progress in quantitative coronary arteriography. Kluwer Academic Publishers, Dordrecht, pp 87–104

Brown BG, Bolson E, Frimer M, Dodge HT (1977) Quantitative coronary arteriography: estimation of dimensions, hemodynamic resistance, and atheroma mass of coronary artery lesions using the arteriogram and digital computation. Circulation 55:329–337

Bruschke AVG, Wijers TS, Kolsters W, Landmann J (1981) The anatomic evolution of coronary artery disease demonstrated by coronary arteriography in 256 nonoperated patients. Circulation 63:527–536

Büchi M, Hess OM, Kirkeeide RL, Suter T, Muser M, Osenberg HP et al. (1990) Validation of a new automatic system for biplane quantitative coronary arteriography. Int J Card Imaging 5:93–103

Chen SJ, Carroll JD (2000) 3-D reconstruction of coronary arterial tree to optimize angiographic visualization. IEEE Trans Med Imaging 19:318–336

de Feyter PJ, Vos J, Reiber JHC, Serruys PW (1993) Value and limitations of quantitative coronary angiography to assess progression and regression. In: Reiber JHC, Serruys PW (eds) Advances in quantitative coronary arteriography. Kluwer Academic Publishers, Dordrecht, pp 255–271

Dijkstra J, Koning G, Reiber JHC (1999) Quantitative measurements in IVUS images. Int J Card Imaging 15:513–522

Geijer H (2002) Radiation dose and image quality in diagnostic radiology. Optimalization of the dose-image quality relationship with clinical experience from scoliosis radiography, coronary intervention and a flat panel digital detector. Acta Radiol Suppl 43:1–43

Glagov S, Weisenberg E, Zarins CK, Stankunavicius R, Kolettis GJ (1987) Compensatory enlargement of human atherosclerotic coronary arteries. N Engl J Med 316:1371–1375

Heintzen P (1971) Roentgen-, cine- and videodensitometry. Georg Thieme Verlag, Stuttgart

Holmes DR Jr, Laskey WK, Wondrow MA, Cusma JT (2004) Flat-panel detectors in the cardiac catheterization laboratory: revolution or evolution – what are the issues? Cathet Cardiovasc Intervent 63:324–330

Ishii Y, van Weert AWM, Hekking E, de Marie K, ter Horst J, Oemrawsingh PV et al. (2001) A novel quantitative method for evaluating diffuse in-stent narrowing at follow-up angiography. Cathet Cardiovasc Intervent 54:309–317

Janssen JP, Koning G, de Koning PJ, Tuinenburg JC, Reiber JHC (2002) A novel approach for the detection of pathlines in X-ray angiograms: the wavefront propagation algorithm. Int J Cardiovasc Imaging 18:317–324

Janssen JP, Koning G, de Koning PJ, Tuinenburg JC, Reiber JH (2004) Validation of a new method for the detection of pathlines in vascular X-ray images. Invest Radiol 39:524–530

Jukema JW, Bruschke AVG, Reiber JHC (1996) Lessons learned from angiographic coronary atherosclerosis trials. In: Reiber JHC, van der Wall EE (eds) Cardiovascular imaging. Kluwer Academic Publishers, Dordrecht/Boston/London, pp 119–132

Kalbfleisch SJ, McGillem MJ, Simon SB, DeBoe SF, Pinto IM, Mancini GB (1990) Automated quantitation of indexes of coronary lesion complexity. Comparison between patients with stable and unstable angina. Circulation 82:439–447

Kirkeeide RL (1991) Coronary obstructions, morphology and physiologic significance. In: Reiber JHC, Serruys PW (eds) Quantitative coronary arteriography. Kluwer Academic Publishers, Dordrecht, pp 229–244

Kirkeeide RL, Fung P, Smalling RW, Gould KL (1982) Automated evaluation of vessel diameter from arteriograms. Computers in Cardiology, 215–218 Los Alamitos, CA, IEEE-Computer Society Press

Lansky AJ, Desai KJ, Bonon R, Koning G, Tuinenburg J, Reiber JHC (2002) Quantitative coronary angiography methodology in vascular brachytherapy II. In: Waksman R, (ed) Vascular brachytherapy, 3rd edn. Futura Publishing Co., Inc Amronk, NY, pp 543–562

Leber AW, Becker A, Knez A, Ziegler F von, Sirol M, Nikolaou K et al. (2006) Accuracy of 64-slice computed tomography to classify and quantify plaque volumes in the proximal coronary system. J Am Coll Cardiol 47:672–677

Lefevre T, Louvard Y, Morice MC, Loubeyre C, Piechaud JF, Dumas P (2001) Stenting of bifurcation lesions: a rational approach. J Interv Cardiol 14:573–585

Lespérance J, Bilodeau L, Reiber JHC, Koning G, Hudon G, Bourassa M (1998) Issues in the performance of quantitative coronary angiography in clinical research trials. In: Reiber JHC, van der Wall EE (eds) What's new in cardiovascular imaging? Kluwer Academic Publishers, Dordrecht, pp 31–46

Nasu K, Tsuchikane E, Katoh O, Vince G, Virmani R, Surmely JF et al. (2006) Accuracy of in vivo coronary plaque morphology assessment: a validation study of in vivo virtual histology compared with in vitro histopathology. J Am Coll Cardiol 47:2405–2412. [Epub 2006 May 30]

Oost E, Koning G, Sonka M, Oemrawsingh PV, Reiber JH, Lelieveldt BP (2006) Automated contour detection in X-ray left ventricular angiograms using multiview active appearance models and dynamic programming. IEEE Trans Med Imaging 25:1158–1171

Pinto TL, Waksman R (2006) Clinical applications of optical coherence tomography. J Interv Cardiol 19:566–573

Reiber JHC (1991) An overview of coronary quantitation techniques as of 1989. In: Reiber JHC, Serruys PW (eds) Quantitative coronary arteriography. Kluwer Academic Publishers, Dordrecht, pp 55–132

Reiber JHC, Serruys PW (1991) Quantitative coronary angiography. In: Marcus ML, Schelbert HR, Skorton DJ, Wolf GL (eds) Cardiac imaging: a companion to Braunwald's Heart Disease. W.B. Saunders Company, Philadelphia, pp 211–281

Reiber JHC, Booman F, Tan H, Slager CJ, Schuurbiers JC, Gerbrands JJ et al. (1978) A cardiac image analysis system. Objective quantitative processing of angiocardiograms. IEEE Comp Cardiol 239–242

Reiber JHC, Serruys PW, Kooijman CJ, Wijns W, Slager CJ, Gerbrands JJ et al. (1985) Assessment of short-, medium-, and long-term variations in arterial dimensions from computer-assisted quantitation of coronary cineangiograms. Circulation 71:280–288

Reiber JHC, Serruys PW, Slager CJ (1986) Quantitative coronary and left ventricular cineangiography: methodology and clinical applications. Martinus Nijhoff, Boston

Reiber JHC, van der Zwet PM, Koning G, von Land CD, van Meurs B, Gerbrands JJ et al. (1993) Accuracy and precision of quantitative digital coronary arteriography: observer-, short-, and medium-term variabilities. Cathet Cardiovasc Diagn 28:187–198

Reiber JHC, von Land CD, Koning G, van der Zwet PM, van Houdt R, Schalij M et al. (1994a) Comparison of accuracy and precision of quantitative coronary arterial analysis between cinefilm and digital systems. In: Reiber JHC, Serruys PW (eds) Progress in quantitative coronary arteriography. Kluwer Academic, Publishers Dordrecht, pp 67–85

Reiber JHC, Koning G, von Land CD, van der Zwet PM (1994b) Why and how should QCA systems be validated? In: Reiber JHC, Serruys PW (eds) Progress in quantitative coronary arteriography. Kluwer Academic Publishers, Dordrecht, pp 33–48

Reiber JHC, Jukema JW, Koning G, Bruschke AVG (1996b) Quality control in quantitative coronary arteriography. In: Bruschke AVG, Reiber JHC, Lie KI, Wellens HJJ (eds) Lipid lowering therapy and progression of coronary atherosclerosis. Kluwer Academic Publishers Dordrecht, pp 45–63

Reiber JHC, Schiemanck L, van der Zwet PM, Goedhart B, Koning G, Lammertsma M et al. (1996a) State of the art in quantitative coronary arteriography as of 1996. In: Reiber JHC, van der Wall EE (eds) Cardiovascular imaging. Kluwer Academic Publishers, Dordrecht, pp 39–56

Reiber JHC, Koning G, Dijkstra J, Wahle A, Goedhart B, Sheehan FH et al. (2001) Angiography and intravascular ultrasound. In: Sonka M, Fitzpatrick JM (eds) Handbook of medical imaging – vol. 2: medical image processing and analysis. SPIE Press Belligham, WA, pp 711–808

Schaar JA, Regar E, Mastik F, McFadden EP, Saia F, Disco C et al. (2004) Incidence of high-strain patterns in human coronary arteries: assessment with three-dimensional intravascular palpography and correlation with clinical presentation. Circulation 109:2716–9. [Epub 2004 May 24]

Schaar JA, van der Steen AF, Mastik F, Baldewsing RA, Serruys PW (2006) Intravascular palpography for vulnerable plaque assessment. J Am Coll Cardiol 47[8 Suppl]:C86–91

Sonka M, Reddy GK, Winniford MD, Collins SM (1997) Adaptive approach to accurate analysis of small-diameter vessels in cineangiograms. IEEE Trans Med Imaging 16:87–95

Spahn M, Heer V, Freytag R (2003) Flat-panel detectors in X-ray systems. Radiologe 43:340–350

Stiel GM, Stiel LS, Schofer J, Donath K, Mathey DG (1989) Impact of compensatory enlargement of atherosclerotic coronary arteries on angiographic assessment of coronary artery disease. Circulation 80:1603–1609

Tardif JC, Lee H (1998) Applications of intravascular ultrasound in cardiology. In: Reiber JHC, van der Wall EE (eds) What's new in cardiovascular imaging. Kluwer Academic Publishers, Dordrecht, pp 133–148

Tsapaki V, Kottou S, Kollaros N, Dafnomilli P, Koutelou M, Vano E et al. (2004) Comparison of a conventional and flat-panel digital system in interventional cardiology procedures. Br J Radiol 77:562–577

Tuinenburg JC, Koning G, Hekking E, Desjardins C, Harel F, Bilodeau L et al. (2002) One core lab at two international sites, is that feasible? An inter-core lab and intra-observer variability study. Cathet Cardiovasc Intervent 56:333–340

Tuinenburg JC, Koning G, Seppenwoolde Y, Reiber JHC (2006) Is there an effect of flat-panel-based imaging systems on quantitative coronary and vascular angiography? Cathet Cardiovasc Intervent 68:561–566

van der Zwet PM, Reiber JHC (1994) A new approach for the quantification of complex lesion morphology: the gradient field transform; basic principles and validation results. J Am Coll Cardiol 24:216–224

van der Zwet PM, Meyer DJ, Reiber JHC (1995) Automated and accurate assessment of the distribution, magnitude, and direction of pincushion distortion in angiographic images. Invest Radiol 30:204–213

Wahle A, Wellnhofer E, Mugaragu I, Sauer HU, Oswald H, Fleck E (1995) Assessment of diffuse coronary artery disease by quantitative analysis of coronary morphology based upon 3D reconstruction from biplane angiograms. IEEE Trans Med Imaging 14:230–241

2.3 Clinical Intracoronary Ultrasound

Jurgen Ligthart and Pim J. de Feyter

CONTENTS

J. Ligthart, BSc
University Hospital Rotterdam, Thoraxcenter Bd 410, P.O. Box 2040, 3000 CA Rotterdam, The Netherlands
P. J. de Feyter, MD, PhD
University Hospital Rotterdam, Thoraxcenter Bd 410, P.O. Box 2040, 3000 CA Rotterdam, The Netherlands

2.3.1 Introduction

Intravascular ultrasound (IVUS) imaging is unique and provides a clinical method to directly visualize coronary atherosclerosis and other pathological conditions within the wall of the coronary arteries. Ultrasound penetrates below the luminal surface of the coronary artery wall and thus provides tomographic images not just from the arterial wall but also of the coronary atherosclerotic plaques. In the mid 1980s various catheter systems were designed that could be used to study blood vessels and into late eighties intracoronary ultrasound was used in humans (Yock et al. 1988; Mallery et al. 1990; Gussenhoven et al. 1989; Pandian et al. 1988; Potkin et al. 1990; Hodgson et al. 1989; Nissen et al. 1990).

2.3.2 Intracoronary Ultrasound Catheters

Catheter-based intracoronary imaging produces real-time high resolution cross-sectional tomographic images from lumen, plaque, and vessel wall.

Current intracoronary ultrasound catheters typically range in size from 2.6 to 3 F (0.87–1.17 mm in diameter) and can therefore only be safely used in the proximal and mid segments of the coronary arteries and in the presence of less severe coronary stenoses. They can be placed in the coronary tree through a 6-F guiding catheter. An ultrasound investigation of a severe stenosis should only be performed in the setting of a scheduled intervention because crossing with the catheter may cause damage, and obstruction of the coronary blood flow may, depending on the existence of collateral circulation, cause severe ischemia.

The images obtained with the currently used high-frequency (20–50 MHz) transducers are of high quality with an axial resolution which is depth dependent but ranges from 150 to 200 µm and a lateral resolution of 200–400 µm. The images are produced at 20–30 frames/s so that they appear as "real-time" images.

There are two types of intravascular ultrasound devices:

1. A mechanical device with a single transducer which is rotated at 1800 revolutions/min to generate a 360° beam (Fig. 2.3.1a).
2. A solid state device consisting of five integrated circuits and an array of 64 transducer elements in a cylindrical pattern which are activated consecutively to generate a 360° beam (Fig. 2.3.1b).

The measurements of lumen and wall with ultrasound are very accurate and precise because the velocity of sound in soft tissue represents a constant distance, allowing the construction of a calibrated scale across the image (Fig. 2.3.2a,b), which is quite unlike the catheter calibration scale used in quantitated coronary angiography, which may induce errors more readily (Fig. 2.3.3a,b).

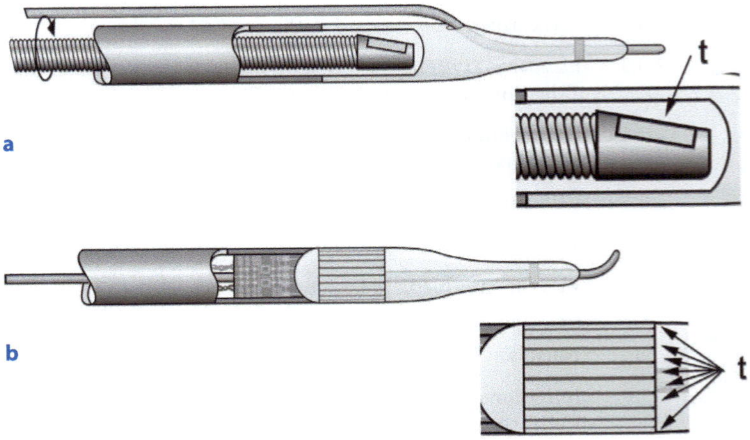

Fig. 2.3.1a,b. Two types of intravascular ultrasound devices: mechanical device (**a**): single transducer (*t*) rotates at 1800 RPM to generate a 360° beam. Solid state device (**b**): 64 transducer elements (*t*) activated consecutively to generate a 360° beam. (Courtesy of Maud van Nierop/N. Bom University Hospital Rotterdam Dijkzigt/Erasmus University Rotterdam)

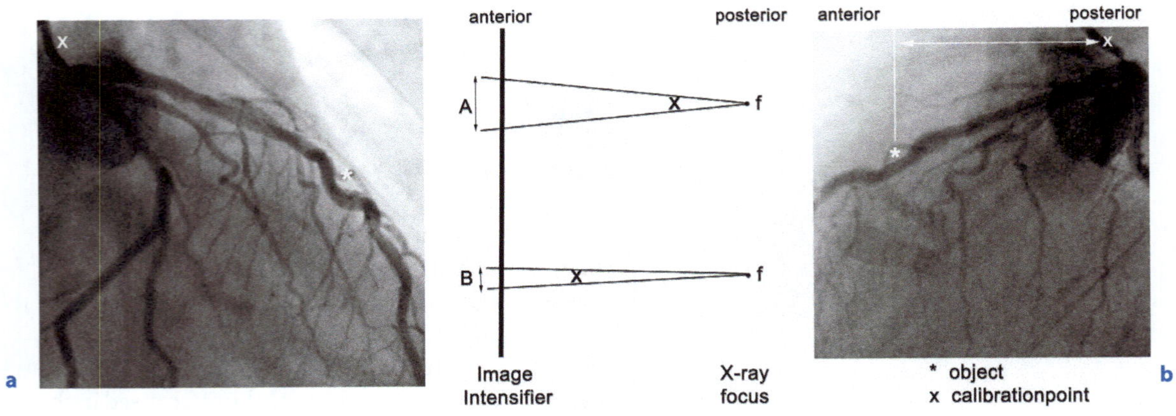

Fig. 2.3.2. a Right anterior oblique angiogram of the left coronary artery. To perform quantitative coronary analyses of the segment marked by an *asterisk*, catheter calibration has to be done at point **x**. **b** Due to this calibration method, errors may be induced. **b** The same left coronary artery from (a) in lateral view, with the segment to analyse marked by an *asterisk* and the calibration point **x**. In a frontal projection the image intensifier is positioned at the anterior side of the patient, while the X-ray tube is (under the table) posterior from the patient. The catheter tip (**x**), used as a calibration marker has a greater distance to the image intensifier than the object to analyse (*asterisk*). The drawing to the left illustrates that the calibration marker (*A*) is enlarged, compared to the object (*B*). Using this calibration in a frontal projection, the size of the object will be underestimated. This may result in the choice of undersized material such as stents or PTCA balloons

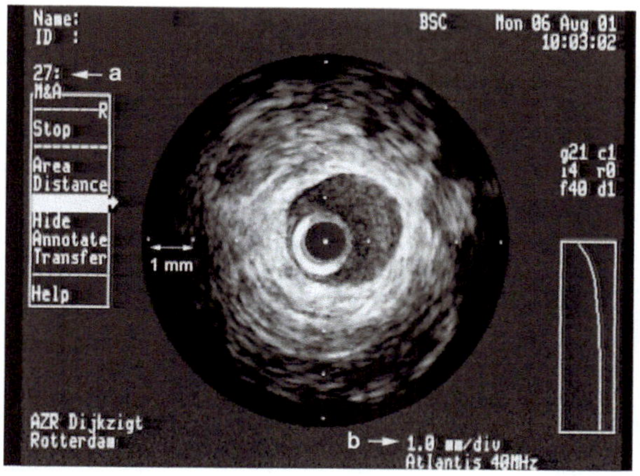

Fig. 2.3.3. Because the velocity of sound represent a constant distance it is possible to construct a calibrated scale across the image. This IVUS cross section shows such a scale with a distance of 1 mm between the points, indicated in the *bottom right* part of image (*b*). Also, when the operator chooses not to have this calibration grid in the image, measurements still can be performed due to the known calibration number of the IVUS system (*a*). Calibration numbers may vary among different types of IVUS machines

Imaging studies are usually recorded on high resolution video tape, but digital recording has recently become possible.

The ultrasound images are usually obtained using a motorized pullback device that withdraws the catheter at a constant speed (usually 0.5 mm/s).

Sidebranches, calcified plaques and perivascular landmarks facilitate interpretation and are necessary for adequate sequential examinations (Yock et al. 1988).

The perivascular landmarks including the coronary veins, pericardium and myocardium can be used as references for both axial position or tomographic orientation within the coronary artery (Figs. 2.3.4, 2.3.5).

These extravascular landmarks provide unique reference points in each coronary artery, which is illustrated in typical examples of imaging the left circumflex (Fig. 2.3.6), left anterior descending (Fig. 2.3.7) and right coronary arteries (Fig. 2.3.8).

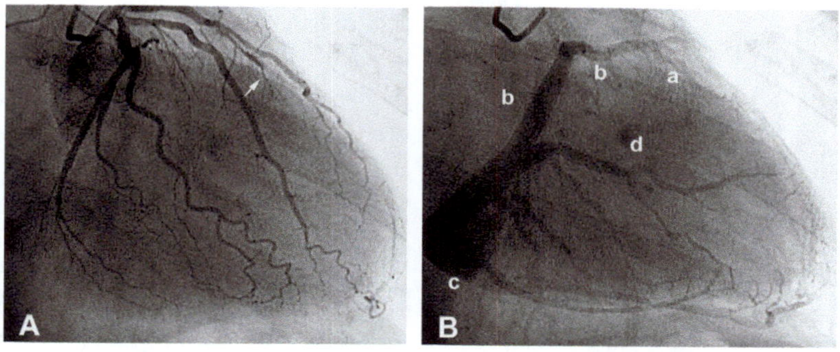

Fig. 2.3.4A,B. Right anterior oblique angiogram of the left coronary artery showing the arterial filling (**A**) and the venous filling (**B**). In this example the left anterior descending artery (LAD) is totally occluded (*arrow*). The veins will often be visible on the IVUS images as landmarkings: Anterior interventricular veins (*a*) joining the great cardiac vein (*b*) which is visible during IVUS pullback of the distal to mid LAD. During IVUS pullback, the great cardiac vein "joins" the mid and proximal LAD. In the case of a balanced or left dominant coronary system the great cardiac vein also joins the circumflex artery. During IVUS pullback side branches emerging from the circumflex artery opposite the vein are marginal branches. Emerging branches at the site of the vein are atrial (*d*). The coronary sinus (*c*) is only visible at the very distal part of the circumflex artery

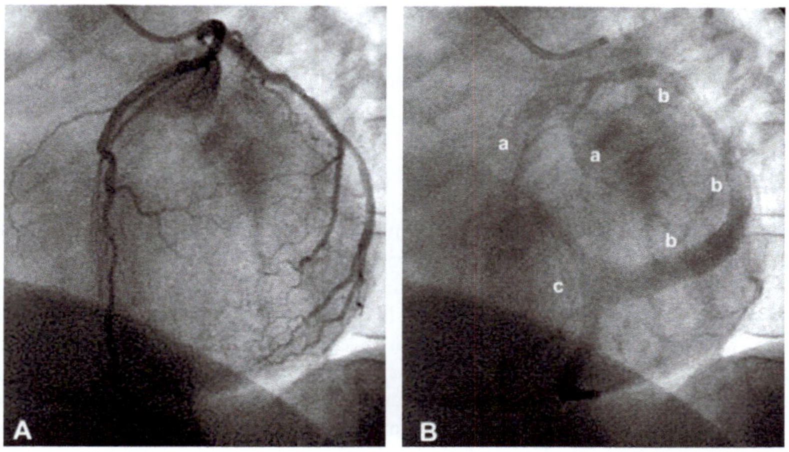

Fig. 2.3.5A,B. Left anterior oblique angiogram of the left coronary system (**A**) and venous system (**B**). The veins will often be visible during IVUS pullback as landmarks: the two anterior interventricular veins (*a*) joining together at the great cardiac vein (*b*). The coronary sinus (c) is visible at the very distal part of the circumflex artery

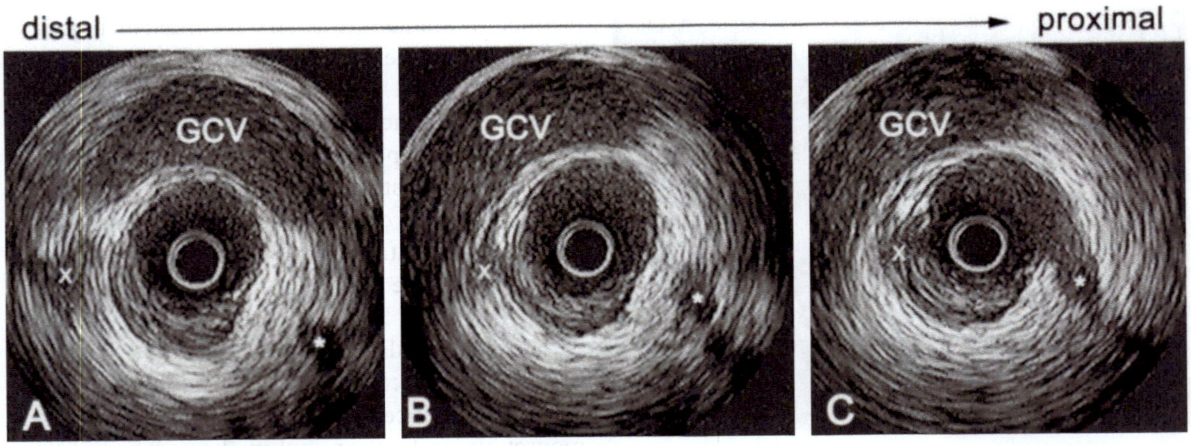

Fig. 2.3.6A–C. Part of a pullback through a circumflex artery of a balanced or left dominant system, starting at cross section *A* through *C*. The great cardiac vein (*GCV*) is imaged at 12 o'clock. Two side branches emerge from this part of the left circumflex artery. Due to the GCV it is possible to determine that side branch ***x*** is an atrial branch, because it emerges from the side of the GCV, while the branch marked by an *asterisk* is a small marginal branch. Marginal branches emerge from the opposite side of the GCV (see Fig. 2.3.4)

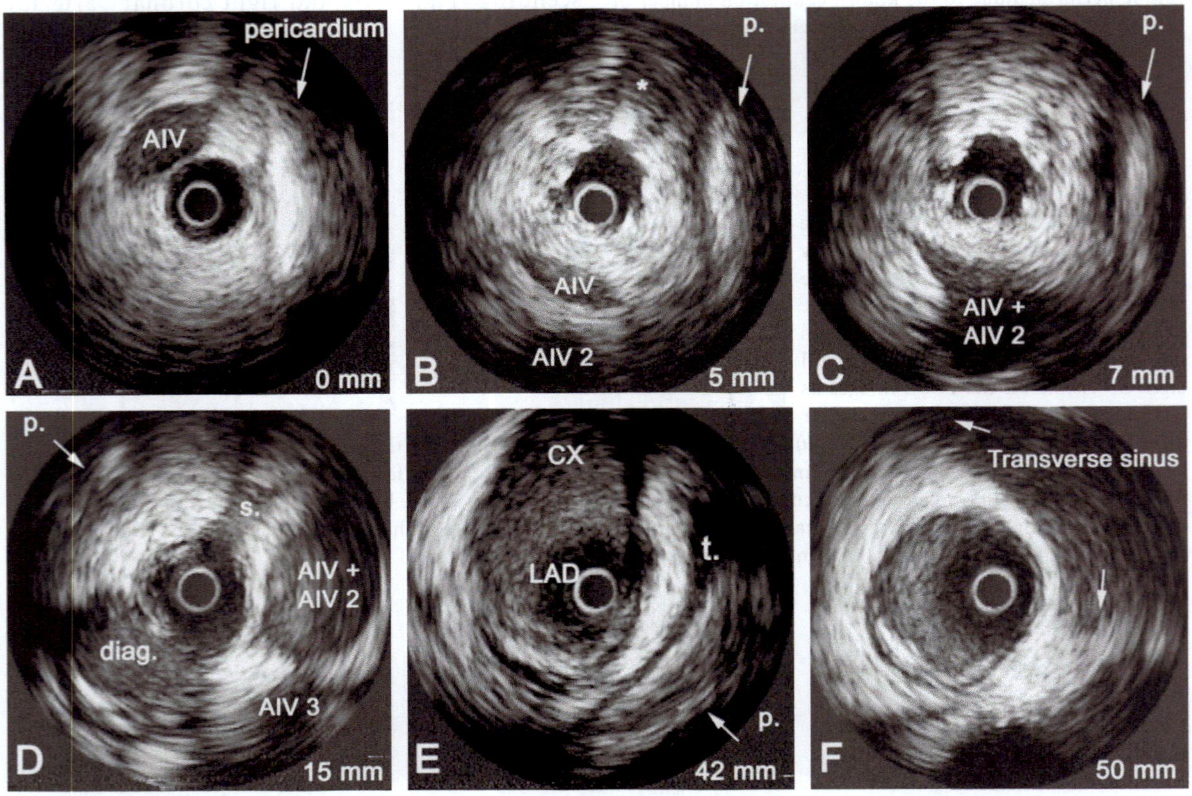

Fig. 2.3.7A–F. Pullback through the descending anterior artery, starting from cross section **A** through **F**. The pullback distances are indicated at the *bottom right* corner of each panel. **A** The cross section of the distal left anterior descending artery (LAD), with the white pericardial line at 3 o'clock. The pericardial effusion is seen at 3 o'clock between the pericardial line and the vessel. The anterior interventricular vein (AIV) is seen at 11 o'clock. While progressing the pullback the AIV rotates counter clockwise to 7 o'clock and behind this vein a second AIV appears. Opposite, a diagonal branch emerges at almost 90° left from the pericardial layer. **C** The two AIV veins joining at 6 o'clock. More proximally (**D**), the joined AIV (*2*) veins rotated further counter clockwise, with a third AIV appearing from 5 o'clock. Also the pericardial layer rotated to 11 o'clock. At 7 o'clock, 90° away from this pericardium a bigger diagonal branch emerges and a septal branch (*s*) emerges at the side of the AIV. Reaching the proximal LAD, at the bifurcation with the circumflex artery (*CX*) (**E**), the triangle of Brock and Mouchet (*t*) is visible. This triangle is described by the trajectory of the GCV together with the LAD-LCX geometry and, although it may vary in size, it is consistently found on IVUS. Reaching the proximal left main (**F**) at 1 o'clock, the transverse sinus is visible

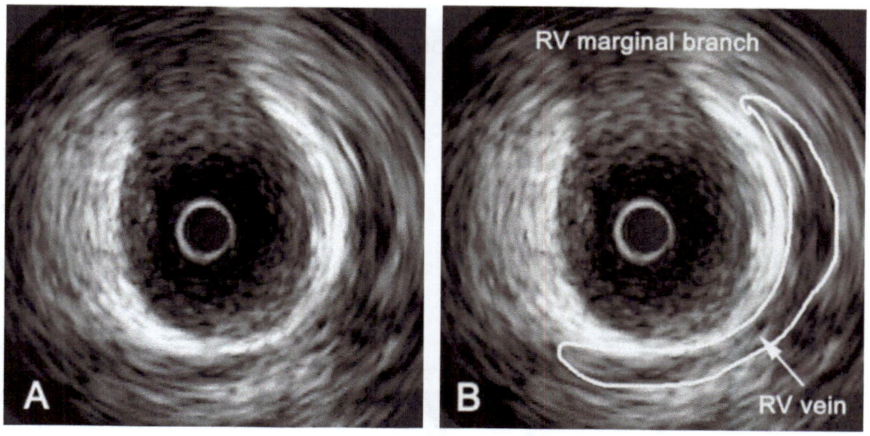

Fig. 2.3.8A,B. IVUS cross section of the mid-right coronary artery (RCA). At 12 o'clock the right ventricular marginal branch emerges. At the opposite the right ventricular vein drapes around the artery in (**A**), typical of IVUS images of the RCA veins, "horseshoe" pattern. **B** The same vein indicated by a *white line*

2.3.3 Intracoronary Imaging of the Normal Coronary Artery

Flowing blood has a typical echogenic appearance of finely textured echoes moving in a swirling pattern: "blood speckle" (Fig. 2.3.9).

The interpretation of coronary IVUS images relies on the fact that the layers of coronary arterial wall can be identified separately. An ultrasound reflection is generated at a tissue interface if there is an abrupt change in acoustic impedance. Two interfaces are observed in the coronary arteries: one at the border between blood and leading edge of the intima and one at the leading edge of the external elastic membrane at the media-adventitia border (Fig. 2.3.10; Table 2.3.1.)

The media stands out as a dark band compared with the intima and adventitia. Ultrasonic exami-

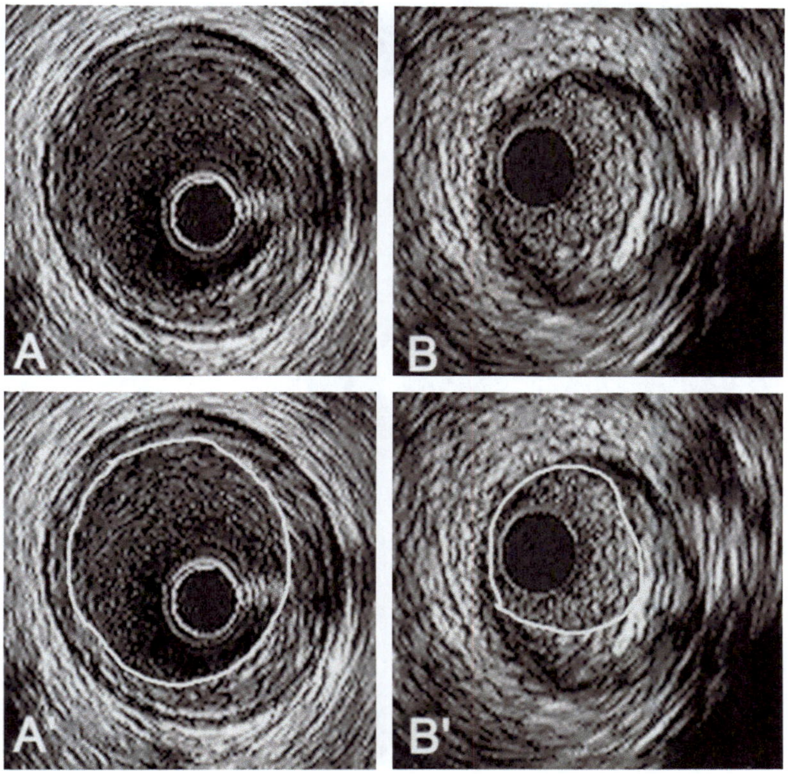

Fig. 2.3.9A,B. Example of different flow patterns on IVUS: *panel A* shows an IVUS cross section with a concentric soft plaque. The lumen indicated in *panel A'* shows dark grey speckling, indicating sufficient blood flow at the location of the cross section . *Panel B* shows an IVUS cross section with an eccentric mixed plaque with a superficial spot of calcium at 5 o'clock. The lumen indicated in *panel B'* shows a bright speckling, caused by slow- or not moving blood. This is often seen near a stenosis that is totally occluded by the IVUS catheter

Medium	Density (kg/mm³)	Sound velocity (m/sec)	Acoustic impedance (Ns/mm³)
Air	1.20	330	3.96 * 10^2
Water	1.00 * 10^3	1480	1.48 * 10^6
Blood	1,03 * 10^3	1570	1.62 * 10^6
Muscle	1.07 * 10^3	1585	1.70 * 10^6
Bone (calcium)	1.91 * 10^3	4080	7.79 * 10^6

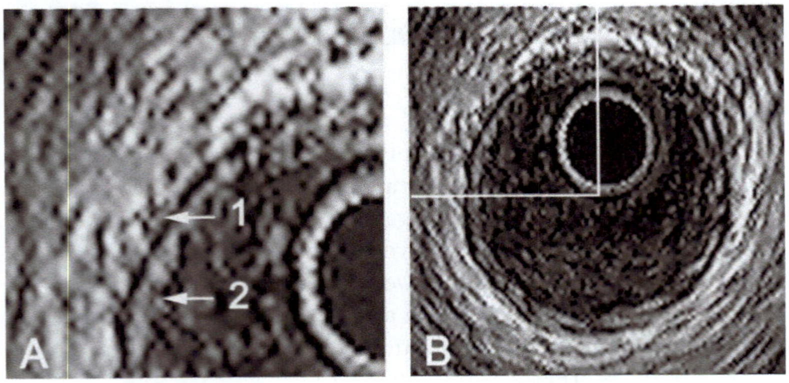

Fig. 2.3.10A,B. The *top panel* shows the difference of acoustic impedance in different media in table form. The acoustic impedance is the product of the density and the sound velocity in a certain medium. The amount of sound reflection and thus the strength of the returned ultrasound signal depends on the difference in acoustic impedance and the length of the soundwave. Although, for example, the sound velocity through calcium is very high, due to its large difference in acoustic impedance with other media, most of the ultrasound signal will be reflected at the edge of the calcium and will not get through the calcium. This is seen on the IVUS image as an "acoustic shadow". **A** An enlargement of the *top left* part of the IVUS cross section in (**B**). The borders of the external elastic membrane with the adventitia (*1*) and the border of the leading edge with the blood (*1*) is clearly visible due to changes in acoustic impedance

Table 2.3.1. Velocity of sound in air, water and various tissues

Medium	Density (kg/mm³)	Sound velocity (m/s)	Acoustic impedance (Ns/mm³)
Air	1.20	330	3.96 * 10^2
Water	1.00 * 10^3	1480	1.48 * 10^6
Blood	1.03 * 10^3	1570	1.62 * 10^6
Muscle	1.07 * 10^3	1585	1.70 * 10^6
Bone (calcium)	1.91 * 10^3	4080	7.79 * 10^6

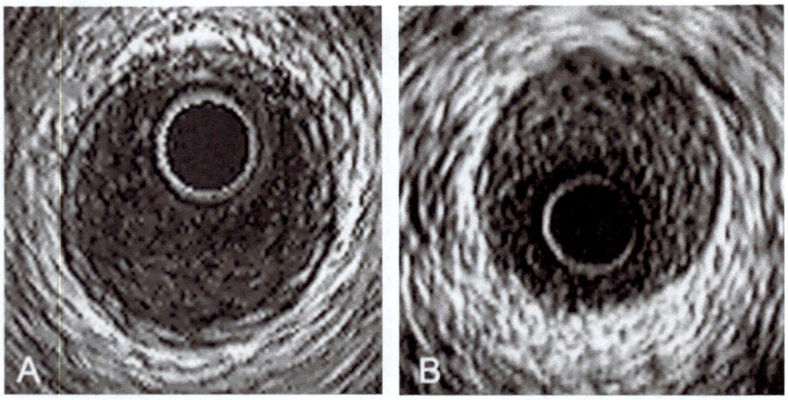

Fig. 2.3.11. A An IVUS cross section of a vessel with a normal intima visible due to an intimal thickness of approximately 0.25 mm. Note the thin echolucent media which appears as a *thin black line* between the intima and the adventitia. **B** The cross section in (**B**) shows an example of an intima with a thickness < 160 μm. It is not possible to determine the intima although the media is visible as a concentric thin black.

nation of the normal coronary wall of adult patients typically reveals a three-layered appearance (bright-dark-bright) corresponding to the components of three wall layers: the intima, the media and the adventitia, which possess a variable echogenicity (Fitzgerald et al. 1998; Potkin et al. 1990; Tobis et al. 1991; Lockwood et al. 1992; St. Goar et al. 1992; Fitzgerald et al. 1992) (Fig. 2.3.11a). The three-layered ultrasound appearance depends on two factors. First, the intima must be of sufficient thickness to be detectable by current ultrasound transducers; the threshold is around 160 μm. Second, there must be a sufficient acoustic interface between the media and the adventitia. It has been shown that there is a progressive increase in the thickness of the intimal layer with age (Nissen et al. 1995). The "normal" intima in "adult patients" is reported to have a maximal thickness of an average 0.15 ± 0.07 mm, and an upper limit of normal of 0.25–0.30 mm (i.e. 2 SD above "normal"). If the intima is thin or poorly reflective, the three-layered appearance is not seen and only a monolayered appearance is displayed (Fitzgerald et al. 1992) (Fig. 2.3.11b).

The media is apparent as a thin middle layer and typically is echolucent. The normal thickness of the media ranges from 125–350 μm (mean 200 μm). The external layer represents the adventitia and peri-adventitial tissues, principally composed of fibrous tissue ranging from 300–350 μm in thickness and exhibiting a characteristic "onion-skin" pattern (Fig. 2.3.12).

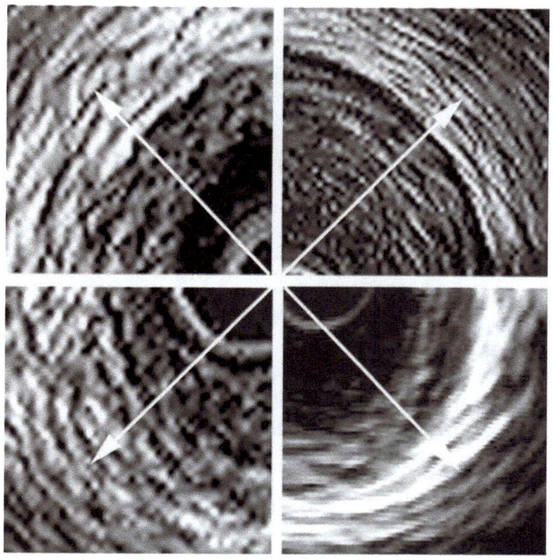

Fig. 2.3.12. Four different IVUS cross sections showing characteristic "onion skin" pattern of adventitia and peri-adventitial layers

2.3.4 Intracoronary Ultrasound of Coronary Atherosclerosis

Ultrasound provides unique insights into the composition of the coronary plaque in humans. Differences in acoustic properties of plaque components provide the capability to discriminate between several plaques types.

Coronary plaques are schematically classified into three categories: soft (echolucent), fibrous (echobright) or calcified (echobright with shadowing) according to plaque echogenicity (Hodgson et al. 1993; de Feyter et al. 1995). Plaques are soft if they are less echogenic than the surrounding adventitia. Comparative histologic studies have shown that these plaques consist either of loose fibrous tissue, lipid accumulations, or necrotic debris (Pasterkamp et al. 1995, 1996; Wong 1995; Ge et al. 1995; Hausmann et al. 1996; Kimura et al. 1996; Fuster and Lewis 1994; Schoenhagen et al. 2000) (Fig. 2.3.13).

Fibrous plaques exhibit an echodensity similar to that of the adventitia and correlative histology has shown that these plaques contain dense fibrous tissue (Tobis et al. 1991; Lockwood et al. 1992; de Feyter et al. 1995; Pasterkamp et al. 1996; Wong 1995; Ge et al. 1995; Hausmann et al. 1996; Kimura et al. 1996; Fuster and Lewis 1994; Schoenhagen et al. 2000; Gussenhoven et al. 1989; Bartorelli et al. 1992; Di Mario et al. 1992; Peter et al. 1994; Hiro et al. 1997) (Fig. 2.3.14).

Calcified plaques have similar or more echodensity than the adventitia but, because calcium does not allow transmission of the ultrasonic beam, there is acoustic shadowing of the deeper wall structures. The calcium may be distributed in the plaque in several ways: as a superficial rim at the luminal surface, as a deeper deposit at the intima-media border or as a concretion with a plaque (Nissen et al. 1995; Mintz et al. 1992; Friedrich et al. 1994) (Fig. 2.3.15).

Lipid depositions within a plaque are poorly echoreflective and may be suspected when an echolucent zone is clearly "visible" within an echoreflective plaque (Fig. 2.3.16).

However, with the current level of technology it is usually not possible to clearly discriminate lipid pools (de Feyter et al. 1995).

Measurements of coronary plaques are obtained from the two ultrasound interfaces: the leading intimal edge and the elastic external membrane (EEM) (see Table 2.3.2). By convention the media is included

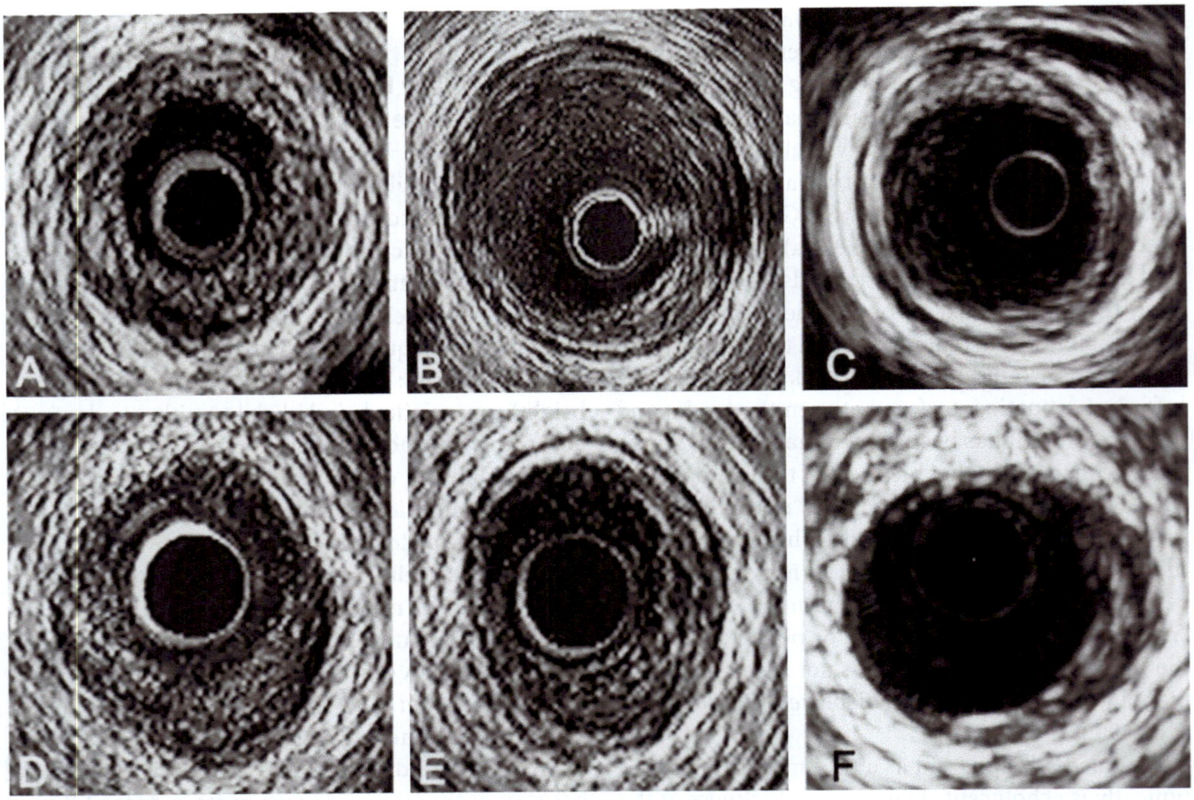

Fig. 2.3.13. A–F Different appearances of soft plaque. **A–C** Concentric soft plaque. **D–F** Eccentric soft plaque. Note how the soft plaque is always darker than the adventitia

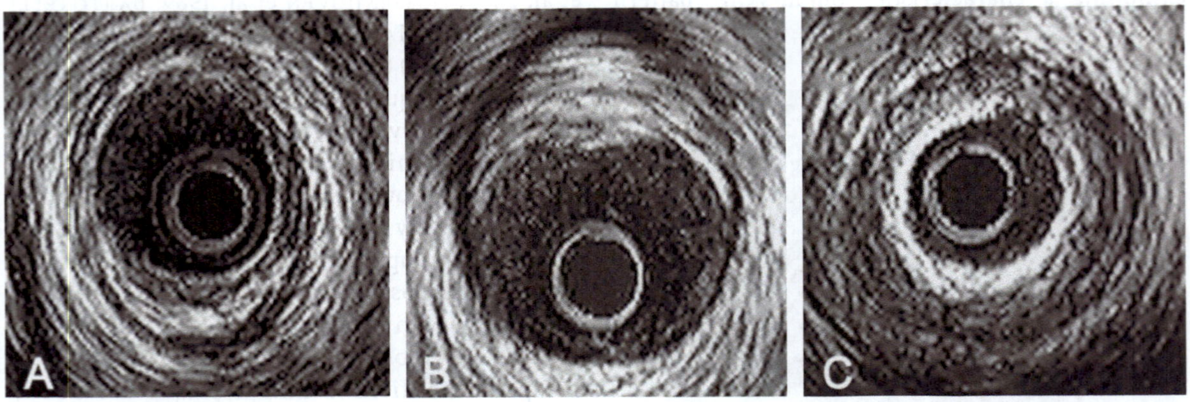

Fig. 2.3.14A–C. Examples of fibrous plaques, appearing as tissue with a density equal to the adventitia. **A** An IVUS cross section with an eccentric fibrous plaque from 3 to 8 o'clock. **B** An eccentric fibrous plaque from 9 to 3 o'clock with some calcification, determined by the acoustic shadow at 12 o'clock. **C** A concentric fibrous ring on top of a concentric soft plaque

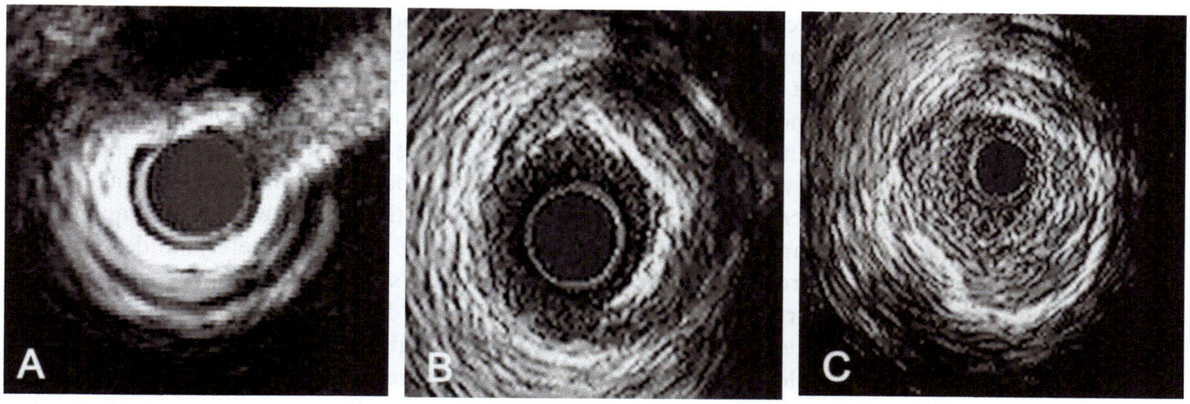

Fig. 2.3.15A,B. Calcium, due to its very high acoustic impedance compared with other tissue, returns most of the ultrasound signal, creating a bright reflex and acoustic shadowing. **A** An IVUS cross section with an almost 360° concentric superficial calcified plaque ("napkin ring") at the ostium of a right coronary artery. The aorta entrance is visible at 1 o'clock. **B** A 180° superficial calcified plaque from 12 to 6 o'clock. **C** 270° Deep calcium from 12 to 8 o'clock. Soft tissue is present on the calcium. Note the reverberation artefact at 1 o'clock

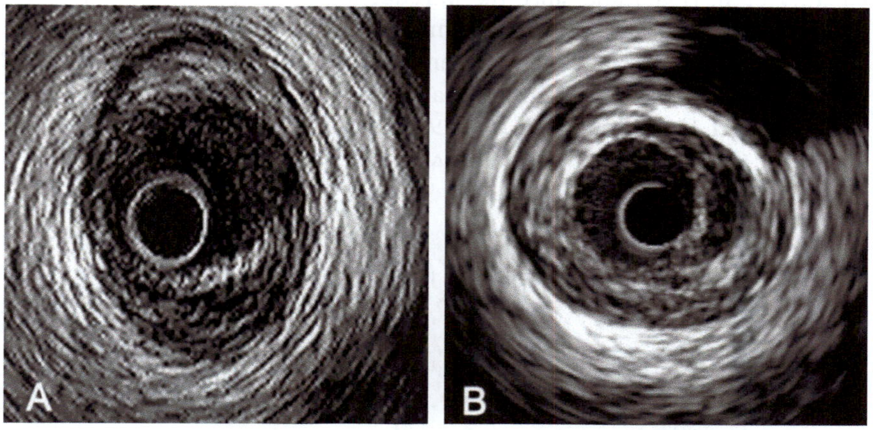

Fig. 2.3.16A,B. Two examples of suspect lipid deposits within a plaque. **A** A fibrous cap is visible from 4 to 8 o'clock, covering a small echolucent zone at 6 o'clock. **B** A cross-sectional image with a concentric mixed plaque. At 1 o'clock 45° of calcium is visible. From 12 to 5 o'clock a thin fibrous cap with an echolucent zone is visible

Table 2.3.2. Commonly used coronary ultrasound measurements as approved by both the European Society of Cardiology (Di Mario et al. 1998; Mintz et al. 2001)

Measurement	Units	Definition
Lumen area	mm^2	Area inside the intimal leading edge
EEM area (total vessel area)	mm^2	Area inside the leading edge of the adventitia
Stent area	mm^2	Area inside the stent struts
Plaque plus media area	mm^2	Difference between EEM area and lumen area in a corresponding cross section
In-stent neointimal area	mm^2	Difference between stent area and lumen area in images acquired late after stent deployment
Percentage plaque area	%	Percentage of EEM area occupied by plaque and calculated as: (EEM area – lumen area)/EEM area × 100
Percentage intimal volume in-stent	%	(Stent area – lumen area)/stent area × 100

EEM, external elastic membrane

into the plaque measurements because the media cannot always be distinguished as a sono-lucent layer, the trailing edge of the intima may be unsharp due to "blooming" of the ultrasound signal into the media, and the media is often "thinned" due the atherosclerotic process itself. Coronary atherosclerosis can be quantified in individual cross sections to provide area-measurements and three-dimensional reconstructed imaging obtained from a motorized IVUS pullback to provide volumetric measurement (Figs. 2.3.17 and 2.3.18). A significant limitation of quantification is the presence of calcium with its attendant shadowing which precludes detection of the outer border of the calcific plaque (Fig. 2.3.19).

Cross-sectional imaging of the coronary lumen and wall perfectly allow to investigate the complex interplay of plaque growth, lumen, lumen narrowing and vessel wall remodelling.

Vessel wall remodeling was initially described by Glagov et al. (1987) and since the introduction of IVUS into the clinical area this phenomenon has invariably been demonstrated to be present in all parts of the coronary tree (Fitzgerald et al. 1998; Pasterkamp et al. 1995; Hermiller et al. 1993; Losordo et al. 1994; Gerber et al. 1994; Nishioka et al. 1996).

Positive remodeling is the compensatory enlargement of the vessel wall associated with the accumulation of the plaque to maintain the "normal" cross-sectional area of the coronary lumen at the coronary plaque (Figs. 2.3.20, 2.3.21). This phenomenon occurs in particular in the earlier stages of the disease and is the reason why angiography (only visualizing the lumen) severely underestimates the extent and severity of coronary atherosclerosis (Topol and Nissen 1995). Indeed, ultrasound imaging of angiographically "normal" appearing coronary segments often demonstrates already diseased vessel wall in symptomatic high risk patients (Wong et al. 1995; Ge et al. 1995; Hausmann et al. 1996; Kimura et al. 1996; Mintz et al. 1995) (Fig. 2.3.22a–c).

At more advanced stages of the disease this compensatory enlargement falls short and lumen obstruction commences. IVUS studies have further increased our knowledge of remodeling of the coronary wall by demonstrating also the phenomenon of vessel negative remodeling of shrinkage, i.e. at diseased sites the total vessel area (EEM) actually decreases in size, contributing to the luminal obstruction (Pasterkamp et al. 1995) (Fig. 2.3.23).

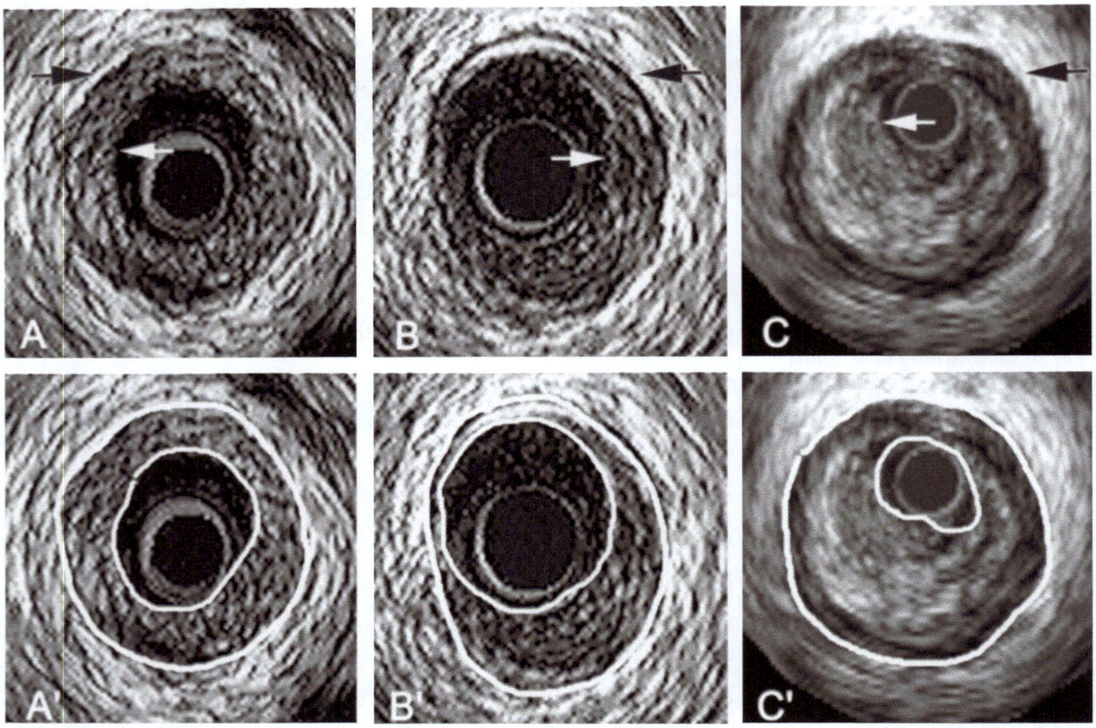

Fig. 2.3.17A–C. IVUS cross sections where the leading edges of the intima are indicated by *white arrows*, while the *black arrows* indicate the external elastic membrane. *Panels A', B' and C'* show the measuring lines of the lumen and total vessel. Note the thin media in *A'* and the unsharp trailing edge of the intima in *C'*

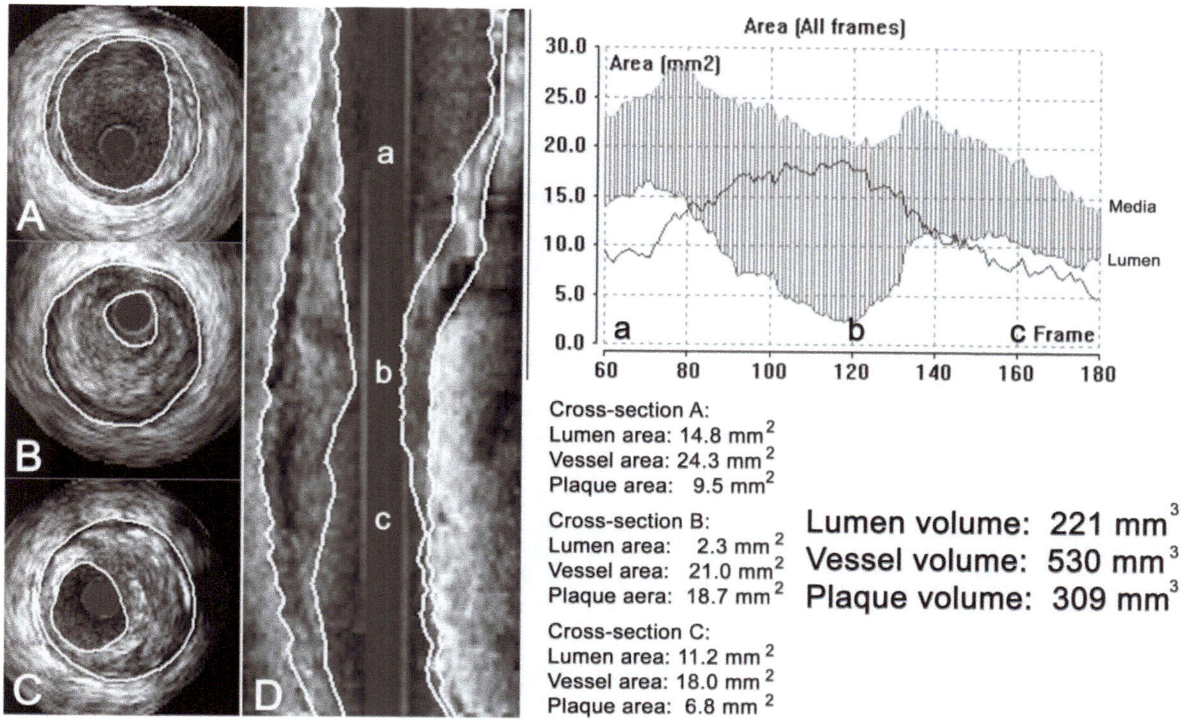

Fig. 2.3.18A–D. Example of a volumetric analysis of a vessel segment. The cross-sectional images were digitally grabbed during a motorized pullback through a vessel segment, creating a longitudinal reconstruction (**D**). After measuring the total vessel area (external elastic membrane) and lumen area of each cross-sectional image a graphic reproduction of the values can be made (*top right panel*) and the volumes of the lumen, total vessel and plaque can be calculated with the determined length of the analysed vessel segment. **B** The cross section with the minimal luminal area. **A,B** Distal and proximal locations, respectively, from cross section (**C**). The total vessel, luminal and plaque areas of these cross sections are given

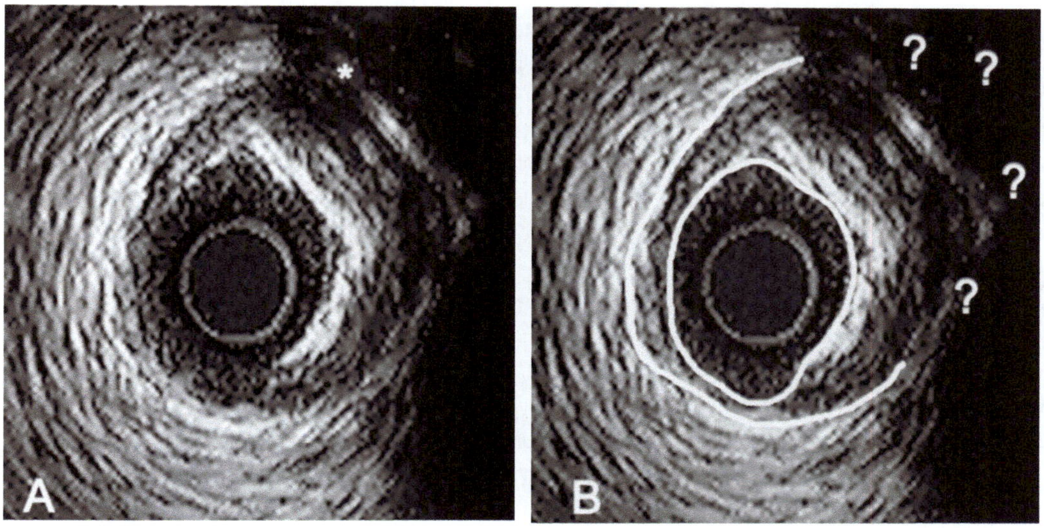

Fig. 2.3.19A,B. Calcium may be a limitation for measurements. **A** A cross-sectional image with an eccentric superficial calcified plaque from 12 to 6 o'clock. A reverberation artefact is visible at the *asterisk*, creating a double image of this plaque. The vessel lumen is easy to determine (**B**); however, it is not possible to measure a reliable total vessel area due to the presence of an almost 180° acoustic shadow at 3 o'clock

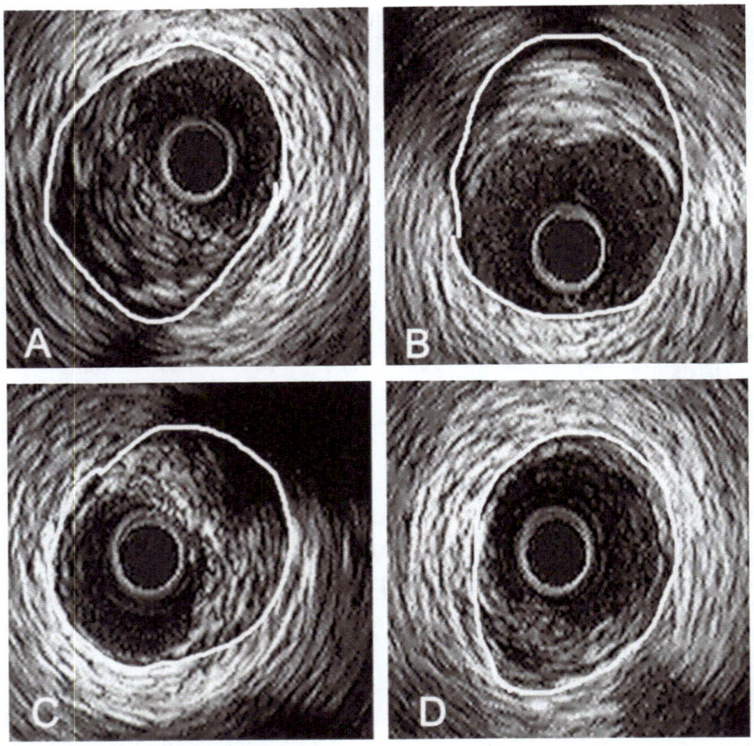

Fig. 2.3.20. A Compensatory enlargement by accumulating of the plaque to maintain a "normal" cross-sectional area. **A–D** Note the oval shape of the external elastic membrane, indicated by the *white line* in all images. The lumen remains more or less circular

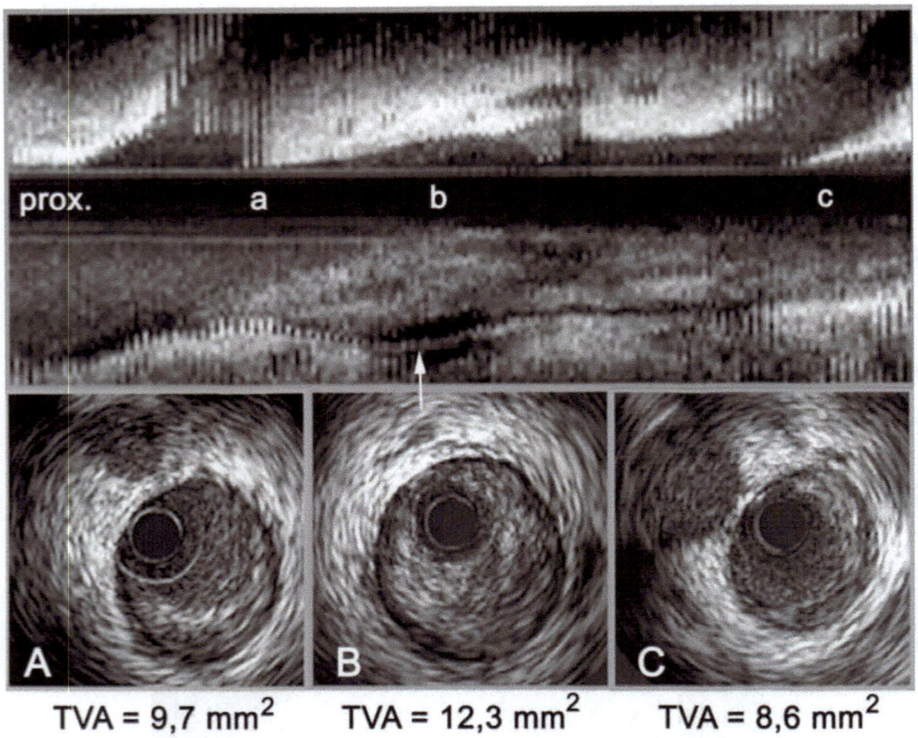

Fig. 2.3.21A–C. Positive remodelling in the proximal anterior descending artery. The *top panel* shows a longitudinal reconstruction. A long soft plaque is extending between *a* and *c* at the lower part of this reconstruction. The *arrow* points to an enlargement of the outer vessel wall, indicating positive remodelling. Cross sections **A–C** (located in the longitudinal reconstruction by the corresponding characters) show an eccentric soft plaque from 3 to 8 o'clock (**A**), an eccentric soft plaque from 12 to 10 o'clock with a small lumen (**B**) and an eccentric soft plaque from 12 to 6 o'clock (**C**), respectively. **C** The first diagonal branch at 11 o'clock. Proximal total vessel area (TVA) is 9.7 mm^2 (**A**). TVA at the stenosis is 12.3 mm^2 (**B**) and the distal TVA (**C**) is 8.6 mm^2. Note the larger TVA of (**B**) compared to the TVA at the proximal (**A**) indicating positive remodelling

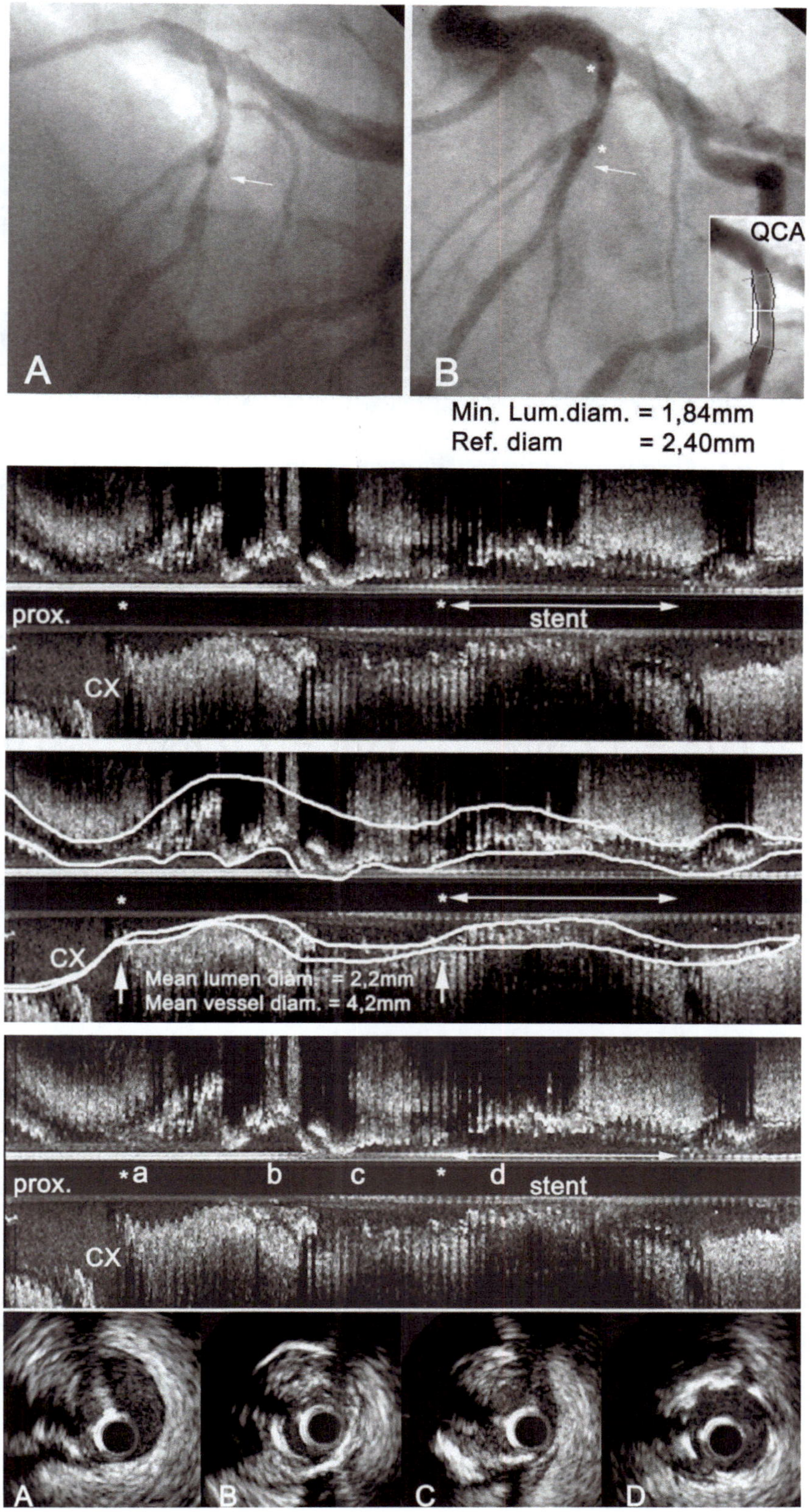

Fig. 2.3.22. A Left coronary angiogram in left superior oblique. *Panel A* shows a short lesion in the mid left anterior descending artery (LAD) (*arrow*). *Panel B* shows a good angiographic result post implantation of a 3.0×13 mm stent. The quantitative analyses of the proximal LAD (*insert*) shows a minimal luminal diameter of 1.85 mm with a reference vessel size of 2.4 mm (between *asterisks*). **B** Longitudinal reconstruction of an IVUS pullback in the same vessel described in (**A**), showing a diffusely diseased, calcified LAD. The *arrow* indicates the implanted stent. The *white lines* in the *bottom panel* indicate the lumen and vessel wall. The average diameters in the segment indicated by an *asterisk* are 2.2 mm for the lumen, matching the size measured by quantitative coronary arteriography (**A**) and 4.2 mm (!) for the total vessel diameter, indicating that angiography underestimated the extent and severity of the disease in this vessel segment. **C** The same longitudinal reconstruction as in (**B**), completed with the matching IVUS cross sections in *panels A–D*. The cross section in *panel A* is located in the proximal LAD. Two guidewires are visible at 9 and 11 o'clock. One guidewire was placed to protect the first diagonal branch, the second guidewire is to guide the IVUS catheter (Boston Scientific 40-Mhz Atlantis short monorail system). From 6 to 12 o'clock a mixed plaque is visible with a spot of superficial calcium at 7 o'clock. *Panel B* shows 20° of superficial calcium at 7 o'clock and from 9 till 1 o'clock deep calcium covered with soft material. *Panel C* shows eccentric mixed plaque from 6 to 1 o'clock. *Panel D* shows the implanted stent covering an eccentric calcified plaque. Note the small lumina in *panels B* and *C* indicating that very short narrowings can be missed by angiography

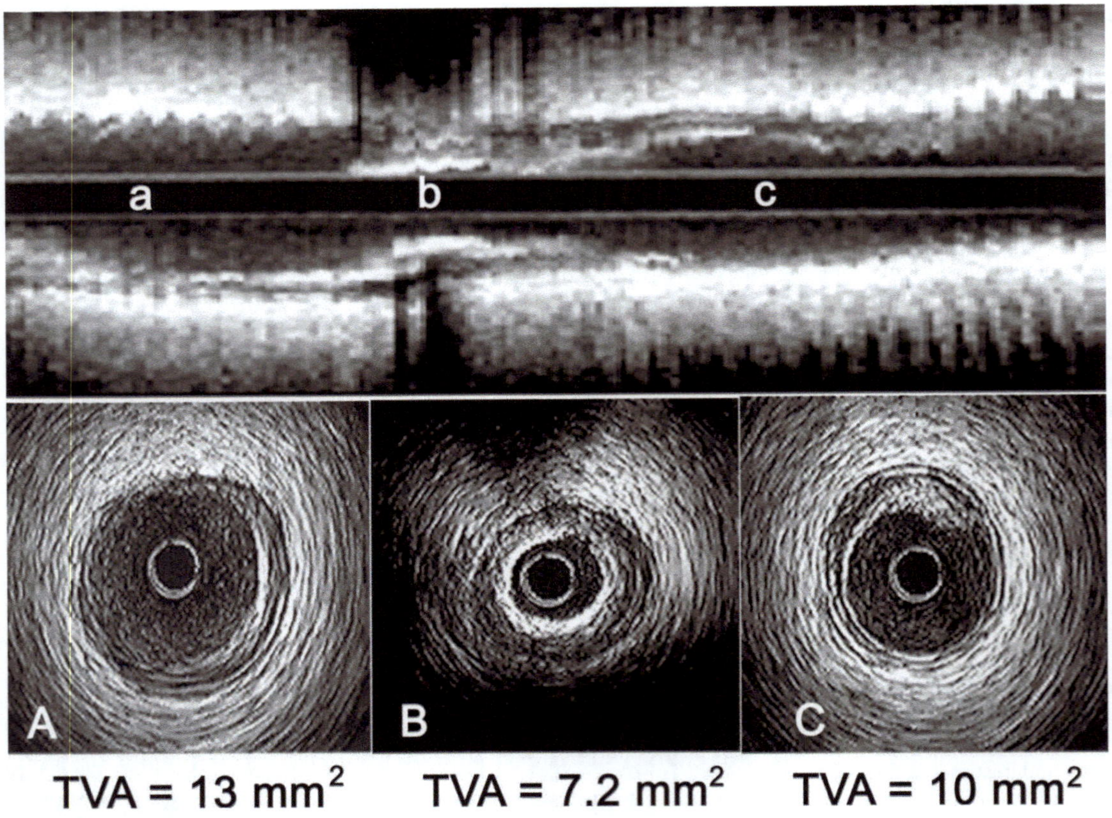

Fig. 2.3.23A–C. Negative remodelling or shrinkage of a diseased segment. The *top panel* shows a longitudinal reconstruction of an IVUS pullback. The location of the IVUS cross sections (**A, B** and **C**) in the reconstruction corresponds to *a*, *b* and *c*. **B** A concentric plaque with a fibrous ring. The total vessel area (TVA) at this point is 7.2 mm^2, while the distal reference segment (**C**) has a TVA of 10 mm^2 and the proximal reference segment has a TVA of 13 mm^2. The fact that the TVA of the diseased segment is smaller than the TVA of the distal reference segment indicates negative remodelling

2.3.5 IVUS and Vulnerable Plaque

The underlying pathology of acute coronary syndromes is plaque rupture or erosion with intracoronary thrombus formation, which may be either occlusive or subocclusive (Fuster and Lewis 1994). Vulnerable plaques are considered to be plaques prone to rupture. Vulnerable plaques have several morphologic and functional markers (see Table 3.2.3) (Fig. 3.2.4). A prominent lipid core is associated with echolucent zones on IVUS images; however, although this is nowadays considered as a lipid core one should keep in mind that this cannot be distinguished from thrombus, bleeding or necrotic tissue. Unfortunately a prominent feature of the vulnerable plaque is a thin and inflamed fibrous cap which cannot be detected by intracoronary ultrasound. Recently, it has been shown with IVUS that unstable plaques exhibit more positive remodeling than stable plaques (Schoenhagen et a. 2000).

Table 2.3.3. Morphologic and functional markers of vulnerable plaques and the role of intracoronary ultrasound.

Morphology	Intracoronary ultrasound
Eccentric, long lesions	+
Prominent lipid core	+ ?
Thin fibrous cap (< 60 µm)	–
Presence of inflammation	–
Remodelling (positive)	+

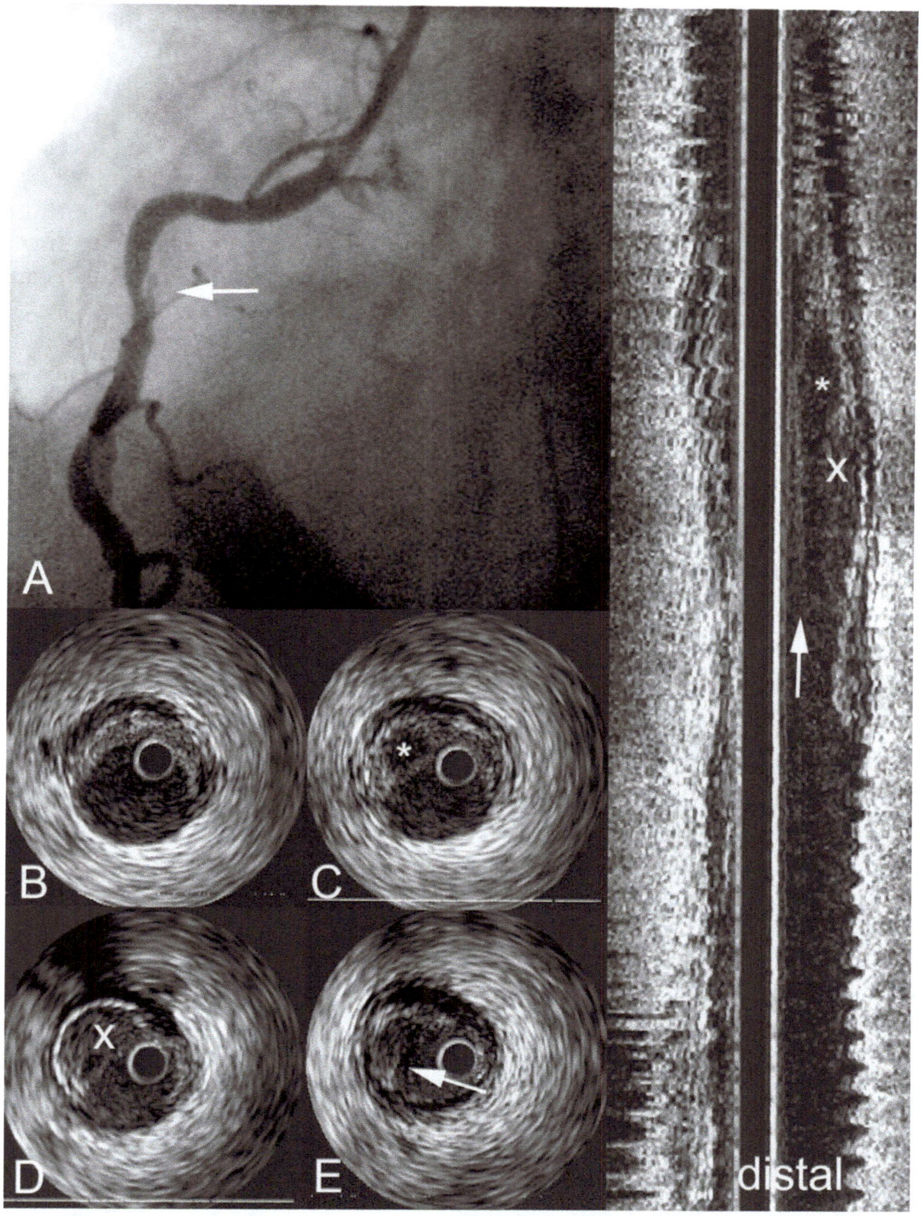

Fig. 2.3.24. A,B Ruptured plaque: Left anterior oblique angio of the right coronary artery shows an irregular shape of the lumen (*arrow*), the appearance fits with a dissection. IVUS shows a ruptured plaque. The "double lumen", indicated by an *asterisk* and *x*, is visible at cross sections (**C**) and (**D**) and at the longitudinal reconstruction. Cross section (**E**) shows the loose flap at the ruptured area (*arrow*). The *arrow* in the longitudinal reconstruction shows the loose flap

Improved radio frequency analysis, such as integrated back scatter analyses and attenuation slope mapping may distinguish between fibrous, necrotic or fatty plaque (Bridal et al. 1997) and using angle dependent echo intensity variation colour mapping it may be possible to more accurately determine the thickness of the fibrous cap (Hiro et al. 2001). Yamagishi et al. (2000) considered an echolucent eccentric plaque with remodelling as a dangerous plaque and they demonstrated that during follow-up of 2 years these plaques were more frequently associated with the occurrence of an acute coronary syndrome. Ruptured plaques can be recognized by ultrasound, but these features occur only infrequently (Kearney et al. 1996; Kotani et al. 2003).

2.3.6 IVUS for In-Stent Restenosis

The most widespread application of IVUS in interventional cardiology is in conjunction with coronary stenting. The metal struts of stents are intensely echoreflective and provide a distinctive ultrasound appearance (Fig. 2.2.25). It has been shown that in-stent thrombosis (early and late) (Fig. 2.3.26) or in-stent restenosis is often related to incomplete stent deployment, incomplete apposition or asymmetric expansion of the stent (Fig. 2.3.27) to the wall, all of which phenomena can be relatively easily detected by IVUS (Colombo et al. 1995). Although, according to these data, the usefulness of IVUS to guide stent-implantation may seem obvious, this could not be confirmed in a large randomized trial. The OPTICUS-trial (optimization with IVUS to reduce stent restenosis) randomized 550 patients to examine if IVUS-guided stent implantation would reduce in-stent restenosis. However, there was no difference between IVUS guided stent-implantation compared to angiographic guided stent-implantation (Mudra et al. 2001). Also, in-stent restenosis following implantation of drug-eluting stents is associated with gross stent underexpansion and a threshold of minimal luminal cross-sectional area within the stent of 4.0 mm^2 has been advocated to minimize or even prevent in-stent restenosis.

IVUS may be useful in case of in-stent restenosis which occurs after drug-eluting stent-implantation because it offers knowledge about underexpansion, hyperplasia, edge problems, incomplete lesion coverage, all of which may be helpful to select size and length of a new drug-eluting stent.

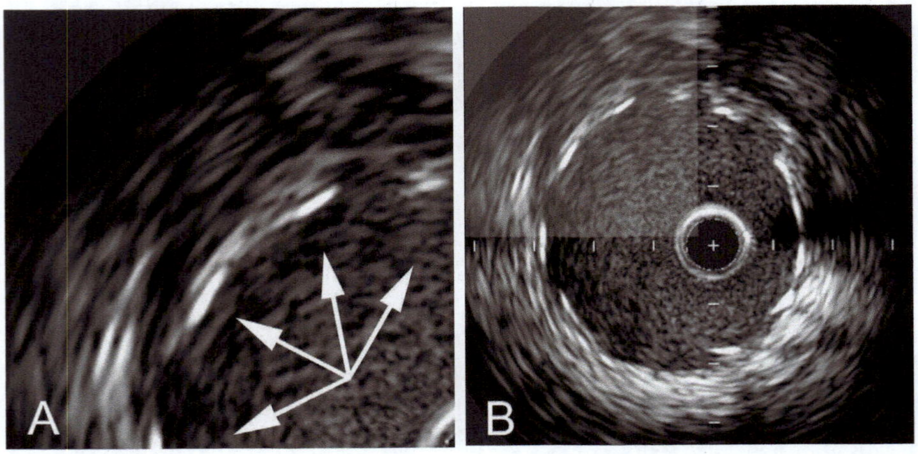

Fig. 2.3.25A,B. Distinctive appearance of stent struts. **A** Enlarged highlighted square as shown in the cross section of (**B**). The *arrows* indicate the echoreflective stent struts of a metal stent

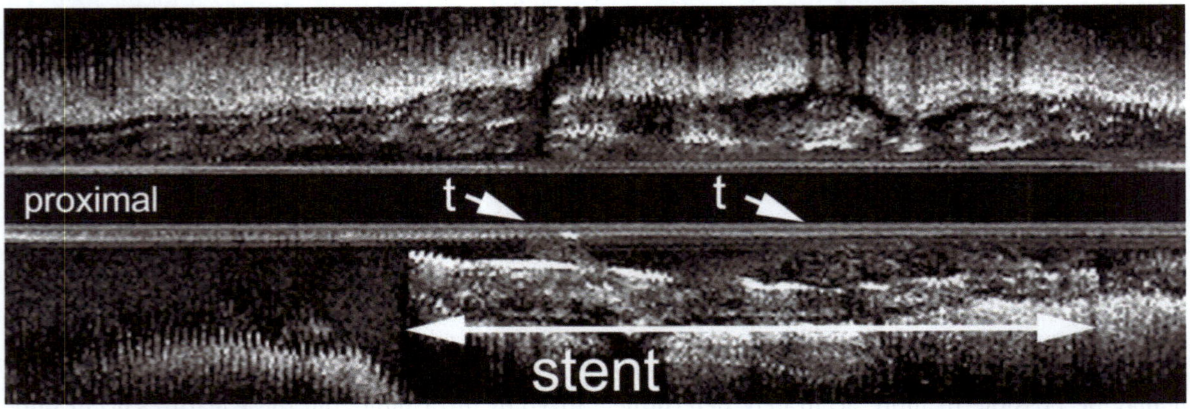

Fig. 2.3.26. Longitudinal IVUS reconstruction showing stent thrombosis in an underdeployed stent. Thrombus is indicated by the *arrowheads*

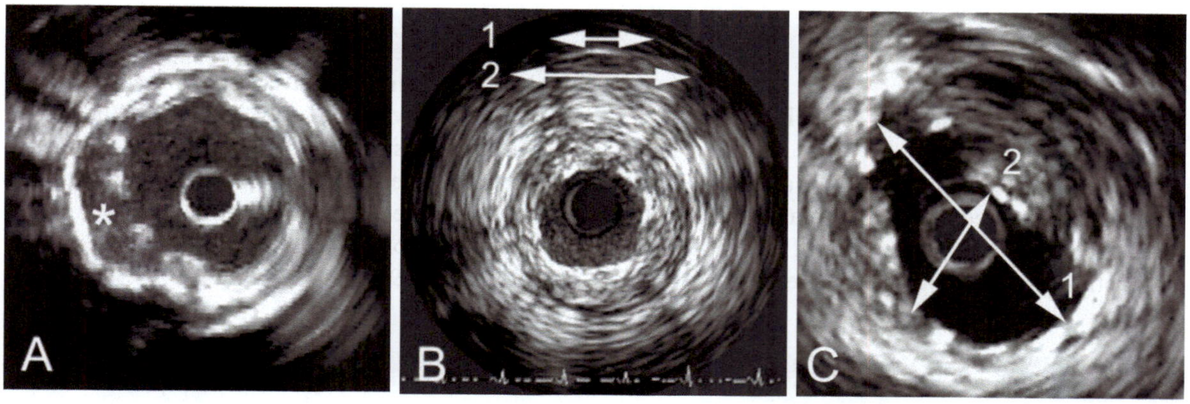

Fig. 2.3.27A–C. Three possible risks for in-stent thrombosis or in-stent restenosis. **A** Stent malapposition. The free space between the lumen wall and the stent is indicated by an *asterisk*. **B** An underdeployed, but well apposed stent. *Arrow 1* indicates the stent diameter (2.45 mm), *arrow 2* indicates the size of the vessel wall (4.1 mm). In this case the stent could be expanded to 3.5 mm. **C** An asymmetrically expanded stent. *Arrow 1* is the maximum stent diameter in this cross section (3.9 mm), *arrow 2* shows the minimum stent diameter (1.39 mm)

2.3.7 IVUS for Intermediate Lesions

It is sometimes difficult to determine from angiography whether a lesion is flow limiting and requires percutaneous coronary intervention. IVUS may then be useful and an intervention may be carried out if the lumen cross-sectional area is 4.0 mm^2 or less in the native coronary segments of the right coronary artery, left circumflex artery and left descending coronary artery (Abizaid et al. 1999) (Fig. 2.3.28). However, a threshold of <5.9 mm^2 (<2.8 mm diameter) is recommended for percutaneous treatment of the left main coronary artery (Jasti et al. 2004).

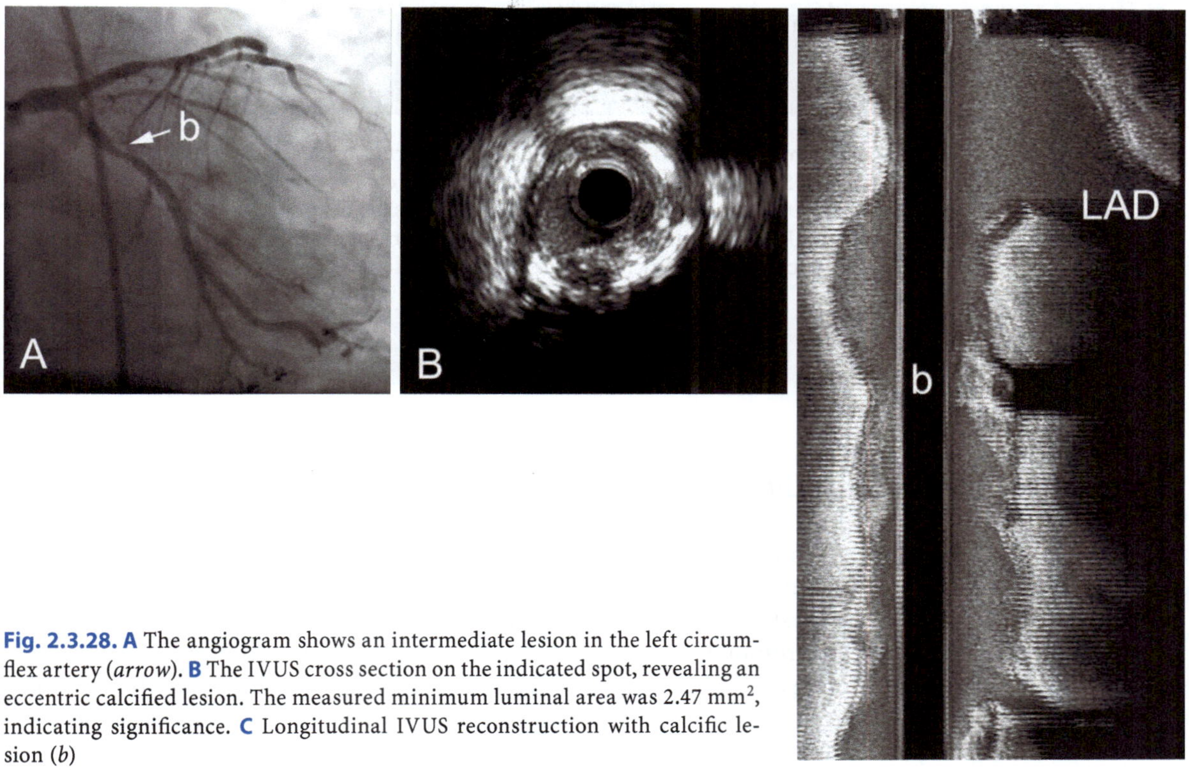

Fig. 2.3.28. A The angiogram shows an intermediate lesion in the left circumflex artery (*arrow*). **B** The IVUS cross section on the indicated spot, revealing an eccentric calcified lesion. The measured minimum luminal area was 2.47 mm^2, indicating significance. **C** Longitudinal IVUS reconstruction with calcific lesion (*b*)

2.3.8
IVUS and Transplant Coronary Artery Disease

Diagnostic angiography is the mainstay of diagnosis of accelerated vascular disease in transplant patients. But the diffuse nature of the disease significantly limits angiographic detection of the exact extent and severity of the disease and abnormal thickening of the intima is seen more frequently using IVUS (Pinto et al. 1994) (Fig. 2.3.29).

IVUS is well suited to documenting the presence of coronary atherosclerosis in young donor hearts. In one study the mean donor age was 32 years and the frequency of atherosclerotic lesions was 56% (Yeung et al. 1995).

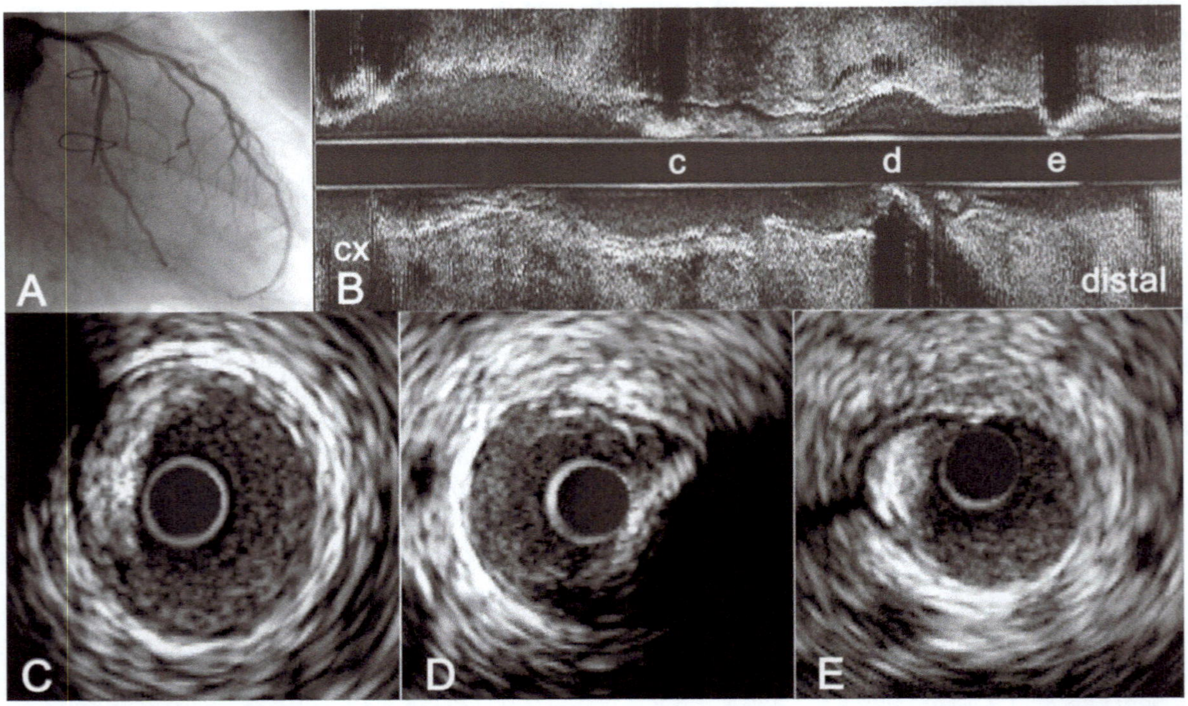

Fig. 2.3.29. A The left coronary angiography in RAO of a patient 14 days post heart transplant. The donor age was 38 years. The angiogram showed no disease. IVUS pullback through the left anterior descending artery (*LAD*), however, exhibited extensive disease, as shown in the longitudinal reconstruction (**B**). Disease is visible near *c* (mixed plaque), *d* (calcified) and *e* (calcified). The corresponding IVUS cross-sectional images show an eccentric fibro-calcific plaque (**C**, 9 o'clock), 90° superficial calcium (**D**, 3 o'clock) and eccentric fibro-calcific plaque with compensatory remodelling (**E**, 10 o'clock)

2.3.9
Limitations of Intracoronary Ultrasound

The safety of IVUS is well documented (Hausmann et al. 1995; Peters et al. 1997). Transient spasm due to catheter manipulation is the most frequently occurring complication which often responds rapidly to intracoronary nitroglycerin (Figs. 2.3.30, 2.3.31).

Occasionally a major complication (dissection or even vessel closure) may occur due to intracoronary ultrasound examination, usually in the setting of an interventional procedure during attempts to cross a severe obstruction. This is usually remedied by balloon angioplasty or stent implantation without the occurrence of adverse sequelae. There is no evidence that instrumentation with IVUS catheters leads to accelerated progression of coronary atheroma.

Intracoronary ultrasound has two distinct limitations that negatively affect image quality. First: non-uniform rotational distortion (NURD), caused by mechanical friction of the catheter drive shaft, may cause distortion of images which, in particular, may occur in tortuous calcified vessels. The image appears to be "circumferentially stretched" on one part of the wall, and it is compressed at the contra-lateral wall (Fig. 2.3.32). This image distortion occurs only with the mechanical device. Second: a transducer ring-down artefact, inherent to all ultrasound devices, which arises from acoustic oscillations in the piezo-electric transducer material adversely affects the "near field" of the image (Fig. 2.3.33a,b).

This makes "the acoustic size" of the transducer slightly larger than its physical size and creation of an image of structures immediately adjacent to the transducer is impossible.

Distortion of images may occur due to mal alignment of the catheter in the vessel, so that the normally round structure of the coronary vessel appears ellipsoid (Fig. 2.3.33c).

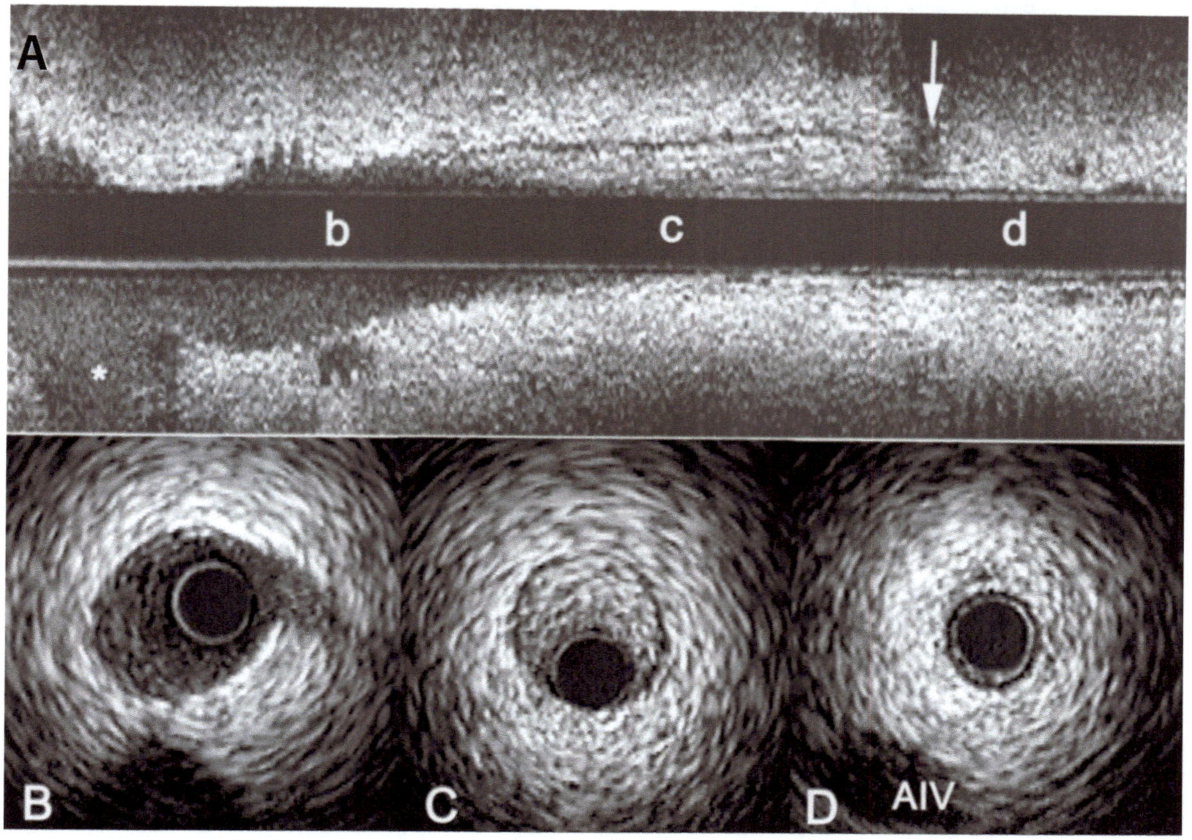

Fig. 2.3.30. A A longitudinal reconstruction of an IVUS pullback through a distal anterior descending artery. The *asterisk* indicates the second diagonal branch. **B–D** IVUS cross-sectional images located at *b*, *c* and *d* in the longitudinal reconstruction. The vessel itself is normal; however, in the distal left anterior descending artery there is an abrupt decrease in the size of the vessel wall (*arrow*). **D** The cross-sectional image of this area, with the vessel wall "crimped" around the IVUS catheter. Due to this spasm the IVUS catheter occludes the lumen, which causes an area of slow or non-moving blood proximal to this occlusion (**A**, (*c*) and **C**). **B** More proximal location, showing normal blood flow due to the presence of a side branch

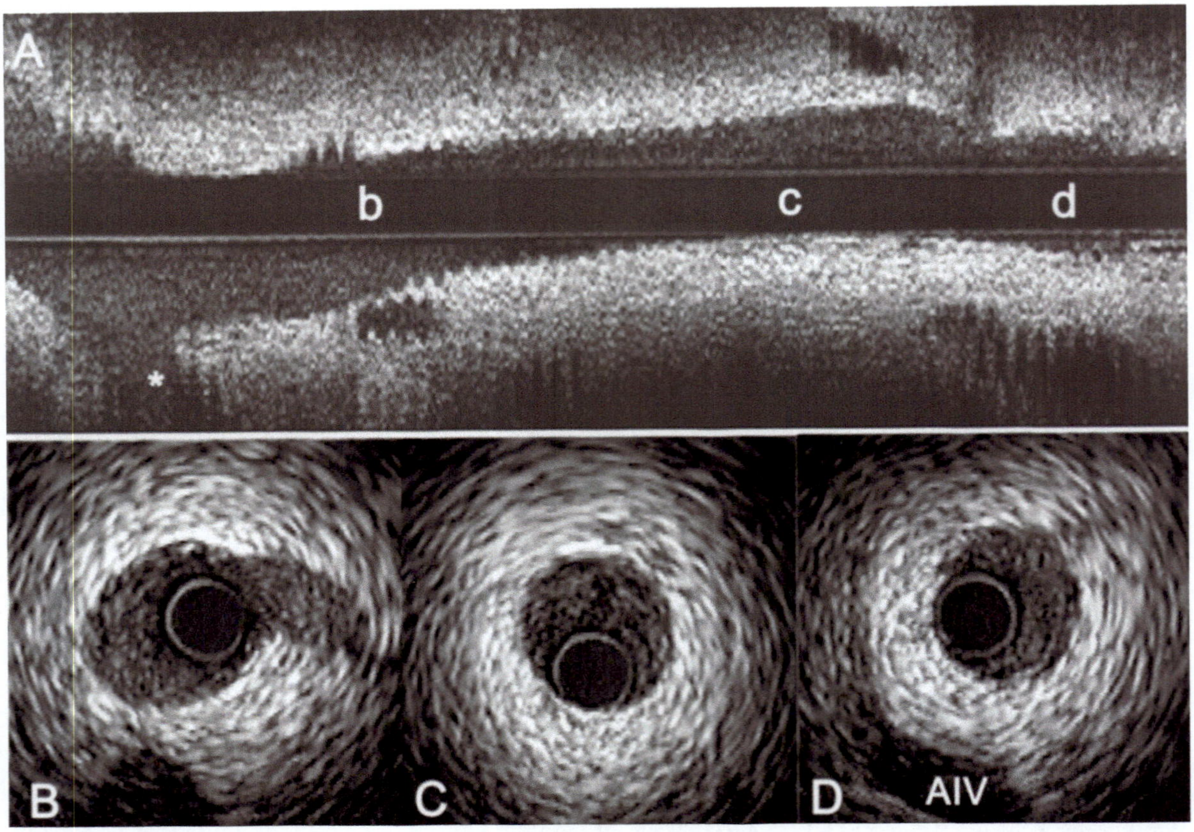

Fig. 2.3.31A–D. Identical figure to Fig.2.3.24 after the intracoronary admission of 3 mg of Isosorbine Dinitrate . The IVUS cross section in (**D**) shows the vessel wall after relaxation, allowing sufficient blood flow. [Compare (**C**) with Fig. 2.3.24]. The longitudinal reconstruction (**A**) shows a normal aspect of the lumen at location *c* compared to Fig. 2.3.24

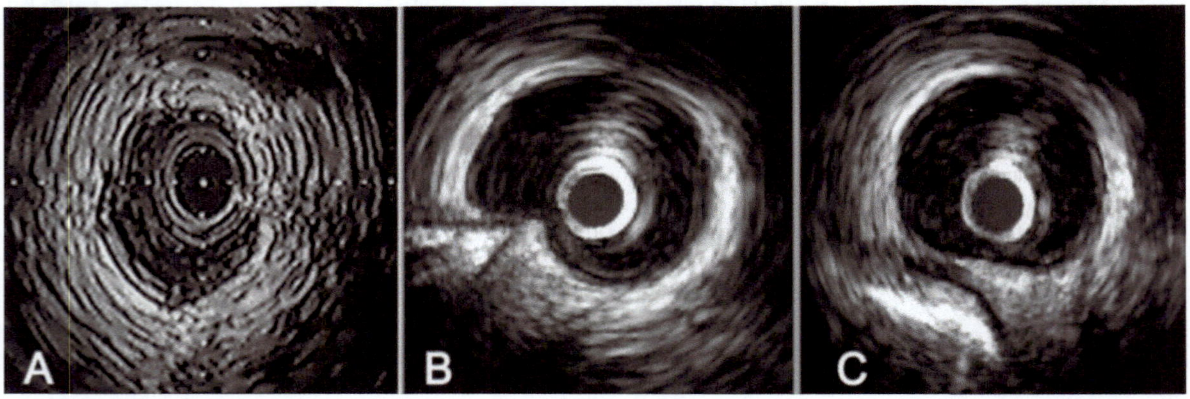

Fig. 2.3.32A–C. Non-uniform rotational distortion (NURD). The classic appearance of this distortion is visible in (**A**). A "smearing" effect is visible due to irregular (slower) rotation of the catheter from 6 to 3 o'clock. Another effect of NURD is visible in (**B**). The "arrow shaped" structure at 8 o'clock is the image of the epicardial line. At that point, due to the sudden release after some friction, the catheter abruptly accelerates in rotational speed (jump) for a short period. **C** The situation after resolution of the problem by stretching the catheter outside of the patient. The epicardial line can be recognized again at 7 o'clock

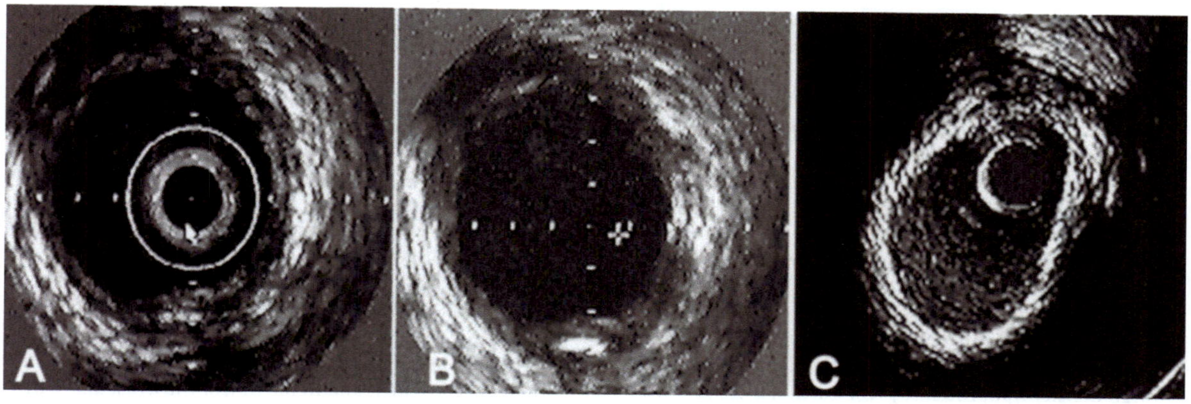

Fig. 2.3.33. A A typical ring-down artefact, caused by acoustic oscillations in the piezo-electric transducer. **B** The same image after hiding the ring-down artefact by means of digital subtraction. **C** The effect of misalignment of the IVUS catheter. This almost 360° calcified vessel appears ellipsoid instead of showing a normal round structure

2.3.10 Conclusion

IVUS has dramatically improved our understanding of coronary atherosclerosis and its response to therapeutic (pharmacological or mechanical) interventions.

IVUS is accurate in determining the dimensions of vessel wall structures, is able to crudely distinguish between tissue components and is uniquely suitable to assess vessel wall remodeling. Unfortunately, IVUS is not able to accurately identify vulnerable plaque.

Future developments in catheter miniaturization, image quality, tissue characterization and 3D reconstruction (Peters et al. 1997; Roelandt et al. 1994; Mintz et al. 2001), will further increase our insights into progression/regression of coronary atherosclerosis.

References

Abizaid AS, Mintz GS, Mehran R et al. (1999) Long-term follow-up after percutaneous transluminal coronary angioplasty was not performed based on intravascular ultrasound findings: importance of lumen dimensions. Circulation 100:256–261

Bartorelli AL, Neville RF, Keren G et al. (1992) In vitro and in vivo intravascular ultrasound imaging. Eur Heart J 13:102–108

Bridal SL, Fornes P, Bruneval P et al. (1997) Parametric (integrated backscatter and attenuation) images constructed using backscattered radio frequency signal (25–56 MHz) from human aortae in vitro. Ultrasound Med Biol 23:215–29

Colombo A, Hall P, Nakamura S et al. (1995) Intracoronary stenting without anticoagulation accomplished with intravascular ultrasound guidance. Circulation 91:1676–1688

de Feyter PJ, Ozaki Y, Baptista J et al. (1995) Ischemia-related lesion characteristics in patients with stable or unstable angina. A study with intracoronary angioscopy and ultrasound. Circulation 92:1408–1413

Di Mario C, The SH, Madretsma S et al. (1992) Detection and characterization of vascular lesions by intravascular ultrasound: an in vitro study correlated with histology. J Am Soc Echocardiogr 5:135–146

Di Mario C, Görge C, Peters R et al. (1998) Clinical application and image interpretation in intracoronary ultrasound. Study Group on Intracoronary Imaging of the Working Group of Coronary Circulation and of the Subgroup on Intravascular Ultrasound of the Working Group of Echocardiography of the European Society of Cardiology. Eur Heart J 19:207–229

Fitzgeral PJ, St Goar FG, Connolly AJ et al. (1992) Intravascular ultrasound imaging of coronary arteries. Is three layers the norm? Circulation 86:154–158

Fitzgerald PJ, Yock C, Yock PG (1998) Orientation of intracoronary ultrasonography: looking beyond the artery. J Am Soc Echocardiogr 11:13–19

Friedrich GJ, Moes NY, Mühlberger VA et al. (1994) Detection of intralesional calcium by intracoronary ultrasound depends on the histologic pattern. Am Heart J 128:435–441

Fuster V, Lewis A (1994) Conner Memorial Lecture. Mechanisms leading to myocardial infarction: insights from studies of vascular biology. Circulation 90:2126–2146

Ge J, Liu F, Görge G et al. (1995) Angiographically 'silent' plaque in the left main coronary artery detected by intravascular ultrasound. Coron Artery Dis 6:805–810

Gerber TC, Erbel R, Görge G et al. (1994) Extent of atherosclerosis and remodeling of the left main coronary artery determined by intravascular ultrasound. Am J Cardiol 73:666–671

Glagov S, Weisenberg E, Zarins CK et al. (1987) Compensatory enlargement of human atherosclerotic coronary arteries. N Engl J Med 316:1371–1375
Gussenhoven EJ, Essed CE, Lancee CT et al. (1989) Arterial wall characteristics determined by intravascular ultrasound imaging: an in vitro study. J Am Coll Cardiol 14:947–952
Hausmann D, Erbel R, Alibelli-Chemarin MJ et al. (1995) The safety of intracoronary ultrasound. A multicenter survey of 2207 examinations. Circulation 91:623–630
Hausmann D, Johnson JA, Sudhir K et al. (1996) Angiographically silent atherosclerosis detected by intravascular ultrasound in patients with familial hypercholesterolemia and familial combined hyperlipidemia: correlation with high density lipoproteins. J Am Cardiol 27:1562–1570
Hermiller JB, Tenaglia AN, Kisslo KB et al. (1993) In vivo validation of compensatory enlargement of atherosclerotic coronary arteries. Am J Cardiol 71:665–668
Hiro T, Leung CY, De Guzman S et al. (1997) Are soft echoes really soft? Intravascular ultrasound assessment of mechanical properties in human atherosclerotic tissue. Am Heart J 133:1–7
Hiro T, Fujii T, Yasumoto K et al. (2001) Detection of fibrous cap in atherosclerotic plaque by intravascular ultrasound by use of color mapping of angle-dependent echo-intensity variation. Circulation 103:1206–1211
Hodgson JM, Reddy KG, Suneja R et al. (1993) Intracoronary ultrasound imaging: correlation of plaque morphology with angiography, clinical syndrome and procedural results in patients undergoing coronary angioplasty. J Am Coll Cardiol 21:35–44
Hodgson JM, Graham SP, Savakus AD et al. (1989) Clinical percutaneous imaging of coronary anatomy using an over-the-wire ultrasound catheter system. Int J Card Imaging. 4:187–193
Jasti V, Ivan E, Yalamanchili V, Wongpraparut N, Leesar MA (2004) Correlations between fractional flow reserve and intravascular ultrasound in patients with an ambiguous left main coronary artery stenosis. Circulation 110:2831–2836
Kearney P, Erbel R, Rupprecht HJ et al. (1996) Differences in the morphology of unstable and stable coronary lesions and their impact on the mechanisms of angioplasty. An in vivo study with intravascular ultrasound. Eur Heart J 17:721–730
Kimura BJ, Russo RJ, Bhargava V et al. (1996) Atheroma morphology and distribution in proximal left anterior descending coronary artery: in vivo observations. J Am Coll Cardiol 27:825–831
Kotani J, Mintz GS, Castagna MT et al. (2003) Intravascular ultrasound analysis of infarct-related and non-infarct-related arteries in patients who presented with an acute myocardial infarction. Circulation 107:2889–2893
Lockwood GR, Ryan LK, Gotlieb AI et al. (1992) In vitro high resolution intravascular imaging in muscular and elastic arteries. J Am Coll Cardiol 20:153–160
Losordo DW, Rosenfield K, Kaufman J et al. (1994) Focal compensatory enlargement of human arteries in response to progressive atherosclerosis. In vivo documentation using intravascular ultrasound. Circulation 89:2570–2577
Mallery JA, Tobis JM, Griffith J et al. (1990) Assessment of normal and atherosclerotic arterial wall thickness with an intravascular ultrasound imaging catheter. Am Heart J 119:1392–1400
Mintz GS, Douek P, Pichard AD et al. (1992) Target lesion calcification in coronary artery disease: an intravascular ultrasound study. J Am Coll Cardiol 20:1149–1155
Mintz GS, Painter JA, Pichard AD et al. (1995) Atherosclerosis in angiographically "normal" coronary artery reference segments: an intravascular ultrasound study with clinical correlations. J Am Coll Cardiol 25:1479–1485
Mintz GS, Nissen SE, Anderson WD, Bailey SR, Erbel R, Fitzgerald PJ, Pinto FJ, Rosenfield K, Siegel RJ, Tuzcu EM, Yock PG (2001) American College of Cardiology Clinical Expert Consensus Document on Standards for Acquisition, Measurement and Reporting of Intravascular Ultrasound Studies (IVUS). A report of the American College of Cardiology Task Force on Clinical Expert Consensus Documents. J Am Coll Cardiol 37:1478–1492
Mudra H, di Mario C, de Jaegere P, Figulla HR, Macaya C, Zahn R, Wennerblom B, Rutsch W, Voudris V, Regar E, Henneke KH, Schachinger V, Zeiher A (2001) OPTICUS (OPTimization with ICUS to reduce stent restenosis) Study Investigators. Randomized comparison of coronary stent implantation under ultrasound or angiographic guidance to reduce stent restenosis (OPTICUS Study). Circulation 104:1343–1349
Nishioka T, Luo H, Eigler NL et al. (1996) Contribution of inadequate compensatory enlargement to development of human coronary artery stenosis: an in vivo intravascular ultrasound study. J Am Coll Cardiol 27:1571–1576
Nissen SE, Grines CL, Gurley JC, Sublett K, Haynie D, Diaz C, Booth DC, DeMaria AN (1990) Application of a new phased-array ultrasound imaging catheter in the assessment of vascular dimensions. In vivo comparison to cineangiography. Circulation 81:660–666
Nissen SE, De Franco AC, Tuzcu EM et al. (1995) Coronary intravascular ultrasound: diagnostic and interventional applications. Coron Artery Dis 6:355–367
Pandian NG, Kreis A, Brockway B et al. (1988) Ultrasound angioscopy: real-time, two-dimensional, intraluminal ultrasound imaging of blood vessels. Am J Cardiol 62:493–494
Pasterkamp G, Wensing PJ, Post MJ et al. (1995) Paradoxical arterial wall shrinkage may contribute to luminal narrowing of human atherosclerotic femoral arteries. Circulation 91:1444–1449
Pasterkamp G, Borst C, Post MJ et al. (1996) Atherosclerotic arterial remodeling in the superficial femoral artery. Individual variation in local compensatory enlargement response. Circulation 93:1818–1825
Peters RJ, Kok WE, Havenith MG et al. (1994) Histopathologic validation of intracoronary ultrasound imaging. J Am Soc Echocardiogr 7(3 Pt 1):230–241
Peters RJ, Kok WE, Di Mario C, Serruys PW, Bar FW, Pasterkamp G, Borst C, Kamp O, Bronzwaer JG, Visser CA, Piek JJ, Panday RN, Jaarsma W, Savalle L, Bom N (1997) Prediction of restenosis after coronary balloon angioplasty. Results of PICTURE (Post-IntraCoronary Treatment Ultrasound Result Evaluation), a prospective multicenter intracoronary ultrasound imaging study. Circulation 95:2254–2261
Pinto FJ, Chenzbraun A, Botas J et al. (1994) Feasibility of serial intracoronary ultrasound imaging for assessment of

progression of intimal proliferation in cardiac transplant recipients. Circulation 90:2348–255
Potkin BN, Bartorelli AL, Gessert JM, Neville RF, Almagor Y, Roberts WC, Leon MB (1990) Coronary artery imaging with intravascular high-frequency ultrasound. Circulation 81:1575–1585
Roelandt JR, di Mario C, Pandian NG et al. (1994) Three-dimensional reconstruction of intracoronary ultrasound images. Rationale, approaches, problems and directions. Circulation 90:1044–1055
Schoenhagen P, Ziada KM, Kapadia SR et al. (2000) Extent and direction of arterial remodeling in stable versus unstable coronary syndromes: an intravascular ultrasound study. Circulation 101:598–603
St. Goar FG, Pinto FJ, Alderman EL et al. (1992) Detection of coronary atherosclerosis in young adult hearts using intravascular ultrasound. Circulation 86:756–763
Tobis JM, Mallery J, Mahon D et al. (1991) Intravascular ultrasound imaging of human coronary arteries in vivo. Analysis of tissue characterizations with comparison to in vitro histological specimens. Circulation 83:913–926
Topol EJ, Nissen SE (1995) Our preoccupation with coronary luminology. The dissociation between clinical and angiographic findings in ischemic heart disease. Circulation 92:2333–2342
von Birgelen C, de Vrey EA, Mintz GS et al. (1997) ECG-gated three-dimensional intravascular ultrasound: feasibility and reproducibility of the automated analysis of coronary lumen and atherosclerotic plaque dimensions in humans. Circulation 96:2944–2952
Wong CB, Porter TR, Xie F et al. (1995) Segmental analysis of coronary arteries with equivalent plaque burden by intravascular ultrasound in patients with and without angiographically significant coronary artery disease. Am J Cardiol 76:598–601
Yamagishi M, Terashima M, Awano K, Kijima M, Nakatani S, Daikoku S, Ito K, Yasumura Y, Miyatake K (2000) Morphology of vulnerable coronary plaque: insights from follow-up of patients examined by intravascular ultrasound before an acute coronary syndrome. J Am Coll Cardiol. 35:106–111
Yeung AC, Davis SF, Hauptman PJ et al. (1995) Incidence and progression of transplant coronary artery disease over 1 year: results of a multicenter trial with use of intravascular ultrasound. Multicenter Intravascular Ultrasound Transplant Study Group. J. Heart Lung Transplant 14(6 Pt 2):S215–20
Yock PG, Johnsen EL, Linker DT (1988) Intravascular ultrasound: development and clinical potential. Am J Card Imaging 2:185–93

2.4 Quantitative Coronary Ultrasound (QCU)

Nico Bruining, Ronald Hamers, Sebastiaan de Winter, and Jos R. T. C. Roelandt

CONTENTS

2.4.1 Introduction

Why use three-dimensional (3D) reconstruction techniques for quantitative analysis of intracoronary ultrasound (ICUS) images? In clinical practice an ICUS catheter is used to examine and interrogate a segment of a coronary vessel by moving the catheter manually forwards and backwards. Since ICUS images show only very thin cross-sectional slices of the coronary vessel (lateral image width approximately 200 µm), it is difficult for the observer to mentally build up a 3D representation of the investigated segment. Digitization of a stack of two-dimensional (2D) cross-sectional images (e.g. a tomographic image data set) makes it possible to create a 3D reconstruction using the computer memory. From this 3D reconstruction several 2D cut-planes through the coronary vessel can be computed, also known as longitudinal views (L-views) (Rosenfield et al. 1991; Di Mario et al. 1995; Roelandt et al. 1994; von Birgelen et al. 1995a; Mintz et al. 1993). The role of ICUS for serial studies and quantitative measurements is well appreciated (Sousa et al. 2001; Nissen and Yock 2001; Slager et al. 2000; Takagi et al. 1999). An L-view also makes it easier to re-study and analyze segments in follow-up studies. Furthermore, measurements of the target area (lesion and stent lengths) are easily obtained from L-views.

2.4.2 ICUS Image Acquisition

The analysis of a coronary segment with ICUS requires a pullback with the ICUS catheter and faithful reconstruction. In recent years, several pullback systems have been developed:

- Manual pullback
- Manual pullback with the ICUS catheter shaft placed in a catheter displacement-sensing device (van Egmond et al. 1994).
- Motorized pullback by a constant speed velocity motor, applying a pullback speed of 1 or 0.5 mm/s^2.
- Motorized pullback at a constant speed of 0.5 mm/s in combination with an electrocardiogram (ECG) labelling device. This enables selection of only the end-diastolic cross-sections for subsequent analysis ("pseudo-gating") (von Birgelen et al. 1995b).

N. Bruining, PhD, FESC
S. de Winter, BSc
J. R. T. C. Roelandt, MD, Professor
Department of Cardiology (Thoraxcenter), Erasmus MC, Dr. Molewaterplein 40, 3015 GD Rotterdam, The Netherlands
R. Hamers, PhD
Department of Cardiology, Department of Radiology, Erasmus MC, Dr. Molewaterplein 40, 3015 GD Rotterdam, The Netherlands

These 3D systems are based on an image acquisition with a pullback device that withdraws the ICUS catheter at a constant speed (0.5 mm/s). However, artifacts and inaccurate measurements of the 3D reconstruction may result from the systolic-diastolic changes of the vascular dimensions, cardiac motion, the respiration and the cyclic axial and rotational movement of the catheter (Roelandt et al. 1994; Bruining et al. 1996). This problem can be solved by using an ECG-gated acquisition system of an ICUS study (Bruining et al. 1995).

- Motorised ECG-gated pullback using a stepping-motor and a dedicated workstation (Bruining et al. 1995, 1996, 1998, 1999; von Birgelen et al. 1997a,b).

Another method to perform gating is the recently developed image-based gating method at the Thoraxcenter called Intelligate.

- Image based retrospective selection of near end-diastolic generated ICUS frames from a non-gated data set (De Winter et al. 2004).

2.4.2.1 Interventional Laboratory "Hardware" Set-Up

In the interventional laboratory only an ICUS console is necessary to perform an ICUS examination. However, for an ECG-gated study an extra 3D workstation is needed (Fig. 2.4.1). Currently, there are two major ICUS ultrasound console and catheter manufacturers (CVIS, Sunnyvale, CA, USA) and VolcanoTherapeutics (Santa Clara, CA, USA). The CVIS catheters are 30- or 40-MHz mechanical rotating element systems. The VolcanoTherapeutics system is made of an electronic circular 20-MHz phased array transducer. Both manufacturers are delivering constant speed pullback devices with their ultrasound consoles.

We have developed a custom-made pullback device for ECG-gated studies at the Thoraxcenter, which is controlled by the EchoScan system of TomTec (TomTec GmbH, Unterschleissheim, Germany). The mechanical rotating element catheters have an external echo-transparent sheath with an independent imaging cable inside and are routinely used for ECG-gated studies. This design guarantees that a pullback over a defined distance in a coronary segment at the proximal end of the catheter results in an equivalent movement of the tip of the catheter. The pulses to activate the stepping motor are generated by the steering logic in the 3D workstation where the scan distance, longitudinal step resolution, ECG and, optionally, the respiration intervals can be set (Bruining et al. 1996; von Birgelen et al. 1997b,c).

2.4.2.2 Image Acquisition

Constant pullbacks: the non-ECG-gated pullbacks by the constant speed motorized devices at 0.5 mm/s require a time of 20 s per cm pullback. Although the images are mostly stored today on CD-ROM, there

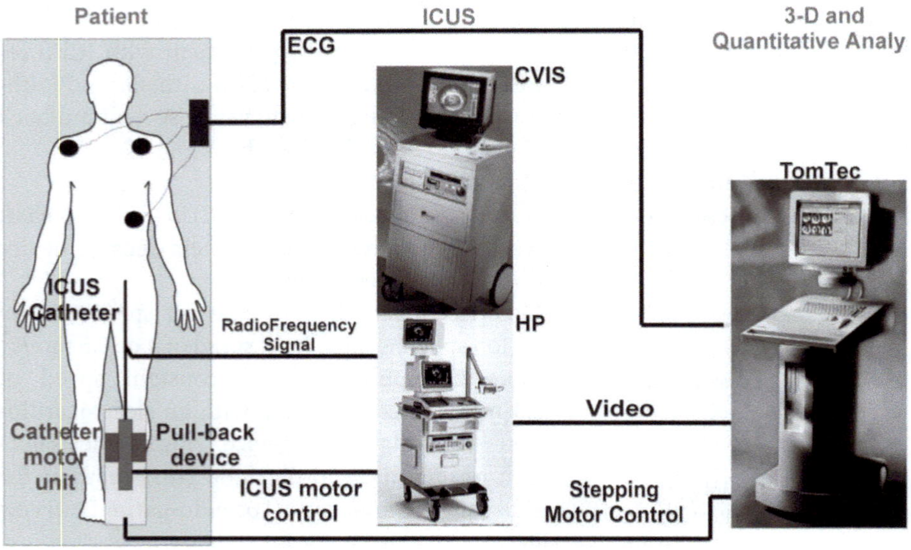

Fig. 2.4.1. The setup in an interventional laboratory. For an electrocardiogram (ECG)-gated acquisition a 3D image acquisition workstation (Echoscan, TomTec GmbH) is used (displayed at the right-hand side). This 3D reconstruction station receives and digitizes the analog video output of the ICUS console and the patient's ECG signal to control the stepping motor. The ICUS images are digitized on-line

may still be some systems which store the data on S-VHS videotape for off-line processing. However, the process of translating the digital video images to analog videotape and subsequently digitizing them again for off-line quantitative analysis deteriorates image quality.

Today, the latest generation ultrasound consoles are capable of building up an L-view in real-time for direct on-line analysis.

ECG-gated: the time to acquire longitudinal discrete intervals of 0.2 mm over 1 cm of axial vessel length is about 1 min. The ICUS images are digitized in real-time and are saved in a 4D (3D + time) tomographic data set (Fig. 2.4.1). The image resolution is 256 × 256 pixels with 8 bits per pixel, and a maximum of 25 images per R-R cycle is acquired. In practice it is possible to acquire almost every consecutive heartbeat. This results in a pullback time, at a heart rate of 70, of 70 × 0.2 mm = 14 mm/min.

2.4.3 Quantitative Analysis

The most simple way of performing cross-sectional and volumetric analysis is by analyzing a stack of 2D cross-sectional images (e.g. to draw the lumen, stent and vessel areas on the ICUS console), to note the outcome of the area measurement and to forward the videotape with 2 s, assuming the catheter was pulled back over 2 s × 0.5 mm/s = 1 mm. Accumulating all the found areas for a final calculation of volumetric parameters gives:

$$V = \sum_{i=1}^{n} iA \times H$$

where V = volume; A = area of EEM boundary, lumen or stent in a given cross-sectional ultrasound image; H = the thickness of the coronary artery slice that is represented by this digitized cross-sectional ICUS image; and n = the number of digitized cross-sectional images encompassing the volume to be measured.

Other more sophisticated approaches use dedicated computer-assisted software packages for quantitative analysis. Videotape-stored studies needs to be digitized applying a computer equipped with a frame grabber before they can be analyzed. There are only a few commercial software packages available to help identify the lumen, stent and external elastic membrane (EEM) boundary contours. This process is known as image segmentation and is mostly done in a or semi-automatic fashion. The software packages are based on a mix of 2D contour detection in the L-views and in the cross-sectional slices.

However, analyzing in the L-views of non-gated ICUS data sets is difficult, not to say impossible. The catheter displacement during the cardiac cycle causes a saw-tooth shape appearance of the coronary vessel wall (Fig. 2.4.2b). This also prohibits ac-

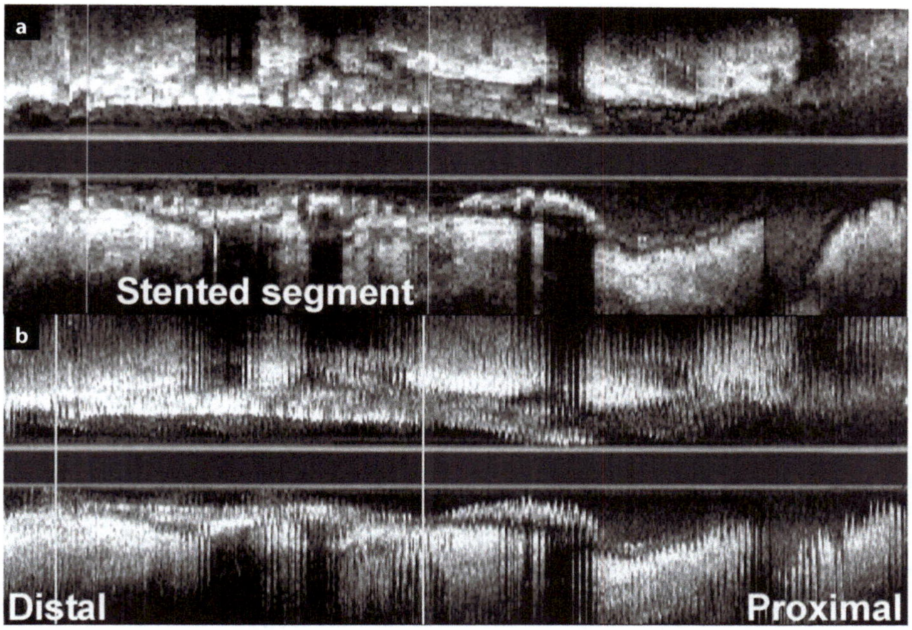

Fig. 2.4.2. a A longitudinal (L-view) reconstructed from an electrocardiogram (ECG)-gated data set is presented. **b** The longitudinal reconstruction of the same segment is presented, but obtained with a non-ECG-gated image acquisition. This results in a saw-tooth shape appearance of the vessel wall. This makes it difficult, or even impossible, to perform an automated detection in these L-views

curate automatic contour detection in the L-views, which is a pity, since all the individual cross-sections must now be analyzed individually. This can be a very time-consuming process, since thousands of frames can be present in a pullback since 30 frames per second are generated. A gating method, on-line hardware gated (Bruining et al. 1998) or off-line retrospectively gated, can solve this problem (De Winter et al. 2004).

Contour detection: The QCU approach developed at the Thoraxcenter by Li et al. (1994) and von Birgelen et al. (1996, 1997d) is based on a two-step analysis approach, and modified versions are now commonly used. After loading the images in the computer memory, two perpendicular L-views of the coronary vessel are displayed (Fig. 2.4.3). With help of a semi-automated lumen and EEM contour detection algorithm, the observer must identify and indicate the lumen and EEM boundaries in these two L-views. The second step is the detection of the lumen and EEM boundaries in each individual cross section, for which the minimum-cost algorithm is applied. The contours are forced to go through the four-contour points, which were transposed from the L-views on the individual cross sections. After automated detection, the observer can inspect all individual cross sections and is able to manually correct them in case the automated contour detection was imprecise. This package makes it possible to analyze up to a maximum of 200 individual cross-sectional images.

2.4.3.1 QCU Developments

Developments of quantitative software addressing new clinical needs are currently underway at a small number of companies and a few research institutes. We developed and validated a new quantitative software package at the Thoraxcenter in collaboration with CURAD (Curad B.V., Wijk bij Duurstede, Netherlands) (Fig. 2.4.4). The set-up of the analysis process differs from earlier described methods. The basic idea behind most QCU programs is to manually trace, or to use semi-automatic software to detect, areas in a stack of 2D cross-sectional ICUS images, with or without an L-view as a reference. Thus different contours of corresponding structures must be traced, or corrected, in many frames resulting in a time-consuming procedure. In order to be more efficient, our novel approach exploits a semi-automatic contour tracing method in several reconstructed L-view displays. The L-view images augment the feasibility to recognize relevant tissue structures,

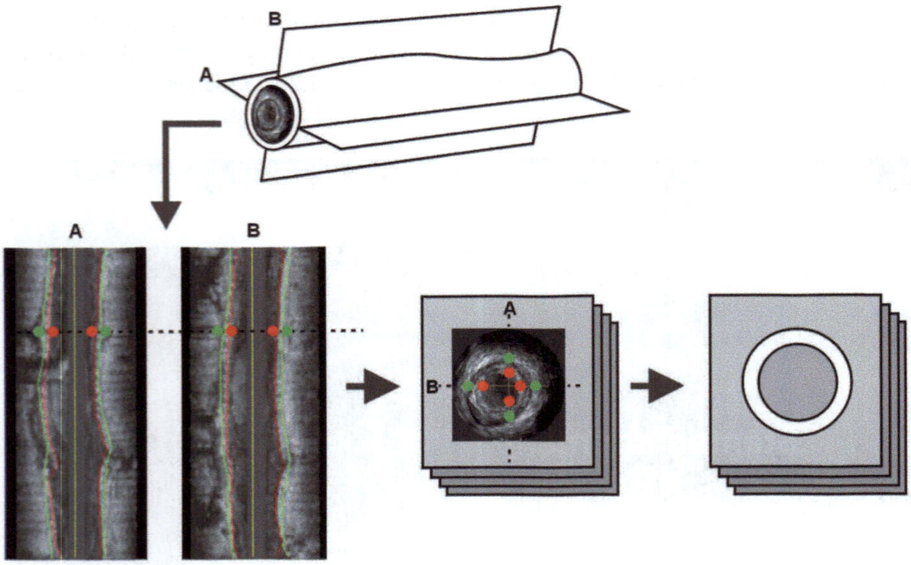

Fig. 2.4.3. Contour detection by Li. et al. (1994). From the tomographic image data set (*top*), two reconstructed longitudinal views are created (*left*). The intima leading edge and the external elastic contour of the vessel are interactively detected in these planes (minimum-cost algorithm). The contour information, using the four-edge points derived from the longitudinal contours (*A* and *B*) is used to guide detection in the individual cross sections (*right*). Contour detection is then performed in the individual cross-sectional images. The result of this automated contour detection can be checked and corrected by the observer

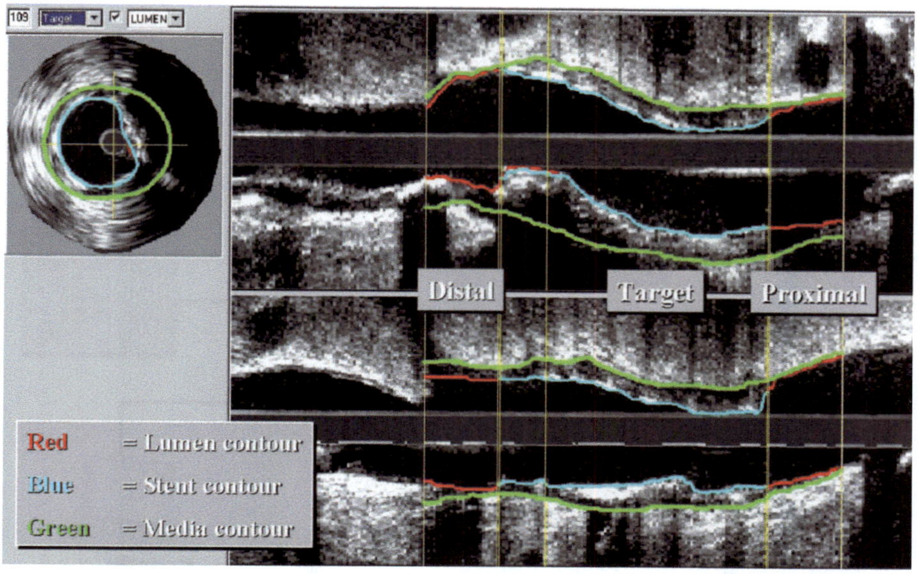

Fig. 2.4.4. This is a screenshot of the new quantitative coronary ultrasound program. The investigated coronary segment can be divided in multiple parts to make later statistical analysis more convenient. Here the segment is divided into a distal, target and proximal part. The contour detection in the cross-sectional images can be checked in the panel at the *top left side*. However, the idea is not to make changes in these individual 2D cross-sectional images, but only in the longitudinal reconstructed images (called L-views)

especially when an ECG-gated acquisition is used. For non-gated data, the method allows the use of data sets consisting of many frames (> 1000), which enhances structure recognition (due to a higher temporal resolution) and minimizes the discontinuities caused by catheter motion, without prolonging analysis time. The edge-detection method uses a digital filter that reduces noise and enhances true boundaries. The identified contour points are subsequently mapped to the individual 2D images, serving as control points for a fitted analytical spline representation of contours in the 2D images. For each structure, quantities of interest, such as 2D areas, are calculated from the mathematical contour description (Fig. 2.4.4). Although as many as 72 L-views can be used, the optimal performance in terms of accuracy and analysis time has been reached by tracing eight to nine contour lines in four to five L-views. 2D images are displayed simultaneously to help navigate through the data set and inspect the results, and are not used for correction in the 2D cross-sectional contours. This software package translates both videotaped and digitally acquired images (such as the ECG-gated sets) to images complying with the DICOM medical image standard (Fig. 2.4.5). The image data set is stored on an ICUS image server connected to the hospital network, which incorporates a database containing the quantitative results. On quantitative workstations throughout the Thoraxcenter, the QCU software can import these data sets for further analysis. Results with this software package did not show loss in accuracy and the speed of analysis is greatly improved. A time of less than 20 min to complete an analysis of an ECG-gated data set was found, independent of the total of individual cross sections included.

As already pointed out, the non-ECG-gated pullback can suffer from artifacts resulting in inaccurate measurements (Bruining et al. 1996, 1998; von Birgelen et al. 1997a,b). The motion of the catheter with respect to its longitudinal position to the coronary vessel (the z-axis) results in typical saw-tooth (or parabolic) shaped appearances of the coronary vessel wall in L-views. This makes it difficult to develop a robust contour-detecting algorithm. In Figure 2.4.2, the differences in L-view appearance of both acquisition methods (gated and non-gated) are presented. The methodology applied for contour detection is similar to the non-gated approach. The use of ECG-gated ICUS image data sets is thus of particular interest when potentially small volumetric changes, such as those expected in progression-

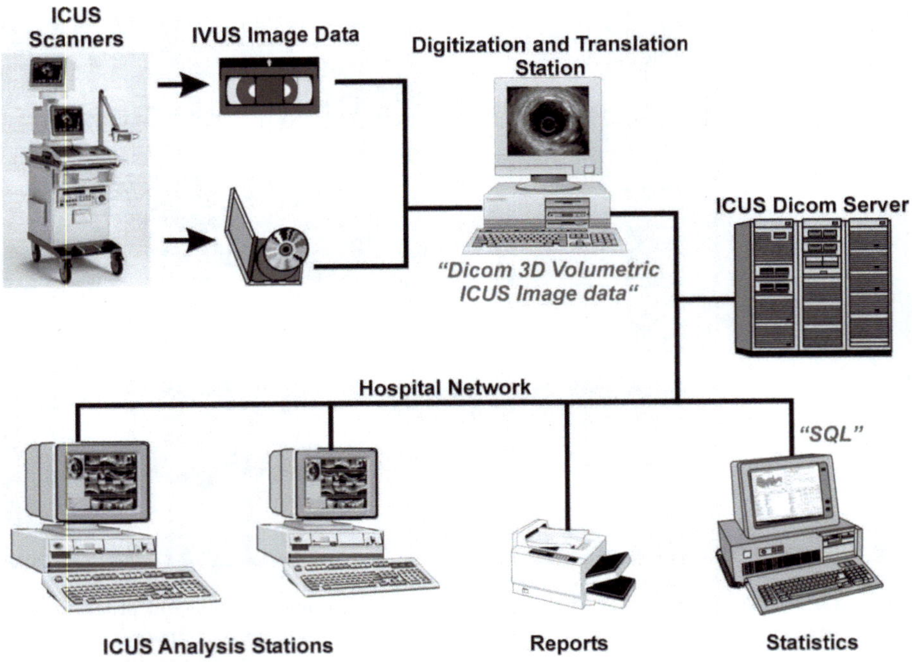

Fig. 2.4.5. This is a schematic overview of our intracoronary ultrasound (ICUS) image data flow. The pullback information is either delivered digitized by the ICUS console itself or digitized later by a workstation from S-VHS videotape. Both image modalities are translated into the DICOM image standard and are stored on an ICUS DICOM server connected to the hospital network. Analysis stations can retrieve the data from this server for further quantitative coronary ultrasound analysis. Statistics can be performed by retrieving numerical data via the standard query language (SQL)

regression studies of atherosclerosis, are being investigated. In addition to the display of the smooth appearance of the EEM boundary being closer to reality, there is a significantly reduced analysis time. It was demonstrated that there is improved accuracy in quantitative results (von Birgelen 1997a,b; Bruining et al. 1998).

Currently there are four QCU soft- and hardware packages commercially available:

- Indec, for add-on equipment for "on-line" analysis of non-ECG-gated data sets plus QCU software for off-line analysis. The add-on equipment can be of interest for institutes not wanting to buy a complete new ICUS console but wishing to refurbish their existing equipment. The system shows an on-line non-ECG-gated L-view, for analysis in the cathlab, and can store analyzed data digitally. However, the method is based on analysis of a stack of 2D images and is not a true 3D based system.
- Medis (Medis, Leiden, The Netherlands) for off-line analysis.
- Tomtec, a 3D workstation for acquisition and on- and off-line analysis of ECG-gated data sets.
- CURAD (Pie Medical Imaging BV, Maastricht, Netherlands), the described CURAD/Thoraxcenter approach.

2.4.4 Limitations

Potential pitfalls in the described QCU software packages are:

- Curvatures of the coronary segment are not taken into account and an artificially straightened L-view is produced. In a curve of the vessel the ICUS slices are no longer parallel to each other due to the fact that the catheter is no longer perpendicular to the vessel wall. This results in a distortion of the volumetric analysis since volume segments at the inner side of the vessel, related to its curvature, will be overestimated and fragments at the outer side underestimated. However, the resulting error seems to be rather small (Schuurbiers et al. 2000). Visualization of the true curvature of the coronary artery segment can only be accomplished by combining bi-plane angiography with the 3D ICUS image data sets (Slager et al. 2000).

- ECG-gated acquisition time takes longer when compared to constant velocity pullbacks.
- In still ICUS frames it is sometimes difficult to determine the exact luminal border, especially when there is an area of slow blood flow and presence of echolucent tissue. A rule in software engineering is that if one is not able to identify a contour by eye, it is not possible to develop a software algorithm for it. This requires that experienced observers still correct for flaws in the automated software detectors. Therefore, most QCU programs are called semi-automated.
- It is not possible to look behind a calcified area of the vessel and thus see and detect the EEM boundary with ICUS; interpolation of the EEM contour is necessary in this situation.
- Due to the nature of the ultrasound beam and its interaction with the struts of stents, they have a very bright (e.g. blooming) appearance on the ICUS images. For this reason it can be difficult to precisely determine the correct stent contours. An eccentric catheter position can also cause false strut image appearances.

2.4.5 Future Developments

The industry is constantly working to improve their catheters (higher frequencies, > 40 MHz), ultrasound consoles (digital imaging, storage and image transfer, on-line analysis), add-on equipment (improved and smaller pullback devices) and software for imaging, image acquisition, analysis and 3D reconstruction. Disadvantages, such as occluding the vessel by means of the catheter, could be prevented by using an imaging guide-wire or a forward scanning catheter (Evans et al. 1994; Ng et al. 1994; Degewa et al. 2001). In this case the site of the stenosis is not occluded during an acquisition. Further improvements could be found in improved on-line quantification and incorporation of ECG-gating functionality in the ultrasound consoles.

2.4.6 Conclusion

Quantitative ICUS is an important analysis tool for the assessment of coronary vessels being treated with new pharmaceutical agents or interventional techniques. The feasibility of ECG-gating, hard- and/or software based, makes it possible to obtain high-quality image data sets with smooth contours suitable for accurate quantitative analysis.

References

Bruining N, von Birgelen C, Di Mario C et al. (1995) Dynamic three-dimensional reconstruction of ICUS images based on an ecg-gated pull-back device. Paper presented at: Computers In Cardiology, Vienna

Bruining N, von Birgelen C, Mallus MT et al. (1996) ECG-gated ICUS image acquisition combined with a semi-automated contour detection provides accurate analysis of vessel dimensions. Paper presented at: Computers In Cardiology, Indianapolis

Bruining N, von Birgelen C, de Feyter PJ et al. (1998) ECG-gated versus nongated three-dimensional intracoronary ultrasound analysis: implications for volumetric measurements. Cathet Cardiovasc Diagn 43:254–260

Bruining N, Sabate M, de Feyter PJ et al. (1999) Quantitative measurements of in-stent restenosis: a comparison between quantitative coronary ultrasound and quantitative coronary angiography. Catheter Cardiovasc Interv 48:133–142

De Winter SA, Hamers R, Degertekin M et al. (2004) Retrospective image-based gating of intracoronary ultrasound images for improved quantitative analysis: The intelligate method. Catheter Cardiovasc Interv 61:84–94

Degawa T, Yagami H, Takahashi K et al. (2001) Validation of a novel wire-type intravascular ultrasound imaging catheter. Catheter Cardiovasc Interv 52:127–133

Di Mario C, von Birgelen C, Prati F et al. (1995) Three-dimensional reconstruction of intracoronary ultrasound: clinical of research tool? Br Heart J 73[Suppl 2]:26–32

Evans JL, Ng KH, Vonesh MJ et al. (1994) Arterial imaging with a new forward-viewing intravascular ultrasound catheter, I. Initial studies. Circulation 89:712–717

Li W, von Birgelen C, Di Mario C et al. (1994) Semi-automated contour detection for volumetric quantification of intracoronary ultrasound. Paper presented at: Computers in cardiology, Washington

Mintz GS, Pichard AD, Satler LF et al. (1993) Three-dimensional intravascular ultrasonography: reconstruction of endovascular stents in vitro and in vivo. J Clin Ultrasound 21:609–615

Ng KH, Evans JL, Vonesh MJ et al. (1994) Arterial imaging with a new forward-viewing intravascular ultrasound catheter, II. Three-dimensional reconstruction and display of data. Circulation 89:718–723

Nissen SE, Yock P (2001) Intravascular ultrasound: novel pathophysiological insights and current clinical applications. Circulation 103:604–616

Roelandt JR, di Mario C, Pandian NG et al. (1994) Three-dimensional reconstruction of intracoronary ultrasound images. Rationale, approaches, problems, and directions. Circulation 90:1044–1055

Rosenfield K, Losordo DW, Ramaswamy K et al. (1991) Three-dimensional reconstruction of human coronary and peripheral arteries from images recorded during two-dimensional intravascular ultrasound examination. Circulation 84:1938–1956

Schuurbiers JC, von Birgelen C, Wentzel JJ et al. (2000) On the IVUS plaque volume error in coronary arteries when neglecting curvature. Ultrasound Med Biol 26:1403–1411

Slager CJ, Wentzel JJ, Schuurbiers JC et al. (2000) True 3-dimensional reconstruction of coronary arteries in patients by fusion of angiography and IVUS (ANGUS) and its quantitative validation. Circulation 102:511–516

Sousa JE, Costa MA, Abizaid A et al. (2001) Lack of neointimal proliferation after implantation of sirolimus-coated stents in human coronary arteries: a quantitative coronary angiography and three-dimensional intravascular ultrasound study. Circulation 103:192–195

Takagi A, Tsurumi Y, Ishii Y et al. (1999) Clinical potential of intravascular ultrasound for physiological assessment of coronary stenosis: relationship between quantitative ultrasound tomography and pressure-derived fractional flow reserve. Circulation 100:250–255

van Egmond FC, Li W, Gussenhoven EJ et al. (1994) Catheter displacement sensing device. Thoraxcentre J (6):9–12

von Birgelen C, Erbel R, Di Mario C et al. (1995a) Three-dimensional reconstruction of coronary arteries with intravascular ultrasound. Herz 20:277–289

von Birgelen C, Di Mario C, Prati F et al. (1995b) Intracoronary ultrasound: three-dimensional reconstruction techniques. In: de Feyter PJ, Di Mario C, Serruys PW (eds) Quantitative coronary imaging. Barjesteh, Meeuwse & Co., Rotterdam, pp 181–197

von Birgelen C, van der Lugt A, Nicosia A et al. (1996) Computerized assessment of coronary lumen and atherosclerotic plaque dimensions in three-dimensional intravascular ultrasound correlated with histomorphometry. Am J Cardiol 78:1202–1209

von Birgelen C, de Vrey EA, Mintz GS et al. (1997a) ECG-gated three-dimensional intravascular ultrasound: feasibility and reproducibility of the automated analysis of coronary lumen and atherosclerotic plaque dimensions in humans. Circulation 96:2944–2952

von Birgelen C, Mintz GS, Nicosia A et al. (1997b) Electrocardiogram-gated intravascular ultrasound image acquisition after coronary stent deployment facilitates on-line three-dimensional reconstruction and automated lumen quantification. J Am Coll Cardiol 30:436–443

von Birgelen C, Mintz GS, de Feyter PJ et al. (1997c) Reconstruction and quantification with three-dimensional intracoronary ultrasound. An update on techniques, challenges, and future directions. Eur Heart J 18:1056–1067

von Birgelen C, de Feyter PJ, de Vrey EA et al. (1997d) Simpson's rule for the volumetric ultrasound assessment of atherosclerotic coronary arteries: a study with ECG-gated three- dimensional intravascular ultrasound. Coron Artery Dis 8:363–369

Non-Invasive Coronary Imaging

3

3.1 Multi-Detector Row Computed Tomography – Technical Principles, New System Concepts, and Clinical Applications

Thomas Flohr and Bernd Ohnesorge

CONTENTS

T. Flohr, PhD
Siemens Healthcare, Computed Tomography Division, Siemensstrasse 1, 91301 Forchheim, Germany
and
Institute for Diagnostic Radiology, Eberhard-Karls-University, Tübingen, Germany
B. Ohnesorge, PhD
Siemens Limited China, Healthcare, Siemens International Medical Park, 278, Zhou Zhu Road, SIMZ, Nanhui District, Shanghai 2013118, P.R. China

3.1.1 Introduction

Coronary artery imaging is a demanding application for any non-invasive imaging modality. On the one hand, high temporal resolution is needed to virtually freeze the cardiac motion and to avoid motion artifacts in the images. On the other hand, sufficient spatial resolution – at best sub-millimeter – is required to adequately visualize small and complex anatomical structures such as the coronary arteries. The complete coronary artery tree has to be examined within one short breath-hold time to avoid breathing artifacts and to limit the amount of contrast agent if necessary. In 1984, electron beam computed tomography (EBCT) was introduced as a non-invasive imaging modality for the diagnosis of coronary artery disease (Boyd and Lipton 1982; Agatston et al. 1990; Achenbach et al. 1998, Becker et al. 2000a). The temporal resolution of 100 ms allowed for motion-free imaging of the cardiac anatomy in the diastolic heart phase even at higher heart rates. Due to the restriction to non-spiral scanning in electrocardiogram (ECG)-synchronized cardiac examinations, a single breath-hold scan of the heart required slice widths not smaller than 3 mm. The resulting through-plane (z-axis) resolution was limited and not adequate for 3D visualization of the coronary arteries. Initial attempts to use 3rd generation single-slice CT systems, based on the mechanical rotation of X-ray tube and detector, for cardiac imaging were not convincing due to poor temporal resolution and insufficient volume coverage with thin slices (Becker et al. 2000b; Bahner et al. 1999). Since 1999, four-slice CT systems with higher volume coverage speed and improved temporal resolution of 250 ms and less owing to shorter gantry rotation times (0.5 s) have been clinically used for ECG-triggered or ECG-gated multi-detector row CT (MDCT) examinations at low to moderate heart rates (Ohnesorge et al. 1999, 2000, 2002; Klingenbeck et al. 1999; Kachelriess et al. 2000). Due to the increased scan speed with four simultaneously acquired slices, coverage of the entire heart volume with thin slices (i.e. 4 × 1 mm or 4 × 1.25 mm collimation) within one breath-hold became feasible. The improved through-plane resolution allowed for high-resolution CT imaging of the heart and the coronary arteries (Knez 2000, 2001; Nieman et al. 2001, Kopp et al. 2002; Becker et al. 2002). First clinical studies demonstrated MDCT's potential to not only detect but to some degree also characterize non-calcified and calcified atherosclerotic plaques in the coronary arteries based on their CT attenuation (Schröder et al. 2001). Despite all promising advances, challenges and limitations with respect to motion artifacts in patients with higher heart rates, limited spatial resolution and long breath-hold times up to 40 s remained for four-slice cardiac CT (Nieman et al. 2001). In 2000, shorter examination times for coronary CT angiography (CTA) were realized with an MDCT offering 8 × 1.25 mm collimation. Introduced in 2001, 16-slice CT systems with sub-millimeter collimation (16 × 0.5 mm, 16 × 0.625 mm, 16 × 0.75 mm) and gantry rotation times down to 0.375 s provided improved spatial and temporal resolution compared with four-slice and eight-slice scanners, while examination times were considerably reduced to about 15–18 s (Flohr 2002a,b). Detection and characterization of coronary plaques, even in the presence of calcifications, benefited from the increased robustness of 16-slice technology (Nieman et al. 2002a; Ropers et al. 2003; Mollet et al. 2004, 2005a; Kuettner et al. 2004a; Hoffmann et al. 2005).

Available since 2004, 64-slice CT systems are a further leap in integrating coronary CTA into routine clinical algorithms. Two different scanner concepts were introduced by the different vendors: the "volume concept" pursued by GE, Philips and Toshiba aims at a further increase in volume coverage speed by using 64 detector rows instead of 16, thus providing 32 mm–40 mm z-coverage, without changing other physical parameters of the scanner compared with the respective 16-slice version. The "resolution concept" pursued by Siemens uses 32 physical detector rows in combination with double z-sampling, an advanced z-sampling technique enabled by a periodic motion of the focal spot in the z-direction, to simultaneously acquire 64 overlapping 0.6 mm slices with the goal of pitch-independent increase of through-plane resolution and reduction of spiral artifacts (Flohr et al. 2004, 2005). The 64-slice CT systems provide further improved temporal resolution (165 ms and less with multi-segment reconstruction) due to gantry rotation times down to 0.33 s. The wider coverage with thinner slices has shortened the examination time to 6–12 s, which is an adequate breath-hold time even for dyspneic patients. Figure 3.1.1 demonstrates the improvement in image

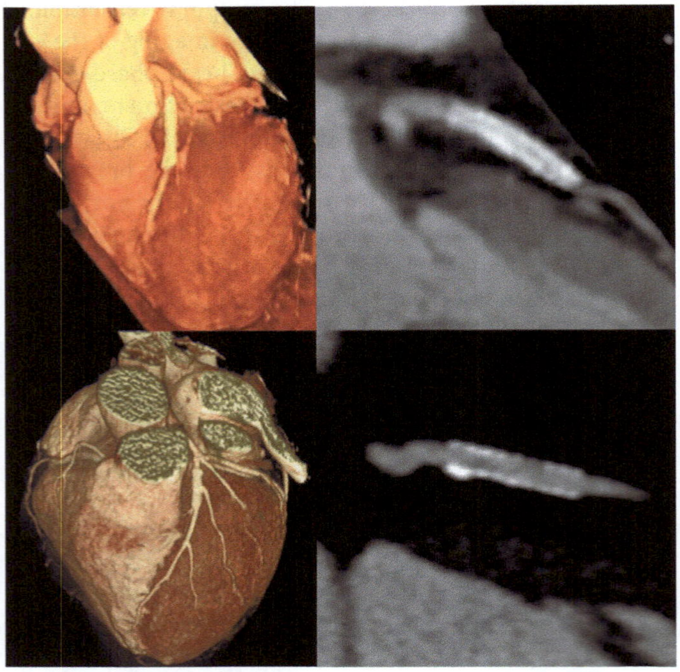

Fig. 3.1.1. Patient examples depicting similar clinical situations (a stent in the proximal left anterior descending artery) to compare the clinical performance of ECG-gated cardiac CT with a four-slice CT system (4 × 1 mm collimation, 500 ms rotation time) and a 64-slice CT system (32 × 0.6 mm collimation with double z-sampling, 330 ms rotation time). With the 64-slice system (*bottom*), the in-stent lumen can be evaluated (four-slice case courtesy of Hopital de Coracao, Sao Paulo, Brasil; 64-slice case courtesy of PUMC, Beijing, China)

quality, in particular with regard to spatial resolution, from four-slice to 64-slice CT systems. While image quality at higher heart rates and robustness of the method in clinical routine seem to be significantly improved with 64-slice CT systems compared with previous generations of MDCT, most authors still propose the administration of beta-blockers for patients with higher heart rates (e.g. LEBER et al. 2005; RAFF et al. 2005; MOLLET et al. 2005b).

In 2005, a dual source CT (DSCT) system, i.e. a CT system with two X-ray tubes and two corresponding detectors offset by 90°, was introduced by one vendor (FLOHR et al. 2006). The key benefit of DSCT for cardiac scanning and coronary CT angiography is improved temporal resolution. A scanner of this type provides temporal resolution of a quarter of the gantry rotation time (in this case 83 ms), independent of the patient's heart rate. First clinical studies have meanwhile demonstrated the potential of DSCT to enable clinically robust cardiac examinations in patients with high and irregular heart rates (ACHENBACH et al. 2006; JOHNSON et al. 2006, SCHEFFEL et al. 2006). Scanners of this type also show promising properties for general radiology applications, such as the potential of dose accumulation for the examination of obese patients by simultaneously using both X-ray tubes, or the potential of dual energy acquisitions for tissue characterization, calcium quantification, and quantification of the local blood volume in contrast-enhanced scans.

In this chapter, we present the technical principles and clinical applications of MDCT in cardiac imaging. We discuss technology and clinical performance of 16-slice CT, 64-slice CT and DSCT equipment, as well as CT systems with area detector technology, and we give a brief overview on clinical applications of ECG-synchronized cardiac CT scanning.

3.1.2 Technical Principles of ECG-Synchronized Cardiac Scanning with MDCT

3.1.2.1 Technology Overview

Electron beam CT (EBCT) was the first cross-sectional non-invasive imaging modality that could visualize the cardiac anatomy and the coronary arteries (BOYD and LIPTON 1982). In EBCT, an electron beam is emitted from a powerful electron gun and magnetically deflected to hit a semi-circular anode surrounding the patient. The magnetic deflection sweeps the electron beam over the target, thus generating an X-ray source that virtually rotates around the patient (Fig. 3.1.2). Given the absence of mechanically moving parts a sweep can be accomplished in 50–100 ms, in this way providing images with excellent temporal resolution. The technical principles of EBCT have been discussed elsewhere (MCCOLLOUGH and ZINK 1994; MCCOLLOUGH et al. 1994, 1999).

EBCT suffers from inherent disadvantages of the measurement principle which have prevented a more widespread use of these systems in cardiology or general radiology. Due to the restriction to non-spiral, sequential scanning, a single breath-hold scan of the entire heart requires slice widths not smaller than 3 mm. The resulting limited through-plane resolution is sufficient for Ca scoring; it is, however, not adequate for three-dimensional visualization of the coronary arteries and for the reliable detection of non-calcified atherosclerotic plaques. Image quality is degraded by scattered radiation due to missing anti-scatter collimator blades on the detector, with typical artifacts presenting as hypodense zones in the mediastinum. A fixed beam current of about 640 mA is used, limiting the exposure to 32–64 mAs per slice (STANFORD and RUMBERGER 1992). As a consequence, signal-to-noise ratio is at least problematic, if not insufficient

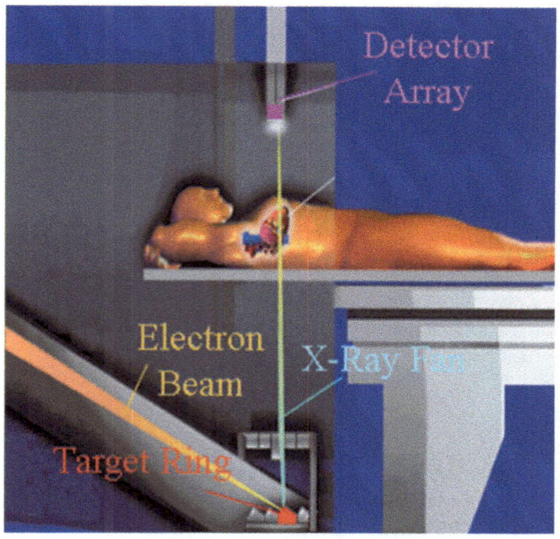

Fig. 3.1.2. The electron beam CT (EBCT) principle. An electron beam is magnetically deflected to hit a semi-circular anode surrounding the patient (angular coverage 210°). The electron beam is swept over the target in 50–100 ms, thus generating an X-ray source that virtually rotates around the patient. The temporal resolution of EBCT images is 50–100 ms

for larger patients. An EBCT system intended to overcome some of these limitations, the Imatron e-speed (General Electric, Milwaukee, USA), had been installed at several research sites, but was never commercially introduced. In summary, the EBCT principle is currently not considered adequate either for state-of-the-art cardiac imaging or for general radiological applications.

Since 1998, third-generation MDCT systems with simultaneous acquisition of 4 (1998), 8 (2000), 16 (2001) and 64 slices (2004), and minimum rotation times of 500 ms (1998), 420 ms (2001), 375 ms (2002) and 330 ms (2004) have been used for ECG-synchronized examinations of the heart and coronary arteries. Third-generation CT scanners employ the so-called "rotate/rotate" geometry, in which both X-ray tube and detector are mounted onto a rotating gantry and rotate about the patient (Fig. 3.1.3). In a MDCT system, the detector comprises several rows of 700 and more detector elements which cover a scan field of view (SFOV) of usually 50 cm. The X-ray attenuation of the object is measured by the individual detector elements. All measurement values acquired at the same angular position of the measurement system are called a "projection" or "view". Typically 1000 projections are measured during each 360° rotation. A suitable MDCT detector must provide different slice widths to adjust the optimum

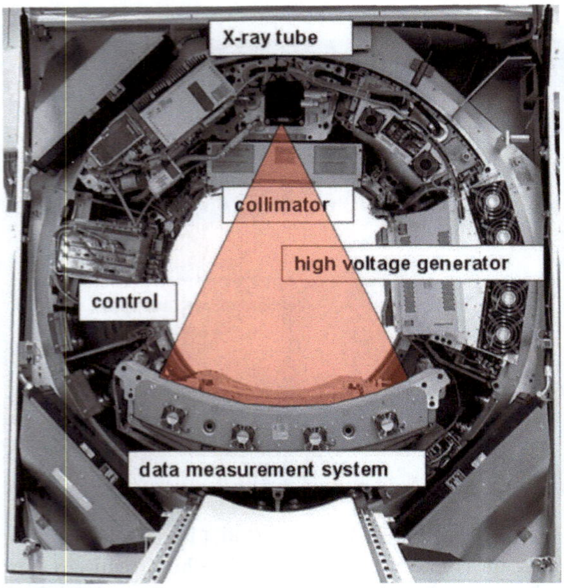

Fig. 3.1.3. Basic system components of a modern 3rd generation CT system, in which both X-ray tube and detector are mounted onto a rotating gantry and rotate around the patient

scan speed, through-plane resolution and image noise for each application. Different manufacturers of MDCT scanners have introduced different detector designs: the fixed array detector consists of detector elements with equal sizes in the through-plane (z-axis) direction, while the adaptive array detector comprises detector rows with different sizes in the through-plane direction. In order to be able to select different slice widths, all scanners electronically combine several detector rows to a smaller number of slices according to the selected beam collimation and the desired slice width. Figure 3.1.4 gives an overview on the detector designs of three generations of MDCT scanners.

The 64-slice systems by GE, Philips and Toshiba utilize detectors with 64 rows providing 32 mm–40 mm z-coverage, and aim at a further increase in volume coverage speed without changing other physical parameters of the scanner compared with the respective 16-slice version (Fig. 3.1.4, bottom right). The Siemens Sensation 64 scanner (Siemens Medical Solutions, Forchheim, Germany) utilizes a detector with 32 collimated 0.6-mm rows (Fig. 3.1.4, bottom left) in combination with a periodic motion of the X-ray focal spot in the through-plane direction (z-flying focal spot) to double the number of simultaneously acquired slices and to improve data sampling along the z-axis (Flohr et al. 2004, 2005). By permanent electromagnetic deflection of the electron beam in the X-ray tube the focal spot is wobbled between two different positions on the anode plate. The amplitude of the periodic z-motion is adjusted such that two subsequent readings are shifted by half a collimated slice width in the patient's z-axis direction (Fig. 3.1.5). Therefore, the measurement rays of two subsequent readings interleave in the z-direction, and two subsequent 32-slice readings with 0.6-mm collimated slice-width are combined to one 64-slice projection with a sampling distance of 0.3 mm at the iso-center. With this technique, 64 overlapping 0.6-mm slices per rotation are acquired, and the sampling scheme is similar to that of a 64 × 0.3 mm detector. The clinical benefits of optimized z-sampling with the z-flying focal spot technique are improved through-plane resolution at any pitch (Fig. 3.1.6) and suppression of spiral artifacts. Typical spiral artifacts result from insufficient data sampling along the z-axis and present as hyper- or hypo-dense "windmill" structures surrounding z-inhomogeneous high-contrast objects such as bones or contrast filled vessels (e.g. vena cava), which rotate when scrolling through a stack of images.

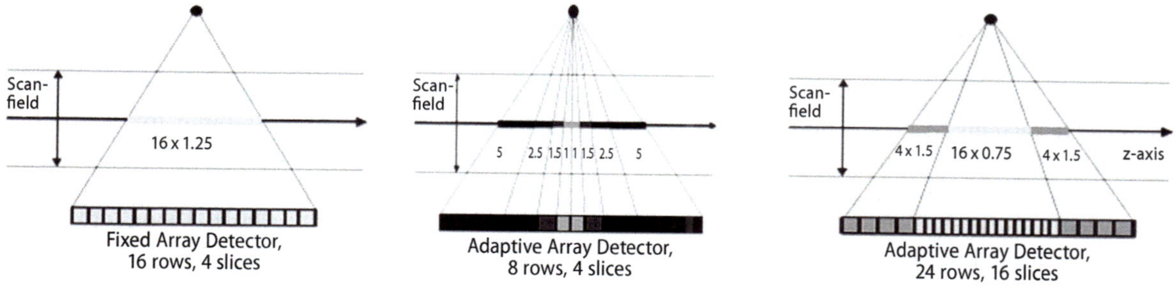

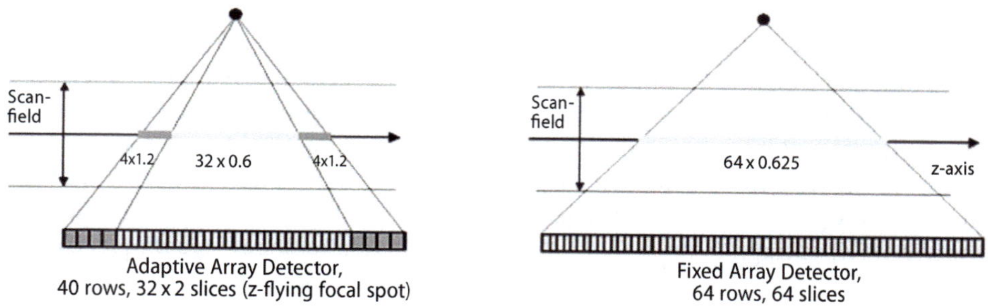

Fig. 3.1.4. Examples of fixed array detectors and adaptive array detectors used in commercially available four-, 16- and 64-slice systems

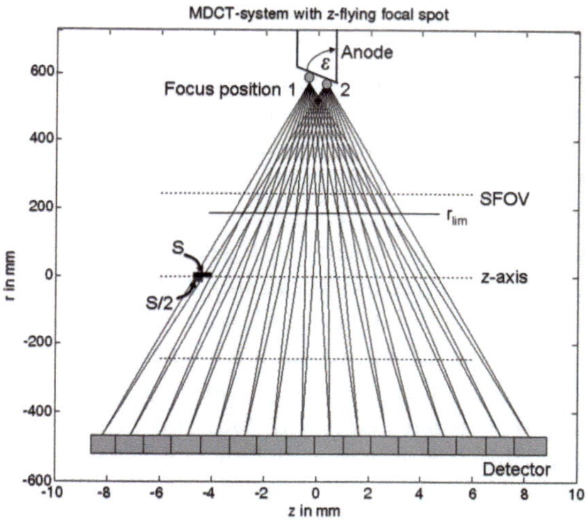

Fig. 3.1.5. Principle of improved z-sampling with the z-flying focal spot technique. Due to a periodic motion of the focal spot in the z-direction two subsequent 32-slice readings are shifted by half a collimated slice-width S/2 at the iso-center and can be interleaved to one 64-slice projection. Improved z-sampling is not only achieved at the iso-center, but maintained in a wide range of the scan field of view (*SFOV*), which can be defined by a "limiting" radius r_{lim}. The distances of both focal spot and detector from the iso-center and the widths of the detector rows are true to scale

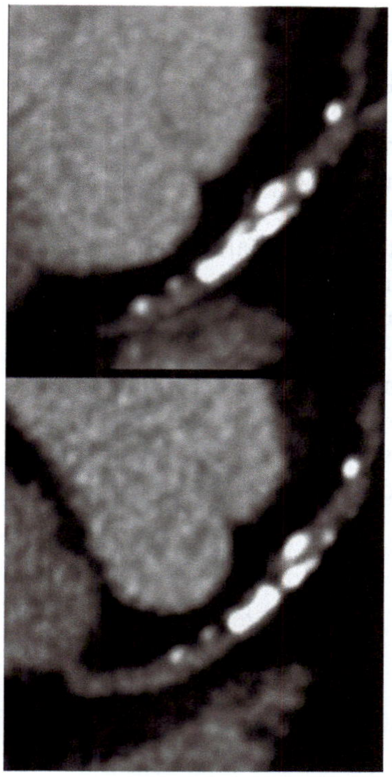

Fig. 3.1.6. Improvement of through-plane resolution with the z-flying focal spot technique. Scan data for a patient with severe calcifications in the left anterior descending artery was acquired on a CT system with a detector comprising 32 collimated 0.6-mm rows. *Top*, reconstruction without z-flying focal spot, slice-width ~ 0.8 mm. *Bottom*, reconstruction with z-flying focal spot, slice-width ~ 0.6 mm. Ca-blooming is significantly reduced. (Images courtesy of Dr. A. Küttner, Tübingen University, Germany)

A key requirement for the mechanical design of the gantry is the stability of both focal spot and detector position during rotation, in particular with regard to the rapidly decreasing rotation times of modern CT systems (from 750 ms in 1994 to 330 ms in 2004). Hence, the mechanical support for X-ray tube, tube collimator and data measurement system (DMS) has to be designed such as to withstand the high gravitational forces associated with fast gantry rotation (~ 17 G for 0.42 s rotation time, ~ 28 G for 0.33 s rotation time). Rotation times of less than 0.25 s (mechanical forces > 45 G) appear to be beyond today's mechanical limits.

Currently, two different techniques are employed to synchronize data acquisition and image reconstruction to the patient's ECG in cardiac CT scanning, namely prospective ECG-triggering and retrospective ECG-gating.

3.1.2.2 ECG-Triggered Sequential MDCT Scanning and Image Reconstruction

The most basic approach for ECG-synchronized CT data acquisition is prospectively ECG-triggered axial scanning, which was previously introduced with EBCT and single-slice spiral CT (Boyd and Lipton 1982; Achenbach et al. 1998; Becker et al. 2000a). The patient's ECG signal is monitored during examination, and axial scans are started with a pre-defined temporal offset relative to the R-waves which can be either relative (given as a certain percentage of the RR-interval time) or absolute (given in milliseconds) and either forward or reverse (Ohnesorge et al. 1999) (see Fig. 3.1.7). Data acquisition is therefore "triggered" by the R-waves of the patient's ECG signal. Usually, partial scan data intervals consisting of 180° of data plus the total fan angle plus a transition angle for smooth data weighting (in total 240–260° of data) are acquired. The partial scan data interval is then used as input for a modified half-scan reconstruction which extracts 180° of scan data in parallel geometry (Ohnesorge et al. 2000; Flohr and Ohnesorge 2001). Using optimized half-scan reconstruction algorithms with adequate data weighting, a temporal resolution up to half the gantry rotation time per image (165 ms for 330 ms gantry rotation) can be achieved in a sufficiently centered region of interest. The number of images acquired with every scan corresponds to the number of active detector slices. In between the individual axial scans the table moves to the next z-position, the heart volume is therefore covered by a "step-and-shoot" technique. Due to the time necessary for table motion, typically every second heart beat can be used for data acquisition (Fig. 3.1.8).

Prospective ECG-triggering combined with "step-and-shoot" acquisition of axial slices is the most dose-efficient way of ECG-synchronized scanning as only the very minimum of scan data needed for image reconstruction is acquired in the previously selected heart phase. As a drawback, reconstruction of images in different phases of the cardiac cycle for functional evaluation is not possible, and the method encounters its limitations for patients with severe arrhythmia, since ECG-triggered axial scanning depends on a reliable prediction of the patient's next RR-interval by using the mean of the preceding RR-intervals.

While ECG-triggered axial scanning was abandoned for coronary CTA with four-slice, eight-slice and 16-slice CT systems due to long acquisition times with thin slices, the method has recently been

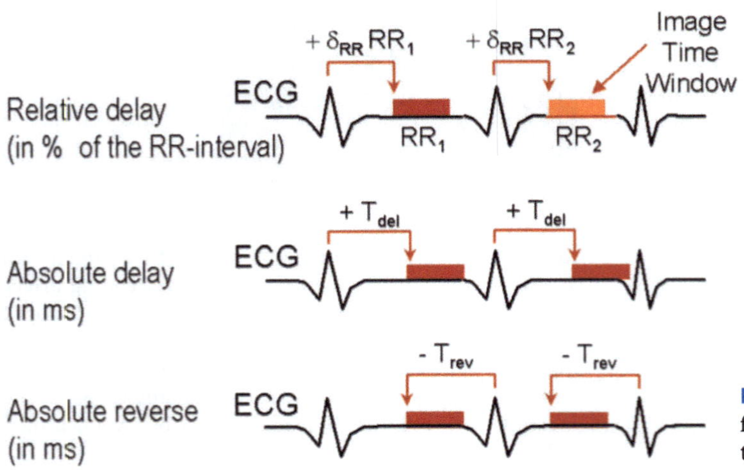

Fig. 3.1.7. Absolute and relative phase setting for ECG-synchronized CT examinations of the heart

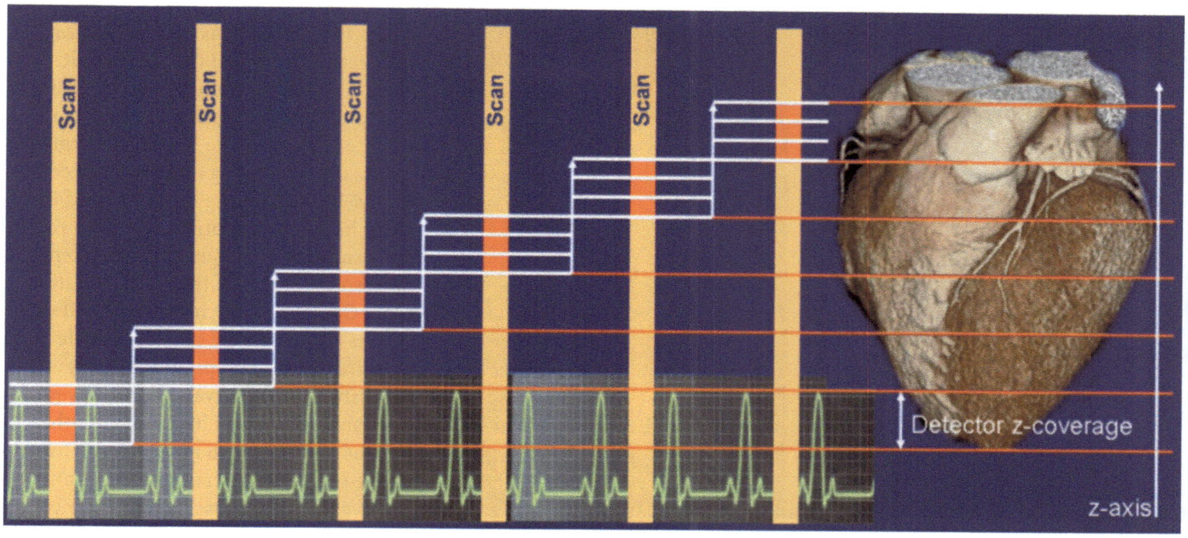

Fig. 3.1.8. Sequential volume coverage with prospectively ECG-triggered multi-detector row CT scanning. Multiple images corresponding to the number of active detector slices (in this case four slices) are acquired with a user-selectable delay after a detected R-wave. The images (marked as *orange blocks*) cover a z-range of the heart that equals the detector z-width at the iso-center. Partial scans with optimized image reconstruction are performed to provide a temporal resolution of half the gantry rotation time. Due to the necessary table movement from one stationary position to the next, a scan can typically be acquired in every other heart cycle

re-introduced for 64-slice CT systems. They make it possible to cover the entire heart with 0.6-mm or 0.625-mm slices within a reasonable breath-hold time at very low radiation dose to the patient (Hsieh et al. 2006).

3.1.2.3 ECG-Gated Spiral MDCT Scanning and Image Reconstruction

With retrospective ECG-gating, the heart volume is covered continuously by a spiral scan. The patient's ECG signal is recorded simultaneously to allow for a retrospective selection of the data segments used for image reconstruction (Ohnesorge et al. 2000, 2002; Kachelriess et al. 2000). Phase-consistent coverage of the heart requires highly overlapping spiral acquisition at low table feed that has to be adapted to the patient's heart rate to avoid gaps between image stacks reconstructed at the same relative phase in consecutive heart cycles (Fig. 3.1.9).

Image reconstruction for ECG-gated multi-slice spiral scanning consists of two parts: multi-slice spiral interpolation to compensate for the continuous table movement and to obtain scan data at the desired image z-position, followed by a partial scan reconstruction of the axial data segments. A "single-slice" partial scan data segment is generated for each image using a partial rotation of the multi-slice spiral scan which covers the given z-position. For each projection angle within the multi-slice data segment an interpolation is performed between the data of those two detector slices that are in closest proximity to the desired image plane z_{ima} (Fig. 3.1.10). The temporal resolution is constant and equals half the gantry rotation time of the scanner using optimized partial scan reconstruction techniques as described above. For 330-ms gantry rotation, temporal resolution can be as good as 165 ms.

At higher heart rates temporal resolution can be improved by dividing the partial scan data segment used for image reconstruction into N=2–4 sub-segments acquired in subsequent heart cycles ("segmented" reconstruction). Each sub-segment is generated by using data from one heart period, and there are temporal gaps between the multi-slice data segments used for image reconstruction (Fig. 3.1.11) (Kachelriess et al. 2000; Flohr and Ohnesorge 2001). For each projection angle an interpolation is performed between the data of those two detector slices that are in closest proximity to the desired image plane. The result are N single-slice partial scan sub-segments located at the given image z-position z_{ima} (Fig. 3.1.11), which can be put together to build up the partial scan data segment. With this technique, the patient's heart-rate and the

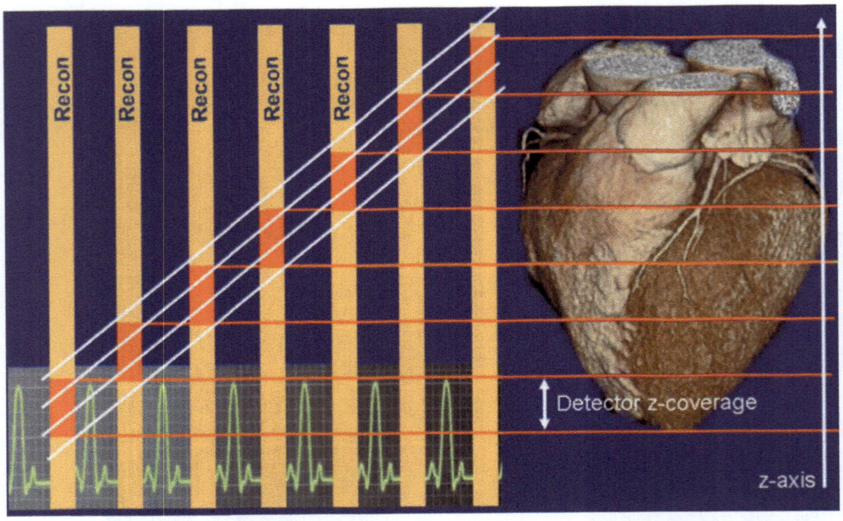

Fig. 3.1.9. Continuous volume coverage with retrospectively ECG-gated multi-detector row CT scanning for the example of a four-slice CT system. A spiral scan with continuous table feed is performed. Stacks of overlapping images (marked as orange blocks) can be reconstructed in every heart cycle. Optimized image reconstruction techniques provide a temporal resolution of half the gantry rotation time. Continuous 3D imaging in different phases of the cardiac cycle is feasible by shifting the start points of image reconstruction relative to the R-waves. The table feed has to be adapted to the patient's heart rate to avoid gaps between image stacks reconstructed at the same relative phase in consecutive heart cycles

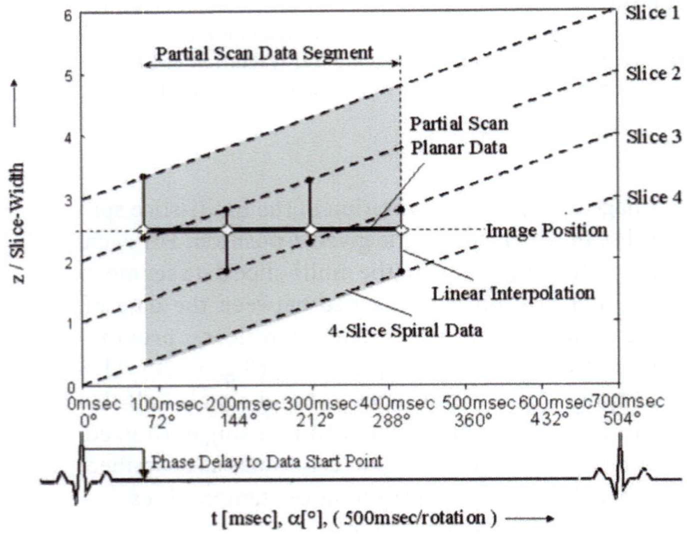

Fig. 3.1.10. Principle of retrospectively ECG-gated spiral scanning with single-segment reconstruction. The patient's ECG signal is indicated as a function of time on the horizontal axis, and the position of the detector slices relative to the patient is shown on the vertical axis (in this example for a four-slice CT system with 0.5-s gantry rotation time). The table moves continuously, and continuous spiral scan data of the heart volume are acquired. Only scan data acquired in a pre-defined cardiac phase, usually the diastolic phase, are used for image reconstruction (indicated as a *grey shaded box*). The spiral interpolation is illustrated for some representative projection angles α

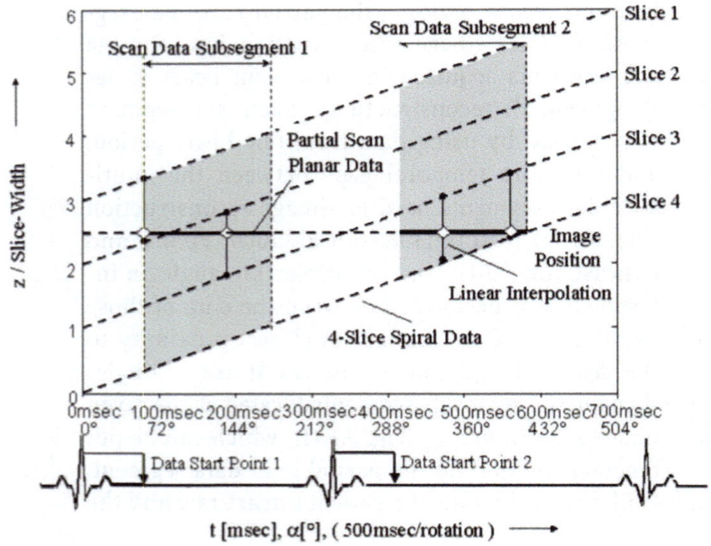

Fig. 3.1.11. Principle of retrospectively ECG-gated spiral scanning with multi-segment reconstruction. Spiral interpolation scheme for the example of a four-slice scanner using N=2 sub-segments of multi-slice data from consecutive heart periods for image reconstruction (compare to Fig. 3.1.10). Both sub-segments have to fit together to build up a partial scan data interval. The spiral interpolation is indicated for some representative projection angles α

gantry rotation time of the scanner have to be properly de-synchronized to allow for improved temporal resolution. Two requirements have to be met: first, start- and end-projection angles of the sub-segments have to fit together to build up a full partial scan interval. As a consequence, the start projections of subsequent sub-segments have to be shifted relative to each other. Second, all sub-segments have to be acquired in the same relative phase of the patient's heart cycle to reduce the total time interval contributing to an image. If the patient's heart beat and the rotation of the scanner are completely synchronous, the two requirements are contradictory. For instance, for a heart-rate of 60 beats per minute (bpm) and a 360° rotation time of 500 ms, the same heart phase always corresponds to the same projection angle segment, and a partial scan interval cannot be divided into smaller sub-segments acquired in successive heart periods. Then no better temporal resolution than half the gantry rotation time is achieved. In the best case, when the patient's heart beat and the rotation of the scanner are optimally de-synchronized, the entire partial scan interval can be divided into N sub-segments of equal length, and each sub-segment is restricted to a data time interval of 1/(2N) times the rotation time within the same relative heart phase. Generally, depending on the relation of rotation time and patient heart rate, temporal resolution is not constant but varies between one half and 1/(2N) times the gantry rotation time. There are "sweet spots", heart rates with optimum temporal resolution, and heart rates where temporal resolution cannot be improved beyond half the gantry rotation time (Fig. 3.1.12). Multi-segment approaches rely on a complete periodicity of the heart motion, and they encounter their limitations for patients with arrhythmia or patients with changing heart rates during examination. With increased N better temporal resolution can be achieved, but at the expense of reduced volume coverage within one breath-hold time or loss of through-plane resolution. To maintain good through-plane resolution and thin-slice images, every z-position of the heart has to be seen by a detector slice at every time during the N heart cycles. As a consequence, the larger N and the lower the patient's heart rate is, the more the spiral pitch has to be reduced, resulting in increased examination times and increased radiation dose to the patient. If the pitch is too high, certain z-positions will not be covered by a detector slice in the desired phase of the cardiac cycle. To obtain images at these z-positions, far-reaching spiral interpolations have to be performed, which degrade slice sensitivity profiles (SSPs) and reduce through-plane resolution.

In general, clinical practice suggests the use of N = 1 segment at lower heart rates and N = 2 segments at higher heart rates. It has been demonstrated that multi-segment reconstruction approaches are clinically useful only up to a maximum of two segments for imaging of cardiac and coronary anatomy (Greuter et al. 2007). In some CT scanners, the partial scan data segment is automatically divided into one or two sub-segments depending on the patient's heart rate during examination [adaptive cardio volume, ACV, algorithm (Flohr and Ohnesorge 2001)]. At heart rates below a certain threshold, one sub-segment of consecutive multi-slice spiral data from the same heart period is used. At higher heart rates, two sub-segments from adjacent heart cycles contribute to the partial scan data segment (Fig. 3.1.12). In some other CT scanners, the single-segment partial scan images are reconstructed prospectively as

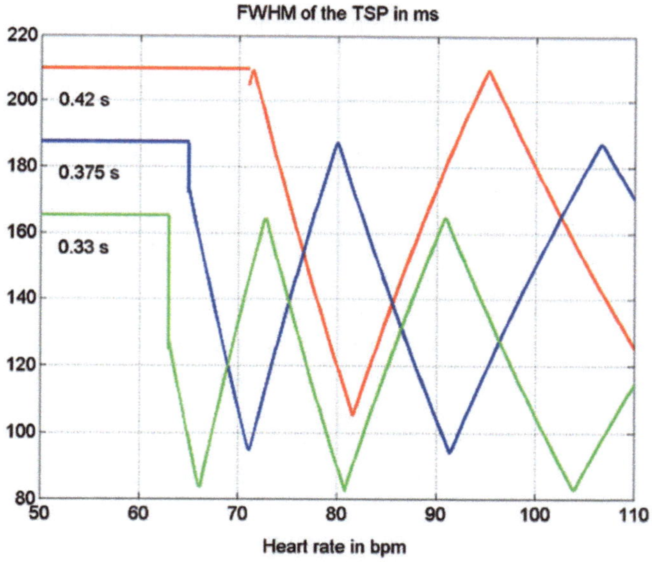

Fig. 3.1.12. Temporal resolution [full width at half maximum (*FWHM*) of the temporal sensitivity profile (*TSP*)] as a function of the heart rate for the adaptive cardio volume approach with 0.42-s, 0.375-s and 0.33-s gantry rotation time. For lower heart rates, a single-segment reconstruction with constant temporal resolution is performed. At higher heart rates, data from two consecutive heart cycles are used for image reconstruction, and the temporal resolution depends on the heart rate. For 0.42-s rotation time, the temporal resolution reaches its optimum of 105-ms at 82 bpm. For 0.375-s rotation time, "sweet spots" with optimum temporal resolution of 94 ms are 71 bpm and 92 bpm. For 0.33-s rotation time, the best possible temporal resolution of 83 ms is achieved at 66 bpm, 81 bpm and 104 bpm

base-line images, followed by a two-segment reconstruction retrospectively for a potential gain of temporal resolution for higher heart rates.

By using ECG-gated spiral acquisition images are reconstructed in every heart beat, hence faster volume coverage than with prospective ECG-triggering is possible. Moreover, the continuous spiral acquisition enables reconstruction of overlapping image slices, and a through-plane spatial resolution about 20% below the effective slice-width can be achieved. Image reconstruction during different heart phases is feasible by shifting the start points of the data segments used for image reconstruction relative to the R-waves. This allows for a retrospective selection of reconstruction phases that provide best image quality in an individual patient and for anatomy with special motion patterns (Hong et al. 2001; Kopp et al. 2001). Besides the morphological information that is in most cases derived from images reconstructed in diastole, additional reconstructions of the same scan data in different phases of the cardiac cycle enable analysis of global cardiac function parameters such as end-diastolic volume, end-systolic volume and ejection fraction. In case of arrhythmia and premature beats, retrospective ECG-editing can help to still achieve diagnostic image quality by discarding certain RR intervals for image reconstruction or by shifting the reconstruction phases individually in different heart cycles, while such techniques are not yet fully available for ECG-triggered acquisitions (Cademartiri et al. 2006).

As a drawback, relatively high radiation exposure is involved with retrospectively ECG-gated spiral imaging of the heart due to continuous X-ray exposure and overlapping data acquisition at low table feed. To maintain the benefits of ECG-gated spiral CT but reduce patient dose ECG-controlled dose-modulation ("ECG-pulsing") has been developed (Jakobs et al. 2002). During the spiral scan, the output of the X-ray tube is modulated according to the patient's ECG. It is kept at its nominal value during a user-defined phase of the cardiac cycle, in general the mid- to end-diastolic phase. During the rest of the cardiac cycle, the tube output is reduced. Clinical studies with four-slice CT systems and ECG-controlled reduction of the tube current to 20% of its nominal value have demonstrated dose reduction by 30%–50% depending on the patient's heart rate (Jakobs et al. 2002). The image quality of the high-dose images for morphological evaluation is not affected, while the low dose images are still sufficient for functional evaluation. If functional evaluation is not required, further reduction of the tube current outside the desired cardiac phases (e.g. to 4% of its nominal value), can reduce the radiation dose by additional 20%. Similar to ECG-triggered sequential scanning, ECG-controlled dose modulation relies on a prediction of the patient's next RR-interval by analyzing the preceding RR-intervals. Therefore, conventional ECG-pulsing approaches encounter their limitations for patients with arrhythmia, which has so far prevented a more widespread use in clinical practice. Recently, a more versatile ECG-pulsing algorithm has been introduced which reacts flexibly to arrhythmia and ectopic beats and has the potential to considerably enhance the clinical application spectrum of ECG-controlled dose modulation.

3.1.2.4
Evaluation of Spatial Resolution

While in-plane spatial resolution did not significantly change from four-slice CT to 64-slice CT, through-plane resolution considerably improved. The progress in through-plane resolution from four-slice CT to 64-slice CT can best be demonstrated with a z-resolution phantom, which consists of a Lucite plate with rows of cylindrical holes with different diameters aligned in the through-plane (z-axis) direction (Fig. 3.1.13): while the four-slice system can resolve the 1-mm cylinders in an ECG-gated spiral scan mode with 4 · 1-mm collimation (reconstruction slice width ~ 1.3 mm), the 16-slice system depicts the 0.6 mm cylinders with 16 · 0.75 mm collimation (reconstruction slice width ~ 0.85 mm), and the 64-slice system can even differentiate the 0.4 mm cylinders thanks to 32 · 0.6 mm collimation in combination with z-flying focal spot (double z-sampling) for the simultaneous acquisition of 64 overlapping 0.6 mm slices (reconstruction slice width 0.65 mm).

A further significant increase in spatial resolution for routine cardiac scanning, however, is unlikely. Increased spatial resolution goes hand in hand with increased pixel noise in the images. Consequently, to maintain a given signal-to-noise ratio, one has to increase the applied radiation dose. If spatial resolution is to be doubled in all three dimensions without increasing the pixel noise, e.g. to perform routine examinations at 0.2-mm isotropic resolution comparable to catheter angiography instead of 0.4 mm, the dose needs to be increased 16-fold. It is not expected that radiation dose to the patient can be increased

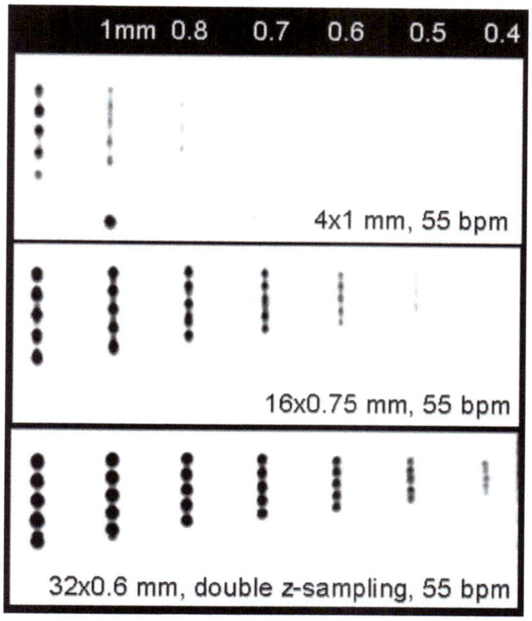

Fig. 3.1.13. Evaluation of the spatial resolution in the z-axis direction for ECG-gated cardiac spiral CT with four-, 16- and 64-slice equipment using a through-plane resolution phantom at rest. The phantom comprises air-filled cylinders with 0.4–3.0 mm diameter that can be examined with multiplanar reformation cuts along the scan direction. A maximum through-plane resolution of 1.0 mm is achieved with four-slice CT and 4 · 1 mm collimation. 16-Slice CT provides up to 0.6-mm through-plane resolution based on 16 · 0.75 mm collimation. 64-Slice CT with 32 · 0.6 mm collimation and z-flying focal spot enables the visualization of objects down to 0.4-mm diameter

this much for routine applications. If – on the other hand – spatial resolution is increased without corresponding increase in radiation dose, excess image noise can severely degrade the visualization of small coronary arteries and atherosclerotic plaques, such that the gain in spatial resolution will not necessarily translate in improved image quality and clinical benefit (Fig. 3.1.14).

3.1.2.5 Evaluation of Temporal Resolution

The temporal resolution at a certain point in the SFOV is determined by the acquisition time window of the data contributing to the reconstruction of that particular image point. Similar to SSPs, temporal resolution may be characterized by time sensitivity profiles (TSPs). The temporal resolution ΔT_{ima} assigned to an image is the full width at half maximum (FWHM) of the TSP. For a direct measurement of temporal resolution, a thin aluminum cylinder mounted on a rotating device can be used. The cylinder performs a rotation with a fixed radius of e.g. 5 cm around the iso-center of the scanner. The rotation speed of the cylinder and the gantry rotation speed of the CT system have to be exactly synchronized. For every projection angle α the cylinder is then seen by the same fan angle (the same detector channel), and the rotating cylinder is depicted as an arc of a circle in the CT image. The length of the arc corresponds to the length of the data interval used for image reconstruction. Figure 3.1.15 shows an image of the rotating cylinder phantom acquired at 0.42-s gantry rotation time and reconstructed using an artificial ECG-signal with 55 bpm (left). On the right side, the normalized CT values of the image along a circular path matching the trajectory of the cylinder as indicated by the dashed line are shown, which represent the TSP. The measured FWHM of the TSP is $\Delta T_{ima} = 208$ ms; this is in good agreement with the theoretically expected value and confirms that modified partial scan reconstruction approaches can provide a temporal resolution of half the gantry rotation time close to the iso-center (Flohr et al. 2003).

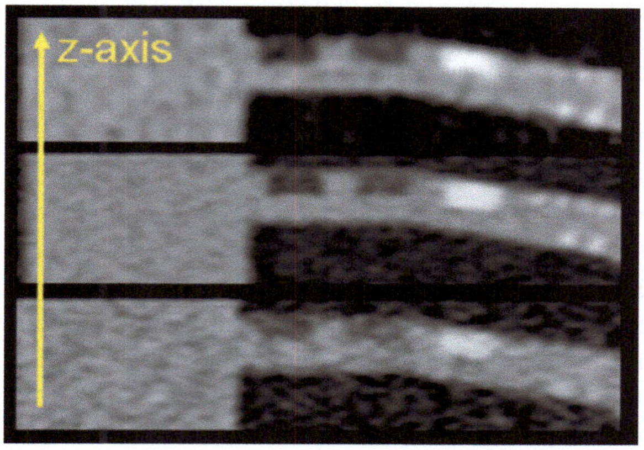

Fig. 3.1.14. Multiplanar reformations in the z-direction for a computer-simulated left coronary artery phantom with calcified and non-calcified plaques. *Top*, 0.75-mm slice width, image noise corresponding to 120 kV, 185 mAs. *Center*, improved through-plane resolution with 0.3-mm slice width and correspondingly increased radiation dose to maintain the image noise level (120 kV, 460 mAs). *Bottom*, 0.3-mm slice width without radiation dose adaptation (120 kV, 185 mAs). In this case, the gain in spatial resolution does not translate into improved image quality. Hence, a further significant increase in spatial resolution for routine cardiac scanning is unlikely

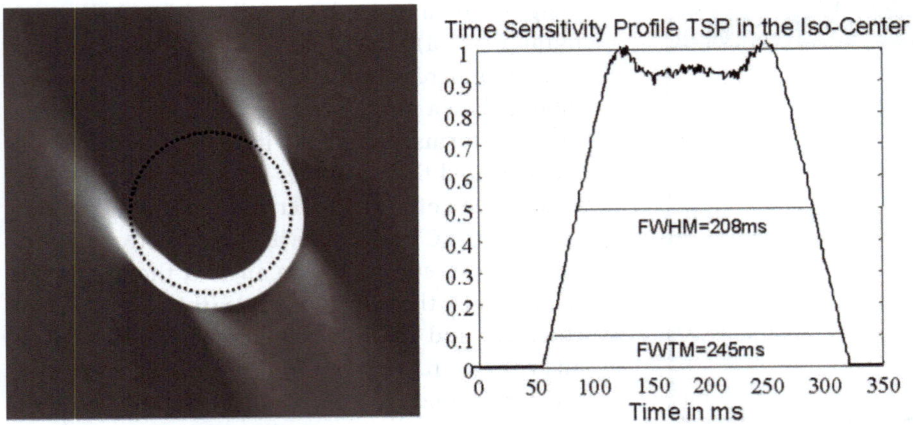

Fig. 3.1.15. Direct evaluation of temporal resolution. Scan data for a cylinder phantom rotating at a radius of 5 cm were acquired at 0.42-s gantry rotation time and reconstructed using an artificial ECG signal with 55 bpm (*left*). Normalized CT values of the image along a circular path matching the trajectory of the cylinder are shown on the *right side*. They represent the time sensitivity profile *TSP*. The measured full width at half maximum (*FWHM*) of the TSP is the temporal resolution ΔT_{ima} = 208 ms, in good agreement with the theoretically expected value

3.1.3 New System Concepts

3.1.3.1 CT Systems with Area Detectors

With today's available detector z-coverage of up to 40 mm, a retrospectively ECG-gated volume image of the heart still consists of several image slabs reconstructed from data acquired in multiple consecutive heart beats (Figs. 3.1.8 and 3.1.9). As a consequence of insufficient temporal resolution and variations of the heart motion from one cardiac cycle to the next – in particular in case of arrhythmia – these image slabs can be blurred or shifted relative to each other, resulting in banding artifacts in multiplanar reconstructions (MPRs) or volume rendering techniques (VRTs). The width of an image slab originating from one heart beat is proportional to the detector z-coverage. With increasing detector z-coverage the number of heart beats contributing to the volume image decreases, and so does the number of steps in case of artifacts. However, as a downside of increasing detector width larger portions of the data can be distorted if an ectopic beat occurs during the scan. A new level of clinical performance can probably be expected from CT scanners with area detectors that are wide enough in the z-direction to cover the entire cardiac anatomy in a single heart beat without movement of the table (Mori et al. 2004, 2006a,b; Kondo et al. 2005). With area-detector CT scanners high-resolution imaging of the cardiac morphology, as well as dynamic and functional assessment through repeated scanning of the same scan range, may become possible.

Meanwhile, a CT scanner with 320 · 0.5 mm collimation has been introduced by one vendor (Toshiba Medical Systems), after a long evaluation phase using a prototype with 256 · 0.5-mm collimation. Due to effects related to the cone-beam geometry of the X-ray beam, the scanner can cover a volume of approximately 140 mm in the z-direction with one rotation, the resulting volume images have an isotropic resolution of about 0.5–0.8 mm (Mori et al. 2006a). All scan data are acquired in the same RR-cycle, and stairstep artifacts between slabs of images from different heart cycles can be avoided. The diagnostic quality of this one shot that covers the entire heart, however, depends on the available temporal resolution, which is 175 ms for single-segment reconstruction at the fastest gantry rotation time of 0.35 s. In the worst case, the entire scan will suffer from reduced image quality if it is acquired in a short RR-cycle with insufficient temporal resolution. Ectopic beats that would otherwise only degrade the image quality of a single image slab and could in many cases be corrected for by ECG-editing (deletion of the corresponding R-peak; see Cademartiri et al. 2006) can now render the entire examination nondiagnostic.

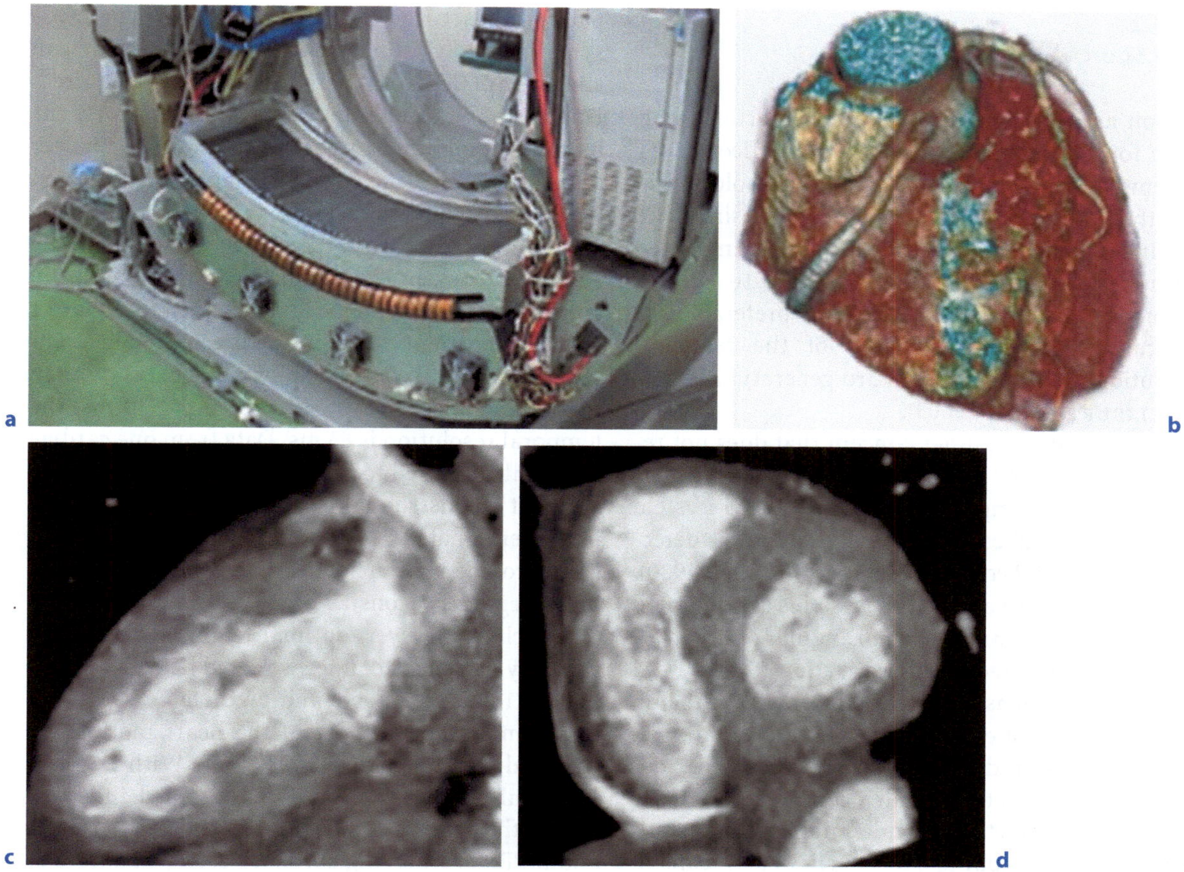

Fig. 3.1.16a–d. Prototype of an area-detector CT system with 256 × 0.5-mm collimation (**a**) and preliminary in-vivo patient results. A four-dimensional data set of the heart and the coronary arteries can be acquired from scans without table-feed. The prototype system covers a z-range of about 100 mm in one rotation. Volume rendered visualization of a volunteer's heart (**b**), multiplanar reformation of the left ventricle in a long axis (**c**) and short axis (**d**) view. (Data courtesy of Ehime University, Japan)

Another potential advantage of CT scanners with area detectors is the ability to evaluate perfusion defects, e.g. due to coronary artery narrowing, in the entire myocardium. Today only limited ranges of the myocardium (3–4 cm depending on the CT scanner type and its detector z-coverage) can be covered with sequential ECG-controlled scan protocols without table movement to study dynamic contrast enhancement. CT imaging of the myocardial perfusion is conceptually promising, yet it has to compete with other well-established modalities (in particular magnetic resonance imaging MRI), and a number of obstacles have to be overcome to prove clinical feasibility. For clinically relevant diagnostic information stress perfusion testing at elevated heart rates (e.g. after the administration of Adenosine) is mandatory, which requires excellent temporal resolution – at best below 50–100 ms. The expected CT density changes in the myocardium are very small, hence CT scan and reconstruction techniques will have to be carefully optimized to reliably detect these subtle changes in the presence of partial scan artifacts and other artifacts. Most important, the radiation dose to the patient has to be limited for this special acquisition protocol requiring multiple irradiations of the same cardiac volume.

Meanwhile, the scanner and its image reconstruction have been technically evaluated (Mori et al. 2004, 2006a) and first in-vitro studies and clinical images of pigs have been presented (Mori et al. 2006b). First patient studies using the prototype 256-slice version of the scanner (Kondo et al. 2005) have demonstrated its potential to visualize the cardiac anatomy and to assess cardiac function (Fig. 3.1.16). In a preliminary clinical report (Kido et al. 2007), 90.9% of the AHA coronary segments 1–3, 5–7, 9 and 11 could be evaluated in five patients.

3.1.3.2
Dual Source CT (DSCT)

Motion artifacts remain the most important challenge for coronary CTA even with 64-slice MDCT systems. Further improved temporal resolution of less than 100 ms at all heart rates is desirable to eliminate the need for heart rate control. Increased gantry rotation speed rather than multi-segment reconstruction approaches appears preferable for clinically robust improvement of the temporal resolution with conventional 3rd generation MDCT (Halliburton et al. 2003).

An alternative scanner concept that does not require faster gantry rotation, but provides considerably enhanced temporal resolution is a CT system with multiple tubes and the corresponding detectors (Robb and Ritman 1979; Ritman et al. 1980). In a DSCT, the two acquisition systems are mounted onto the rotating gantry with an angular offset of 90° (Fig. 3.1.17). In a technical realization (SOMATOM Definition, Siemens Medical Solutions, Forchheim, Germany), one detector covers the entire scan field of view (50 cm in diameter), whereas the other detector is restricted to a smaller, central field of view (26 cm). Both detectors provide simultaneous acquisition of 64 overlapping 0.6 mm slices by means of double z-sampling (z-flying focal spot technology). The gantry rotation time is 330 ms (Flohr et al. 2006).

The key benefit of DSCT for cardiac scanning is improved temporal resolution equivalent to a quarter of the gantry rotation time, independent of the patient's heart rate (Flohr et al. 2006). For ECG-synchronized CT image reconstruction, a halfscan sinogram of CT data in parallel geometry is required. Due to the 90° angle between both detectors, the halfscan sinogram can be split up into two quarter scan sinograms which are simultaneously acquired by the two acquisition systems in the same relative phase of the patient's cardiac cycle and at the same anatomical level (Fig. 3.1.18). With this approach, constant temporal resolution equivalent to a quarter of the gantry rotation time $t_{rot}/4$ is achieved in a centered region of the scan field of view that is covered by both acquisition systems. For $t_{rot} = 330$ ms, the temporal resolution is 83 ms. Data from one cardiac cycle only are used to reconstruct an image (single-segment reconstruction). This is a major difference to conventional MDCT systems, which can theoretically provide similar temporal resolution by using multi-segment reconstruction. With multi-segment approaches, however, optimal temporal resolution can only be achieved at few selected heart rates (see Fig. 3.1.12), and a stable and predictable heart rate and complete periodicity of the heart motion are required for adequate performance. With DSCT, a temporal resolution of $t_{rot}/4$ is obtained independent of the heart rate. Figure 3.1.19 shows axial slices and MPRs of a moving coronary artery phantom at 70 bpm (left) and at 90 bpm (right), both for the DSCT system (top) and for a comparable 64-slice single-source CT system (bottom). The phantom simulates realistic coronary artery motion, based on published values for the coronary arteries (Achenbach et al. 2000). The images at 70 bpm show only slight

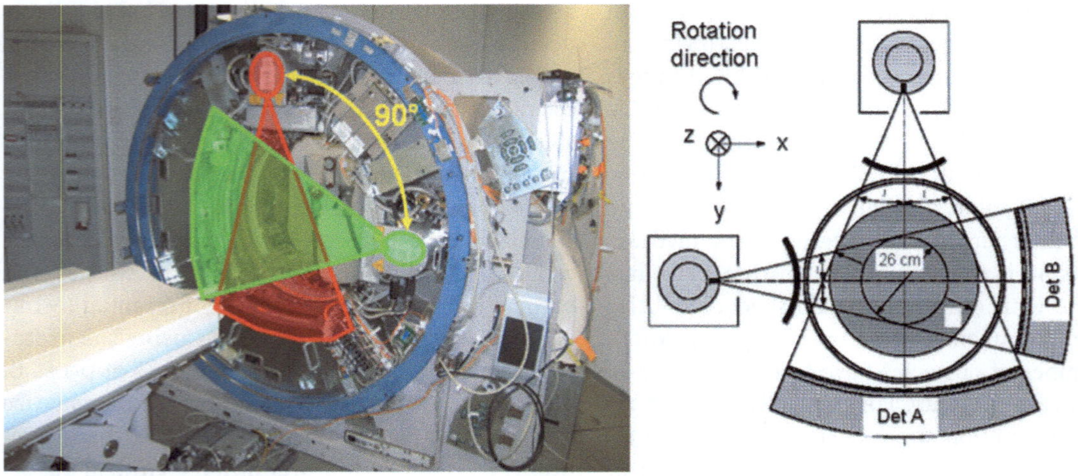

Fig. 3.1.17. A dual-source CT using two tubes and two corresponding detectors offset by 90° (*left*). In a technical realization, one detector (*A*) covers the entire scan field of view with a diameter of 50 cm, while the other detector (*B*) is restricted to a smaller, central field of view (*right*)

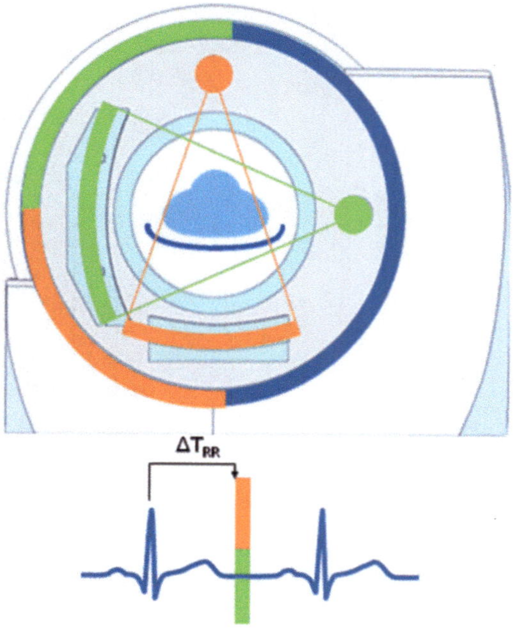

Fig. 3.1.18. With a dual-source CT scanner the halfscan data segment necessary to reconstruct an image at a certain phase within the patient's cardiac cycle (e.g. at a time ΔT_{RR} after the R-peak) can be split up into two quarter scan segments (indicated in *green* and *orange*) that are acquired by both measurement systems simultaneously. A scanner of this type provides temporal resolution equivalent to a quarter of the gantry rotation time, independent of the patient's heart rate

motion artifacts with the single-source CT, since its temporal resolution with two-segment reconstruction (140 ms) is sufficient to adequately visualize the moving phantom if the reconstruction phase is carefully optimized. At 90 bpm, the single-source CT images show increased motion artifacts. Image quality is degraded by blurring as a consequence of the insufficient temporal resolution of 160 ms at this heart rate. With the DSCT system, the depiction of the moving coronary artery phantom is nearly free of artifacts both at 70 bpm and at 90 bpm, thereby allowing for a reliable evaluation of the in-stent lumen at both heart rates. Figure 3.1.20 shows a comparison of MDCT single-segment and multi-segment reconstruction and DSCT single-segment reconstruction for the same patient with arrhythmia.

Multi-segment approaches can also be applied to DSCT systems to further improve temporal resolution for advanced functional evaluations of the heart, such as the detection of wall motion abnormalities, or the determination of parameters such as peak ejection fraction. With two-segment reconstruction, temporal resolution varies between 42 ms and 83 ms.

Several clinical studies have meanwhile demonstrated that DSCT can provide diagnostic results in coronary CT angiography examinations irrespective of the patients' heart rate (Achenbach et al. 2006;

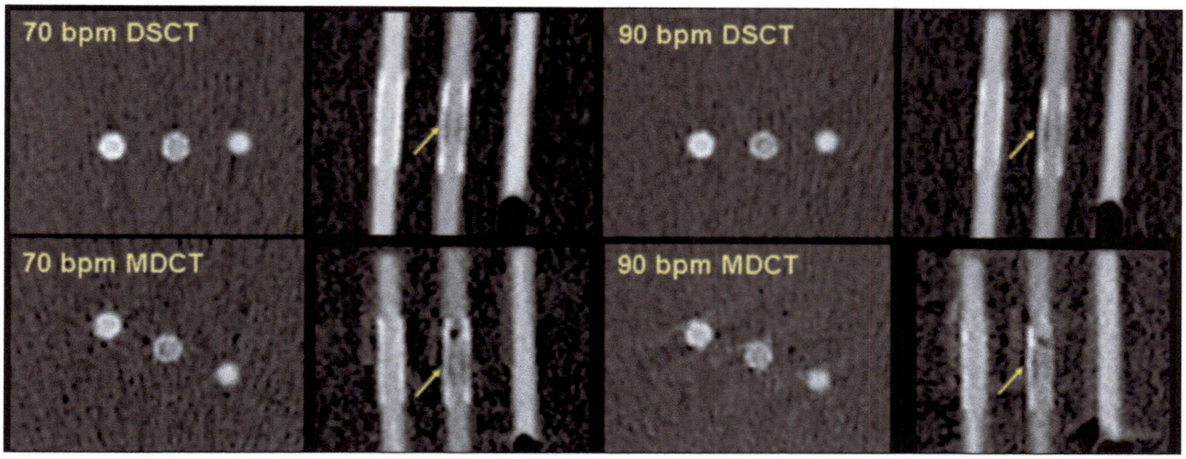

Fig. 3.1.19. Axial slices and multiplanar reformations of a moving coronary artery phantom at 70 bpm (*left*) and at 90 bpm (*right*), for the dual-source CT (*DSCT*) system (*top*) and for a comparable 64-slice single-source CT system (*bottom*), both at 330-ms gantry rotation time. The phantom consisted of three contrast-filled Lucite tubes with a lumen of 4 mm. Coronary artery stents were inserted in two of the tubes. One of the stents contained an artificial 50% stenosis within the stent. The tubes were immersed in a water bath and moved in a periodic manner by a computer-controlled robot arm at an angle of 45° relative to the scan plane to simulate heart motion. The temporal resolution of the DSCT is 83 ms, the temporal resolution of the multi-detector row CT (*MDCT*) using two-segment reconstruction is 140 ms at 70 bpm and 160 ms at 90 bpm. The in-stent stenosis (*arrow*) can be clearly appreciated on the DSCT images both for 70 bpm and 90 bpm, while the MDCT images suffer from image quality degradation at 90 bpm due to motion artifacts

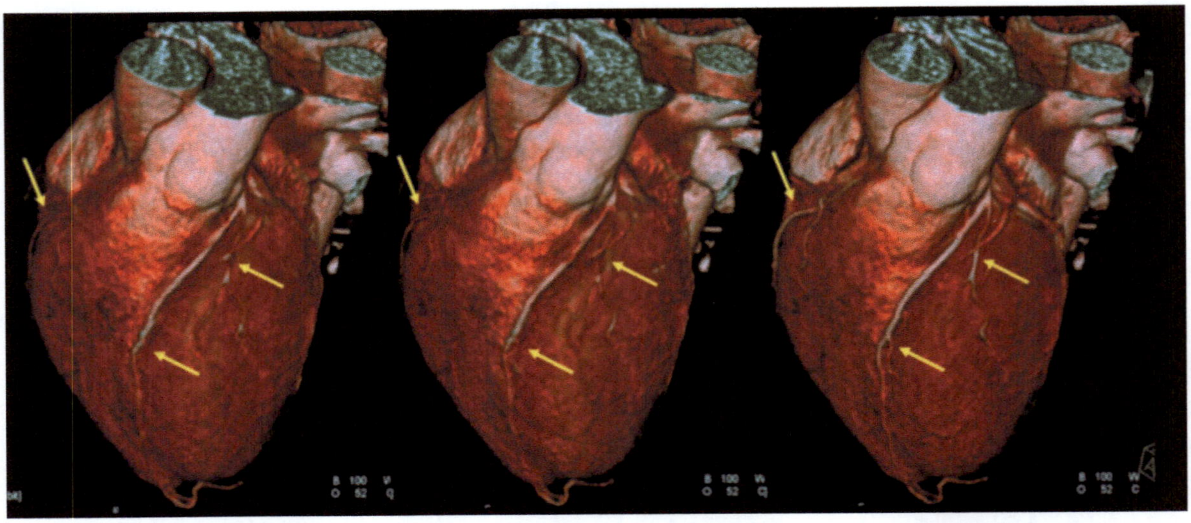

Fig. 3.1.20. Volume rendered visualizations of the heart of a patient with severe arrhythmia (varying heart rate from 86 bpm to 122 bpm) during scan data acquisition on a dual-source CT system. *Left*, reconstruction by using data from only one of the two measurement systems. This corresponds to a scan acquired on a conventional 64-slice single-source multi-detector row CT system with a temporal resolution of 165 ms and single-segment reconstruction. Discontinuities in the coronary arteries and blurring (*arrows*) are caused by insufficient temporal resolution. *Center*, two-segment reconstruction applied to the data from one measurement system only. As a consequence of the rapidly varying heart rate, temporal resolution is not consistently improved by the multi-segment technique. The visualization still suffers from artifacts. *Right*, reconstruction by using data from both measurement systems in a single-segment reconstruction (temporal resolution 83 ms). The coronary arteries are now almost free of motion artifacts, despite the patient's arrhythmia

Johnson et al. 2006; Scheffel et al. 2006). With DSCT, image quality seems to be much less dependent on heart rate variations than with MDCT, hence clinically robust image quality in patients with high and irregular heart rate during the scan can be achieved (Fig. 3.1.21). Imaging of the coronary arteries is possible both in systole and in diastole (Fig. 3.1.22). Diagnostic accuracy can also be improved in patients at low and normal heart rates. First clinical experience indicates that the elimination of cardiac motion due to the improved temporal resolution significantly reduces Ca-blooming (Fig. 3.1.23), which has so far been an obstacle in the assessment of coronary artery disease in patients with significant calcifications in the coronary arteries.

DSCT systems make use of several mechanisms to reduce the radiation dose to the patient in an ECG-synchronized examination: as a consequence of the single-segment reconstruction approach the table feed in ECG-gated spiral examinations can be significantly increased at elevated heart rates (see Fig. 3.1.9), thereby reducing both the examination time and the radiation dose to the patient. An efficient mechanism for ECG-controlled modulation of the X-ray tube output (ECG-pulsing) minimizes the length of the high dose intervals, while it reacts flexibly to ectopic beats and heart rate variations.

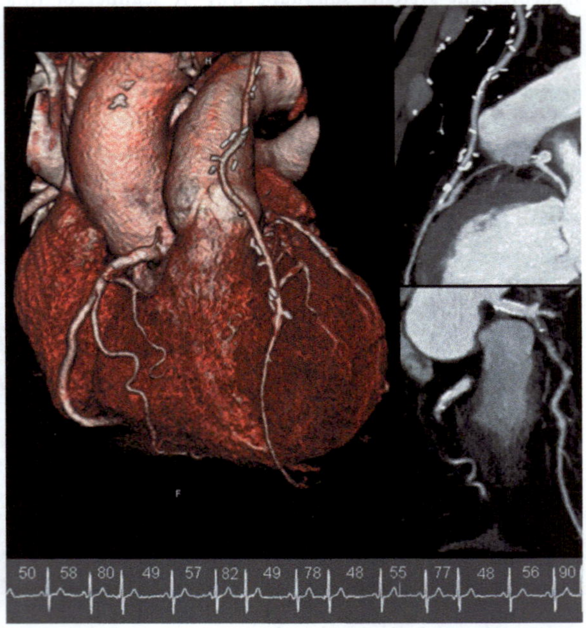

Fig. 3.1.21. Evaluation of a left internal mammary artery (LIMA) graft on a dual-source CT in a patient with rapidly varying heart rate. No beta-blocker was used for heart rate control. The patient's heart rate during the scan varied between 48 bpm and 90 bpm, an excerpt of the ECG is shown at the *bottom*. The anastomosis of the LIMA graft can be clearly evaluated (*top right*), as well as a stent in the proximal RCA (*bottom right*). (Images courtesy of Dr. S. Achenbach, Erlangen University, Germany)

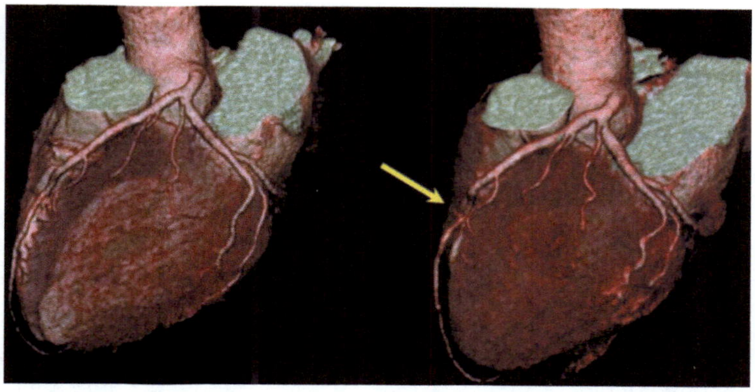

Fig. 3.1.22. Case study illustrating the potential of dual-source CT to provide diagnostic cardiac images both in diastole and systole. Evaluation of a myocardial bridge (*arrow*) in diastole (*left*) and end-systole (*right*). (Images courtesy of Dr. C. Becker, Klinikum Großhadern, LMU Munich, Germany)

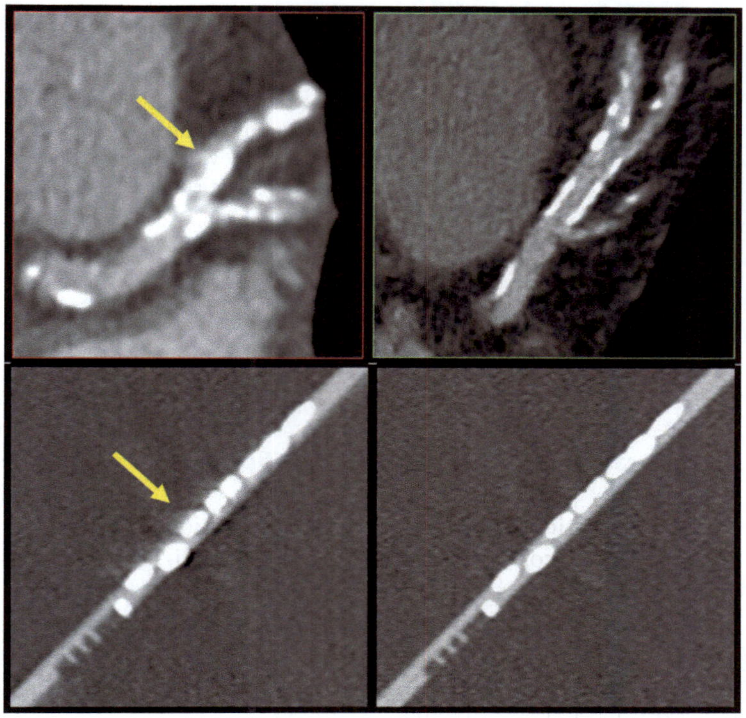

Fig. 3.1.23. Improved visualization of calcified plaques (reduced "blooming" artifact) at lower heart rates due to improved temporal resolution. A comparable clinical situation (calcified left anterior descending artery) is shown both for a conventional 64-slice CT system with 165-ms temporal resolution (*top left*) and a dual-source CT system with 83-ms temporal resolution (*top right*). The spatial resolution of both systems is similar (images courtesy of Dr. S. Achenbach, Erlangen University, Germany). At least part of the blooming artifact is caused by residual coronary artery motion (*arrow*). This clinical result is supported by a computer simulation study of a moving coronary artery at identical spatial resolution, but different temporal resolution (165 ms, *bottom left*, versus 83 ms, *bottom right*)

ECG-gated spiral cardiac examinations with DSCT systems result in radiation dose values that are for low heart rates similar and for higher heart rates less than those obtained with comparable MDCT systems (McCollough et al. 2007). Another means to reduce radiation dose is the use of ECG-triggered sequential acquisitions instead of spiral scans for patients with sufficiently stable heart rate (Fig. 3.1.24).

DSCT can also be utilized for general purpose CT imaging taking advantage of the high power reserves of 160 kW for long scan ranges and obese patients. The possibility of dual-energy acquisition by operating both X-ray tubes at different kV-settings has the potential to open a new era of clinical applications. The evaluation of dual energy CT data can in principle add functional information to the mere morphological information based on different X-ray attenuation coefficients that is usually obtained in a CT examination. Dual-energy acquisition can support the automatic differentiation of vessels and bone and might become useful to differentiate vascular lesions or to better quantify myocardial enhancement to visualize and evaluate myocardial perfusion defects. Clinical research will be needed to evaluate the potential of dual energy CT for relevant cardio-vascular applications.

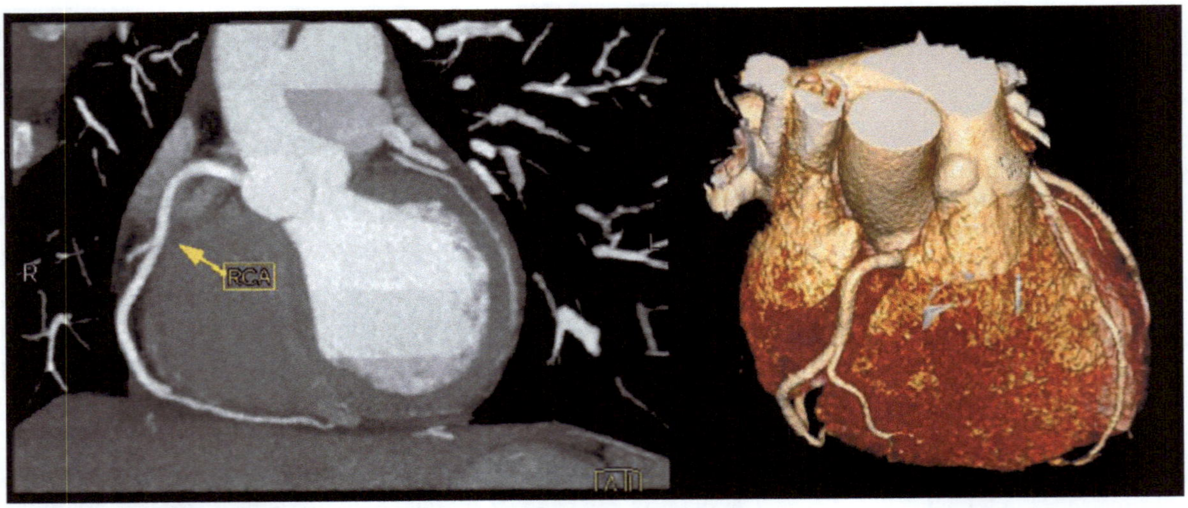

Fig. 3.1.24. Case study illustrating the performance of ECG-triggered sequential acquisition ("step and shoot" scanning) for coronary CT angiography on a dual-source CT system with 83-ms temporal resolution. A 43-year old woman with a family history of coronary artery disease, heart rate during data acquisition 72 bpm. ECG-triggered sequential scanning is a means to reduce radiation dose to the patient, provided the heart rate is stable. In this case, 100 kV instead of 120 kV were used for further dose reduction, resulting in a patient dose of about 1.5 mSv. (Images courtesy of Cedars-Sinai Medical Center, Los Angeles, USA)

3.1.4 Clinical Applications

3.1.4.1 Quantification of Coronary Artery Calcification

The quantification of coronary artery calcification by MDCT ("Ca-scoring") is a growing clinical application as it has been included as a useful test in the guidelines of several leading societies (Mieres et al. 2005; De Backer et al. 2003; Silber and Richartz 2005). Ca-scoring will be covered in a separate chapter of this book, hence it will be omitted here.

3.1.4.2 CT Angiography of the Coronary Arteries

Non-invasive coronary CT angiography poses high requirements on spatial resolution, low-contrast detectability and temporal resolution, hence optimization of the examination protocols is of critical importance for best examination results.

The first clinical CTA studies of the coronary arteries were performed with four-slice CT scanners with gantry rotation times down to 0.5 s (Ohnesorge et al. 2000; Achenbach et al. 2000, Nieman et al. 2001). They proved the feasibility of coronary CTA with MDCT systems, yet the performance parameters in terms of spatial resolution, temporal resolution and breath-hold times were too limited for regular clinical use. Improvement of diagnostic accuracy could be demonstrated for 16-slice CT technology with sub-millimeter collimation and rotation times of less than 0.4 s (Kuettner et al. 2005; Mollet et al. 2005a). Currently, 16-slice systems are considered as the entry level for coronary CTA. The further enhanced spatial resolution, temporal resolution and reduced breath-hold times of recent 64-slice CT scanners resulted in improved image quality at higher heart rates and considerably increased robustness of the method in clinical routine (Raff et al. 2005; Leschka et al. 2005). The availability of a 64-slice CT scanner is a prerequisite for imaging of coronary stents and analysis of coronary plaques (Fig. 3.1.25). Nevertheless, the majority of all studies using four-, 16- and 64-slice CT for coronary CT angiography agree that image quality degrades with increasing heart rate and increasing heart rate variability (e.g. Hoffmann et al. 2005; Leschka et al. 2006, Wintersperger et al. 2006). As a consequence, the administration of beta-blockers to lower and stabilize the patients' heart rate has become routine clinical practice. Even with 64-slice CT systems, most authors still propose the administration of beta-blockers for patients with higher heart rates (e.g. Leber et al. 2005,

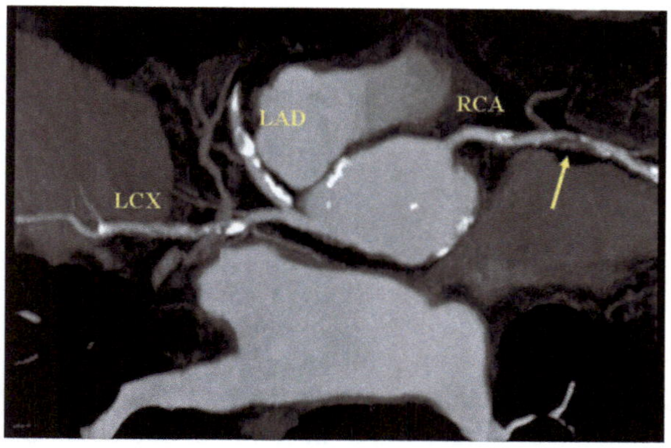

Fig. 3.1.25. Coronary CT angiography examination of a patient with chest pain, illustrating the performance of 64-slice CT with 32 × 0.6-mm detector collimation, simultaneous acquisition of 64 slices by means of a z-flying focal spot and 330-ms gantry rotation time. A thin-slab maximum intensity projection visualizes the main coronary artery segments and reveals multiple calcified, non-calcified and mixed lesions. The non-calcified stenosis in the right coronary (*RCA*) can be readily assessed (*arrow*). *LCX*, left circumflex artery; *LAD*, left anterior descending artery. (Images courtesy of Dr. U. J. Schoepf, MUSC, Charleston, South Carolina, USA)

Raff et al. 2005; Mollet et al. 2005b). First clinical studies with DSCT have meanwhile demonstrated the potential of this technique to provide diagnostic results in coronary CT angiography examinations irrespective of the patients' heart rate (Achenbach et al. 2006; Johnson et al. 2006; Scheffel et al. 2006). With DSCT, the use of beta-blockers can be avoided.

If the administration of beta-blockers for patient preparation is planned, contra-indications [bronchial asthma, AV block, severe congestive heart failure, aortic stenosis, etc. (Ryan et al. 1996)] have to be ruled out and informed consent must be obtained from the patient. Depending on the patient's initial heart rate, 50–200 mg of Metoprololtartrat may be administered orally 30–90 min prior to the investigation. Alternatively, 5–20 mg of Metoprololtartrat can be administered intravenously (Ryan et al. 1996) immediately prior to CT scanning.

A homogenous and sufficiently high vascular lumen enhancement is essential for coronary MDCT angiography. However, dense contrast material in the right atrium may result in streak artifacts arising from the right atrium and interfering with the right coronary artery (Fig. 3.1.26, left). Coronary atherosclerosis is commonly associated with calcifications that may be obscured by dense contrast material and hamper the assessment of the residual lumen. While a contrast medium flow rate of typically 1 g/s iodine (e.g. 300 mg/ml administered at 3.3 ml/s) by peripheral venous injection in an ante-cubital vein was commonly used with four-slice CT systems, resulting in an enhancement of approximately 250–300 HU (e.g. Schröder et al. 2001), a much higher flow rate of up to 2 g/s iodine is recommended for 64-slice CT and DSCT. Mollet et al. (2005b) use 400 mg/ml iodine at a mean flow rate of 5 ml/s for 64-slice CT, while Johnson et al. (2006) use 370 mg/ml iodine at a mean flow rate of 5.3 ml/s for DSCT.

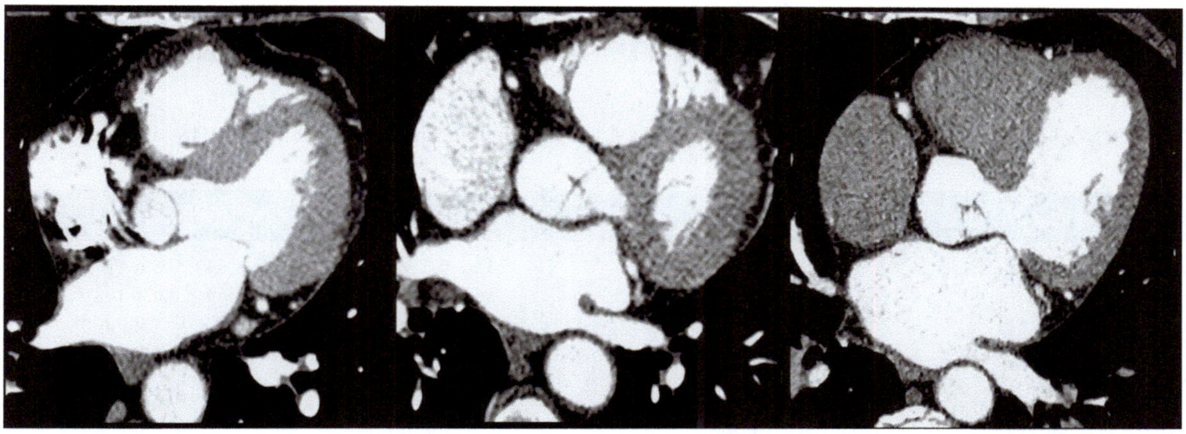

Fig. 3.1.26. Streak artifacts can arise from dense contrast material in the right atrium and interfere with the right coronary artery in the case of sub-optimal timing of the contrast bolus. This was a severe problem with four-slice CT scanners due to long acquisition times (*left*). Complete and homogenous enhancement of the left ventricle and the coronary arteries can be achieved with a dedicated contrast media protocol in 16-slice and 64-slice CT (*center*, 16-slice CT). A flush with saline can result in a wash out of the contrast medium from the right ventricle (*right*, 64-slice CT). (Images courtesy of the Dr. C. Becker, Klinikum Großhadern, LMU Munich, Germany)

A saline flush is often used to maintain a compact bolus. The sequential injection of contrast medium and saline allows for selective enhancement of the left ventricular system with a wash out of contrast in the right ventricular system (Fig. 3.1.26, right).

The final vessel enhancement will depend on the patient's cardiac output. In patients with low cardiac output, e.g. under beta-blocker medication, the contrast medium will accumulate in the cardiac chambers and lead to a higher enhancement than in patients with high cardiac output and corresponding faster dilution of the contrast agent. The patient's circulation time can either be determined by a test bolus of e.g. 20 ml contrast material followed by a saline flush at the level of the ascending aorta, or the MDCT scan can be started by a bolus tracking approach.

The cranio-caudal size of the heart to be covered by the CT scan is in the range 10–14 cm. The typical acquisition protocols for coronary CTA with four-slice, 16-slice and 64-slice CT scanners are listed in Table 3.1.1. Today's 16- to 64-slice CT scanners provide a z-axis resolution of 0.6–0.8 mm, based on 0.8- to 1.0-mm effective slice-width. For special high-resolution reconstructions of stented or heavily calcified coronary artery segments down to 0.6 mm effective slice width, corresponding to 0.4 mm z-axis resolution, can be achieved with 64-slice CT systems that apply a flying focal spot in the z-direction (see Fig. 3.1.13). In order to maximize the iodine contrast-to-noise ratio a kV setting of 120 kV rather than 140 kV has been established as the clinical standard. Lower kV settings, e.g. 100 kV, have the potential to provide further improved contrast-to-noise ratio at reduced radiation dose to the patient (Hohl et al. 2006; Hausleiter et al. 2006); however, the evaluation of these protocols is still on-going. In general, they are better suited for small and medium-sized patients.

Optimization of scan protocols with regard to radiation exposure is particularly important for contrast-enhanced CT imaging of the coronary arteries. Various publications are available that discuss the radiation exposure of MDCT in cardiac applications (Hunold et al. 2003; McCollough 2003; Morin et al. 2003; Hausleiter et al. 2006). Considerable disagreement of dose values can be found in the literature, mainly due to a lack of standardization of scan protocols and related parameters such as slice-thickness, in-plane resolution, image noise, and scan ranges. Table 3.1.2 summarizes estimates of the effective patient dose for ECG-gated coronary CTA protocols with 16-slice and 64-slice CT systems, using the Siemens 16 and 64 scanners as representative examples. Calculations of the effective patient dose for the standard protocols recommended by the manufacturer were performed with WinDose (Kalender et al. 1999). The scan range assumed for the dose calculations was 12 cm. The effective patient dose is directly related to the scan range. Increasing the scan range from 12 cm to 14 cm as an example will increase the dose by a factor 14/12 = 1.17. The mAs value is calculated from the applied mA value and the rotation time and determines the signal-to-noise ratio in the axial image slices ($mAs = mA \times t_{Rot}$). Some manufacturers such as Siemens have introduced an "effective" mAs-concept for spiral scanning which includes the factor 1/pitch into the mAs definition, i. e. they take the dose accumulation with decreasing spiral pitch (the spi-

Table 3.1.1. Typical acquisition parameters for coronary CT angiography examinations with four-, 16- and 64-slice CT systems

	Four slices	16 Slices	64 Slices
Collimation	4 × 1 mm/ 4 × 1.25 mm	16 × 0.5 mm/ 16 × 0.625 mm/ 16 × 0.75 mm	64 × 0.5 mm/ 64 × 0.625 mm/ 2 × 32 × 0.6 mm (double z-sampling)
Slice width/ spatial resolution	1.3 mm/ 1 mm	0.8–1 mm/ 0.6–0.8 mm	0.6–0.8 mm/ 0.4–0.6 mm
Rotation time/ Temporal resolution	0.5 s/ 250 ms	0.375–0.42 s/ 188–210 ms	0.33–0.4 s/ 165–200 ms
Scan time to cover the heart volume	40 s	15–20 s	6–12 s
Contrast protocol (typical)	~ 150 ml @ 3.5 ml/s	~ 110 ml @ 4 ml/s	~ 80 ml @ 5 ml/s

ral pitch is defined as the ratio of the total detector z-width at the iso-center and the table feed per rotation) into account (effective mAs = mA x t_{Rot} / pitch). Some other manufacturers, such as Toshiba and GE, stay with the conventional mAs-definition, and the user has to perform the pitch correction by himself. When comparing the scan parameters for CT systems of different manufacturers, the underlying mAs definition has to be taken into account. Due to the small pitch values used in ECG-gated cardiac scanning (typically $0.2 \leq \text{pitch} \leq 0.4$) the difference is significant.

The effective patient dose for cardio-thoracic examinations can be estimated by simply multiplying the product of $CTDI_w$ (in milliGray) and scan range (in centimeters) with the conversion factor 0.017 mSv/(mGy cm), if software tools such as WinDose are not available. This conversion is averaged between male and female models, but it is only valid for standard sized patients. It will underestimate radiation dose for small and pediatric patients.

Hausleiter et al. (2006) assessed the effective radiation dose of ECG-gated spiral coronary CTA in 1035 patients. They found an average dose of 10.6 mSv and 6.4 mSv for 16-slice CT without and with ECG-controlled dose modulation, respectively, and 14.8 mSv and 9.4 mSv for 64-slice CT without and with ECG-controlled dose modulation, respectively, in good agreement with the values given in Table 3.1.2. Use of 100 kV instead of 120 kV further reduced the average radiation dose to 5.4 mSv for 64-slice CT with ECG-controlled dose modulation. In a first study using DSCT, Stolzmann et al. (2007) found an average dose of 8.8 mSv at a tube voltage of 120 kV when using ECG-controlled dose modulation with tube current reduction to 20% outside the pulsing window. Using a protocol with tube current reduction to 4% outside the pulsing window, average estimated radiation dose was 7.8 mSv at 120 kV. The mean scan range (z) in this study was 127 mm. All patients were in sinus rhythm with a mean heart rate of 68 ± 17 bpm. First radiation dose values were reported for the prototype scanner with 256 × 0.5 mm collimation (Toshiba Medical Systems). Mori et al. (2007) estimate a radiation dose of 14.1 mSv for coronary CTA with the 256-slice system in a cine scan mode with 1.5-s total scan time.

Recently, the use of ECG-triggered sequential "step and shoot" scanning for coronary CTA was re-introduced (Hsieh et al. 2006). With this technique the entire heart can be covered with sub-millimeter slices within reasonable breath-hold times with 64-slice CT systems. The method is restricted to patients with low and regular heart rates, and functional evaluation is not possible. Nevertheless, radiation dose values can be very low. Scheffel et al. (2008) performed ECG-triggered coronary CTA with DSCT in 120 patients at an average radiation dose of 2.5±0.8 mSv.

Table 3.1.2. Scan parameters and radiation dose estimates for 16- and 64-slice ECG-gated spiral coronary CT angiography, using the Siemens 16 and 64 scanners as representative examples. Calculations of the effective patient dose for the standard protocols recommended by the manufacturer were performed with WinDose. The dose estimates are only valid for standard sized patients

	ECG-gated coronary CTA			
	Siemens 16-slice		Siemens 64-slice	
Collimation (mm)	16 × 0.75		64 × 0.6 (double z-sampling)	
Reconstructed slice (mm)	0.75/1		0.6/0.75	
Rotation time (s)	0.42	0.375	0.375	0.33
kV	120	120	120	120
mA	370	413	435	467
mAs	155	155	163	154
Pitch	0.28	0.25	0.24	0.20
Table feed (mm/s)	8	8	12.3	11.7
Eff. mAs	555	620	680	770
$(CTDI_w)_n$ (mGy/mAs)	0.078	0.078	0.077	0.077
$CTDI_w$ (mGy)	43.3	48.4	52.4	59.3
Eff. patient dose (mSv), male without ECG-pulsing Scan range 12 cm	9.5	10.7	11.5	13.0
Eff. patient dose (mSv), female without ECG-pulsing Scan range 12 cm	13.3	14.9	16.2	18.2
Eff. patient dose (mSv), male with ECG-pulsing Scan range 12 cm	4.8–6.6	5.4–7.4	5.8–8.0	6.5–9.1
Eff. patient dose (mSv), female with ECG-pulsing Scan range 12 cm	6.7–9.4	7.4–10.4	8.2–11.3	9.1–12.7

3.1.4.3 Detection of Coronary Artery Stenosis

Significant coronary artery stenosis may cause a hemo-dynamically relevant blood flow reduction that may lead to myocardial ischemia with clinical symptoms such as angina pectoris. Figure 3.1.27 is a visualization of the cardiac anatomy with volume rendering views obtained from a coronary CTA examination. Coronary artery segments can be numbered according to the model suggested by the American Heart Association (Austen et al. 1975) (Fig. 3.1.28). A scoring system for lumen narrowing (Schmermund et al. 1998) can be used to describe different grades of coronary artery stenosis: A, angiographically normal segment (0% stenosis); B, non-obstructive disease (1%–49% lumen diameter stenosis); C, significant (50%–74%) stenosis; D, high-grade (75%–99%) stenosis; E, total occlusion (100% stenosis).

Table 3.1.3 summarizes the key results of 36 clinical studies on the detection of significant coronary artery

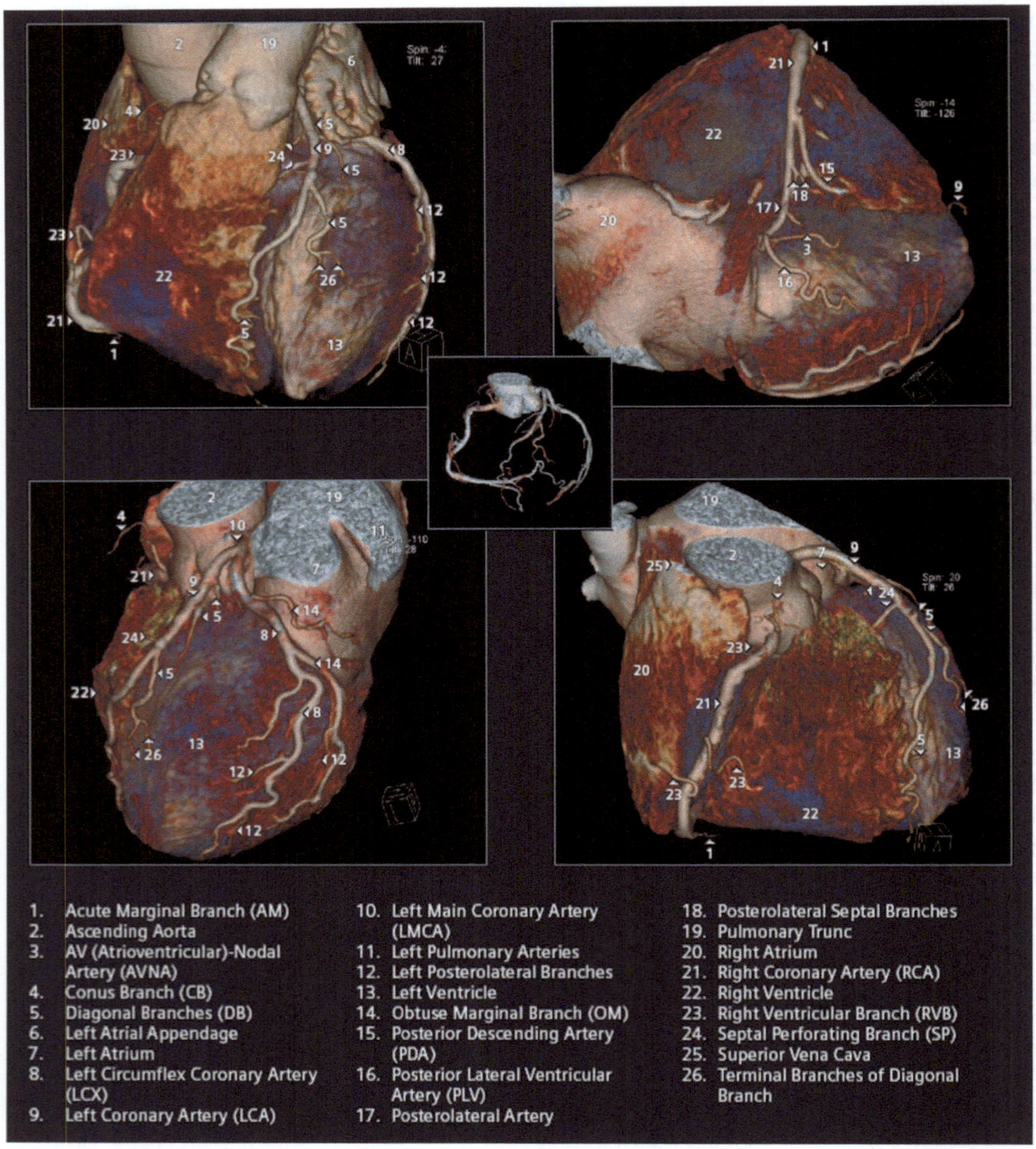

Fig. 3.1.27. Visualization of the cardiac anatomy with volume rendering views obtained from a coronary CT angiography examination. (Images courtesy of the Dr. C. Becker, Klinikum Großhadern, LMU Munich, Germany, graphics courtesy of Siemens Healthcare, Forchheim, Germany)

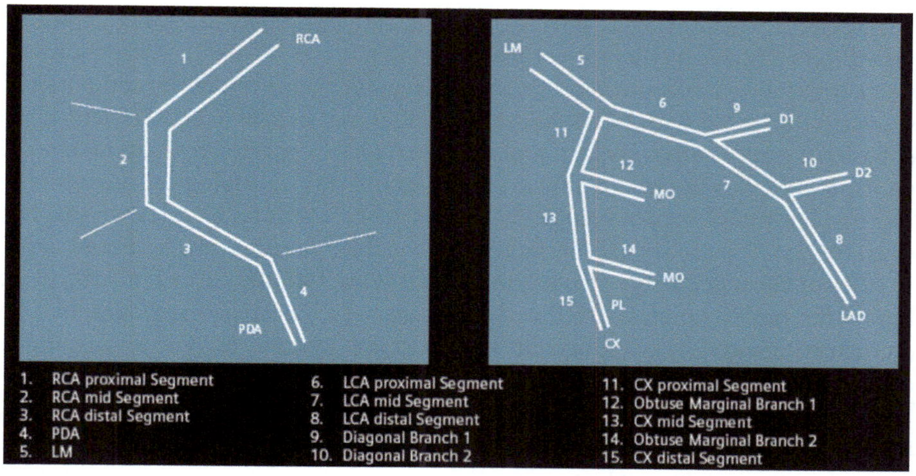

Fig. 3.1.28. Coronary artery segment classification according to the American Heart Association scheme (Austen et al. 1975)

stenosis (> 50% in diameter) with the different generations of CT systems in comparison with conventional catheter angiography (for details see Appendix). While specificity was high even with four-slice cardiac CT, there is a significant increase both in sensitivity and in the percentage of evaluable coronary artery segments from one scanner generation to the next. Interestingly, the mean heart rate in studies performed with 16-slice and 64-slice CT systems is lower than in the initial four-slice studies, probably due to the more frequent use of beta-blockers. This may be one reason for the significantly increased percentage of evaluable coronary artery segments, together with the improved temporal and spatial resolution of those systems. In most studies, coronary artery segments were excluded from evaluation because of small size and poor image quality, mainly due to motion artifacts. The first comparison using a dual source CT system (Scheffel et al. 2006) indicates further improved sensitivity and specificity at higher mean heart rate. No beta-blockers were administered in this study; the result, however, is preliminary due to the low number of evaluated coronary artery segments in comparison with the four-, 16- and 64-slice studies.

Because of the still limited spatial resolution in coronary CTA the definite assessment of the degree of coronary artery stenosis remains problematic even with 64-slice CT systems (Leber et al. 2005). Extensive calcifications may hamper the detection of coronary artery stenosis. In patients with diffuse, severe disease, such as in some patients with diabetes, the diagnostic value of coronary CTA may be limited due to insufficient spatial resolution. Patients with a high clinical likelihood of disease, with typical angina or obvious myocardial ischemia on exercise testing, and patients with known CAD are generally better approached by catheter angiography with the option to perform percutaneous coronary intervention in the same session. The interpretation of coronary CTAs is limited by missing visualization of contrast run-off and retrograde filling of coronary arteries. Furthermore, the hemodynamic relevance of coronary artery stenosis cannot reliably be determined without wall motion or perfusion information about the myocardium under rest and under exercise. Limitations have also been seen in patients with a body mass index above 30 (Raff et al. 2005) and absolute arrhythmia (Herzog et al. 2002).

Table 3.1.3. Weighted average values for sensitivity, specificity (both per segment), percentage of evaluable segments and mean heart rate during examination, derived from 36 clinical studies on the detection of significant coronary artery stenosis with the different generations of CT systems in comparison with conventional catheter angiography

CT system (number of slices)	Sensitivity	Specificity	Evaluable segments	Mean heart rate
4	78%	94%	79% (4368/5521)	64.5 bpm
16	87%	93%	95% (10538/11136)	62.0 bpm
64	89%	94%	98% (6472/6602)	62.6 bpm
Dual source (preliminary)	96%	98%	100% (420/420)	70.3 bpm

In conclusion, 64-slice MDCT can consistently provide good image quality for coronary CTA in patients with low to moderate heart rates when regular sinus rhythm is present. DSCT has the potential to enhance the application spectrum of cardiac CT to patients with high and irregular heart rates. According to recently published official guidelines (Hendel et al. 2006), CT coronary angiography is reasonable to rule out coronary artery stenosis in patients with low to intermediate pretest likelihood of disease. CT coronary angiography is appropriate for the examination of symptomatic patients who have an uninterpretable or equivocal stress test result, who have an uninterpretable ECG or are unable to exercise. CT coronary angiography can be used for the examination of patients with acute chest pain and intermediate pretest probability of CAD, but normal ECG and negative serial enzymes. A further application is the evaluation of suspected coronary anomalies.

3.1.4.4 Evaluation of Atherosclerotic Plaque

While catheter angiography can only visualize the contrast filled vessel lumen, MDCT as a cross-sectional modality is able to also display the coronary artery wall. Coronary calcifications, which represent an advanced stage of atherosclerosis, can easily be assessed without application of contrast media. However, different stages of coronary atherosclerosis may be present at the same time, and the extent of coronary atherosclerosis will be underestimated by only assessing coronary calcifications (Wexler et al. 1996). With contrast enhancement, MDCT is able to detect (and possibly characterize) also non-calcified atherosclerotic plaques (Fig. 3.1.29), first reported by Becker et al. (2000b).

Histological and intravascular ultrasound (IVUS) studies have shown that high atherosclerotic plaque burden can be found even in the absence of high-grade coronary artery stenosis on conventional coronary angiography. The correlation between acute cardiac events and high-grade coronary artery stenosis is poor. It has been reported that 68% of the patients who received coronary angiography by incidence prior to their acute cardiac event did not show any significant coronary artery stenosis (Ziada et al. 1999). On the other hand, a recent study showed that patients with nonobstructive plaques in the coronary arteries had a higher cardiovascular event rate than patients without any plaque (Pundziute et al. 2007). In early stages of CAD, the coronary arteries may undergo a process of positive remodeling that compensates for the coronary wall thickening and keeps the inner lumen of the vessel rather unchanged (Glagov et al. 1987). The underlying type of coronary artery disease may be a fibrous cap atheroma with accumulation of cholesterol. In case of inflammatory processes the fibrous cap of an atheroma may become thinned, putting the plaque at risk for rupture and consecutive thrombosis (Virmani et al. 2000).

The current gold standard to assess coronary atherosclerosis in vivo is IVUS. Recent studies (Achenbach et al. 2004; Leber et al. 2004, 2005)

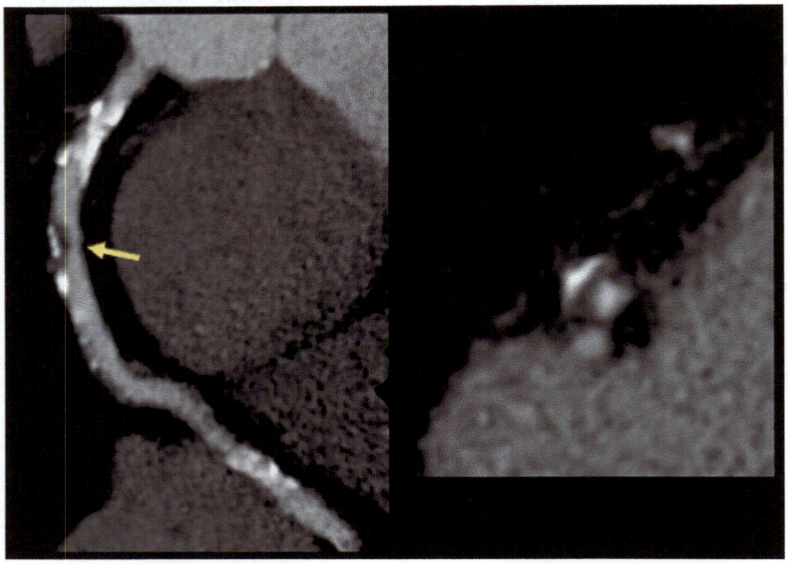

Fig. 3.1.29. Coronary CT angiography examination of a patient with severe three-vessel disease, acquired on a 64-slice CT with 32 × 0.6-mm detector collimation, simultaneous acquisition of 64 slices by means of a z-flying focal spot and 330-ms gantry rotation time. Curved multiplanar reformation along the right coronary artery (RCA) (*left*) and cross section perpendicular to the centerline of the RCA at the position of the arrow (*right*) for the analysis of a mixed plaque with lipid and calcified components. (Images courtesy of Dr. J. Breen, Mayo Clinic Rochester, Minnesota, USA)

found sensitivities of 78%–84% and specificities of 87%–92% for the detection of non-calcified plaques with 16-slice CT and 64-slice CT compared with IVUS. Since lipid rich plaques are assumed to have a higher risk of rupture, researchers have tried to differentiate plaque types based on their CT attenuation (Schröder et al. 2001; Becker et al. 2003; Caussin et al. 2004; Leber et al. 2003a, 2006; Carrascosa et al. 2006; Pohle et al. 2007). These studies demonstrated that lipid-rich plaques have lower CT attenuation values than fibrous plaques (mean attenuation values 14–71 HU versus 91–121 HU). Unfortunately, the measurement values show a large variability, probably due to insufficient spatial resolution, and only limited conclusions concerning plaque characterization can currently be drawn from MDCT attenuation measurements. Other clinically relevant indicators such as the amount of remodeling and the plaque volume, however, are readily available with MDCT.

3.1.4.5 Evaluation of Cardiac Function

Any contrast-enhanced retrospectively ECG-gated MDCT data set that has been acquired to visualize the cardiac anatomy can be re-used for the assessment of cardiac function (Kopp et al. 2005). Measurement of global cardiac function and of some regional function parameters by MDCT is possible through image reconstruction of the heart in different phases of the cardiac cycle. Global cardiac function is represented by end-diastolic volume, end-systolic volume, ejection fraction and left ventricular stroke volume, which can be derived from reconstructions of the left ventricle in the end-diastolic and end-systolic phase of the cardiac cycle. These reconstructions can also serve for the determination of regional function parameters such as wall thickness and systolic wall thickening. Image reconstruction at multiple equidistant time points throughout the cardiac cycle can reveal additional information about regional wall motion. The functional diagnosis of the myocardium may be complemented by first pass perfusion information that is included in the initial contrast-enhanced study of the cardiac morphology. Furthermore, late enhancement of infarcted myocardium can be analyzed with MDCT (Kopp et al. 2005; Paul et al. 2005). The evaluation of late enhancement requires an additional retrospectively ECG-gated low-dose acquisition with a 3- to 5-min delay after the initial contrast administration.

First studies with four-slice and 16-slice CT scanners demonstrated good agreement of global cardiac function parameters derived from MDCT measurements with the gold standard modalities catheter-ventriculography, echocardiography and MRI in patients with suspected or manifest coronary heart disease (Juergens et al. 2002, 2004; Heuschmid 2003, 2005, 2006). However, a systematic overestimation of the end-systolic volume was reported by several researchers, probably as a consequence of limited temporal resolution (Mahnken et al. 2003; Juergens et al. 2004; Kopp et al. 2005). This overestimation resulted in a systematic underestimation of the left ventricular ejection fraction (EF) by 1%–7%. 64-slice CT scanners with rotation times down to 330 ms provide improved temporal resolution for a more accurate assessment of global cardiac function parameters, and they also enable the detection of regional wall motion abnormalities (Kopp et al. 2005). The use of multi-segment reconstruction can increase temporal resolution and can thus provide significantly better end-systolic image quality (Juergens et al. 2005; Mahnken et al. 2006) (Fig. 3.1.30). Protocols that enable image reconstruc-

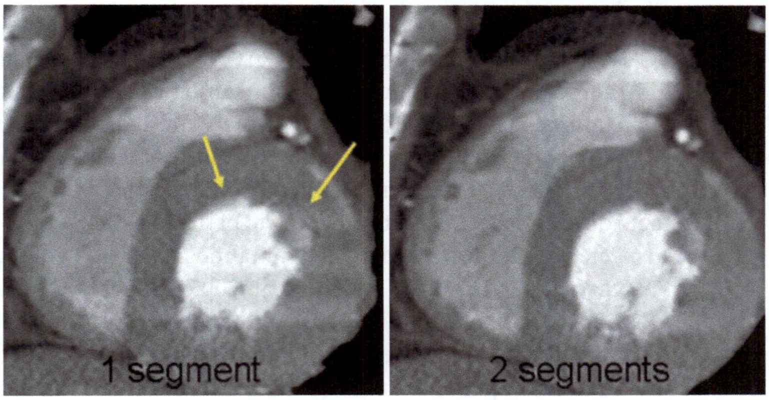

Fig. 3.1.30. CT angiographic study of a patient with a heart rate of 101–108 bpm during examination. Scan data were acquired on a 64-slice CT with 32 × 0.6-mm detector collimation, simultaneous acquisition of 64 slices by means of a z-flying focal spot and 330-ms gantry rotation time. The images were reconstructed in end-systole for functional evaluation. The temporal resolution was 165 ms for single-segment reconstruction and 83–105 ms for two-segment reconstruction, resulting in sharper delineation of the myocardial wall and a reduction of blurring caused by cardiac motion. (Case courtesy of Dr. C. Becker, Klinikum Großhadern, LMU, Munich, Germany)

tion with more than two segments, however, are usually not recommended as they require scanning with reduced pitch values resulting in increased radiation exposure. A first phantom study using DSCT (Mahnken et al. 2007) demonstrates a smaller deviation from the phantom's real volumes with DSCT than with single-source CT due to better temporal resolution. Comparing dual-source data reconstruction with single-source data reconstruction, the percent deviation from the phantom's real volumes for EF was 0.7% (dual-source, single-segment) and 4.3% (single-source). More importantly, there was no correlation between heart rate and EF for dual-source data reconstruction, whereas a relevant correlation was observed for single-source data reconstruction. The authors conclude that DSCT allows reliable quantification of global ventricular function independent of the heart rate, and that multi-segment image reconstruction is not needed for DSCT assessment of global ventricular function.

Both left and right ventricular function parameters can be derived from the original axial slices or from MPRs orthogonal to the ventricular axes. In order to minimize the total amount of reconstructed slices in a study it is sufficient to use a slice width of about 2 mm with a slice increment between 1 mm and 2 mm for reconstruction of axial slices or MPRs that are used as an input for cardiac function analysis. In the case of retrospectively ECG-gated image acquisition with ECG-controlled dose modulation the evaluation of cardiac function parameters is still feasible despite the reduced radiation dose and higher image noise during systole. Functional evaluation is not possible for ECG-triggered sequential coronary CTA, since the scan data cannot be reconstructed in systole and diastole.

3.1.4.6 Cardio-thoracic Examinations

ECG-synchronized imaging of the heart and the cardio-thoracic vessels with one CT scan can be useful for comprehensive diagnosis in patients with chest pain, in patients before and after cardio-thoracic intervention or surgery, in a variety of cardio-thoracic diseases and in adult or pediatric patients with suspected or known cardio-thoracic abnormalities (Ohnesorge et al. 2005; Gaspar et al. 2005; White et al. 2005; Ghersin et al. 2006). With 16-slice CT scanners a reasonable breath-hold time below 30 s to cover the required scan range of about 300 mm can only be achieved with protocols that apply slice collimations between 1.0 and 1.5 mm. With these protocols visualization of the cardiac anatomy is feasible, but diagnosis of the coronary arteries will be compromised. However, 64-slice CT scanners can overcome these limitations, since they are able to cover the entire chest in an ECG-gated mode with sub-millimeter collimation for comprehensive diagnosis of the cardio-thoracic vessels including the coronary arteries. Thus 64-slice CT enables the rapid triage of patients in the emergency room who present with equivocal chest pain, non-diagnostic ECG, and negative serum markers. Such patients usually undergo a period of observation with repeated assessment of ECG and cardiac markers and further work-up. Inclusion of 64-slice CT into the diagnostic algorithm allows for rapid diagnosis of common causes of acute chest pain, such as pulmonary embolism, aortic dissection, aortic and pulmonary aneurysm or significant coronary artery disease (Schoepf 2007) (Fig. 3.1.31). However, retrospectively ECG-gated multi-slice spiral scanning with high resolution and long scan ranges can result in considerable radiation exposure which is of particular concern in patients with low likelihood of disease. Therefore, scan techniques and protocols for ECG-synchronized CT angiography of the chest have to be carefully selected according to the clinical indication. Some 64-slice CT systems are equipped with special protocols for ECG-gated examinations of the chest that utilize higher pitch values up to 0.3 for increased scan speed and reduced radiation exposure (Johnson et al. 2007). Even if image reconstruction is then limited to single-segment algorithms, the shorter examination time and reduced radiation exposure are clinically beneficial. In combination with the use of ECG-controlled dose modulation radiation exposure can be limited to about 12 mSv for a scan range of 300 mm (Fig. 3.1.32).

Dedicated contrast media protocols and accurate timing of the contrast bolus are required to enable the visualization of both pulmonary arterial and systemic arterial circulation of the chest with a single injection. In general, more contrast material than for pure heart examinations is required since the bolus enhancement has to be extended over a longer scan time. While 120–150 ml of contrast agent are adequate for 16- to 40-slice CT scanners, the contrast volume can be limited to 100–120 ml with 64-slice CT scanners. Flow rates of 4 ml/s seem to be feasible for all scanner types. The use of a saline chaser bolus is recommended. Shorter delay times of 18–20 s are normally used to balance the contrast enhancement

Fig. 3.1.31. 64-Slice CT as a triage tool in the emergency room allows for rapid diagnosis of common causes of acute chest pain, such as pulmonary embolism, aortic dissection, or significant coronary artery disease. (Courtesy of Dr. H. Alkadhi, University Hospital Zurich, Switzerland)

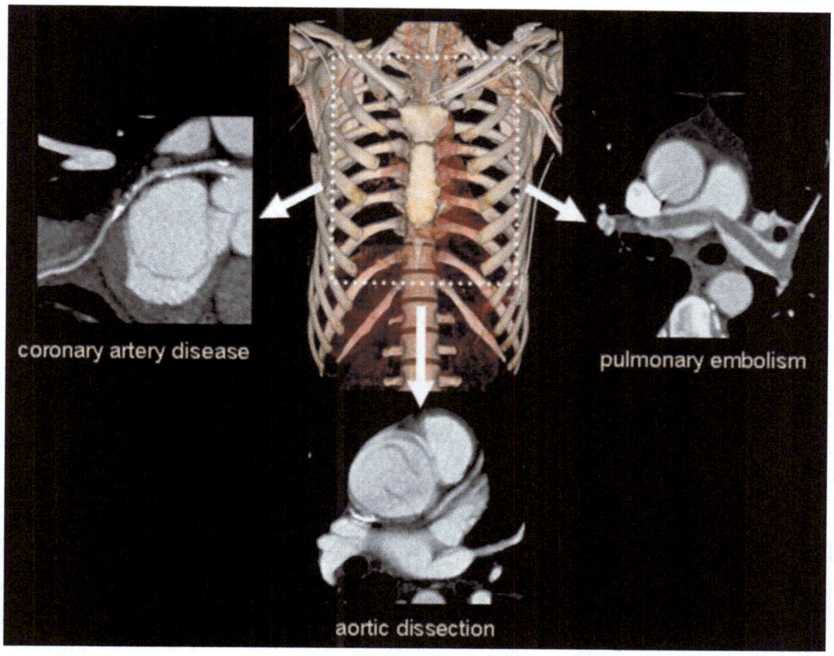

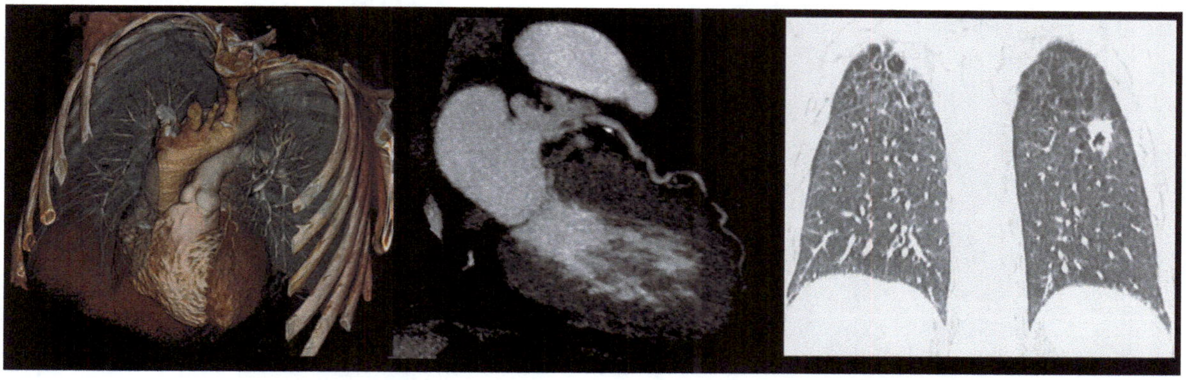

Fig. 3.1.32. ECG-gated acquisition of the chest in a 52-year-old man with a smoking history of 25 pack years who presented in the emergency department with acute chest pain but had negative serum markers. Scan data were acquired on a 64-slice CT with 32 · 0.6-mm detector collimation, simultaneous acquisition of 64 slices by means of a z-flying focal spot, 330-ms gantry rotation time and pitch 0.3. Focused reconstruction of the coronary arteries showed mildly obstructive atherosclerotic plaque in the left anterior descending artery (*center*). Lung-window reconstruction of the entire chest revealed incidental squamous cell carcinoma of the left upper lobe of the lung (*right*). (Images courtesy of Dr. U. J. Schoepf, MUSC, Charleston, South Carolina, USA)

of thoracic aorta, heart chambers, pulmonary arteries, and coronary arteries.

3.1.5 Advanced Image Post-Processing

In addition to the on-going refinement of CT acquisition technology with the goal of integrating cardiac CT into routine clinical protocols, advanced visualization and evaluation tools have been developed. They provide the user with optimized clinical workflow solutions, e.g. for vessel segmentation and vessel analysis, and detailed reporting functionality. These advanced application packages make use of all available 3D post-processing techniques such as MPRs, MIPs and VRTs to simplify and streamline the clinical workflow. Typically, MPRs and VRTs of a coronary CTA image data set are shown for a first orientation, with the rib cage automatically removed. Vessels can then be automatically segmented to calculate curved MPRs or curved MIPs along the respective center lines. Two different types of vessel segmentation are currently used. In a vessel probe approach, a marker (mouse click) is placed in the vessel of interest. A centerline extending on both sides of the marker is calculated, and the corresponding vessel segment is displayed as a curved MPR. In a vessel segmentation approach, the entire coronary artery tree is segmented as a first step. Arteries or branches that are not initially recognized by the segmentation algorithm can usually be appended by marking them with a mouse click. The user can then define centerlines between two arbitrary points on that tree as a basis for further evaluation. MPRs on straight planes perpendicular to the centerline of the vessel are shown in addition to curved MPRs to facilitate the comprehensive evaluation of coronary stenosis and plaques. In some of these advanced application packages, the degree of a stenosis has to be manually measured (e.g. by a length measurement using an electronic ruler), in some others, it is automatically determined by calculating area ratios of the vessel's cross sections. Figure 3.1.33 shows a screenshot of a comprehensive cardiac evaluation tool (syngo Circula-

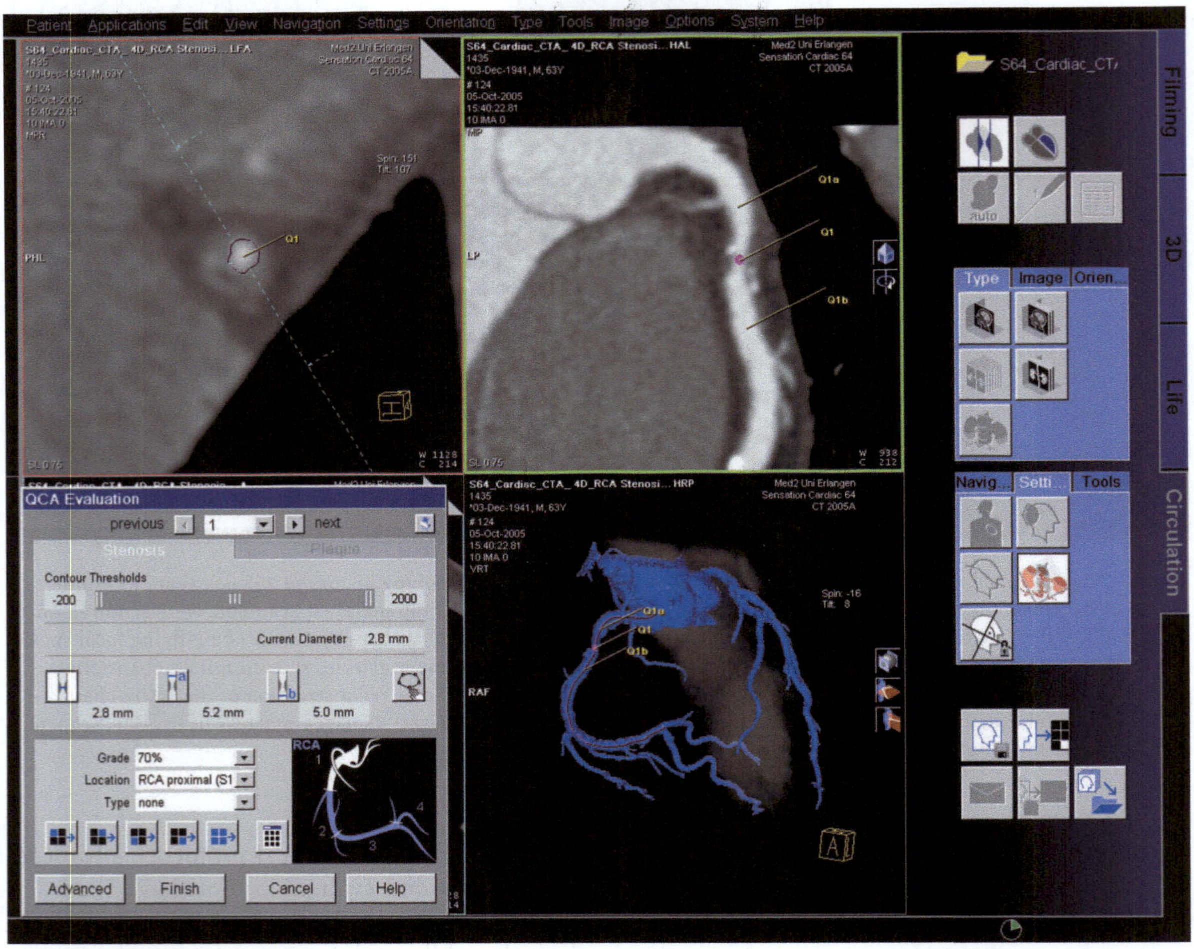

Fig. 3.1.33. Case study demonstrating advanced vessel analysis in a patient with a significant stenosis in the right coronary artery (RCA) (courtesy of Dr. S. Achenbach, Erlangen University, Germany). The images are processed using an advanced cardiac evaluation package (syngo Circulation, Siemens, Forchheim, Germany). Segmented coronary artery tree with a centerline along the RCA and three markers indicating the high-grade stenosis (*bottom right*), curved multiplanar reformation along the RCA following the centerline (*top right*) and cross section perpendicular to the centerline of the RCA (*top left*). The *red dot* marks the position of the cross-sectional image. Cross sections perpendicular to the centerline of a vessel are helpful for an evaluation of the vessel, in this case for the grading of the stenosis

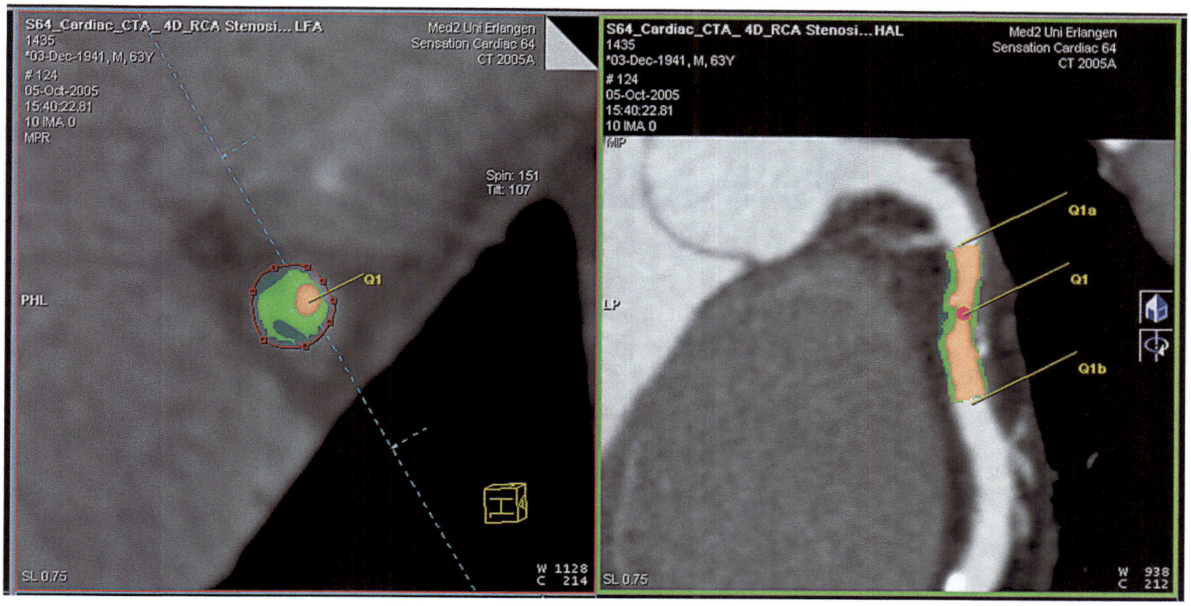

Fig. 3.1.34. Plaque evaluation tool, assigning different colors to voxels within different ranges of CT numbers. In this example, a stenosis in the right coronary artery is evaluated (see also Fig. 3.1.33). *Dark green* is used for voxels with CT numbers between -25 HU and 50 HU (potential "lipid" plaques), *light green* is used for voxels with CT numbers between 50 HU and 150 HU (potential "fibrous" plaques), *orange* is used for voxels between 150 HU and 500 HU (contrast filled lumen), and *pink* is used for voxels with CT numbers > 500 HU (calcifications)

tion, Siemens, Forchheim, Germany). The bottom right image represents a VRT of the segmented coronary artery tree with a centerline (indicated in red) along the RCA. Three markers indicate a high-grade stenosis in the RCA. The top right image shows a curved MPR along this centerline. The top left image shows a cross section perpendicular to the centerline at the position indicated by the red dot in the top right image.

As an addition to vessel segmentation approaches the development of advanced evaluation tools is ongoing that help visualize and quantify plaques in the coronary arteries. Figure 3.1.34 shows a curved MPR along the RCA and a cross-sectional image perpendicular to the centerline for the same patient as in Fig. 3.1.33. Using a plaque-evaluation tool, the voxels belonging to four different ranges of CT numbers, that may represent different types of plaques, are color-coded. The volume of the compartments can be calculated, and an individual "plaque burden" can be derived for the patient. Clinical studies are needed to evaluate the potential and the clinical relevance of these plaque quantification tools. Ideally, they could, for example, be used to monitor the therapy response of patients undergoing medical treatment aimed at reducing their total plaque burden.

Finally, new post-processing tools enable an automatic volumetric segmentation of the contrast-enhanced cardiac chambers and the calculation of global cardiac function parameters such as EF or stroke volume.

Appendix. Meta-analysis of 36 clinical studies on the detection of significant coronary artery stenoses (> 50% in diameter) with the different generations of CT systems in comparison with conventional catheter angiography, on a per-segment basis. The mean values for the respective CT systems (4-, 16-, 64-slices) are weighted by the corresponding numbers of evaluable segments

Reference	CT (slices)	Prevalence CAD	Sensitivity Specificity	Assessed segments	Minimum diameter	Mean HR	Beta-blocker prior to scan
Nieman et al. (2001)	4			73% 173/237			
Achenbach et al. (2001)	4		91% 84%	68% 174/256	2 mm		
Knez et al. (2001)	4	70%	78% 98%	94% 358/387	2 mm	65 ± 7	
Becker et al. (2002)	4	64%	81% 90%	95% 187/196	1.5 mm	58 ± 8	No, patients < 74.5 bpm only
Vogl et al. (2002)	4		75% 99%	100% 1039	1.8 mm	64.2	Yes, > 70 bpm
Nieman et al. (2002b)	4	62%	82% 93%	70% 358/512	2 mm		No
Nieman et al. (2002c)	4	75%	84% 95%	68% 505/741	2 mm	68 ± 12.1	No
Leber et al. (2003b)	4	67%	82% 96%	80% 653/795	2 mm	64 ± 7	Yes, > 70 bpm
Morghan-Hughes et al. (2003)	4		72% 86%	68% 140/206	Proximal/ mid only	64 ± 12	No, patients < 75 bpm only
Kuettner et al. (2004b)	4	100%	66% 98%	57% 487/858	all	67.2 ± 11.3	
Gerber et al. (2005)	4	81%	79% 71%	100% 294	1.5 mm	60 ± 7	Yes
Weighted mean four-slices			78% 94%	79% (4368/5521)		64.5	
Nieman et al. (2002a)	16	86%	95% 86%	100% 231	2 mm	56 ± 6	Yes, > 65 bpm
Ropers et al. (2003)	16	53%	92% 93%	88% 270/308	1.5 mm	62 ± 10	Yes, > 60 bpm
Mollet et al. (2004)	16	83%	92% 95%	100% 1384	2 mm	57.7 ± 7.7	Yes, > 65 bpm
Hoffmann et al. (2004)	16	67%	63% 96%	100% 530	all	60 ± 7	Yes, > 65 bpm
Dewey et al. (2004)	16		88% 94%	98% 133/136			No
Küttner et al. (2004a)	16	60%	72% 97%	100% 780	all	63.5 ± 10.3	Yes
Martuscelli et al. (2004)	16	67%	89% 98%	84% 613/729	1.5 mm	59 ± 5	Yes

Reference	CT (slices)	Prevalence CAD	Sensitivity Specificity	Assessed segments	Minimum diameter	Mean HR	Beta-blocker prior to scan
Hoffmann et al. (2005)	16	56%	95% 98%	93.6 1296/1384	1.5 mm	68.7 ± 12	Yes, > 75 bpm
Schuijf (2005)	16	98%	98% 97%	94% 298/317		65 ± 7	
Mollet et al. (2005a)	16	63%	95% 98%	100% 610	2 mm	57.1 ± 1	Yes, > 70 bpm
Achenbach et al. (2005)	16	54%	94% 96%	96% 635/663	1.5 mm	58 ± 6	Yes, > 60 bpm
Dorgelo et al. (2005)	16	100%	94% 96%	98% 257/262	2 mm	64.3 ± 9.1	Yes, > 70 bpm
Kuettner et al. (2005)	16	50%	82% 98%	100% 936	all	64.1 ± 9.2	Yes, > 65 bpm
Dewey et al. (2006)	16	52%	82% 90%	93% 402/430	1.5 mm	70 ± 11	
Morgan-Hughes et al. (2005)	16	56%	83% 97%	100% 675	all	64 ± 15	
Coles et al. (2006)	16	74%	92% 55%	78% 970/1243	all	60 ± 5	Yes, > 65 bpm
Kefer et al. (2007)	16	54%	67% 99%	100% 518	1.5 mm	61 ± 8	
Weighted mean 16-slices			87% 93%	95% (10538/11136)		62.0	
Raff et al. (2005)	64		95% 86%	88% 935/1065	all	65 ± 10	Yes, > 65 bpm
Mollet et al. (2005b)	64		99% 95%	100% 725	all	57.8 ± 5.8	Yes, >70 bpm
Leber et al. (2005)	64		73% 97%	100% 798	all	62 ± 13	Yes, > 70 bpm
Leschka et al. (2005)	64		94% 97%	100% 1005	1.5 mm	66.3 ± 14.7	No
Ghostine et al. (2006)	64		72% 99%	100% 990	all	67 ± 13	Yes, > 70 bpm
Pugliese et al. (2006)	64	71%	99% 96%	100% 494	all	58 ± 6	Yes, > 70 bpm
Meijboom et al. (2007)	64	85%	92% 91%	100% 1525	all	60 ± 8	Yes, > 65 bpm
Weighted mean 64-slices			89% 94%	98% (6472/6602)		62.6	
Scheffel et al. (2006)	DSCT		96.4% 97.5%	100% 420	1.5 mm	70.3 ± 14.2	No

References

Achenbach S, Moshage W, Ropers D, Nössen J, Daniel WG (1998) Value of electron-beam computed tomography for the non-invasive detection of high-grade coronary artery stenoses and occlusions. N Engl J Med 339:1964–71

Achenbach S, Ropers D, Holle J et al. (2000) In-plane coronary arterial motion velocity: measurement with electron beam CT. Radiology 216:457–463

Achenbach S, Giesler T, Ropers D, Ulzheimer S, Derlien H, Schulte C, Wenkel E, Moshage W, Bautz W, Daniel WG, Kalender WA, Baum U (2001) Contrast-enhanced, retrospectively electrocardiographically-gated, multislice spiral computed tomography. Ciculation 103:2535–2538

Achenbach S, Moselewski F, Ropers D, Ferencik M, Hoffmann U, MacNeill B, Pohle K, Baum U, Anders K, Jang IK, Daniel WG, Brady TJ (2004) Detection of calcified and noncalcified coronary atherosclerotic plaque by contrast-enhanced, submillimeter multidetector spiral computed tomography: a segment-based comparison with intravascular ultrasound. Circulation 109:14–17

Achenbach S, Ropers D, Pohle FK, Raaz D, von Erffa J, Yilmaz A, Muschiol G, Daniel WG (2005) Detection of coronary artery stenoses using multi-detector CT with 16×0.75 collimation and 375 ms rotation. Eur Heart J 26:1978–1986

Achenbach S, Ropers D, Kuettner A, Flohr T, Ohnesorge B, Bruder H, Theessen H, Karakaya M, Daniel WG, Bautz W, Kalender WA, Anders K (2006) Contrast-enhanced coronary artery visualization by dual-source computed tomography – initial experience. Eur J Radiol 57:331–335

Agatston AS, Janowitz WR, Hildner FJ, Zusmer NR, Viamonte M, Detrano R (1990) Quantification of coronary artery calcium using ultrafast computed tomography. JACC 15:827–832

Austen WG, Edwards JE, Frye RL, Gensini GG, Gott VL, Griffith LS, McGoon DC, Murphy ML, Roe BB (1975) A reporting system on patients evaluated for coronary artery disease. Report of the Ad Hoc Committee for Grading of Coronary Artery Disease, Council on Cardiovascular Surgery, American Heart Association. Circulation 51[4 Suppl]:5–40

Bahner ML, Böse J, Lutz A, Wallschläger H, Regn J, van Kaick G (1999) Retrospectively ECG-gated spiral CT of the heart and lung. Eur Radiol 9:106–109

Becker CR, Jakobs TF, Aydemir S, Becker A, Knez A, Schöpf UJ, Brüning R, Haberl R, Reiser MF (2000a) Helical and single-slice conventional CT versus electron beam CT for the quantification of coronary artery calcification. AJR Am J Roentgenol 174:543–547

Becker CR, Knez A, Ohnesorge B, Schoepf UJ, Reiser MF (2000b) Imaging of noncalcified coronary plaques using helical CT with retrospective ECG-gating. AJR Am J Roentgenol 175:423–444

Becker CR, Knez A, Leber A, Treede H, Ohnesorge B, Schoepf UJ, Reiser MF (2002) Detection of coronary artery stenoses with multislice helical CT angiography. JCAT 26:750–755

Becker CR, Nikolaou K, Muders M, Babaryka G, Crispin A, Schoepf UJ, Loehrs U, Reiser MF (2003) Ex vivo coronary atherosclerotic plaque characterization with multi-detector-row CT. Eur Radiol 13:2094–2098

Boyd DP, Lipton MJ (1982) Cardiac computed tomography. Proceedings of the IEEE, 71:298–307

Cademartiri F, Mollet NR, Runza G, Baks T, Midiro M, McFadden EP, Flohr TG, Ohnesorge B, de Feyter PJ, Krestin GP (2006) Improving diagnostic accuracy of MDCT coronary angiography in patients with mild heart rhythm irregularities using ECG editing. AJR Am J Roentgenol 186:634–638

Carrascosa PM, Capunay CM, Garcia-Merletti P, Carrascosa J, Garcia MF (2006) Characterization of coronary atherosclerotic plaques by multidetector computed tomography. Am J Cardiol 97:598–602

Caussin C, Ohanessian A, Ghostine S, Jacq L, Lancelin B, Dambrin G, Sigal-Cinqualbre A, Angel CY, Paul JF (2004) Characterization of vulnerable nonstenotic plaque with 16-slice computed tomography compared with intravascular ultrasound. Am J Cardiol 94:99–100

Coles DR, Wilde P, Oberhoff M, Rogers CA, Karsch KR, Baumbach A (2006) Multislice computed tomography coronary angiography in patients admitted with a suspected acute coronary syndrome. Int J Cardiovascular Imag (published online)

De Backer G, Ambrosioni E, Borch-Johnsen K et al. (2003) European guidelines on cardiovascular disease prevention in clinical practice – third joint task force of European and other societies (executive summary). Eur Heart J 24:1601–1610

Dewey M, Laule M, Krug L et al. (2004) Multisegment and halfscan reconstruction of 16-slice computed tomography for detection of coronary artery stenoses. Invest Radiol 39:223–229

Dewey M, Telge F, Schnapauff D, Laule M, Borges AC, Wernecke KD, Schink T, Baumann G, Rutsch W, Rogalla P, Taupitz M, Hamm B (2006) Noninvasive detection of coronary artery stenoses with multislice computed tomography or magnetic resonance imaging. Ann Intern Med 145:407–415

Dorgelo J, Willems TP, Geluk CA, van Ooijen PMA, Zijlstra F, Oudkerk M (2005) Multidetector computed tomography guided treatment strategy in patients with non-ST elevation acute coronary syndromes: a pilot study. Eur Radiol 15:708–713

Endo M, Mori S, Kandatsu S, Tanada S, Sugihara N, Saito Y, Adachia A, Miyazaki H (2005) Development of real 4D CT with real-time reconstruction and display. IEEE Nuclear Science Symposium Conference Record, vol. 5:2603–2606

Flohr T, Ohnesorge B (2001) Heart rate adaptive optimization of spatial and temporal resolution for ECG-gated multi-slice spiral CT of the heart. JCAT 25:907–923

Flohr T, Stierstorfer K, Bruder H, Simon J, Schaller S (2002a) New technical developments in multislice CT, part 1: approaching isotropic resolution with sub-mm 16-slice scanning. Fortschr Röntgenstr 174:839–845

Flohr T, Stierstorfer K, Bruder H, Simon J, Schaller S, Ohnesorge B (2002b) New technical developments in multislice CT, part 2: sub-millimeter 16-slice scanning and increased gantry rotation speed for cardiac imaging. RöFo Fortschr Röntgenstr 174:1022–1027

Flohr T, Ohnesorge B, Bruder H, Stierstorfer K, Simon J, Suess C, Schaller S (2003) Image reconstruction and performance evaluation for ECG-gated spiral scanning with a 16-slice CT system, Med Phys 30:2650–2662

Flohr T, Stierstorfer K, Raupach R, Ulzheimer S, Bruder H (2004) Performance evaluation of a 64-slice CT-system

with z-flying focal spot. Röfo Fortschr Geb Röntgenstr Neuen Bildgeb Verfahr 176:1803–1810
Flohr TG, Stierstorfer K, Ulzheimer S, Bruder H, Primak AN, McCollough CH (2005) Image reconstruction and image quality evaluation for a 64-slice CT scanner with z-flying focal spot. Med Phys 32:2536–2547
Flohr TG, McCollough CH, Bruder H, Petersilka M, Gruber K, Süß C, Grasruck M, Stierstorfer K, Krauss B, Raupach R, Primak AN, Küttner A, Achenbach S, Becker C, Kopp A, Ohnesorge BM (2006) First performance evaluation of a dual-source CT (DSCT) system. Eur Radiol 16:256–268
Gaspar T, Halon D, Rubinshtein R, Peled N (2005) Clinical applications and future trends in cardiac CTA. Eur Radiol 15[Suppl 4]:D10–D14
Gerber BL, Coche E, Pasquet A, Ketelslegers E, Vancraeynest D, Grandin C, van Beers BE, Vanoverschelde JLJ (2005) Coronary artery stenosis: direct comparison of four-section multi-detector row CT and 3D navigator MR imaging for detection – initial Results. Radiology 234:98–108
Ghersin E, Litmanovich D, Dragu R, Rispler S, Lessick J, Amos O, Brook OR, Grubergc L, Beyar R, Engel A (2006) 16-MDCT coronary angiography versus invasive coronary angiography in acute chest pain syndrome: a blinded prospective study (2006). AJR Am J Roentgenol 186:177–184
Ghostine S, Caussin C, Daoud B, Habis M, Perrier E, Pesenti-Rossi D, Sigal-Cinqualbre A, Angel CY, Lancelin B, Capderou A, Paul JF (2006) Non-invasive detection of coronary artery disease in patients with left bundle branch block using 64-slice computed tomography. JACC 48:1929–1934
Glagov S, Weisenberg E, Zarins C, Stankunavicius R, Kolettis G (1987) Compensatory enlargement of human atherosclerotic coronary rteries. N Engl J Med 316:1371–1375
Greuter MJW, Flohr T, van Ooijen PMA, Oudkerk M (2007) A model for temporal resolution of multidetector computed tomography of coronary arteries in relation to rotation time, heart rate and reconstruction algorithm. Eur Radiol 17:784–812
Haage P, Schmitz-Rode T, Hubner D, Piroth W, Gunther RW (2000) Reduction of contrast material dose and artifacts by a saline flush using a double power injector in helical CT of the thorax. AJR Am J Roentgenol 174:1049–53
Halliburton SS, Stillman AE, Flohr T, Ohnesorge B, Obuchowski N, Lieber M, Karim W, Kuzmiak S, Kasper JM, White RD (2003) Do segmented reconstruction algorithms for cardiac multi-slice computed tomography improve image quality? Herz 28:20–31
Hausleiter J, Meyer T, Hadarnitzky M, Huber E, Zankl M, Martinoff S, Kastrati A, Schömig A (2006) Radiation dose estimates from cardiac multislice computed tomography in daily practice. Circulation 113:1305–1310
Hendel RC, Patel MR, Kramer CM, Poon M et al. (2006) ACCF/ACR/SCCT/SCMR/ASNC/NASCI/SCAI/SIR 2006 appropriateness criteria for cardiac computed tomography and cardiac magnetic resonance imaging: a report of the American College of Cardiology Foundation Quality Strategic Directions Committee Appropriateness Criteria Working Group, American College of Radiology, Society of Cardiovascular Computed Tomography, Society for Cardiovascular Magnetic Resonance, American Society of Nuclear Cardiology, North American Society for Cardiac Imaging, Society for Cardiovascular Angiography and Interventions, and Society of Interventional Radiology. JACC 48:1475–1497
Herzog C, Abolmaali N, Balzer JO, Baunach S, Ackermann H, Dogan S, Britten MB, Vogl TJ (2002) Heart-rate-adapted image reconstruction in multidetector-row cardiac CT: influence of physiological and technical prerequisite on image quality. Eur Radiol 12:2670–8
Heuschmid M, Küttner A, Schröder S et al. (2003) Left ventricular functional parameters using ECG-gated multidetector spiral CT in comparison with invasive ventriculography. Fortschr Röntgenstr 175:1349–1354
Heuschmid M, Rothfuss J, Schröder S et al. (2005) Left ventricular functional parameters: comparison of 16-slice spiral CT with MRI. Fortschr Röntgenstr 177:60–66
Heuschmid M, Rothfuss JK, Schroeder S, Fenchel M, Stauder N, Burgstahler C, Franow A, Kuzo RS, Kuettner A, Miller S, Claussen CD, Kopp AF (2006) Assessment of left ventricular myocardial function using 16-slice multidetector-row computed tomography: comparison with magnetic resonance imaging and echocardiography. Eur Radiol 16:551–559
Hittmair K, Fleischmann D (2001) Accuracy of predicting and controlling time dependent aortic enhancement from a test bolus injection. J Comput Assist Tomogr 25:287–94
Hoffmann U, Moselewski F, Cury RC, Ferencik M, Jang I, Diaz LJ, Abbara S, Brady TJ, Achenbach S (2004) Predictive value of 16-slice multidetector spiral computed tomography to detect significant obstructive coronary artery disease in patients at high risk for coronary artery disease. Circulation 110:2638–2643
Hoffmann MHK, Shi H, Schmitz BL, Schmid FT, Lieberknecht M, Schulze R, Ludwig B, Kroschel U, Jahnke N, Haerer W, Brambs HJ, Aschoff AJ (2005) Noninvasive coronary angiography with multislice computed tomography. JAMA 293:2471–2478
Hohl C, Mühlenbruch G, Wildberger JE, Leidecker C, Süss C, Schmidt T, Günther RW, Mahnken AH (2006) Estimation of radiation exposure in low-dose multislice computed tomography of the heart and comparison with a calculation program. Eur Radiol 16:1841–6
Hong C, Becker CR, Huber A, Schöpf UJ, Ohnesorge B, Knez A, Brüning R, Reiser MF (2001) ECG-gated reconstructed multi-detector row CT coronary angiography: effect of varying trigger delay on image quality. Radiology 220:712–717
Hopper KD, Mosher TJ, Kasales CJ, Ten Have TR, Tully DA, Weaver JS (1997) Thoracic spiral CT: delivery of contrast material pushed with injectable saline solution in a power injector. Radiology 205:269–71
Hsieh J, Londt J, Vass M, Li J, Tang X, Okerlund D. (2006) Step-and-shoot data acquisition and reconstruction for cardiac x-ray computed tomography. Med Phys 33:4236–48
Hunold P, Vogt FM, Schmermund A, Debatin JF, Kerkhoff G, Budde T, Erbel R, Ewen K, Barkhausen J (2003) Radiation exposure during cardiac CT: effective doses at multi-detector row CT and electron-beam CT. Radiology 226:145–152
Jakobs T, Becker CR, Ohnesorge B, Flohr T, Schoepf UJ, Reiser MF (2002) Reduction of radiation exposure with ECG-controlled tube current modulation for retrospectively ECG-gated helical scans of the heart. Eur Radiol 12:1081–1086

Johnson TRC, Nikolaou K, Wintersperger BJ, Leber AW, von Ziegler F, Rist C, Buhmann S, Knez A, Reiser MF, Becker CR (2006) Dual source cardiac CT imaging: initial experience. Eur Radiol 16:1409–1415

Johnson TR, Nikolaou K, Wintersperger BJ, Knez A, Boekstegers P, Reiser MF, Becker CR (2007) ECG-gated 64-MDCT angiography in the differential diagnosis of acute chest pain. AJR Am J Roentgenol 188:76–82

Juergens KU, Grude M, Fallenberg EM et al. (2002) Using ECG-gated multidetector CT to evaluate global left ventricular myocardial function in patients with coronary artery disease. AJR Am J Roentgenol 179:1545–1550

Juergens KU, Maintz D, Grude M et al. (2004) Semiautomated analysis of left ventricular function using 16-slice multidetector-row computed tomography (MDCT) of the heart in comparison to steady-state-free-precession (SSFP) cardiac magnetic resonance imaging. Eur Radiol 14:S2–272

Juergens KU, Maintz D, Grude M, Boese JM, Heimes B, Fallenberg EM, Heindel W, Fischbach R (2005) Multi-detector row computed tomography of the heart: does a multi-segment reconstruction algorithm improve left ventricular volume measurements? Eur Radiol 15:111–117

Kachelrieß M, Ulzheimer S, Kalender WA (2000) ECG-correlated image reconstruction from subsecond multi-row spiral CT scans of the heart. Med Phys 27:1881–1902

Kalender WA, Schmidt B, Zankl M, Schmidt M (1999) A PC program for estimating organ dose and effective dose values in computed tomography. Eur Radiol 9:555–562

Kefer JM, Coche E, Vanoverschelde JLJ, Gerber BL (2007) Diagnostic accuracy of 16-slice multidetector-row CT for detection of in-stent restenosis vs detection of stenosis. Eur Radiol 17:87–96

Kido T, Kurata A, Higashino H, Sugawara Y, Okayama H, Higaki J, Anno H, Katada K, Mori S, Tanada S, Endo M, Mochizuki T (2007) Cardiac imaging using 256-detector row four-dimensional CT: preliminary clinical report. Radiat Med 25:38–44

Klingenbeck K, Schaller S, Flohr T, Ohnesorge B, Kopp AF, Baum U (1999) Subsecond multi-slice computed tomography : basics and applications. Eur J Radiol 31:110–124

Knez A, Becker CR, Leber A, Ohnesorge B, Reiser MF, Haberl R (2000) Non-invasive assessment of coronary artery stenoses with multidetector helical computed tomography. Circulation 101:e221–e222

Knez A, Becker CR, Leber A, Ohnesorge B, Becker A, White C, Haberl R, Reiser MF, Steinbeck G (2001) Usefulness of multislice spiral computed tomography angiography for determination of coronary artery stenoses. Am J Cardiol 88:1191–1194

Kondo C, Mori S, Endo M, Kusakabe K, Suzuki N, Hattori A, Kusakabe M (2005) Real-time volumetric imaging of human heart without electrocardiographic gating by 256-detector row computed tomography: initial experience. J Comput Assist Tomogr 29:694–698

Kopp AF, Schröder S, Küttner A, Heuschmid M, Georg C, Ohnesorge B, Kuzo R, Claussen CD (2001) Coronary arteries: retrospectively ECG-gated multi-detector row CT angiography with selective optimization of the reconstruction window. Radiology 221:683–688

Kopp AF, Schröder S, Küttner A, Baumbach A, Heuschmid M, Georg C, Kuzo R, Ohnesorge B, Karsch K, Claussen CD (2002) High resolution multi-slice computed tomography with retrospective gating for angiography in coronary arteries: Results in 102 patients. Eur Heart J 23:1714–1725

Kopp AF, Heuschmid M, Reinmann A et al. (2005) Evaluation of cardiac function and myocardial viability with 16- and 64-slice multidetector computed tomography. Eur Radiol 15[Suppl 4]:D15–D20

Kuettner A, Trabold T, Schroeder S, Feyer A, Beck T, Brueckner A, Heuschmid M, Burgstahler C, Kopp AF, Claussen CD (2004a) Noninvasive detection of coronary lesions using 16-detector multislice spiral computed tomography Technology. JACC 44:1230–1237

Kuettner A, Kopp AF, Schroeder S, Rieger T, Brunn J, Meisner C, Heuschmid M, Trabold T, Burgstahler C, Martensen J, Schoebel W, Selbmann HK, Claussen CD (2004b) Diagnostic accuracy of multidetector computed tomography coronary angiography in patients with angiographically proven coronary artery disease. JACC 43:831–839

Kuettner A, Beck T, Drosch T et al. (2005) Diagnostic accuracy of noninvasive coronary imaging using 16-detector slice spiral computed tomography with 188 ms temporal resolution. J Am Coll Cardiol 45:123–125

Leber AW, Knez A, White CW, Becker A, von Ziegler F, Muehling O, Becker C, Reiser M, Steinbeck G, Boekstegers P (2003a) Composition of coronary atherosclerotic plaques in patients with acute myocardial infarction and stable angina pectoris determined by contrast-enhanced multislice computed tomography. Am J Cardiol 91:714–718

Leber AW, Knez A, Becker C, Becker A, White C, Thilo C, Reiser M, Haberl R, Steinbeck G (2003b) Non-invasive intravenous coronary angiography using electron beam tomography and multislice computed tomography. Heart 89:633–639

Leber AW, Knez A, Becker A, Becker C, von Ziegler F, Nikolaou K, Rist C, Reiser MF, White C, Steinbeck G, Boekstegers P (2004) Accuracy of multidetector spiral computed tomography in identifying and differentiating the composition of coronary atherosclerotic plaques: a comparative study with intravascular ultrasound. JACC 43:1241–1247

Leber AW, Knez A, Ziegler F, Becker A, Nikolaou K, Paul S, Wintersperger B, Reiser MF, Becker CR, Steinbeck G, Boekstegers P (2005) Quantification of obstructive and nonobstructive coronary lesions by 64-slice computed tomography – a comparative study with quantitative coronary angiography and intravascular ultrasound. JACC 46:147–154

Leber AW, Becker A, Knez A, von Ziegler F, Sirol M, Nikolaou K, Ohnesorge B, Fayad ZA, Becker CR, Reiser M, Steinbeck G, Boekstegers P (2006) Accuracy of 64-slice computed tomography to classify and quantify plaque volumes in the proximal coronary system: a comparative study using intravascular ultrasound. J Am Coll Cardiol 47:672–677

Leschka S, Alkadhi H, Plass A, Desbiolles L, Gruenenfelder J, Marincek B, Wildermuth S (2005) Accuracy of MSCT coronary angiography with 64-slice technology: first experience. Eur Heart J 26:1482–1487

Leschka S, Wilfermuth S, Boehm Th, Desbiolles L, Husmann L, Plass A, Koepfli P, Schepis T, Marincek B, Kaufmann Ph, Alkadhi H (2006) Noninvasive coronary angiography with 64-section CT: effect of average heart rate and heart rate variability on image quality. Radiology 241:378–385

Mahnken AH, Spuentrup E, Niethammer M et al. (2003) Quantitative and qualitative assessment of left ventricu-

lar volume with ECG-gated multislice spiral CT: value of different image reconstruction algorithms in comparison to MRI. Acta Radiol 44:604–611
Mahnken AH, Hohl C, Suess C, Bruder H, Mühlenbruch G, Das M, Günther RW, Wildberger JE (2006) Influence of heart rate and temporal resolution on left-ventricular volumes in cardiac multi-slice spiral CT: a phantom study. Invest Radiol 41:429–35
Mahnken AH, Bruder H, Suess C, Muhlenbruch G, Bruners P, Hohl C, Guenther RW, Wildberger JE (2007) Dual-source computed tomography for assessing cardiac function: a phantom study. Invest Radiol 42:491–498
Martuscelli E, Romagnoli A, D'Eliseo A, Razzini C, Tomassini M, Sperandio M, Simonetti G, Romeo F (2004) Accuracy of thin-slice computed tomography in the detection of coronary stenoses. Eur Heart J 25:1043–1048
McCollough CH, Zink FE (1994a) The technical design and performance of ultrafast computed tomography. Radiol Clin North Am 32:521–536
McCollough CH, Zink FE, Morin R (1994b) Radiation dosimetry for electron beam CT. Radiology 192:637–643
McCollough CH, Kanal KM, Lanutti N, Ryan KJ (1999) Experimental determination of section sensitivity profiles and image noise in electron beam computed tomography. Med Phys 26:287–295
McCollough C (2003) Patient dose in cardiac computed tomography. Herz 28:1–6
McCollough CH, Primak AN, Saba O, Bruder H, Stierstorfer K, Raupach R, Suess C, Schmidt B, Ohnesorge BM, Flohr TG (2007) Dose performance of a 64-channel dual-source CT scanner. Radiology 243:775–784
Meijboom WB, Mollet NR, van Mieghem CA, Weustink AC, Pugliese F, van Pelt N, Cademartiri F, Vourvouri E, de Jaegere P, Krestin GP, de Feyter PJ (2007) 64-Slice computed tomography coronary angiography in patients with non-ST elevation acute coronary syndrome. Heart, published online
Mieres JH, Shaw LJ, Arai A et al. (2005) Role of noninvasive testing in the clinical evaluation of women with suspected coronary artery disease. Consensus statement of the American Heart Association. Circulation 111:682–696
Mollet NR, Cademartiri F, Nieman K, Saia F, Lemos PA, McFadden EP, Pattynama PMT, Serruys PW, Krestin GP, de Feyter PJ (2004) Multislice spiral computed tomography coronary angiography in patients with stable angina pectoris. JACC 43:2265–2270
Mollet NR, Cademartiri F, Krestin GP et al. (2005a) Improved diagnostic accuracy with 16-row multi-slice computed tomography coronary angiography. J Am Coll Cardiol 45:128–32
Mollet NR, Cademartiri F, van Mieghem CAG, Runza G, McFadden EP, Baks T, Serruys PW, Krestin GP, de Feyter PJ (2005b) High-resolution spiral computed tomography coronary angiography in patients referred for diagnostic conventional coronary angiography. Circulation 112:2318–2323
Morghan-Hughes GJ, Marshall AJ, Roobottom CA (2003) Multislice computed tomographic coronary angiography: experience in a UK centre. Clin Radiol 58:378–383
Morgan-Hughes GJ, Roobottom CA, Owens PE, Marshall AJ (2005) Highly accurate coronary angiography with submillimetre, 16-slice computed tomography. Heart 91:308–313
Mori S, Endo M, Tsunoo T, Kandatsu S, Tanada S, Aradate H et al. (2004) Physical performance evaluation of a 256-slice CT-scanner for dour-dimensional imaging. Med Phys 31:1348–1356
Mori S, Endo M, Obata T, Tsunoo T, Susumu K, Tanada S (2006a) Properties of the prototype 256-row (cone beam) CT scanner. Eur Radiol 16:2100–2108
Mori S, Kondo C, Suzuki N, Hattori A, Kusakabe M, Endo M (2006b) Volumetric coronary angiography using the 256-detector row computed tomography scanner: comparison in vivo and in vitro with porcine models. Acta Radiol 47:186–191
Mori S, Nishizawa K, Kondo C, Ohno M, Akahane K, Endo M (2007) Effective doses in subjects undergoing computed tomography cardiac imaging with the 256-multislice CT scanner. Eur J Radiol 65:442–448 [Epub ahead of print]
Morin R, Gerber T, McCollough C (2003) Radiation dose in computed tomography of the heart. Circulation 107:917–922
Niemann K, Oudkerk M, Rensing BJ, van Ooijen P, Munne A, van Geuns RJ, de Feyter P (2001) Coronary angiography with multi-slice computed tomography. Lancet 357:599–603
Nieman K, Cademartiri F, Lemos PA, Raaijmakers R, Pattynama PMT, de Feyter PJ (2002a) Reliable noninvasive coronary angiography with fast submillimeter multislice spiral computed tomography. Circulation 106:2051–2054
Nieman K, Rensing BJ, van Geuns RJM et al. (2002b) Usefulness of multislice computed tomography for detecting obstructive coronary artery disease. Am J Cardiol 89:913–918
Nieman K, Rensing BJ, van Geuns RJM, Vos J, Pattynama PMT, Krestin GP, Serruys PW, de Feyter PJ (2002c) Non-invasive coronary angiography with multislice spiral computed tomography: impact of heart rate. Heart 88:470–474
Ohnesorge B, Flohr T, Schaller S, Klingenbeck-Regn K, Becker CR, Schöpf UJ, Brüning R, Reiser MF (1999) Technische Grundlagen und Anwendungen der Mehrschicht CT. Radiologe 39:923–931
Ohnesorge B, Flohr T, Becker CR, Kopp AF, Knez A, Baum U, Klingenbeck-Regn K, Reiser MF (2000) Cardiac imaging by means of electrocardiographically gated multisection spiral CT: initial experience. Radiology 217:564–571
Ohnesorge B, Becker CR, Flohr T, Reiser MF (2002) Multislice CT in cardiac imaging – technical principles, clinical application and future developments. Springer, Berlin Heidelberg New York, ISBN 3-540-42966-2
Ohnesorge BM, Hofmann LK, Flohr TG, Schöpf UJ (2005) CT for imaging coronary artery disease: defining the paradigm for its application. Int J Cardiovasc Imaging 21:85–104
Paul JF, Wartski M, Caussin C, Sigal-Cinqualbre A, Lancelin B, Angel C, Dambrin G (2005) Late defect on delayed contrast-enhanced multi-detector row CT scans in the prediction of SPECT infarct size after reperfused acute myocardial infarction: initial experience. Radiology 236:485–489
Pohle K, Achenbach S, MacNeill B, Ropers D, Ferencik M, Moselewski F, Hoffmann U, Brady TJ, Jang IK, Daniel WG (2007) Characterization of non-calcified coronary atherosclerotic plaque by multi-detector row CT: comparison to IVUS. Atherosclerosis 190:174–180

Pugliese F, Mollet NRA, Runza G, van Mieghem C, Meijboom WB, Malagutti P, Baks T, Krestin GP, de Feyter PJ, Cademartiri F (2006) Diagnostic accuracy of non-invasive 64-slice CT coronary angiography in patients with stable angina pectoris. Eur Radiol 16:575–582

Pundziute G, Schuijf JD, Jukema JW, Boersma E, de Roos A, van der Wall EE, Bax JJ (2007) Prognostic value of multislice computed tomography coronary angiography in patients with known or suspected coronary artery disease. JACC 49:2070–2071

Raff GL, Gallagher MJ, O'Neill WW, Goldstein JA (2005) Diagnostic accuracy of noninvasive coronary angiography using 64-slice spiral computed tomography. JACC 46:552–557

Ritman E, Kinsey J, Robb R, Gilbert B, Harris L, Wood E (1980) Three-dimensional imaging of heart, lungs, and circulation. Science 210:273–280

Robb R, Ritman E (1979) High speed synchronous volume computed tomography of the heart. Radiology 133:655–661

Ropers D, Baum U, Pohle K, Anders K, Ulzheimer S, Ohnesorge B, Schlundt C, Bautz W, Daniel WG, Achenbach S (2003) Detection of coronary artery stenoses with thin-slice multi-detector row spiral computed tomography and multiplanar reconstruction. Circulation 107:664–666

Ryan T, Anderson J, Antman E, Braniff B, Brooks N, Califf R, Hillis L, Hiratzka L, Rapaport E, Riegel B, Russell R, Smith E, Weaver W (1996) ACC/AHA guidelines for the management of patients with acute myocardial infarction. A report of the American College of Cardiology/American Heart Association Task Force on Practice Guidelines (Committee on Management of Acute Myocardial Infarction). J Am Coll Cardiol 28:1328–1428

Scheffel H, Alkadhi H, Plass A, Vachenauer R, Desbiolles L, Gaemperli O, Schepis T, Frauenfelder T, Schertler T, Husmann L, Grunenfelder J, Genoni M, Kaufmann PA, Marincek B, Leschka S (2006) Accuracy of dual-source CT coronary angiography: first experience in a high pretest probability population without heart rate control. Eur Radiol 16:2739–2747

Scheffel H, Alkadhi H, Leschka S, Plass A et al. (2008) Low-dose CT coronary angiography in the step-and-shoot mode: diagnostic performance. Heart [June 2, epub ahead of print]

Schmermund A, Rensing BJ, Sheedy PF, Bell MR, Rumberger JA (1998) Intravenous electron-beam computed tomographic coronary angiography for segmental analysis of coronary artery stenosis. Am J Cardiol 31:1547–1554

Schoepf UJ (2007) Cardiothoracic multi-slice CT in the emergency department. In: Ohnesorge BM, Flohr TG, Becker CR, Knez A, Reiser MF (eds) Multi-slice and dual-source CT in cardiac imaging, 2nd edn. Springer, Berlin Heidelberg New York

Schröder S, Kopp AF, Baumbach A, Küttner A, Georg C, Ohnesorge B, Herdeg C, Claussen CD, Karsch (2001) Non-invasive detection and evaluation of atherosclerotic plaque with multi-slice computed tomography. JACC 37:1430–1435

Schuijf JD, Baxx JJ, Salm LP, Jukema JW, Lamb HJ, van der Wall EE, de Roos A (2005) Noninvasive coronary imaging and assessment of left ventricular function using 16-slice computed tomography. Am J Cardiol 95:571-574

Silber S, Richartz BM (2005) Impact of cardiac CT and cardiac MR on the assessment of coronary risk (German). Z Kardiol 94[Suppl 4]:1–11

Stanford W, Rumberger J (1992) Ultrafast computed tomography in cardiac imaging: principles and practise. Futura Publishing Company, New York

Stolzmann P, Scheffel H, Schertler T, Frauenfelder T, Marincek B, Kaufmann PA, Alkadhi H (2007) Radiation dose estimates in dual-source computed tomography coronary angiography. Submitted for publication

Virmani R, Kolodgie FD, Burke AP, Frab A, Schwartz SM (2000) Lessons from sudden coronary death. A comprehensive morphological classification scheme for atherosclerotic lesions. Arterioscler Thromb Vasc Biol 20:1262–1275

Vogl TJ, Abolmaali ND, Diebold T, Engelmann K, Ay M, Dogan S, Wimmer-Greinecker G, Moritz A, Herzog C (2002) Techniques for the detection of coronary atherosclerosis: multi-detector row CT coronary angiography. Radiology 223:212–220

Wexler L, Brundage B, Crouse J, Detrano R, Fuster V, Maddahi J, Rumberger J, Stanford W, White R, Taubert K (1996) Coronary artery calcification: pathophysiology, epidemiology, imaging methods, and clinical implications. A statement for health professionals from the American Heart Association. Circulation 94:1175–92

White CS, Kuo D, Kelemen M, Jain V, Musk A, Zaidi E, Read K, Sliker C, Prasad R (2005) Chest pain evaluation in the emergency department: can MDCT provide a comprehensive evaluation? AJR Am J Roentgenol 185:533–540

Wintersperger BJ, Nikolaou K, von Ziegler F, Johnson T, Rist C, Leber A, Flohr T, Knez A, Reiser MF, Becker CR (2006) Image quality, motion artifacts, and reconstruction timing of 64-slice coronary computed tomography angiography with 0.33-second rotation speed. Invest Radiol 41:436–442

Ziada K, Kapadia S, Tuzcu E, Nissen S (1999) The current status of intravascular ultrasound imaging. Curr Probl Cardiol 24:541–566

Non-Invasive Coronary Imaging

3

3.2 Developments in MR Coronary Angiography

Robert R. Edelman and Debiao Li

CONTENTS

There are numerous reasons why a safe, non-invasive method for evaluating the coronary arteries would be beneficial. Diagnostic catheter angiography exposes the patient to ionizing radiation, although at a reasonably low dose. More importantly, it is an invasive procedure that involves a small risk of complications such as hemorrhage at the arterial puncture site, coronary dissection, and so forth. Although generally safe and accurate, it would not be suitable as a means to routinely follow the efficacy of medical therapy (e.g. lipid lowering therapy to reduce plaque burden). In cases where the level of clinical suspicion is equivocal, an invasive test would not be justified. Intravascular ultrasound provides an unparalleled view of coronary plaque, but is also invasive and limited in the extent of vessels that can be evaluated. Multi-detector CT (MDCT) angiography is a powerful new tool for diagnosis of coronary artery disease and already has proven accurate for diagnosing native and bypass graft coronary disease (Schoepf et al. 2007). There is little doubt that it will soon become a standard tool for the evaluation of patients with suspected coronary ischemia. Recent evidence suggests that coronary CT angiography can eliminate the need for diagnostic coronary catheterization in many patients at risk of coronary artery disease without any negative impact on patient outcome (Gilard et al. 2007). Nonetheless, significant concerns involve exposure to ionizing radiation, contrast-induced nephropathy in patients with impaired renal function, fast heart rates (at least with single X-ray source systems), and coronary calcification that can make diagnosis of a coronary stenosis problematic.

Magnetic resonance (MR) coronary angiography is a non-invasive procedure that neither requires exposure to ionizing radiation nor use of iodinated contrast agents (Stuber and Weiss 2007). Given the diagnostic tools that are already available, is there a

R. R. Edelman, MD
Department of Radiology G507, Evanston Hospital, 2650 Ridge Ave, Evanston IL 60201, USA
D. Li, PhD
Professor, Department of Radiology, Northwestern University Medical School, 737 N. Michigan Ave Ste 1600, Chicago, IL 60611, USA

niche for MR coronary angiography? The answer is "yes", but only if the accuracy of MR coronary angiography is sufficient to compete with MDCT. This is by no means a trivial task, given that MDCT coronary angiography using 64-slice scanners already has a negative predictive value approaching 100% (Herzog et al. 2007). Moreover, CT scanning is remarkably fast, providing evaluation of the entire coronary tree and other cardiac structures in under 10 s. On the other hand, MR coronary angiography has strengths that are complementary to coronary CT angiography's weaknesses. For instance, it has been shown in some patients with dense coronary calcifications that MR coronary angiography can demonstrate a stenosis not evaluable by coronary CT angiography (Langer et al. 2005; Cheng et al. 2007). The safety advantages of using MR are clear, given the absence of ionizing radiation or risk of contrast-induced nephropathy. Fast heart rates are generally not as limiting for MR as they are for single-source CT. On the other hand, MR coronary imaging techniques which involve the use of gadolinium chelates entail a risk of nephrogenic systemic fibrosis in patients with impaired renal function.

In this chapter, we will review the historical development of MR coronary angiography, starting from the early days of gated two-dimensional (2D) spin-echo, with subsequent developments including breath-hold 2D segmented gradient-echo, breath-hold navigator-gated three-dimensional (3D), whole-heart acquisitions using parallel imaging, and novel contrast agents. Potential future developments will also be considered.

3.2.1 Technical Development

Any attempt to image the coronary arteries must contend with the combined challenges of cardiac pulsation, respiratory motion, and small vessel diameter (typically 2–4 mm). Spin-echo (SE) (and subsequent turbo SE) methods naturally tend to make flowing blood appear dark. This phenomenon occurs because of gradient-induced dephasing as well as outflow of excited spins from the imaging plane before the signals are refocused by the 180° pulse. The first attempts at imaging the coronary arteries using MR involved ECG-gated SE pulse sequences (Paulin et al. 1987). Although the proximal coronary arteries could occasionally be shown, there tended to be marked image degradation from respiration. Scan times were too long to permit data acquisition during a breath-hold. Moreover, each image in a multi-slice acquisition was acquired during a different phase of the cardiac cycle, precluding 3D image processing. Finally, it is generally more difficult to evaluate the patency of small vessels with dark blood than bright blood imaging methods, particularly since there is little contrast between dark blood and dark muscle in the myocardium.

One can make the flowing blood within the heart appear bright using cine gradient-echo imaging techniques (Nayler et al. 1986). Cine imaging is used for a wide variety of clinical applications, such as measurement of ventricular function (Lotan et al. 1989). There are clear advantages to making the flowing blood in the coronary arteries appear bright. Contrast between vessel and myocardium or dense calcification is improved. Image processing is simplified, since a maximum intensity projection or volume rendering technique can be used to make a three-dimensional display of the vessels. Although portions of the coronary arteries are occasionally seen on standard cine gradient-echo scans through the heart, the images are generally too blurred from respiratory motion to permit accurate evaluation. However, two subsequent developments largely overcame the problem of respiratory motion.

The first approach involved "segmenting" or grouping the phase-encoding steps (Atkinson and Edelman 1991; Edelman et al. 1991). Instead of acquiring a single phase-encoding step per phase of the cardiac cycle within each R-R interval, anywhere from 6–12 phase-encoding steps are acquired. The duration of each segment is kept below about 150 ms to minimize blurring from cardiac motion. The acquisition of each segment is timed to occur during mid-to-late diastole when the coronary arteries are most quiescent (although the right coronary artery is sometimes better seen at end-systole). Although the temporal resolution for each phase of the cardiac cycle was reduced, the scan time was decreased by the same factor of 6–12, permitting scans to be completed within a reasonable breath-holding period of 10–20 s. Of course, it is possible to go much faster now with the implementation of parallel imaging techniques (Sodickson 2006; Pruessmann et al. 1999).

With the breath-hold segmented gradient-echo method, a series of 2D images spanning the coronary arteries are acquired over a series of breath-holds. Although image quality is adequate, it is difficult to reliably evaluate a tortuous coronary artery because of image misregistration between different breath-holds. Alternatively, one can acquire a thin slab 3D acquisition ("VCATS") with a limited number of 3D slices within a single breath-hold (van Geuns et al. 2000). Because thin, contiguous slices are acquired within each breath-holding period, coronary evaluation is more straightforward.

The next step in the technical development was the implementation of navigator techniques for coronary artery imaging (Wang and Ehman 2000; Danias et al. 1997; Stuber et al. 1999a; Li et al. 1996). Gating techniques involving an external bellows device to monitor the stage of respiration had been in existence since the early days of MRI (Ehman et al. 1984). However, these methods were unreliable, for instance being unable to monitor respiration in patients who predominant relied on their chest muscles for breathing. Navigator methods involve the detection of a signal at the interface of the dome of the diaphragm and lung tissue. The navigator signal can be produced by a slice-selective 90°–180° radiofrequency (RF) pulse pair, where the rectangular slices excited by each pulse are oriented to produce a diamond-shaped intersection. A more robust approach to producing the navigator signal involves the use of a 2D spiral RF excitation ("pencil beam") that excites a narrow cylinder of tissue.

Irrespective of the method that is used to produce the navigator signal, it allows precise monitoring of the respiratory phase. By selecting a single phase of respiration, one can minimize or eliminate blurring due to respiratory motion. The method is highly effective in most patients, although it is ineffective in a minority of patients with inconsistent breathing patterns. The main drawback of navigator gating is a reduction in scan efficiency and consequent prolongation of scan time, typically by a factor of 2–4. On the other hand, it is typically more efficient than acquiring a series of individual breath-hold scans, and better tolerated by the patient since they merely need to breathe quietly for the duration of the scan. Scan efficiency can be improved by accepting a broader range of the respiratory cycle at the expense of increased blurring. However, the blurring can be largely avoided using slice-following techniques that adjust the slice position by a factor that depends on the diaphragm position (Stuber et al. 1999b).

Using navigator techniques, it is much easier to acquire ECG-triggered 3D data sets that span large portions of the coronary artery tree. Moreover, one can obtain contiguous thin sections with near isotropic spatial resolution, which greatly simplifies the image interpretation. Free-breathing, whole-heart coronary acquisitions can be acquired in just a few minutes using a combination of parallel imaging and partial Fourier techniques (Nehrke et al. 2006). Alternatively, breath-hold whole heart MR coronary angiography can be performed using a high parallel acceleration factor in conjunction with multi-coil arrays having a large number of elements (e.g. 32) (Niendorf et al. 2004). However, the signal-to-noise ratio (SNR) will be lower than with free-breathing techniques.

3.2.2 Pulse Sequences and K-space Trajectories

Most bright blood MR coronary angiography uses gradient-echo pulse sequences whereas dark blood imaging uses turbo SE pulse sequences. Segmented gradient-echo pulse sequences suffer from limited SNR as well as saturation effects, particular when a 3D volume is acquired. More recently, balanced steady-state free precession (also called "trueFISP" or "FIESTA") techniques have been implemented (Deshpande et al. 2001). Because the TR is very short, scan times are reduced. The technique is resistant to flow artifact and provides high SNR. The main drawback is its greater sensitivity to static field inhomogeneities, resulting in banding artifacts that can make an angiogram uninterpretable. Moreover, the sequence uses a combination of very short TR and large flip angles, so that power deposition is high. Power deposition becomes a limiting factor at 3 Tesla.

A variety of k-space trajectories have been tested in an effort to maximize spatial resolution and scan efficiency. Cartesian trajectories (in widespread use for clinical MRI throughout the body) acquire one or a series of phase-encoding lines within each repetition time (or R-R interval for coronary artery imaging). Non-Cartesian trajectories, which include multi-shot echo planar, spiral, and radial, each offer potential advantages and disadvantages. For instance, high quality images of the coronary arteries have been obtained using spiral imaging, which involves simultaneous oscillation of two magnetic field gradients during signal readout (Meyer et al. 1992). Drawbacks include marked sensitivity to off-resonance effects and the need for specialized image reconstruction algorithms. Radial methods acquire a series of phase-encoding lines of data that are oriented in a radial pattern (Stehning et al. 2004). Each radial line of data passes through the center of k-space. Radial imaging methods naturally are resistant to flow-related artifacts. In addition, they are particularly useful for cine and real-time imaging. Despite these innovations, most coronary artery imaging still uses Cartesian acquisition methods.

3.2.3 Image Contrast

The proximal coronary arteries are typically embedded in epicardial fat, whereas the distal vessels are surrounded by myocardium. Several approaches have been devised to maximize contrast between the coronary arteries and the surrounding tissues. These methods include: (a) fat suppression, (b) magnetization transfer contrast (MTC); (c) T2-prep, and (d) administration of MR contrast agents. Fat signals can be suppressed by the application of a frequency-selective RF saturation pulse or by use of a spectral-spatial excitation selective for water signals. Given the static field inhomogeneity caused by nearby lung tissue, fat suppression may be imperfect but is usually adequate over most of the coronary tree.

The distal portions of the coronary arteries are embedded in muscle rather than epicardial fat, so fat suppression is not sufficient to maximize vessel conspicuity. An additional contrast mechanism is to apply a high amplitude RF pulse that is tuned hundreds of Hz away from the Larmor frequency. This technique, called MTC, causes a reduction in the signal intensity of tissues that contain substantial concentrations of macromolecules. MTC improves the conspicuity of the coronary arteries by reducing the signal intensity of myocardium while causing only a slight reduction in the signal intensity of blood within the coronary arteries (Li et al. 1993).

T2-prep is a method for reducing the signal intensity of both the myocardium and coronary veins (Brittain et al. 1995). It does so by introducing a degree of T2 contrast into the image. The method involves magnetization preparation consisting of a 90° RF pulse followed by a series of 180° pulses and finally another 90° RF pulse. Both myocardium and deoxygenated blood in the coronary veins have relatively short T2 relaxation times, which results in a marked loss of signal intensity with T2-prep. There is only a slight loss of signal in the coronary arteries, so that contrast between the coronary arteries and myocardium is improved. However, T2-prep should not be used after administration of a contrast agent since the contrast agent substantially shortens the T2 relaxation time of the blood vessels, in addition to shortening the T1 relaxation time. Examples of coronary artery images acquired on healthy volunteers using various sequences in conjunction with real-time navigator respiratory gating during free breathing are shown in Figure 3.2.1.

Vessel contrast for MR coronary angiography can be further improved by administering a paramagnetic contrast agent (Goldfarb and Edelman 1998). This is routinely done for MR angiography in the body, although without the complicating factors of cardiac motion and requirement for ECG triggering. An inversion pulse can be applied prior to each data acquisition to maximize the contrast between the blood vessel and surrounding tissues (Hofman et al. 1999). Unfortunately, standard gadolinium chelates rapidly redistribute out of the intravascular compartment, so that maximum effect is only obtained during the first pass (<30 s). The short period of peak enhancement is incompatible with navigator-based acquisitions that are several minutes in duration at a minimum. Nonetheless, promising whole-heart MR coronary angiograms have been obtained with navigator gating at 3 Tesla using a slow infusion of gadobenate dimeglumine, a high relaxivity contrast agent (Bi et al. 2007).

Alternatively, MR coronary angiography can be done after administration of a blood pool contrast agent (Li et al. 1998; Huber et al. 2003; Taylor et al. 1999). For instance, the intravascular half-lives for these agents are on the order of many minutes to hours. An example of intravascular contrast-enhanced coronary MRA is shown in Figure 3.2.2. These agents include gadolinium-based macromolecular chelates as well as iron oxide-based ultrasmall particles. Currently, several of these agents are in clinical trials and should be available for routine clinical use within the next few years.

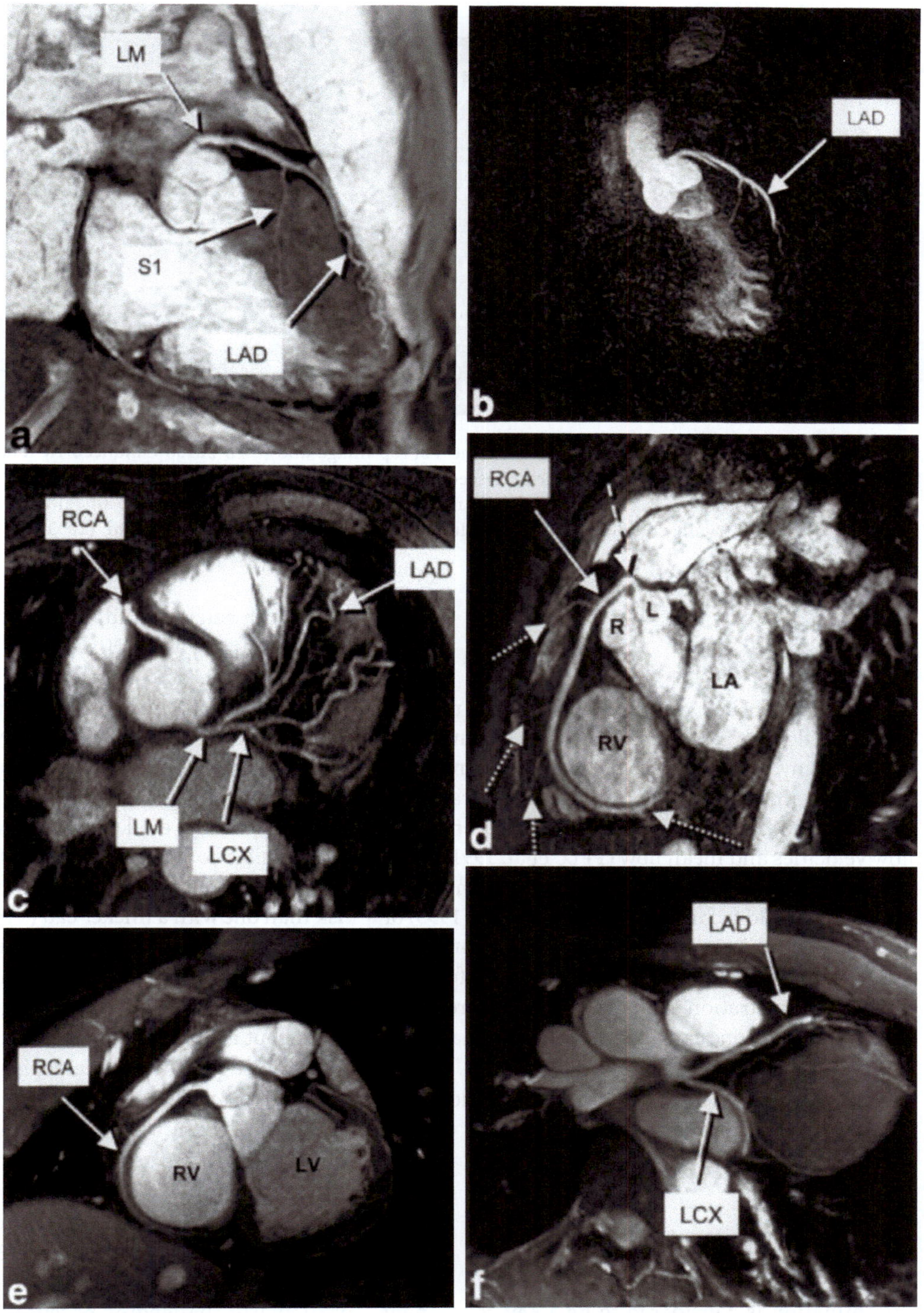

Fig. 3.2.1a–f. Reformatted images of 3D coronary MRA data acquired with real-time navigator technology during free breathing. **a** A video-inverted black-blood coronary MRA is displayed adjacent to a spin-tagged acquisition of (**b**) the left coronary arterial system. **c** An right coronary artery (*RCA*) together with a left coronary arterial system, including the left main coronary artery (*LM*), left anterior descending artery (*LAD*), left circumflex artery (*LCX*), and some smaller-caliber branching segments (using a T2Prep segmented k-space gradient-echo acquisition). **d** An anomalous RCA (*dashed arrow*) from the left coronary cusp (*L*) acquired with a T2Prep SSFP sequence is shown. *R*, right coronary cusp; *RV*, right ventricle; *LA*, left atrium. **e,f** Right and left coronary arterial systems acquired with an interleaved spiral imaging sequence. [Reproduced with permission from Etienne et al. (2002)]

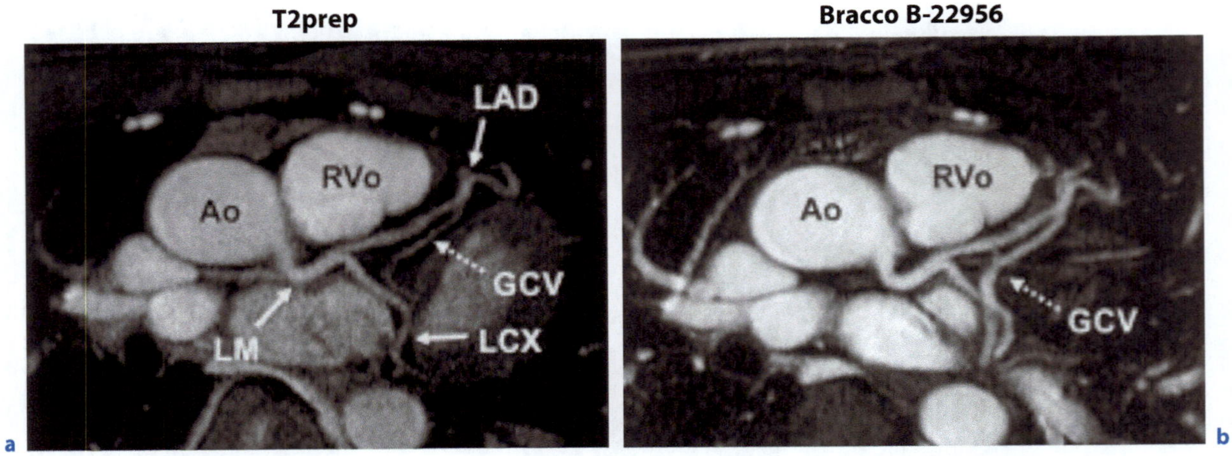

Fig. 3.2.2 a,b. Multiplanar reformatted **(a)** baseline T2Prep image and **(b)** B-22956-enhanced IR image. Improved vessel delineation of the left main (*LM*), left anterior descending (*LAD*), left circumflex (*LCX*) arteries, and great cardia vein (*GCV*) can visually be appreciated. B-22956 is a gadolinium-based blood pool agent from Bracco Imaging S.p.A., Milan, Italy. *Ao*, aorta; *RVo*, right ventricular outflow tract. [Reproduced with permission from Huber et al. (2003)]

3.2.4 Flow Quantification

The above-described techniques have been primarily directed towards delineation of the coronary artery anatomy. It is also possible to obtain functional information through the use of phase-contrast cine imaging techniques, which permit measurement of flow velocities and mean flow (Pelc et al. 1991). Measurement of coronary blood flow can be accomplished with breath-hold techniques (Edelman et al. 1993) or with free-breathing navigator methods (Nagel et al. 1999). If flow measurements are obtained before and during administration of pharmacological stress (e.g. adenosine), then one can determine the coronary flow reserve (Clarke et al. 1995). Measurement of flow reserve can be helpful to predict the physiological significance of a coronary artery stenosis.

3.2.4.1 Coronary Wall Imaging

Inflammation is considered to be a key component in the evolution of the so-called "vulnerable plaque" (Schaar et al. 2004; Ross 1999) Acute coronary syndrome is caused by the rupture of a lipid-rich vulnerable plaque (commonly one that is not hemodynamically significant and is invisible by coronary angiography) or, less often, by erosion of a predominantly fibrous plaque (Fuster 1994; Davies 1995; Burke et al. 1997). Cardiac CT is able to demonstrate both calcified and non-calcified plaque in the coronary artery wall. However, it is not yet able to determine whether a particular plaque is inflamed.

Dark blood MRI has been used to evaluate plaque characteristics in the carotid arteries. For instance, fibrous plaque components appear relatively bright on T2-weighted images whereas the lipid core appears dark (Toussaint et al. 1996; Yuan et al. 2001). It is also possible to measure the thickness of the plaque cap. Presumably a plaque with a thin cap is more at risk than one with a thicker cap (Virmani et al. 2003). Inflammation can be detected on the basis of enhancement with extracellular gadolinium chelates. Another gadolinium chelate, gadofluorine, shows avid plaque uptake but is not suitable for human use (Sirol et al. 2004). Since phagocytic macrophages accumulate in inflamed plaques, uptake of ultra-small iron oxide particles has been used as a biomarker of plaque inflammation (Ruehm et al. 2001; Trivedi et al. 2004).

In principle, these MRI approaches to characterizing plaque can be applied to imaging of the coronary arteries (Stuber et al. 2001; Fayad et al. 2000). However, imaging of the coronary wall is particularly challenging because the wall is so thin compared to that of the carotid artery, in addition to the previously mentioned challenges of overcoming cardiac and respiratory motion. Nonetheless, there are promising early results, in particular using navigator-gated 3D dark blood technique (Fig. 3.2.3) (Kim et al. 2002). Imaging at high field (e.g. 3 Tesla) may be particularly beneficial for this application (Koktzoglou et al. 2005).

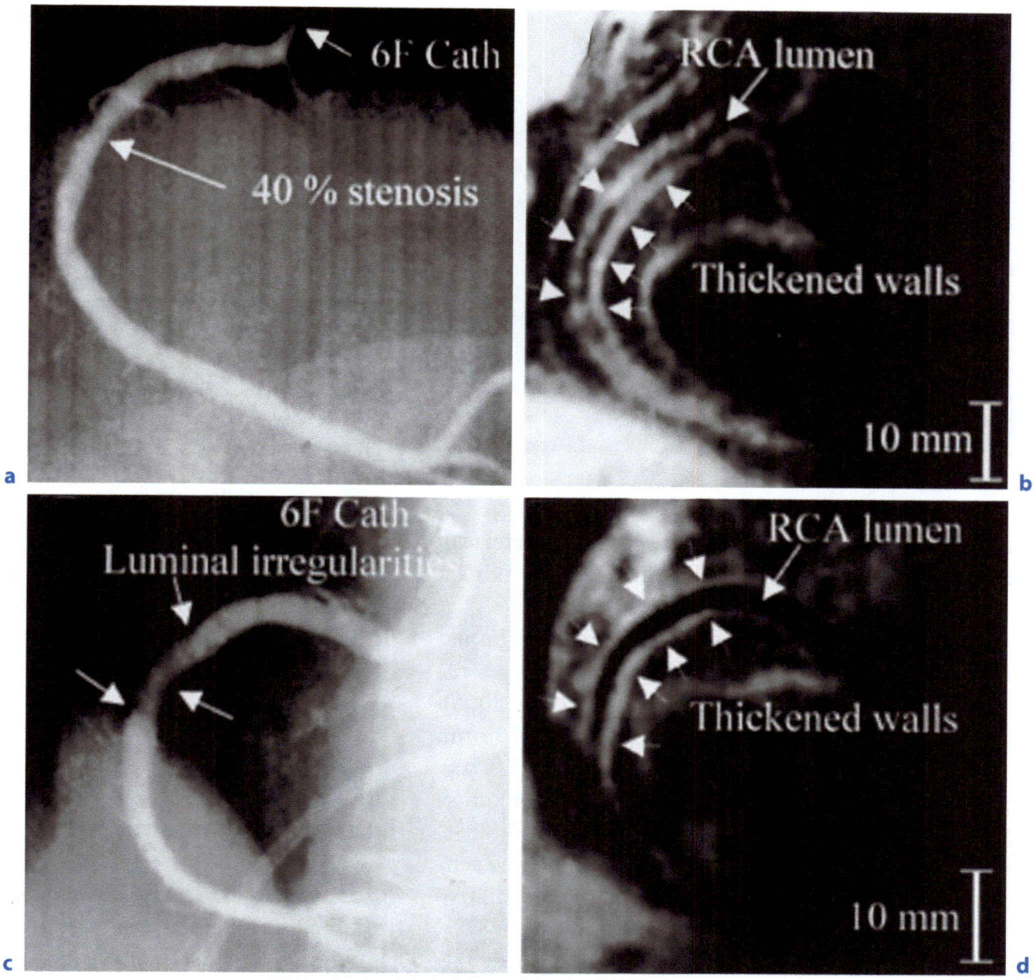

Fig. 3.2.3 a–d. X-ray angiography in two patients with (**a**) a focal 40% stenosis (*white arrow*) and (**c**) minor (≈10% stenoses) luminal irregularities (*white arrows*) of the proximal RCA. The corresponding black-blood 3D CMR vessel wall scans (**b,d**) demonstrate an irregularly thickened right coronary artery (*RCA*) wall (> 2 mm) indicative of an increased atherosclerotic plaque burden. The inner and outer RCA walls are indicated by *white dotted arrows*. The catheter size for the X-ray was 6-F. [Reproduced with permission from Kim et al. (2002)]

3.2.6 Clinical Results

Initial clinical results using breath-hold 2D MR coronary angiography were promising (Fig. 3.2.4) (Manning et al. 1993). However, subsequent single center trials gave variable results (Duerinckx and Urman 1994; Post et al. 1997).

Only one large-scale, multi-center clinical trial has been performed with MR coronary angiography (Kim et al. 2001). This trial was performed in 109 patients recruited from seven centers. Overall accuracy of MR coronary angiography was 72%. The sensitivity, specificity, and accuracy for patients with disease of the left main coronary artery or three-vessel disease were 100%, 85%, and 87%, respectively. The negative predictive values for any coronary artery disease and for left main artery or three-vessel disease were 81% and 100%, respectively. The authors concluded that MR coronary angiography allows for the accurate detection of coronary artery disease of the proximal and middle segments and reliably identifies left main coronary artery or three-vessel disease. These results are promising, but also indicate the need for additional technical development. Ongoing concerns include variable success of navigator gating depending on breathing patterns, inadequate spatial resolution (particularly for the assess-

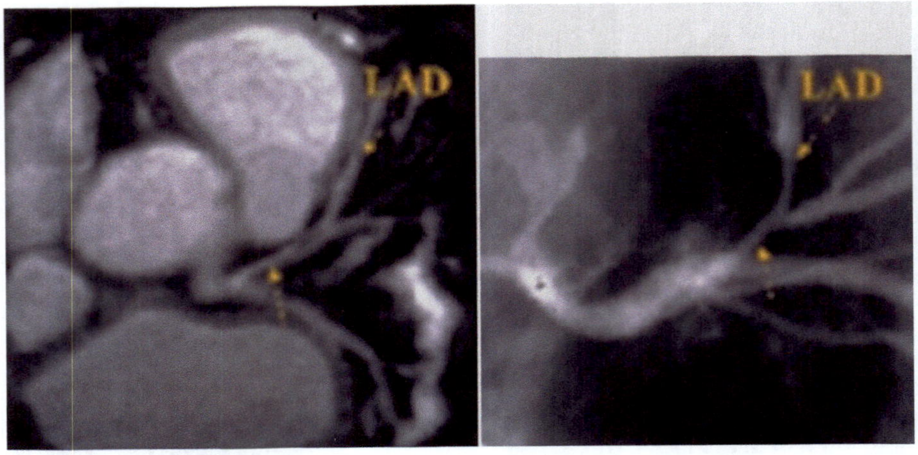

Fig. 3.2.4. Axial coronary MR angiogram (*left*) demonstrates a stenosis of the left anterior descending coronary artery and shows good correlation with the coronary catheterization (*right*). (Images courtesy of Dr. Warren Manning)

ment of distal or non-dominant coronary arteries), arrhythmias, and occasional difficulty identifying a vessel filling from retrograde collateral flow.

Promising clinical results have been obtained in whole-heart MR coronary angiography by a research group in Japan (Sakuma et al. 2005, 2006). Reconstructed voxel size was 0.55×0.55×0.75 mm, comparable to that obtained using 64-slice CT angiography. In this study of 131 patients, the acquisition of MR angiography was completed in 113 (86%) of 131 patients. On a patient-based analysis, the sensitivity, specificity, positive and negative predictive value, and accuracy of MR angiography were 82%, 90%, 88%, 86%, and 87%, respectively. These values in the individual segments were 78%, 96%, 69%, 98%, and 94%. Two examples of coronary MRA in patients are given in Figures 3.2.5 and 3.2.6. Scan time was fairly lengthy, however, averaging 12.9 min. One would anticipate that shorter scan times could be obtained with higher parallel acceleration factors, assuming SNR was sufficient.

3.2.7 Future Developments

Coronary MR imaging has benefited substantially from the improvements in phased array coils, parallel imaging, and fast imaging techniques. It has been shown that 2D parallel imaging with a 32-element receiver-coil array allows an acceleration factor of 4×2 and single breath-hold whole-heart coronary

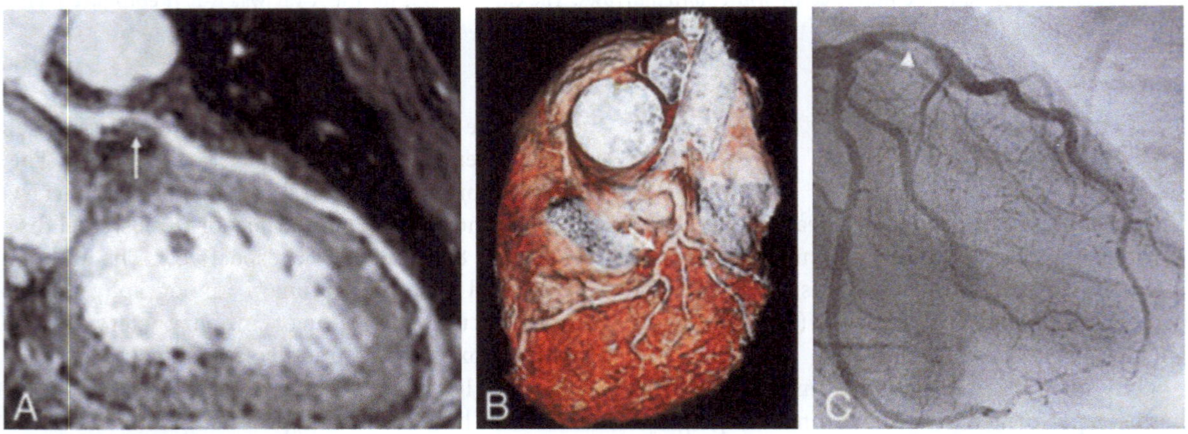

Fig. 3.2.5 A–C. Visualization of a stenosis in the left anterior descending artery (LAD) with whole-heart coronary magnetic resonance angiography. **A** Curved multiplanar reconstruction image shows a stenosis in the LAD (*white arrow*). **B** Volume-rendering method demonstrates a three-dimensional view of the LAD with stenosis (*white arrow*). **C** X-ray coronary angiography reveals a stenosis of the proximal LAD (*arrowhead*). [Reproduced with permission from Sakuma et al. (2006)]

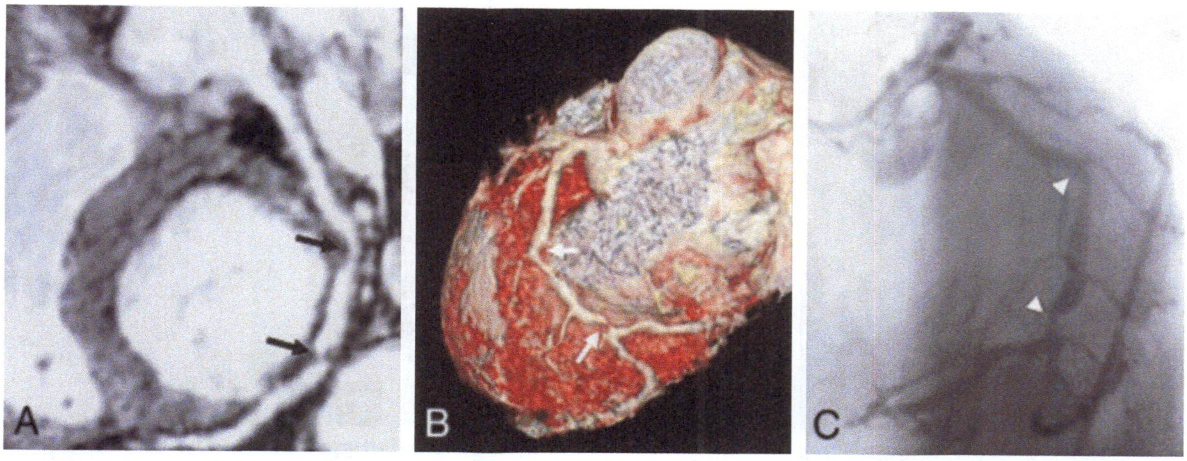

Fig. 3.2.6 A–C. A patient with stenosis in the left circumflex (LCX) artery. **A** Curved multiplanar reconstruction demonstrates stenoses of LCX in two locations (*black arrows*). **B** Volume rendering method shows three-dimensional view of LCX with stenoses (*white arrows*). **C** X-ray coronary angiography of the same artery confirms stenoses of LCX (*arrowhead*). [Reproduced with permission from Sakuma et al. (2006)]

MRA (Niendorf et al. 2006) (Fig. 3.2.7). Imaging at 3 Tesla has the potential to improve coronary SNR by a factor in the range of 50%–100% and promising results have already been demonstrated (Bi et al. 2005; Stuber et al. 2002). However, cardiac imaging at 3 Tesla involves daunting challenges, in particular related to he greater B0 and B1 field inhomogeneity and four-fold higher RF power deposition. Consequently, no convincing advantage for high field MR coronary angiography has been shown to date (Sommer et al. 2005). B0 inhomogeneity causes signal loss and poor fat suppression along the posterior cardiac margin at the interface with lung. In particular, this artifact can degrade the quality of left circumflex coronary artery images. In addition, at 3 Tesla the wavelength of the radiofrequency energy is comparable to the dimensions of the body, resulting in a marked worsening of B1 field inhomogeneity. As a result, the flip angle of the transmitted RF pulse varies widely through the field of view, resulting in variable tissue contrast and loss of SNR. Potential solutions include adiabatic RF pulses (Nezafat et al. 2006), RF shimming, and transmit SENSE (Katscher et al. 2003). The latter technique involves transmitting the RF pulses from different elements of a phased array coil so as to compensate for the B1 field inhomogeneity. Another concern is the increased magnetohydrodynamic effect at 3 Tesla, which causes an artifactual peaking of the T-wave. Although this effect can interfere with the reliability of ECG gating, our experience is that reliable gating is obtained using standard vector ECG gating systems (Fischer et al. 1999). Pulse gating is not affected by field strength and so provides a reliable alternative to ECG gating. A promising approach is contrast-enhanced MRA during slow infusion of a new FDA-approved contrast media (MultiHance; Bracco Imaging SpA, Milan, Italy), which allows whole-heart coronary MRA in approximately 5 min (Fig. 3.2.8) (Fischer et al. 1999). Compared to SSFP which is commonly used at 1.5 Tesla, contrast-enhanced gradient-echo imaging is relatively insensitive to B_0 field inhomogeneities due to its spoiled gradient structure. Both myocardium and epicardial fat signals can be effectively suppressed by a nonselective inversion pulse, which is less sensitive to B_0 and B_1 inhomogeneities than T_2 preparation and the spectrally selective fat saturation conventionally used with SSFP. Therefore, contrast-enhanced gradient-echo imaging is likely to be more tolerant of imperfections in B_0 and B_1 fields, and result in more consistent image quality among subjects at 3 T. In addition, it deposits less power than SSFP because it uses lower flip angles and eliminates T_2 preparation, which requires a composite RF pulse train or high-energy adiabatic refocusing pulses.

Arterial spin labeling (ASL) techniques are particularly well suited to 3 Tesla because the blood has a longer T1 relaxation time, resulting in a more prolonged effective tagging period. The increased SNR is also beneficial. In one study, a 2D tagging pulse was applied to the aortic root for a navigator-gated acquisition. After a suitable delay period for the tagged (dark) blood to enter the coronary artery tree,

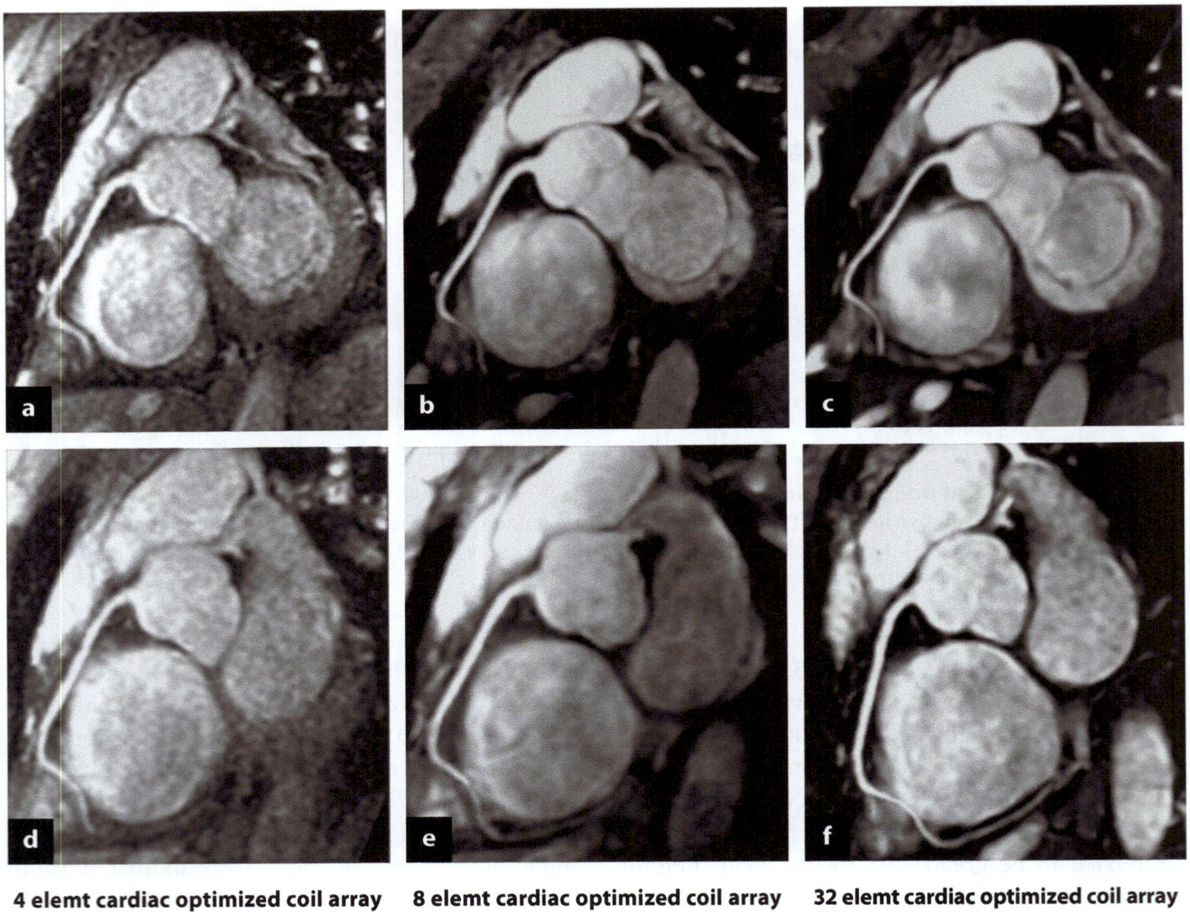

Fig. 3.2.7a–f. MR angiograms of the right coronary artery (RCA) (reformatted MIP, slice thickness = 3 mm) derived from healthy volunteers using (**a**,**d**) a four-element cardiac-optimized coil array, (**b**,**e**) an eight-element cardiac-optimized coil array, and (**c**,**f**) the 32-element coil array. Unaccelerated images were acquired using a short breath-hold, ECG-gated 3D SSFP sequence (matrix size = 256 × 256 × 12) together with thin targeted slabs that were aligned to the RCA. The distal portion of the RCA is clearly visualized in the image from the 32-element array because of the sound-to-noise ratio improvement over images from the four- and eight-element arrays. [Reproduced with permission from Niendorf et al. (2006)]

a 3D data set was acquired. A second 3D data set was also acquired but without the aortic tagging pulse. Subtraction of the two sets of images demonstrated long segments of the coronary arteries without any substantial background signal intensity. Alternatively, the tagging pulse can be applied directly to a coronary artery in order to make the blood appear dark and improve depiction of plaque in the wall of the vessel.

There are also a variety of novel contrast agents under development. These include contrast agents with higher T1 relaxivity that current gadolinium chelates. Contrast agents using hyperpolarized C13 offer the potential of visualizing the coronary arteries while eliminating confounding signals from background tissues (Svensson et al. 2003). Hyperpolarized C13 might also be used to provide perfusion and metabolic information about the myocardium (Kohler et al. 2007).

Many patients with a history of coronary artery disease have undergone stenting. Although these patients can generally be imaged safely with MR, it is impossible to visualize the lumen of the stent so that restenosis cannot be reliably diagnosed. One potential solution is the use of novel stent designs with magnetic susceptibilities similar to water. Preliminary studies in a swine model demonstrated artifact-free visualization of the coronary stent lumen (Buecker et al. 2004).

In conclusion, MR coronary angiography can provide detailed evaluation of the coronary arteries in the large majority of patients. Although spatial resolution needs to be further improved and the accuracy is not yet competitive with coronary CT angiography, it has the potential to be a valuable adjunct in cases where coronary calcification precludes adequate evaluation or iodinated contrast agents are contraindicated. In addition, the capability to image plaque components within the coronary vessel wall has the potential to aid in the detection of vulnerable plaque and enable earlier, more effective intervention.

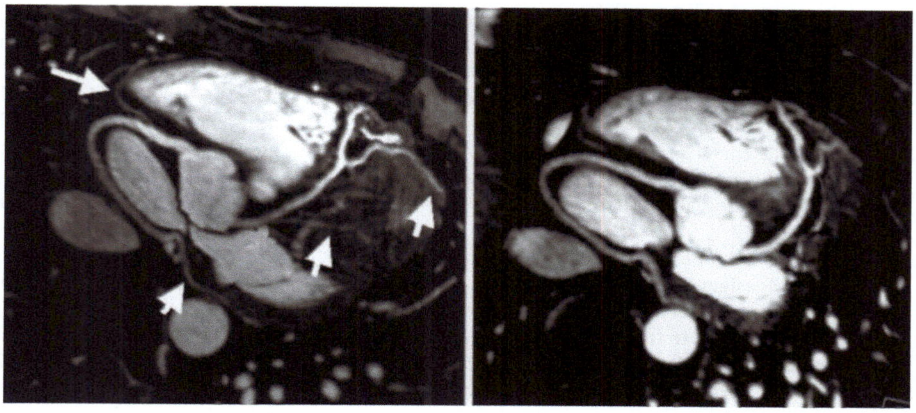

Fig. 3.2.8. Reformatted whole-heart coronary artery images obtained with slow infusion of Gd-BOPTA. Note that the left and right coronary arteries are sharply depicted and the distal segments and small branches are visible, as indicated by *arrows*. [Reproduced with permission from Bi et al. (2007)]

References

Atkinson DJ, Edelman RR (1991) Cineangiography of the heart in a single breath-hold with a segmented turbo-FLASH sequence. Radiology 178:357–60

Bi X, Deshpande V, Simonetti O, Laub G, Li D (2005) Three-dimensional breathhold SSFP coronary MRA: a comparison between 1.5-T and 3.0-T. J Magn Reson Imaging 22:206–212

Bi X, Carr JC, Li D (2007) Whole-heart coronary magnetic resonance angiography at 3 Tesla in 5 minutes with slow infusion of Gd-BOPTA, a high-relaxivity clinical contrast agent. Magn Reson Med 58:1–7

Brittain JH, Hu BS, Wright GA, Meyer CH, Macovski A, Nishimura DG (1995) Coronary angiography with magnetization-prepared T2 contrast. Magn Reson Med 33:689–696

Buecker A, Spuentrup E, Ruebben A et al. (2004) New metallic MR stents for artifact-free coronary MR angiography: feasibility study in a swine model. Invest Radiol 39:250–253

Burke AP, Farb A, Malcom GT, Liang YH, Smialek J, Virmani R (1997) Coronary risk factors and plaque morphology in men with coronary disease who died suddenly. N Engl J Med 336:1276–82

Cheng L, Zhao X, Wang X, Gao Y, Ma L, Sun W (2007) Comparative study of coronary MRA, CTA and X-ray angiography. Proceedings of the International Society for Magnetic Resonance in Medicine, Berlin

Clarke GD, Eckels R, Chaney C et al. (1995) Measurement of absolute epicardial coronary artery flow and flow reserve with breath-hold cine phase-contrast magnetic resonance imaging. Circulation 91:2627–2634

Danias PG, McConnell MV, Khasgiwala VC, Chuang ML, Edelman RR, Manning WJ (1997) Prospective navigator correction of image position for coronary MR angiography. Radiology 203:733–736

Davies MJ (1995) Acute coronary thrombosis – the role of plaque disruption and its initiation and prevention. Eur Heart J 16[Suppl L]:3–7

Deshpande VS, Shea SM, Laub G, Simonetti OP, Finn JP, Li D (2001) 3D magnetization-prepared true-FISP: a new technique for imaging coronary arteries. Magn Reson Med 46:494–502

Duerinckx AJ, Urman MK (1994) Two-dimensional coronary MR angiography: analysis of initial clinical results. Radiology 193:731–738

Edelman RR, Manning WJ, Burstein D, Paulin S (1991) Coronary arteries: breath-hold MR angiography. Radiology 181:641–643

Edelman RR, Manning WJ, Gervino E, Li W (1993) Flow velocity quantification in human coronary arteries with fast, breath-hold MR angiography. J Magn Reson Imaging 3:699–703

Ehman RL, McNamara MT, Pallack M, Hricak H, Higgins CB (1984) Magnetic resonance imaging with respiratory gating: techniques and advantages. AJR Am J Roentgenol 143:1175–1182

Etienne A, Botnar RM, Van Muiswinkel AM, Boesiger P, Manning WJ, Stuber M (2002) „Soap-Bubble" visualization and quantitative analysis of 3D coronary magnetic resonance angiograms. Magn Reson Med 48:658–66

Fayad ZA, Fuster V, Fallon JT et al. (2000) Noninvasive in vivo human coronary artery lumen and wall imaging using black-blood magnetic resonance imaging. Circulation 102:506–10

Fischer SE, Wickline SA, Lorenz CH (1999) Novel real-time R-wave detection algorithm based on the vectorcardiogram for accurate gated magnetic resonance acquisitions. Magn Reson Med 42:361–370

Fuster V (1994) Mechanisms leading to myocardial infarction: insights from studies of vascular biology. Circulation 90:2126–246

Gilard M, Le Gal G, Cornily J-C,Vinsonneau U, Joret C, Pennec PY, Mansourati J, Boschat J (2007) Midterm prognosis of patients with suspected coronary artery disease and normal multislice computed tomographic findings. Arch Intern Med 165:1686–1689

Goldfarb JW, Edelman RR (1998) Coronary arteries: breath-hold, gadolinium-enhanced, three-dimensional MR angiography. Radiology 206:830–834

Herzog C, Zwerner PL, Doll JR, Nielsen CD, Nguyen SA, Savino G, Vogl TJ, Costello P, Schoepf UJ (2007) Significant coronary artery stenosis: comparison on per-patient and per-vessel or per-segment basis at 64-section CT angiography. Radiology 244:112–120

Hofman MBM, Henson RE, Kovacs SJ et al. (1999) Blood pool agent strongly improves 3D magnetic resonance coronary angiography using an inversion pre-pulse. Magn Reson Med 41:360–367

Huber ME, Paetsch I, Schnackenburg B, Bornstedt A, Nagel E, Fleck E, Boesiger P, Maggioni F, Cavagna FM, Stuber M (2003) Performance of a new gadolinium-based intravascular contrast agent in free-breathing inversion-recovery 3D coronary MRA. Magn Reson Med 49:115–121

Katscher U, Borrnert P, Leussler C, van den Brink JS (2003) Transit SENSE. Magn Reson Med 49:144–150

Kim WY, Danias PG, Stuber M et al. (2001) Coronary magnetic resonance angiography for the detection of coronary stenoses. N Engl J Med 345:1863–1869

Kim WY, Stuber M, Bornert P, Kissinger KV, Manning WJ, Botnar RM (2002) Three-dimensional black-blood cardiac magnetic resonance coronary vessel wall imaging detects positive arterial remodeling in patients with nonsignificant coronary artery disease. Circulation 106:296–9

Kohler SJ, Yen Y, Wolber J et al. (2007) In Vivo 13 carbon metabolic imaging at 3-T with hyperpolarized ^{13}C-1-pyruvate. Magn Reson Med 58:65–69

Koktzoglou I, Simonetti OP, Li D (2005) Coronary artery wall imaging: initial experience at 3 Tesla. J Magn Reson Imaging 21:128–132

Langer C, Wiemer M, Peterschröder A, Franzke K, Meyer H, Horstkotte D (2005) Multislice computed tomography and magnetic resonance imaging: complementary use in noninvasive coronary angiography. Circulation 112:e-43–e344

Li D, Paschal CB, Haacke EM, Adler LP (1993) Coronary arteries: three dimensional MR imaging with fat saturation and magnetization transfer contrast. Radiology 187:401–406

Li D, Kaushikkar S, Haacke EM, Woodard PK, Dhawale P, Kroeker RM, Laub G, Kuginuki Y, Gutierrez FR (1996) Coronary arteries: three-dimensional MR imaging with retrospective respiratory gating. Radiology 201:857–863

Li D, Dolan RP, Walovitch RC, Lauffer RB (1998) Three-dimensional MRI of coronary arteries using an intravascular contrast agent. Magn Reson Med 39:1014–1018

Lotan CS, Cranney GB, Bouchard A, Bittner V, Pohost GM (1989) The value of cine nuclear magnetic resonance imaging for assessing regional ventricular function. J Am Coll Cardiol 14:1721–9

Manning WJ, Li W, Edelman RR (1993) A preliminary report comparing magnetic resonance coronary angiography with conventional angiography. N Engl J Med 328:828–832

Meyer CH, Hu BS, Nishimura DG, Macovski A (1992) Fast spiral coronary artery imaging. Magn Reson Med 28:202–213

Nagel E, Bornstedt A, Hug J, Schnackenburg B, Wellnhofer E, Fleck E (1999) Noninvasive determination of coronary blood flow velocity with magnetic resonance imaging: comparison of breath-hold and navigator techniques with intravascular ultrasound. Magn Reson Med 41:544–549

Nayler GL, Firmin DN, Longmore DB (1986) Blood flow imaging by cine magnetic resonance. J Comput Assist Tomogr 10:715–22

Nehrke K, Bornert P, Mazurkewitz P, Winkelmann R, Grasslin I (2006) Free-breathing whole-heart coronary MR angiography on a clinical scanner in four minutes. J Magn Reson Imaging 23:752–756

Nezafat R, Stuber M, Ouwerkerk R, Gharib AM, Desai MY, Pettigrew RI (2006) B1-insensitive T2 preparation for improved coronary magnetic resonance angiography at 3-T. Magn Reson Med 55:858–864

Niendorf T, Sodickson DK, Hardy CJ et al. (2004) Towards whole heart coverage in a single breath-hold: coronary artery imaging using a true 32-channel phased array MRI system. ISMRM, Kyoto, Japan, p 703

Niendorf T, Hardy CJ, Giaquinto RO, Gross P, Cline HE, Zhu Y, Kenwood G, Cohen S, Grant AK, Joshi S, Rofsky NM, Sodickson DK (2006) Toward single breath-hold whole-heart coverage coronary MRA using highly accelerated parallel imaging with a 32-channel MR system. Magn Reson Med 56:167–176

Paulin S, von Schulthess GK, Fossel E, Krayenbuehl HP (1987) MR imaging of the aortic root and proximal coronary arteries. AJR Am J Roentgenol 148:665–670

Pelc NJ, Herfkens RJ, Shimakawa A, Enzmann DR (1991) Phase contrast cine magnetic resonance imaging. Magn Reson Q 7:229–254

Post JC, van Rossum AC, Hofman MB, de Cock CC, Valk J, Visser CA (1997) Clinical utility of two-dimensional magnetic resonance angiography in detecting coronary artery disease. Eur Heart J 18:426–433

Pruessmann K, Weiger M, Scheidegger M, Boesiger P (1999) SENSE: sensitivity encoding for fast MRI. Magn Reson Med 42:952–962

Ross R (1999) Atherosclerosis – an inflammatory disease. N Engl J Med 340:115–126

Ruehm SG, Corot C, Vogt P, Kolb S, Debatin JF (2001) Magnetic resonance imaging of atherosclerotic plaque with ultrasmall superparamagnetic particles of iron oxide in hyperlipidemic rabbits. Circulation 103:415–422

Sakuma H, Ichikawa Y, Suzawa N et al. (2005) Assessment of coronary arteries with total study time of less than 30 minutes by using whole-heart coronary MR angiography. Radiology 237:316–321

Sakuma H, Ichikawa Y, Chino S, Hirano T, Makino K, Takeda K (2006) Detection of coronary artery stenosis with whole-heart coronary magnetic resonance angiography. J Am Coll Cardiol 48:1946–1950

Schaar JA, Muller JE, Falk E et al. (2004) Terminology for high-risk and vulnerable coronary artery plaques. Report of a meeting on the vulnerable plaque, June 17 and 18, 2003, Santorini, Greece. Eur Heart J 25:1077–1082

Schoepf UJ, Zwerner PL, Savino G, Herzog C, Kerl JM, Costello P (2007) Coronary CT angiography. Radiology 244:46–63

Sirol M, Itskovich VV, Mani V et al. (2004) Lipid-rich atherosclerotic plaques detected by gadofluorine-enhanced in vivo magnetic resonance imaging. Circulation 109:2890–2896

Sodickson DK (2006) Parallel imaging methods. In: Clinical magnetic resonance imaging, 3rd edn. Elsevier, Philadelphia, pp 231–248

Sommer T, Hackenbroch M, Hofer U et al. (2005) Coronary MR angiography at 3.0-T versus that at 1.5-T: initial results in patients suspected of having coronary artery disease. Radiology 234:718–725

Stehning C, Bornert P, Nehrke K, Eggers H, Dossel O (2004) Fast isotropic volumetric coronary MR angiography using free-breathing 3D radial balanced FFE acquisition. Magn Reson Med 52:197–203

Stuber M, Weiss RG (2007) Coronary magnetic resonance angiography. J Magn Reson Imaging 26:219–234

Stuber M, Botnar RM, Danias PG, Kissinger KV, Manning WJ (1999a) Breathhold three-dimensional coronary magnetic resonance angiography using real-time navigator technology. J Cardiovasc Magn Reson 1:233–238

Stuber M, Botnar RM, Danias PG, Kissinger KV, Manning WJ (1999b) Submillimeter three-dimensional coronary MR angiography with real-time navigator correction: comparison of navigator locations. Radiology 212:579–587

Stuber M, Botnar RM, Kissinger KV, Manning WJ (2001) Free-breathing black-blood coronary MR angiography: initial results. Radiology 219:278–283

Stuber M, Botnar RM, Fischer SE et al. (2002) Preliminary report on in vivo coronary MRA at 3 Telsa in humans. Magn Reson Med 48:425–429

Svensson J, Månsson S, Johansson E, Petersson JS, Olsson LE (2003) Hyperpolarized 13C MR angiography using true-FISP. Magn Reson Med 50:256–262

Taylor AM, Panting JR, Keegan J, Gatehouse PD, Amin D, Jhooti P, Yang GZ, McGill S, Burman ED, Francis JM, Firmin DN, Pennell DJ (1999) Safety and preliminary findings with the intravascular contrast agent NC100150 injection for MR coronary angiography. J Magn Reson Imaging 9:220–227

Toussaint JF, LaMuraglia GM, Southern JF, Fuster V, Kantor HL (1996) Magnetic resonance images lipid, fibrous, calcified, hemorrhagic, and thrombotic components of human atherosclerosis in vivo. Circulation 94:932–938

Trivedi RA, U-King-Im J-M, Graves MJ et al. (2004) In vivo detection of macrophages in human carotid atheroma: temporal dependence of ultrasmall superparamagnetic particles of iron oxide-enhanced MRI. Stroke 35:1631–1635

van Geuns RJ, Wielopolski PA, de Bruin HG et al. (2000) MR coronary angiography with breath-hold targeted volumes: preliminary clinical results. Radiology 217:270–277

Virmani R, Burke AP, Kolodgie FD, Farb A (2003) Pathology of the thin-cap fibroatheroma: a type of vulnerable plaque. J Interv Cardiol 16:267–272

Wang Y, Ehman RL (2000) Retrospective adaptive motion correction for navigator-gated 3D coronary MR angiography. J Magn Reson Imaging 11:208–214

Yuan C, Mitsumori LM, Ferguson MS, Polissar NL, Echelard D, Ortiz G, Small R, Davies JW, Kerwin WS, Hatsukami TS (2001) In vivo accuracy of multispectral magnetic resonance imaging for identifying lipid-rich necrotic cores and intraplaque hemorrhage in advanced human carotid plaques. Circulation 104:2051–2056

Non-Invasive Coronary Imaging

3

3.3 Clinical Implementation of Coronary Imaging

Hatem Alkadhi, Riksta Dikkers, Christoph R. Becker, Stephan Achenbach, and Valentin E. Sinitsyn

CONTENTS

H. Alkadhi, MD
Institute of Diagnostic Radiology, University Hospital Zurich, Raemisstrasse 100, 8091 Zurich, Switzerland

R. Dikkers, MD, PhD
Department of Radiology, University Medical Center Groningen, University Groningen, Hanzeplein 1, PO Box 30.001, 9700 RB Groningen, The Netherlands

C. R. Becker, MD
Department of Clinical Radiology, Klinikum Grosshadern, University of Munich, Marchioninistr. 15, 81377 Munich, Germany

S. Achenbach, MD, PhD
Department of Internal Medicine II, University of Erlangen, Ulmenweg 18, 91054 Erlangen, Germany

V. E. Sinitsyn, MD, PhD
Professor, Department of Tomography, Cardiology Research Center, Cherepkovskaya 15A, 121 552 Moscow, Russia

3.3.1 Introduction

Coronary heart disease is one of the leading causes of mortality, morbidity, and death in developed countries. Increasing efforts have been undertaken in screening and diagnosing coronary artery disease (CAD) with different imaging modalities such as catheter angiography, ultrasound, or MRI. For a long period of time, electron beam CT with its high temporal resolution of 100 ms was the only CT modality capable of imaging the coronary arteries without motion artifacts. Due to the restriction to a non-spiral scanning mode in ECG-synchronized cardiac investigations, a single breath-hold scan of the heart required slice widths as large as 3 mm. Thus, the resulting transverse resolution was limited and not sufficient for the detailed and diagnostic visualization of the coronary arteries. Multi-slice CT has advanced rapidly in the last decade and 64-slice and dual-source CT scanners are now state-of-the-art scanners for robust imaging of the coronary arteries, myocardium, and cardiac valves with high quality in terms of morphology and even function. In this chapter, we will describe the most important clinical applications of multi-slice CT for coronary artery imaging and we will discuss those areas where cardiac CT can be implemented in the daily clinical setting.

3.3.2 Patient Preparation for Non-invasive Coronary Angiography with CT

Since the introduction of four-slice CT technology in 1999, there has been a growing use of CT for coronary imaging (Ohnesorge et al. 2000).

The development of ECG-synchronized CT scanning and reconstruction techniques has provided fast volume coverage together with a high spatial and temporal resolution being a prerequisite for artefact-free cardiac imaging. However, for obtaining diagnostic image quality, careful preparation of the patient and an optimized scanning protocol is necessary.

The increasing number of detector elements and the increasing width of the detectors in recent years have made it possible to scan larger volumes with thinner slices within a single breath-hold. Especially for cardiac patients who may suffer from dyspnea, maintaining a long breath-hold is often difficult or even impossible to perform. The reduction of the breath-hold time from 40 s for four-slice CT scanners to approximately 10 s for 64-slice CT reduced the occurrence of breathing artefacts enormously.

To prevent artefacts due to rapid motion of the coronary arteries, the average heart rate should be below 65 bpm when using four-slice to 64-slice CT technology. Slow heart rates disproportionately prolong the end-diastolic relaxation and end-systolic contraction phase in which the heart shows only little motion (Husmann et al. 2007). Thus, reconstruction intervals can be placed within these phases and do not contain data from adjacent portions of the heart cycle possibly containing motion (Kerl et al. 2007). With the higher temporal resolution of dual-source CT, heart rate reduction is no longer necessary. Several studies showed a diagnostic image quality with dual-source CT even in patients with heart rates above 100 bpm (Achenbach et al. 2006; Flohr et al. 2006; Johnson et al. 2006; Matt et al. 2007). Besides the average heart rate, the variability of heart rate has been shown to be another important factor limiting the image quality of the examination (Leschka et al. 2006). It appears that the problem of heart rate variability has to do with the type of image reconstruction, in that multi-segment reconstructions are more prone to blurring artifacts caused by heart rate variability as compared to mono-segment reconstructions (Matt et al. 2007).

Beta-receptor antagonists for controlling the patients' heart rate can be safely used.

Patients are screened for medical conditions that may preclude them from receiving beta-blockers, including sinus bradycardia (defined as a heart rate below 60 bpm), systolic blood pressure of less than 100 mmHg, allergy to the medication or its constituents, decompensated cardiac failure, asthma, bronchospasm, and second- or third-degree atrioventricular block (Pannu et al. 2006). In the absence of contraindications, metoprolol tartrate may be administered orally 30–90 min prior to CT. Alternatively, 5 mg of metoprolol tartrate can be given intravenously immediately prior the scan. If the ventricular response is unsatisfactory, and heart rate remains high, additional doses of up to 15 mg can be given (Kerl et al. 2007). There is less experience with alternative heart rate-controlling medications. However, if there are contraindications for the use of beta-blockers, calcium channel blockers may be used via either the intravenous or oral route (Kerl et al. 2007). Monitoring of vital functions, heart rate, and blood pressure is essential when heart rate-controlling medication is used.

Sublingual nitroglycerin has been shown to prevent coronary artery spasm that may mimic coronary stenosis, especially in younger individuals (Hamon and Hamon 2006). Furthermore, it is known to provide better visualization through widening of the coronaries and is routinely given prior to every invasive catheter coronary angiography (Dewey et al. 2006). Although no systematic studies are available to support the use of nitroglycerin for cardiac CT with regard to the diagnostic performance of the examination, it is recommended and should be given in preparation of the CT scan. Nitroglycerin can be administered by using a 0.4-mg tablet sublingually or a sublingual spray. Contraindications for nitroglycerin comprise arterial hypotension, recent myocardial infarction, severe anemia, increased intracranial pressure, and known hypersensitivity to the medication. In addition, nitroglycerin is contraindicated in patients who recently took nitrate-based medication (Viagra, Cialis, Levitra) for erectile dysfunction. It is important to know that the administration of nitroglycerin is in rare cases associated with a reflex tachycardia that may impair the image quality and diagnostic yield of the examination. In general, this tachycardia does not occur when beta-blockers are also administered.

3.3.3 Contrast Media Administration

Intravenous access is preferably established in an antecubital vein. In particular, if a left internal mammary arterial bypass graft is to be evaluated, an access site in the right arm is preferred to prevent streak artifacts arising from undiluted contrast material in the left anonymous or subclavian vein interfering with the origin of the left internal mammary artery (Kerl et al. 2007). Because of the high injection rate of 4–6 ml/s needed for optimal contrast attenuation of the coronary vessels, an 18-Gauge catheter or larger should be used.

The administration of contrast media should be carefully timed to achieve an accurate and homogenous vascular lumen enhancement for diagnostic CT coronary angiography studies. High contrast enhancement is mandatory to identify small coronary branches at CT. High concentration non-ionic contrast agents with a flow rate of 4–6 ml/s should be used to achieve optimal intra-luminal enhancement. It is important to note that the major determinant of intra-luminal contrast enhancement is the iodine flux. A sufficient iodine flux can be achieved through a high injection rate (i.e., 5–6 ml/s) while using "lower" concentrated contrast material (i.e., 300, 320, or 350 mg/ml) or through a "lower" injection rate (4–5 ml/s) while using a higher concentration contrast agent (i.e., 370 or 400 mg/ml). Another factor that should be kept in mind is the dependency of contrast attenuation at CT from the kilovoltage setting. When using only 100 kV in normal weighted or slim patients the total amount of contrast media can be reduced while obtaining a similar contrast attenuation (Lenschka et al. 2008).

Dense contrast media in the right heart chambers and superior vena cava may result in streak artefacts and can interfere with the evaluation of the right coronary artery. A saline bolus chaser is therefore advised to flush the contrast out of the right atrium. This chaser also keeps the contrast bolus compact and prolongs the plateau phase of contrast for coronary artery vessel lumen enhancement (Kerl et al. 2007). For functional analysis of the heart, however, some enhancement of the right ventricle enabling the delineation of the ventricular septum is needed. A biphasic contrast protocol with a saline bolus chaser following the contrast bolus will often result in a good delineation of the left ventricle with clear enhancement of the coronary arteries, but may prevent identification of the structures of the right ventricle. A triphasic contrast protocol ensures high contrast enhancement in the left ventricle and coronary arteries and a less enhanced but clearly visible right ventricle and interventricular septum. For the triphasic protocol the initial iodine contrast bolus is followed by a saline/contrast mixture (for example 80% saline and 20% contrast) that is finally followed by a saline bolus chaser (Kerl et al. 2007). This protocol can be administered by using a dual-syringe injection system.

The timing of the contrast bolus arrival can be done through the test bolus or the bolus tracking technique. For the test bolus technique, determination of the contrast circulation time is performed by injecting a test bolus of 5 g iodine with a flow rate of 1 g/s iodine followed by a saline bolus chaser. A series of consecutive scans is acquired at the level of the aortic root, and the arrival time of the test bolus can be determined by the delay time between the start of the contrast material injection and the peak enhancement in the ascending aorta. For the bolus tracking technique, the beginning of the CT scan is triggered automatically by the arrival of the main contrast bolus. A pre-scan is taken at the level of the aortic root and a region of interest is placed into the ascending aorta. When contrast injection begins, repeated scanning at the same level is performed. If the density in the ascending aorta reaches a certain threshold (e.g. 100–140 HU), the scan is initiated after a predefined delay time. Prior to the initiation of the data acquisition, the patient is instructed to hold his breath in mild inspiration. A delay time of 4–10 s has been shown to suffice for adequate contrast enhancement of the heart. For both contrast timing techniques, the contrast media injection protocol has to be adjusted to the scan duration taking into account the delay time.

The final coronary vessel enhancement will depend on various patient-specific factors, one important factor being the cardiac output of the patient (Husmann et al. 2006). In patients with low cardiac output the contrast media will accumulate in the cardiac chambers and lead to a higher enhancement than in patients with high cardiac output where the contrast agent will be faster diluted by the non-enhanced blood.

3.3.4 Image Post-Processing Technique

Together with the development of new scanners dedicated software tools are being deployed, allowing detailed diagnosis of plaque morphology and quantification of coronary artery stenosis. However, review of the individual transverse source images cannot be abandoned and must be the major part of the diagnostic process in each case. Every post-processing step necessarily and by design reduces the available information for the sake of more intuitive image visualization (Kerl et al. 2007). Artefacts and other pitfalls which can result in reduced image quality and misinterpretation can be missed by not looking at the transverse source images. The most common problems include: motion-related artefacts caused by cardiac, pulmonary, or other body motion; beam-hardening effects caused by metallic implants or severe calcifications; and artefacts resulting from technical errors or limitations (Choi et al. 2004).

Software packages offer CT images to be displayed in different planes and to reconstruct 3D volumes. In the evaluation of cardiac anatomy, especially in the case of coronary anomalies or after coronary artery bypass grafting (CABG) surgery, 3D images can be helpful for quick spatial orientation. Because of isotropic (equal voxel dimensions in x-axis, y-axis, and z-axis) for 64-slice CT and dual-source CT, image data can be rearranged in arbitrary imaging planes with comparable image quality as in the original transverse sections. Multi-planar reformatted (MPR) images serve the purpose of enabling views of coronary artery lesions from different angles and perspectives, which enables better assessment of stenosis severity and residual perfused lumen than can be appreciated by only a single projection. Dedicated cardiac software offers automatic vessel contour and vessel lumen detection generating a cross-sectional MPR image along the centerline of the vessel lumen and provide maximum intensity projection (MIP) images parallel to the long axis of the vessel (Cury et al. 2006; Flohr et al. 2007; Hoffmann et al. 2006; Leber et al. 2005). The 3D representation of the coronary arteries with CT has made it possible to also measure the coronary artery area stenosis next to the traditional coronary artery lumen diameter stenosis assessment. All these extra tools provide a means for rapid analysis of the coronary artery tree for the detection and grading of stenosis. After automatically removing the osseous thoracic cage, the pulmonary veins and surrounding structures, the heart is isolated. In the next (semi-) automatic step the coronary arteries are identified. Each vessel can thereafter be analysed using the MPR and cross-sectional views of the vessel.

One study evaluating the difference in diagnostic accuracy comparing standard projections versus user-interactive post-processing showed that standard projections not always suffice for optimal diagnosis (Cademartiri et al. 2004). All automated measurements of vessel analysis tools should therefore not be trusted blindly, and the experience and acumen of the physician is still required to validate the results in the appropriate clinical context.

3.3.5 Diagnosis of Coronary Artery Disease

The leading indication of cardiac CT has become the non-invasive imaging of the coronary arteries in patients with a low to intermediate risk for CAD.

As impressive as recent technical advancements of CT are, it still falls short of the clinical reference standard, invasive catheter coronary angiography (CA). The spatial resolution of the catheter-based technique is 0.2 mm and thus twice that of cardiac CT, and the temporal resolution of up to 10 ms of CA is still not reached with CT. Of course, CA has also the advantage of being both diagnostic and therapeutic in the same session. On the other hand, CA is cost-extensive and is associated with a low but not negligible risk of morbidity and mortality that is associated with the invasive procedure (Scanlon et al. 1999). In 2002, about 2 million conventional CA procedures were performed in Europe (Maier et al. 2006). Interestingly, only in a third of these procedures was a subsequent percutaneous intervention performed. Thus, CA was mostly used as a purely diagnostic tool. This leads to a high number of invasive diagnostic procedures that could be reduced with a reliable non-invasive filter test.

Since the introduction of CT, a large number of studies have evaluated the diagnostic performance of the non-invasive modality to diagnose CAD. Several meta-analyses have been performed to combine the existing evidence of the accuracy of CT in the detection of CAD compared with CA. One meta-analysis included 15 papers and a total of 944 patients with an intermediate pre-test probability of disease undergoing four-slice or 16-slice CT (van der Zaag-Loonen et al. 2006). The authors found a pooled sensitivity for stenosis detection of 89%, while up to 28% of the patients could not be scanned and up to 32% of all segments could not be evaluated completely due to non-diagnostic image quality. Thus, it was concluded that four-slice and

16-slice CT technology does not suffice to reliably diagnose or to rule out CAD. Another meta-analysis evaluating the diagnostic performance of 16-slice and 64-slice CT found a pooled sensitivity and specificity for CT in the detection of CAD of 83% and 93% in a segment-based analysis, 90% and 87% in a vessel-based analysis, and 91% and 86% in a patient-based analysis (Sun and Jiang 2006). This analysis furthermore showed that 64-slice CT allowed for the evaluation of the entire coronary artery tree in most studies.

Table 3.3.1 lists the results of publications that have analyzed the diagnostic performance of stenosis detection using 64-slice CT and dual-source CT in comparison to the reference standard modality of invasive CA. With dual-source CT, the diagnostic performance appears to be further improved when compared to 64-slice CT. The first experience study with dual-source CT showed a sensitivity of 96% and a specificity of 98%, together with a positive predictive value of 86% and negative predictive value of 99% for the diagnosis of CAD in comparison with invasive CA (Scheffek et al. 2006). These results could be confirmed in subsequent studies with larger populations showing a similar high diagnostic performance of dual-source CT (Johnson et al. 2007a; Leber et al. 2007; Leschka et al. 2007a; Alkadhi et al. 2008; Ropers et al. 2007; Weustink et al. 2007). Importantly, heart rate reduction through the administration of beta receptor antagonists prior to CT was not used in any of these studies. Despite this fact, the rate of non-evaluable coronary segments was very low (1%–2%). In addition, high diagnostic performance could be maintained in patients having a heart rate of more than 70 bpm.

Owing to the high negative predictive value of CT, no further testing is needed when a patient has a completely diagnostic cardiac CT examination showing normal coronary arteries.

3.3.6 Indications for CT Coronary Angiography

Based on these excellent results for non-invasive coronary imaging with CT, various recommendations have emerged from the various societies.

The Task Force on the Management of Stable Angina Pectoris of the European Society of Cardiology has recommended the performance of CT coronary angiography in patients with stable angina, a low pre-test probability of CAD, and a inconclusive exercise ECG or stress imaging test (Fox et al. 2006). The American Heart Association (AHA) stated that, particularly if the symptoms, age, and gender of a patient suggest a low to intermediate probability of hemodynamically relevant stenoses, ruling out these stenoses by CT coronary angiography may be clinically useful and may help avoid invasive CA (Budoff et al. 2006). Finally, a group including various cardiological and radiological societies has recently stated that the use of CT coronary angiography in patients with an intermediate pre-test probability of CAD and an uninterpretable ECG, or who are unable to exercise, is appropriate (Hendel et al. 2006).

Taking these recommendations into account, cardiac CT for coronary imaging can also be implemented in clinical routine as a gatekeeper for CA in patients undergoing cardiac valvular surgery. Echocardiography is the method of choice to diagnose and grade the severity of valvular disease and provides accurate information regarding valve morphology and ventricular function. Current patient management requires the presence of significant coronary artery stenosis to be excluded in patients undergoing cardiac valve surgery with invasive CA. Thus, the opportunity to non-invasively exclude significant CAD provides a compelling rationale for using coronary CT before valve replacement. In fact, a number of studies could demonstrate the high diagnostic performance of 16-slice and 64-slice CT coronary angiography for the assessment of CAD in patients undergoing elective surgery of mitral or aortic valve disease (Gilard et al. 2006; Holmstrom et al. 2006; Meijboom et al. 2006; Scheffel et al. 2007).

It is important to note that cardiac CT is not considered a competitor to CA, but rather as a filter test for patients to decide whether CA should be performe or not, and whether conservative or invasive therapy should be performed. In this respect, cardiac CT can be seen more as a competitor for nuclear or ECG stress tests. In a head-to-head comparison with ECG stress testing, cardiac CT proved to have a significantly higher sensitivity (91% versus 73%) and specificity (83% versus 31%) (Dewey et al. 2007). In addition, far fewer patients were not assessable by CT (8%) than by stress ECG (19%).

Table 3.3.1. Per-segment and per-patient based sensitivity, specificity, positive (PPV) and negative predictive value (NPV) of CT coronary angiography as compared to catheter coronary angiography

Reference	Analysis	Number	Sensitivity (%)	Specificity (%)	PPV (%)	NPV (%)	Mean Heart Rate ± SD (bpm)
Leschka et al. (2005)	Segment-based	1005	94	97	87	99	66 ± 15
	Patient-based	67	100	100	100	100	
Raff et al. (2005)	Segment-based	935	86	95	66	98	65 ± 10
	Patient-based	70	95	90	93	93	
Mollet et al. (2005)	Segment-based	725	99	95	76	100	58 ± 7
	Patient-based	51	100	92	97	100	
Leber et al. (2005)	Segment-based	798	64	97	83	93	62 ± 13
	Patient-based	45	88	85	88	85	
Pugliese et al. (2006b)	Segment-based	494	99	96	78	99	58 ± 6
	Patient-based	35	100	90	96	100	
Ong et al. (2006)	Segment-based[a]	748	85	98	77	99	62 ± 9
	Segment-based[b]	726	78	98	86	96	62 ± 9
Schuijf et al. (2006b)	Segment-based	842	85	98	82	99	60 ± 11
	Patient-based	60	94	97	97	93	
Ropers et al. (2006a)	Segment-based	1083	93	97	56	100	59 ± 9
	Patient-based	81	96	91	83	98	
Ehara et al. (2006)	Segment-based	884	90	94	89	95	72 ± 13
	Patient-based	67	98	86	98	86	
Nikolaou et al. (2006)	Segment-based	923	82	95	72	97	61 ± 9
	Patient-based	68	97	79	86	96	
Meijboom et al. (2006)	Segment-based	1003	94	98	65	100	60 ± 8
	Patient-based	70	100	92	82	100	
Mühlenbruch et al. (2006)	Segment-based	726	87	95	75	98	70 ± 14
	Patient-based	51	98	50	94	75	
Scheffel et al. (2006)	Segment-based	420	96	98	86	99	70 ± 14
	Patient-based	30	93	100	100	94	
Leber et al. (2007)	Segment-based	1216	90	98	81	99	73
	Patient-based	88	95	90	74	99	
Johnson et al. (2007a)	Segment-based	473	88	98	78	99	68
	Patient-based	35	100	89	89	100	
Heuschmid et al. (2007)	Segment-based	663	96	87	61	99	65 ± 14
	Patient-based	51	97	73	90	92	
Leschka et al. (2007a)	Segment-based	1001	95	96	79	99	68 ± 13
	Patient-based	80	97	87	88	97	

[a]Agatston score <142 (68 patients).
[b]Agatston score >142 (66 patients).
SD, standard deviation; bpm, beats per minute.

3.3.7 Coronary Morphology and Myocardial Function

Although CT provides excellent images of the coronary artery tree, it must be noted that its informational value relies – similar to CA – on the pure description of morphology. By that, cardiac CT does not provide information as to the functional relevance of a coronary lesion.

Moreover, the purely anatomical information depicted by both invasive and non-invasive coronary angiography offers only limited functional and prognostic data on which clinical decision-making can be based. In fact, patients with a documented CAD but a normal myocardial perfusion scan are at low risk for major cardiac events, comparable to that in patients without significant CAD.

In a recent comparison between CT and nuclear myocardial perfusion imaging with single-positron emission computed tomography (SPECT) (Schuijf et al. 2006a) in 114 patients with intermediate likelihood of CAD, only 45% of patients with an abnormal CT had abnormal perfusion on SPECT. Even in patients with obstructive lesions on CT, 50% still had a normal SPECT. These findings are in agreement with other studies (Gaemperli et al. 2007; Hong et al. 2007; Sampson et al. 2007) which showed that only a fraction of patients with obstructive coronary lesions demonstrate ischemia on SPECT and positron emission tomography (PET) perfusion imaging. For this reason, although CT is a reliable tool to rule out functionally relevant CAD in a non-selected population with an intermediate pretest likelihood of disease, an abnormal CT coronary angiogram does not necessarily predict the presence of ischemia. In fact, since CT coronary angiography and perfusion imaging provide different and complementary information, their sequential use or hybrid imaging may provide useful incremental information.

Gaemperli et al. (2007) has reported on a study with 100 consecutive patients with an intermediate pretest likelihood of CAD undergoing myocardial perfusion imaging with SPECT and coronary angiography with 64-slice CT. The authors have found an excellent ability of 64-slice CT to rule out functionally relevant CAD as indicated by the high negative predictive value. However, an abnormal 64-slice CT was a poor predictor of functionally relevant coronary stenoses. On the other hand, a normal myocardial perfusion scan does not exclude the presence of CAD for which aggressive cardiovascular risk modification may be warranted.

3.3.8 Evaluation of Coronary Artery Bypass Grafts

Accurate and reliable assessment of CABG is possible with the most recent CT scanners. Table 3.3.2 lists the results of publications that have analyzed the diagnostic performance of patency and stenosis detection of CABG using 16-slice CT and 64-slice CT in comparison to the reference standard modality of invasive CA.

The accuracy for the assessment of the patency of either arterial or venous graft is in the range of 98% (Jones et al. 2007; Malagutti et al. 2006). CT can therefore be useful in patients after bypass surgery suffering from chest pain. Occlusion detection is reliable and not affected by the use of beta-blockers, the symptomatic status, or the postoperative period (Jones et al. 2007). Stenosis assessment within CABG is more difficult and only possible in approximately 88% of the grafts with a sensitivity of 89% (Jones et al. 2007). CT has the advantage for allowing the assessment of CABG and, within the same examination, also of other findings possibly being the cause of chest pain.

On the other hand, the clinical situation often affords knowledge not only of the status of the CABG, but also the distal run-off as well as of the non-grafted coronary arteries. Here – as those native arteries often suffer from advanced atherosclerosis with severe calcifications – cardiac CT interpretation can be challenging and image quality insufficient for diagnostic purposes (Malagutti et al. 2006; Dikkers et al. 2006).

Patients needing to undergo re-operation after bypass graft surgery benefit from cardiac CT due to the concise visualization in relation to surrounding structures, such as the grafts running behind the sternum that are at risk of damage in the case of resternotomy (Aviram et al. 2005). Cardiac CT for this purpose has a clear advantage over CA (Gasparovic et al. 2005).

3.3.9 Evaluation of Coronary Artery Stents

Follow-up imaging in patients after previous placement of coronary stents who present with recurrent

Table 3.3.2. Sensitivity, specificity, positive (PPV) and negative predictive value (NPV) of 16-slice CT and 64-slice CT for the evaluation of coronary artery bypass graft patency and graft stenosis

Reference	Number of patients/grafts	Evaluation	Non-evaluable	Sensitivity (%)	Specificity (%)	PPV (%)	NPV (%)
Nieman et al. (2003)	24/60[a]	Occlusion	0 5	Observer 1: 100 Observer 2: 100	100 98	94 94	100 100
		Stenosis	10 5	Observer 1: 60 Observer 2: 83	88 90	43 63	94 97
Stauder et al. (2006)	20/50	Occlusion	0	100	100	100	100
		Stenosis	12	99	94	92	99
Burgstahler et al. (2006)	13/43	Occlusion	0	100	100	100	100
		Stenosis	5	100	93	33	100
Salm et al. (2005)	25/67	Occlusion	0	100	100	100	100
		Stenosis	NA	100	94	50	100
Ropers et al. (2006b)	50/138	Occlusion	0	100	100	100	100
		Stenosis	0	100	94	92	100
Malagutti et al. (2007)	52/109	Stenosis[b]	0	100	98	98	100

[a]Venous grafts only, [b]including both significant stenoses and occlusion. NA, not applicable.

symptoms is currently performed with invasive CA. Although promising results have been obtained with CT for the detection of coronary artery stenoses in native coronary arteries, results of the evaluation of coronary stents have been less promising. Because of the artifacts from the metallic struts, the visualization of the lumen within coronary artery stents by CT is more challenging than the assessment of the native coronary arteries. Although image quality and diagnostic accuracy improved substantially with 16-slice as compared with four-slice CT, image quality for a relatively large number of stents has been reported to be non-diagnostic, and particularly stents with thicker struts or smaller diameters tended to exhibit degraded image quality.

Table 3.3.3 lists the results of publications that have analyzed the diagnostic performance of in-stent-restenosis detection using 64-slice CT and dual-source CT in comparison to the clinical reference standard modality of invasive CA.

Schuijf et al. (2007) have reported good interpretability of the in-stent lumen with 64-slice CT, and image quality was considered sufficient in 86% of the stents. The reported sensitivity and specificity of 64-slice CT was 100% each for detection of significant (i.e., ≥ 50%) in-stent restenosis. Similar results with 64-slice CT were published by Oncel et al. (2007) showing a sensitivity of 89% and specificity of 95% for the detection of in-stent restenosis and stent occlusion. Pugliese et al. (2007) recently reported good performance in the detection of in-stent restenosis for dual-source CT in patients with recurrent chest pain after stent implantation. The authors found a sensitivity of 100% and a specificity of 100% for the detection of restenosis in stents ≥ 3.5 mm. Thus, stent diameter must be considered an important predictor of the diagnostic performance of the non-invasive technique. When the stent diameter was ≤ 2.75 mm, the technique is associated with frequent false positive findings. However, due to the high negative predictive value, dual-source CT reliably ruled-out in-stent restenosis irrespective of the stent size.

When evaluating stents, the use of a sharp reconstruction filter for better visualization of the stent struts and the in-stent lumen is recommended (Pugliese et al. 2006a). At the same time, evaluation of the vessel segment with a smooth kernel should also be performed since the exclusive use of a sharp kernel leads to misreading because of increased noise.

Table 3.3.3. Sensitivity, specificity, positive (PPV) and negative predictive value (NPV) of 64-slice CT and dual-source CT for the detection of in-stent restenosis

Reference	Number of patients/stents	Not evaluable (%)	Sensitivity (%)	Specificity (%)	PPV (%)	NPV (%)
Rixe et al. (2006)	64/102	42	86	98	86	98
Rist et al. (2006)	25/46	2	75	92	67	94
Oncel et al. (2007)	30/39	0	89	95	94	90
Ehara et al. (2007)	81/125	12	91	93	77	98
Cademartiri et al. (2007c)	182/192	7	95	93	63	99
Pugliese et al. (2007)	100/178	5	94	92	77	98

Sensitivity and specificity are calculated only for evaluable stents.

3.3.10 Plaque Detection

More than displaying the coronary artery lumen only, CT being a cross-sectional imaging modality is able to display the coronary artery wall as well. Catheter CA is not suited to assess the entire extent of coronary atherosclerosis. A study investigating more than 500 segments with CA, intra-vascular ultrasound (IVUS), and 64-slice CT showed that CA dramatically underestimates the overall extent of any type of plaque (Butler et al. 2007). Only about one third of the segments with CAD as detected by CT were positive at CA. Especially the phenomenon of positive remodelling, defined as growth of plaque through expansion of the media and external elastic membrane in early stages of atherosclerosis with preservation of the cross-sectional lumen, may be completely missed by CA (Butler et al. 2007). The current gold standard to assess coronary atherosclerosis in vivo is IVUS. A study comparing IVUS with multi-slice CT has shown that coronary lesions classified as soft, intermediate, and dense as determined by IVUS correspond to plaques with a CT density of 14 ± 26 HU, 91 ± 21 HU, and 419 ± 194 HU, respectively (Schroeder et al. 2001). Heart specimen studies demonstrated that HU densities of non-calcified plaques depend on the ratio between lipid and fibrous tissue and may increase from atheroma (± 50 HU) and fibroatheroma to fibrotic (± 100 HU) lesions. As has been observed in coronary arteries of symptomatic patients, coronary thrombi present as very low density (± 20 HU) and inhomogeneous plaques (Becker et al. 2003). Commonly, spotty calcified plaques may be found at CT coronary angiography that may be associated with minor wall changes in conventional coronary angiography only. However, it is known that such calcified nodules may be the source of unheralded plaque rupture and consecutive thrombosis potentially leading to sudden coronary death (Virmani et al. 2000).

The quantitative assessment of plaque density by CT must be made with caution, however, as several factors such as the degree of intra-luminal attenuation (Cademartiri et al. 2005) as well as the different reconstruction filter (Cademartiri et al. 2007a) significantly alter the absolute attenuation values of the plaques.

Nevertheless, a purely qualitative classification of plaque morphology into noncalcified, mixed, and calcified types is of relevance for the patient. Particularly the presence of mixed plaques - representing less advanced and possibly less stabilized atherosclerosis as compared with calcified lesions – has been shown to be an independent predictor for hard cardiac events (Pundziute et al. 2007).

3.3.11 Radiation Dose

CT represents the most important source of ionizing radiation arising from medical exposures (Yates et al. 2004). As the basic principle of radiation protection, harmful radiation exposure should be kept as low as reasonably achievable (ALARA). This primary principle must be kept in mind for each cardiac CT examination. Unfortunately, the technical improvements in cardiac CT in the past decade were paralleled by an increase in radiation exposure to the patient. This is caused by low helical pitch values that are required for obtaining a high temporal resolution. Another factor causing the increase in radiation exposure is the decrease in detector collimation width that is required to obtain a high spatial resolution. In order to maintain diagnostic image quality, the number of photons getting to the smaller detectors needs to be increased through an increase in tube current.

For these reasons, various dose saving algorithms have been developed. One of the most important ones can be realized with the implementation of ECG-gated dose modulation (so-called ECG-pulsing) (Jakobs et al. 2002). With this approach, the normal tube output is only applied during that phase of the cardiac cycle at which images of coronary arteries will be reconstructed. During the rest of the cardiac cycle, the tube output is reduced to approximately 25% of the normal value. The application of this technique must take into account that the placement of the ECG-pulsing window requires the prediction of reconstruction phases prior to scanning. This means that at higher heart rates, where various phases even in systole must be reconstructed, the width of the ECG-pulsing window must be widened or the technique must be switched off. In addition, the ECG-gated dose modulation technique becomes less effective at higher heart rates because the time period in which the dose is reduced is shorter. Standard 64-slice CT coronary angiography protocols are associated with an effective dose of approximately 15 mSv without, and of 10 mSv with the use of the ECG-pulsing technique (Hausleiter et al. 2006a).

The radiation dose can be further reduced through the adaptation of the pitch to the heart rate, with an increase in pitch at higher heart rates. This adaptation directly leads to a decrease in the patient dose, because the average dose within the scan volume is directly proportional to 1/pitch. With dual-source CT, where the pitch adapts to the patient's heart rate with an increasing table feed at higher heart rates, the radiation dose is significantly reduced as compared to single-source CT scanners (McCollough et al. 2007). Using a standard scan protocol with ECG-pulsing (Leschka et al. 2007b), dual-source CT is associated with an average effective radiation dose of 7–9 mSv (Stolzmann et al. 2007).

This value can be further reduced to 5–7 mSv when applying a tube voltage of 100 kV that is feasible in patients with a body mass index of below 25 kg/m^2 (Leschka et al. 2008).

Another radiation dose saving technique is the use of prospective ECG-triggering, or step-and-shoot mode. In contrast to retrospective ECG-gating, this mode does not obtain continuous helical data but rather acquires data at predefined time points of the cardiac cycle, requiring a regular and relatively low heart rate. The effective radiation dose of cardiac CT using this technique is approximately 1–3 mSv (Scheffel et al. 2008).

The effective radiation dose of invasive CA ranges between 4 and 22 mSv for purely diagnostic invasive procedures (Einstein et al. 2007; Coles et al. 2006). It should be borne in mind, however, that the overall risk of an examination is a weighted summation of the risk contribution of each component of the procedure. When comparing the risk of invasive CA to that of CT coronary angiography, there are risks common to both procedures, such as the adverse effects to iodinated contrast media and radiation, but there are also risks unique to each examination (Zanzonico et al. 2006). Invasive CA implies additional risks to the patient through a major complication rate of 1.7%, yielding a considerable non-radiogenic risk of mortality. This must be superimposed onto the potential risk associated with X-ray radiation of the technique.

3.3.12 Conclusion

CT technology has witnessed a rapid development in recent decades. The time between the introduction of new CT scanner generations with an increasing number of detectors and faster gantry rotation times is only 1,5–2 years on average. The current literature about CT coronary angiography mostly reflects single-center experiences in relatively small patient populations. The role of CT in clinical practice is still growing, and questions remain regarding its appropriate use. Potential risks are related to the intravenous administration of iodinated contrast material and to the inherent radiation exposure associated with the technique. Inappropriate clinical application could lead to unnecessary treatment of low-risk populations and is associated with significant direct and indirect risks to patients. From a current point of view, cardiac CT fits into the clinical environment as a cost-effective filter test, primarily used in patients with a low to moderate likelihood of CAD, to quickly and efficiently decide on the appropriate therapy.

References

Achenbach S (2006) Computed tomography coronary angiography. J Am Coll Cardiol 48:1919–1928

Achenbach S, Ropers D, Kuettner A, Flohr T, Ohnesorge B, Bruder H et al. (2006) Contrast-enhanced coronary artery visualization by dual-source computed tomography – initial experience. Eur J Radiol 57:331–335

Alkadhi H, Scheffel H, Desbiolles L et al. (2008) Dual-source computed tomography coronary angiography: influence of obesity, calcium load, and heart rate on diagnostic accuracy. Eur Heart J 29:766–76

Annuar BR, Liew CK, Chin SP, Ong TK, Seyfarth MT, Chan WL et al. (2007) Assessment of global and regional left ventricular function using 64-slice multislice computed tomography and 2D echocardiography: a comparison with cardiac magnetic resonance. Eur J Radiol 65:112–119

Aviram G, Sharony R, Kramer A, Nesher N, Loberman D, Ben Gal Y et al. (2005) Modification of surgical planning based on cardiac multidetector computed tomography in reoperative heart surgery. Ann Thorac Surg 79:589–595

Becker CR, Nikolaou K, Muders M, Babaryka G, Crispin A, Schoepf UJ et al. (2003) Ex vivo coronary atherosclerotic plaque characterization with multi-detector-row CT. Eur Radiol 13:2094–2098

Brodoefel H, Klumpp B, Reimann A, Fenchel M, Heuschmid M, Miller S et al. (2007) Sixty-four-MSCT in the characterization of porcine acute and subacute myocardial infarction: determination of transmurality in comparison to magnetic resonance imaging and histopathology. Eur J Radiol 62:235–246

Budoff MJ, Achenbach S, Blumenthal RS et al. (2006) Assessment of coronary artery disease by cardiac computed tomography: a scientific statement from the American Heart Association Committee on Cardiovascular Imaging and Intervention, Council on Cardiovascular Radiology and Intervention, and Committee on Cardiac Imaging, Council on Clinical Cardiology. Circulation 114:1761–1791

Burgstahler C, Beck T, Kuettner A et al. (2006) Non-invasive evaluation of coronary artery bypass grafts using 16-row multi-slice computed tomography with 188 ms temporal resolution. Int J Cardiol 106:244--249

Butler J, Shapiro M, Reiber J, Sheth T, Ferencik M, Kurtz EG et al. (2007) Extent and distribution of coronary artery disease: a comparative study of invasive versus noninvasive angiography with computed angiography. Am Heart J 153:378–384

Cademartiri F, Mollet NR, Lemos PA, McFadden EP, Marano R, Baks T et al. (2004) Standard versus user-interactive assessment of significant coronary stenoses with multislice computed tomography coronary angiography. Am J Cardiol 94:1590–1593

Cademartiri F, Mollet NR, Runza G, Bruining N, Hamers R, Somers P et al. (2005) Influence of intracoronary attenuation on coronary plaque measurements using multislice computed tomography: observations in an ex vivo model of coronary computed tomography angiography. Eur Radiol 15:1426–1431

Cademartiri F, de MC, Pugliese F, Mollet NR, Runza G, van der LA et al. (2006) High iodine concentration contrast material for noninvasive multislice computed tomography coronary angiography: iopromide 370 versus iomeprol 400. Invest Radiol 41:349–353

Cademartiri F, La Grutta L, Runza G et al. (2007a) Influence of convolution filtering on coronary plaque attenuation values: observations in an ex vivo model of multislice computed tomography coronary angiography. Eur Radiol 17:1842–1849

Cademartiri F, La GL, Palumbo A, Maffei E, Aldrovandi A, Malago R et al. (2007b) Imaging techniques for the vulnerable coronary plaque. Radiol Med (Torino) 112:637–659

Cademartiri F, Palumbo A, Maffei E et al. (2007c) Diagnostic accuracy of 64-slice CT in the assessment of coronary stents. Radiol Med (Torino) 112:526--537

Caussin C, Ohanessian A, Ghostine S, Jacq L, Lancelin B, Dambrin G et al. (2004) Characterization of vulnerable nonstenotic plaque with 16-slice computed tomography compared with intravascular ultrasound. Am J Cardiol 94:99–104

Centonze M, Del GM, Nollo G, Ravelli F, Marini M, la Sala SW et al. (2005) The role of multidetector CT in the evaluation of the left atrium and pulmonary veins anatomy before and after radio-frequency catheter ablation for atrial fibrillation. Preliminary results and work in progress. Technical note. Radiol Med (Torino) 110:52–60

Choi HS, Choi BW, Choe KO, Choi D, Yoo KJ, Kim MI et al. (2004) Pitfalls, artifacts, and remedies in multi- detector row CT coronary angiography. Radiographics 24:787–800

Chow BJ, Hoffmann U, Nieman K (2005) Computed tomographic coronary angiography: an alternative to invasive coronary angiography. Can J Cardiol 21:933–940

Coles DR, Smail MA, Negus IS et al. (2006) Comparison of radiation doses from multislice computed tomography coronary angiography and conventional diagnostic angiography. J Am Coll Cardiol 47:1840–1845

Coles DR, Smail MA, Negus IS, Wilde P, Oberhoff M, Karsch KR et al. (2006) Comparison of radiation doses from multislice computed tomography coronary angiography and conventional diagnostic angiography. J Am Coll Cardiol 47:1840–1845

Cury RC, Ferencik M, Achenbach S, Pomerantsev E, Nieman K, Moselewski F et al. (2006) Accuracy of 16-slice multidetector CT to quantify the degree of coronary artery stenosis: assessment of cross-sectional and longitudinal vessel reconstructions. Eur J Radiol 57:345–350

Detrano RC, Anderson M, Nelson J, Wong ND, Carr JJ, Nitt-Gray M et al. (2005) Coronary calcium measurements: effect of CT scanner type and calcium measure on rescan reproducibility – MESA study. Radiology 236:477–484

Dewey M, Hamm B (2007) Cost effectiveness of coronary angiography and calcium scoring using CT and stress MRI for diagnosis of coronary artery disease. Eur Radiol 17:1301–1309

Dewey M, Hoffmann H, Hamm B (2006) Multislice CT coronary angiography: effect of sublingual nitroglycerine on the diameter of coronary arteries. Rofo 178:600–604

Dewey M, Dubel HP, Schink T, Baumann G, Hamm B (2007) Head-to-head comparison of multislice computed tomography and exercise electrocardiography for diagnosis of coronary artery disease. Eur Heart J 28:2485–2490

Dikkers R, Willems TP, Tio RA, Anthonio RL, Zijlstra F, Oudkerk M (2006) The benefit of 64-MDCT prior to invasive coronary angiography in symptomatic post-CABG patients. Int J Cardiovasc Imaging 23:369–377

Ehara M, Surmely JF, Kawai M, Katoh O, Matsubara T, Terashima M et al. (2006) Diagnostic accuracy of 64-slice computed tomography for detecting angiographically significant coronary artery stenosis in an unselected consecutive patient population: comparison with conventional invasive angiography. Circ J 70:564–571

Ehara M, Kawai M, Surmely JF et al. (2007) Diagnostic accuracy of coronary in-stent restenosis using 64-slice computed tomography: comparison with invasive coronary angiography. J Am Coll Cardiol 49:951--959

Einstein AJ, Moser KW, Thompson RC et al. (2007) Radiation dose to patients from cardiac diagnostic imaging. Circulation 116:1290–1305

Flohr TG, McCollough CH, Bruder H, Petersilka M, Gruber K, Suss C et al. (2006) First performance evaluation of a dual-source CT (DSCT) system. Eur Radiol 16:256–268

Flohr TG, Schoepf UJ, Ohnesorge BM (2007) Chasing the heart: new developments for cardiac CT. J Thorac Imaging 22:4–16

Fox K, Garcia MA, Ardissino D et al. (2006) Guidelines on the management of stable angina pectoris: executive summary: the Task Force on the Management of Stable Angina Pectoris of the European Society of Cardiology. Eur Heart J 27:1341–1381

Gaemperli O, Schepis T, Koepfli P et al. (2007) Accuracy of 64-slice CT angiography for the detection of functionally relevant coronary stenoses as assessed with myocardial perfusion SPECT. Eur J Nucl Med Mol Imaging 34:1162–1171

Gasparovic H, Rybicki FJ, Millstine J, Unic D, Byrne JG, Yucel K et al. (2005) Three dimensional computed tomographic imaging in planning the surgical approach for redo cardiac surgery after coronary revascularization. Eur J Cardiothorac Surg 28:244–249

Gerber TC, Kuzo RS, Morin RL (2005) Techniques and parameters for estimating radiation exposure and dose in cardiac computed tomography. Int J Cardiovasc Imaging 21:165–176

Gibbons RJ, Chatterjee K, Daley J, Douglas JS, Fihn SD, Gardin JM et al. (1999) ACC/AHA/ACP-ASIM guidelines for the management of patients with chronic stable angina: a report of the American College of Cardiology/American Heart Association Task Force on Practice Guidelines (Committee on Management of Patients With Chronic Stable Angina). J Am Coll Cardiol 33:2092–2197

Gilard M, Cornily JC, Rioufol G, Finet G, Pennec PY, Mansourati J et al. (2005) Noninvasive assessment of left main coronary stent patency with 16-slice computed tomography. Am J Cardiol 95:110–112

Gilard M, Cornily JC, Pennec PY et al. (2006) Accuracy of multislice computed tomography in the preoperative assessment of coronary disease in patients with aortic valve stenosis. J Am Coll Cardiol 47:2020–2024

Goldstein JA, Gallagher MJ, O'Neill WW, Ross MA, O'Neil BJ, Raff GL (2007) A randomized controlled trial of multislice coronary computed tomography for evaluation of acute chest pain. J Am Coll Cardiol 49:863–871

Greenland P, LaBree L, Azen SP, Doherty TM, Detrano RC (2004) Coronary artery calcium score combined with Framingham score for risk prediction in asymptomatic individuals. JAMA 291:210–215

Hamon M, Hamon M (2006) Images in clinical medicine. Asymptomatic coronary-artery spasm. N Engl J Med 355:2236

Hausleiter J, Meyer T, Hadamitzky M, Huber E, Zankl M, Martinoff S et al. (2006a) Radiation dose estimates from cardiac multislice computed tomography in daily practice: impact of different scanning protocols on effective dose estimates. Circulation 113:1305–1310

Hausleiter J, Meyer T, Hadamitzky M et al. (2006b) Radiation dose estimates from cardiac multislice computed tomography in daily practice: impact of different scanning protocols on effective dose estimates. Circulation 113:1305–1310

Hendel RC, Patel MR, Kramer CM, et al. (2006) ACCF/ACR/SCCT/SCMR/ASNC/NASCI/SCAI/SIR 2006 appropriateness criteria for cardiac computed tomography and cardiac magnetic resonance imaging: a report of the American College of Cardiology Foundation Quality Strategic Directions Committee Appropriateness Criteria Working Group, American College of Radiology, Society of Cardiovascular Computed Tomography, Society for Cardiovascular Magnetic Resonance, American Society of Nuclear Cardiology, North American Society for Cardiac Imaging, Society for Cardiovascular Angiography and Interventions, and Society of Interventional Radiology. J Am Coll Cardiol 48:1475–1497

Heuschmid M, Burgstahler C, Reimann A et al. (2007) Usefulness of noninvasive cardiac imaging using dual-source computed tomography in an unselected population with high prevalence of coronary artery disease. Am J Cardiol 100:587--592

Hoffmann U, Millea R, Enzweiler C, Ferencik M, Gulick S, Titus J et al. (2004) Acute myocardial infarction: contrast-enhanced multi-detector row CT in a porcine model. Radiology 231:697–701

Hoffmann U, Moselewski F, Nieman K, Jang IK, Ferencik M, Rahman AM et al. (2006) Noninvasive assessment of plaque morphology and composition in culprit and stable lesions in acute coronary syndrome and stable lesions in stable angina by multidetector computed tomography. J Am Coll Cardiol 47:1655–1662

Holmstrom M, Sillanpaa MA, Kupari M et al. (2006) Eight-row multidetector computed tomography coronary angiography evaluation of significant coronary artery disease in patients with severe aortic valve stenosis. Int J Cardiovasc Imaging 22:703–710

Hong EC, Kimura-Hayama ET, Di Carli MF (2007) Hybrid cardiac imaging: complementary roles of CT angiography and PET in a patient with a history of radiation therapy. J Nucl Cardiol 14:617–620

Husmann L, Alkadhi H, Boehm T et al. (2006) Influence of cardiac hemodynamic parameters on coronary artery opacification with 64-slice computed tomography. Eur Radiol 16:1111–1116

Husmann L, Leschka S, Desbiolles L et al. (2007) Coronary artery motion and cardiac phases: dependency on heart rate – implications for CT image reconstruction. Radiology 245:567–576

Jakobs TF, Becker CR, Ohnesorge B et al. (2002) Multislice helical CT of the heart with retrospective ECG gating: reduction of radiation exposure by ECG-controlled tube current modulation. Eur Radiol 12:1081–1086

Johnson LW, Lozner EC, Johnson S, Krone R, Pichard AD, Vetrovec GW et al. (1989) Coronary arteriography 1984–1987: a report of the Registry of the Society for Cardiac Angiography and Interventions. I. Results and complications. Cathet Cardiovasc Diagn 17:5–10

Johnson TR, Nikolaou K, Wintersperger BJ, Leber AW, von Ziegler F, Rist C et al. (2006) Dual-source CT cardiac imaging: initial experience. Eur Radiol 16:1409–1415
Johnson TR, Nikolaou K, Busch S et al. (2007a) Diagnostic accuracy of dual-source computed tomography in the diagnosis of coronary artery disease. Invest Radiol 42:684–691
Johnson TR, Nikolaou K, Wintersperger BJ, Knez A, Boekstegers P, Reiser MF et al. (2007b) ECG-gated 64-MDCT angiography in the differential diagnosis of acute chest pain. AJR Am J Roentgenol 188:76–82
Jones CM, Athanasiou T, Dunne N, Kirby J, Aziz O, Haq A et al. (2007) Multi-detector computed tomography in coronary artery bypass graft assessment: a meta-analysis. Ann Thorac Surg 83:341–348
Jongbloed MR, Dirksen MS, Bax JJ, Boersma E, Geleijns K, Lamb HJ et al. (2005) Atrial fibrillation: multi-detector row CT of pulmonary vein anatomy prior to radiofrequency catheter ablation – initial experience. Radiology 234:702–709
Juergens KU, Grude M, Fallenberg EM, Opitz C, Wichter T, Heindel W et al. (2002) Using ECG-gated multidetector CT to evaluate global left ventricular myocardial function in patients with coronary artery disease. AJR Am J Roentgenol 179:1545–1550
Kerl JM, Hofmann LK, Thilo C, Vogl TJ, Costello P, Schoepf UJ (2007) Coronary CTA: image acquisition and interpretation. J Thorac Imaging 22:22–34
Kopp AF, Schroeder S, Kuettner A, Heuschmid M, Georg C, Ohnesorge B et al. (2001) Coronary arteries: retrospectively ECG-gated multi-detector row CT angiography with selective optimization of the image reconstruction window. Radiology 221:683–688
Leber AW, Knez A, von Ziegler F, Becker A, Nikolaou K, Paul S et al. (2005) Quantification of obstructive and nonobstructive coronary lesions by 64-slice computed tomography: a comparative study with quantitative coronary angiography and intravascular ultrasound. J Am Coll Cardiol 46:147–154
Leber AW, Becker A, Knez A, von Ziegler F, Sirol M, Nikolaou K et al. (2006) Accuracy of 64-slice computed tomography to classify and quantify plaque volumes in the proximal coronary system: a comparative study using intravascular ultrasound. J Am Coll Cardiol 47:672–677
Leber AW, Johnson T, Becker A et al. (2007) Diagnostic accuracy of dual-source multi-slice CT-coronary angiography in patients with an intermediate pretest likelihood for coronary artery disease. Eur Heart J 28:2354–2360
Leschka S, Alkadhi H, Plass A et al. (2005) Accuracy of MSCT coronary angiography with 64-slice technology: first experience. Eur Heart J 26:1482--1487
Leschka S, Wildermuth S, Boehm T et al. (2006) Noninvasive coronary angiography with 64-section CT: effect of average heart rate and heart rate variability on image quality. Radiology.; 241:378–385
Leschka S, Scheffel H, Desbiolles L et al. (2007a) Combining dual-source computed tomography coronary angiography and calcium scoring: added value for the assessment of coronary artery disease. Heart [Epub ahead of print]
Leschka S, Scheffel H, Desbiolles L et al. (2007b) Image quality and reconstruction intervals of dual-source CT coronary angiography: recommendations for ECG-pulsing windowing. Invest Radiol 42:543–549
Leschka S, Stolzmann P, Schmid FT et al. (2008) Low kilovoltage cardiac dual-source CT: attenuation, noise, and radiation dose. Eur Radiol. Sep; 18(9):1809–17
Maier W, Abay M, Cook S et al. (2006) The 2002 European registry of cardiac catheter interventions. Int J Cardiol 113:299–304
Malagutti P, Nieman K, Meijboom WB, Van Mieghem CA, Pugliese F, Cademartiri F et al. (2006) Use of 64-slice CT in symptomatic patients after coronary bypass surgery: evaluation of grafts and coronary arteries. Eur Heart J 28:1879–1885
Malagutti P, Nieman K, Meijboom WB et al. (2007) Use of 64-slice CT in symptomatic patients after coronary bypass surgery: evaluation of grafts and coronary arteries. Eur Heart J 28:1879--1885
Matt D, Scheffel H, Leschka S et al. (2007) Dual-source CT coronary angiography: image quality, mean heart rate, and heart rate variability. AJR Am J Roentgenol 189:567–573
McCollough CH, Primak AN, Saba O, Bruder H, Stierstorfer K, Raupach R et al. (2007)Dose performance of a 64-channel dual-source CT scanner. Radiology 243:775–784
Meijboom WB, Mollet NR, Van Mieghem CA et al. (2006) Pre-operative computed tomography coronary angiography to detect significant coronary artery disease in patients referred for cardiac valve surgery. J Am Coll Cardiol 48:1658–1665
Mollet NR, Cademartiri F, van Mieghem CA et al. (2005) High-resolution spiral computed tomography coronary angiography in patients referred for diagnostic conventional coronary angiography. Circulation 112:2318--2323
Mühlenbruch G, Seyfarth T, Soo CS et al. (2007) Diagnostic value of 64-slice multi-detector row cardiac CTA in symptomatic patients. Eur Radiol 17:603--609
Nieman K, Pattynama PM, Rensing BJ, Van Geuns RJ, De Feyter PJ (2003) Evaluation of patients after coronary artery bypass surgery: CT angiographic assessment of grafts and coronary arteries. Radiology 229:749--756
Nikolaou K, Knez A, Rist C et al. (2006) Accuracy of 64-MDCT in the diagnosis of ischemic heart disease. AJR Am J Roentgenol 187:111--117
Ohnesorge B, Flohr T, Becker C, Kopp AF, Schoepf UJ, Baum U et al. (2000) Cardiac imaging by means of electrocardiographically gated multisection spiral CT: initial experience. Radiology 217:564–571
Oncel D, Oncel G, Karaca M (2007) Coronary stent patency and in-stent restenosis: determination with 64-section multidetector CT coronary angiography – initial experience. Radiology 242:403–409
Ong TK, Chin SP, Liew CK et al. (2006) Accuracy of 64-row multidetector computed tomography in detecting coronary artery disease in 134 symptomatic patients: influence of calcification. Am Heart J 151:1323, e1321--1326
Pannu HK, Alvarez W, Jr., Fishman EK (2006) Beta-blockers for cardiac CT: a primer for the radiologist. AJR Am J Roentgenol 186:S341–345
Park JM, Choe YH, Chang S, Sung YM, Kang SS, Kim MJ et al. (2004) Usefulness of multidetector-row CT in the evaluation of reperfused myocardial infarction in a rabbit model. Korean J Radiol 5:19–24
Pohle K, Achenbach S, MacNeill B, Ropers D, Ferencik M, Moselewski F et al. (2007) Characterization of non-calcified coronary atherosclerotic plaque by multi-detector row CT: comparison to IVUS. Atherosclerosis 190:174–180

Pugliese F, Cademartiri F, van Mieghem C et al. (2006a) Multidetector CT for visualization of coronary stents. Radiographics 26:887–904

Pugliese F, Mollet NR, Runza G et al. (2006b) Diagnostic accuracy of non-invasive 64-slice CT coronary angiography in patients with stable angina pectoris. Eur Radiol 16:575--582

Pugliese F, Weustink AC, Van Mieghem C et al. (2007) Dual-source coronary computed tomography angiography for detecting in-stent restenosis. Heart 94:848–854

Pundziute G, Schuijf JD, Jukema JW et al. (2007) Prognostic value of multislice computed tomography coronary angiography in patients with known or suspected coronary artery disease. J Am Coll Cardiol 49:62–70

Raff GL, Gallagher MJ, O'Neill WW, Goldstein JA (2005) Diagnostic accuracy of noninvasive coronary angiography using 64-slice spiral computed tomography. J Am Coll Cardiol 46:552--557

Rasouli ML, Shavelle DM, French WJ, McKay CR, Budoff MJ (2006) Assessment of coronary plaque morphology by contrast-enhanced computed tomographic angiography: comparison with intravascular ultrasound. Coron Artery Dis 17:359–364

Reimann AJ, Rinck D, Birinci-Aydogan A, Scheuering M, Burgstahler C, Schroeder S et al. (2007) Dual-source computed tomography: advances of improved temporal resolution in coronary plaque imaging. Invest Radiol 42:196–203

Rist C, von Ziegler F, Nikolaou K et al. (2006) Assessment of coronary artery stent patency and restenosis using 64-slice computed tomography. Acad Radiol 13:1465--1473

Rixe J, Achenbach S, Ropers D et al. (2006) Assessment of coronary artery stent restenosis by 64-slice multi-detector computed tomography. Eur Heart J 27:2567--2572

Ropers D, Rixe J, Anders K et al. (2006a) Usefulness of multidetector row spiral computed tomography with 64- × 0.6-mm collimation and 330-ms rotation for the noninvasive detection of significant coronary artery stenoses. Am J Cardiol 97:343--348

Ropers D, Pohle FK, Kuettner A et al. (2006b) Diagnostic accuracy of noninvasive coronary angiography in patients after bypass surgery using 64-slice spiral computed tomography with 330-ms gantry rotation. Circulation 114:2334--2341; quiz 2334

Ropers U, Ropers D, Pflederer T et al. (2007) Influence of heart rate on the diagnostic accuracy of dual-source computed tomography coronary angiography. J Am Coll Cardiol 50:2393-2398

Russo V, Gostoli V, Lovato L, Montalti M, Marzocchi A, Gavelli G et al. (2006) Clinical value of multidetector CT coronary angiography as a pre-operative screening test before noncoronary cardiac surgery. Heart 93:1591–1598

Salm LP, Bax JJ, Jukema JW et al. (2005) Comprehensive assessment of patients after coronary artery bypass grafting by 16-detector-row computed tomography. Am Heart J 150:775--781

Sampson UK, Dorbala S, Limaye A et al. (2007) Diagnostic accuracy of rubidium-82 myocardial perfusion imaging with hybrid positron emission tomography/computed tomography in the detection of coronary artery disease. J Am Coll Cardiol 49:1052–1058

Scanlon PJ, Faxon DP, Audet AM, Carabello B, Dehmer GJ, Eagle KA et al. (1999) ACC/AHA guidelines for coronary angiography. A report of the American College of Cardiology/American Heart Association Task Force on practice guidelines (Committee on Coronary Angiography). Developed in collaboration with the Society for Cardiac Angiography and Interventions. J Am Coll Cardiol 33:1756–1824

Scheffel H, Alkadhi H, Plass A et al. (2006) Accuracy of dual-source CT coronary angiography: First experience in a high pre-test probability population without heart rate control. Eur Radiol 16:2739–2747

Scheffel H, Leschka S, Plass A et al. (2007) Accuracy of 64-slice computed tomography for the preoperative detection of coronary artery disease in patients with chronic aortic regurgitation. Am J Cardiol 100:701–706

Scheffel H, Alkadhi H, Leschka S et al. (2008) Low-dose CT coronary angiography in the step-and-shoot mode: diagnostic performance. Heart [Epub ahead of print]

Schmermund A, Mohlenkamp S, Berenbein S, Pump H, Moebus S, Roggenbuck U et al. (2006) Population-based assessment of subclinical coronary atherosclerosis using electron-beam computed tomography. Atherosclerosis 185:177–182

Schoenhagen P, Stillman AE, Garcia MJ, Halliburton SS, Tuzcu EM, Nissen SE et al. (2006) Coronary artery imaging with multidetector computed tomography: a call for an evidence-based, multidisciplinary approach. Am Heart J 151:945–948

Schroeder S, Kopp AF, Baumbach et al. (2001) Noninvasive detection and evaluation of atherosclerotic coronary plaques with multislice computed tomography. J Am Coll Cardiol 37:1430–1435

Schuijf JD, Wijns W, Jukema JW et al. (2006a) Relationship between noninvasive coronary angiography with multi-slice computed tomography and myocardial perfusion imaging. J Am Coll Cardiol 48:2508–2514

Schuijf JD, Pundziute G, Jukema JW et al. (2006b) Diagnostic accuracy of 64-slice multislice computed tomography in the noninvasive evaluation of significant coronary artery disease. Am J Cardiol 98:145--148

Schuijf JD, Pundziute G, Jukema JW et al. (2007) Evaluation of patients with previous coronary stent implantation with 64-section CT. Radiology 245:416–423

Stauder NI, Kuttner A, Schroder S et al. (2006) Coronary artery bypass grafts: assessment of graft patency and native coronary artery lesions using 16-slice MDCT. Eur Radiol 16:2512-2520

Stolzmann P, Scheffel H, Schertler T et al. (2007) Radiation dose estimates in dual-source computed tomography coronary angiography. Eur Radiol 18:592–599

Sun Z, Jiang W (2006) Diagnostic value of multislice computed tomography angiography in coronary artery disease: a meta-analysis. Eur J Radiol 60:279–286

Taylor AJ, Bindeman J, Feuerstein I, Cao F, Brazaitis M, O'Malley PG (2005) Coronary calcium independently predicts incident premature coronary heart disease over measured cardiovascular risk factors: mean three-year outcomes in the Prospective Army Coronary Calcium (PACC) project. J Am Coll Cardiol 46:807–814

van der Zaag-Loonen HJ, Dikkers R, de Bock GH, Oudkerk M (2006) The clinical value of a negative multi-detector computed tomographic angiography in patients suspected of coronary artery disease: a meta-analysis. Eur Radiol 16:2748–2756

Virmani R, Kolodgie FD, Burke AP et al. (2000) Lessons from sudden coronary death: a comprehensive morphological classification scheme for atherosclerotic lesions. Arterioscler Thromb Vasc Biol 20:1262–1275

Weustink AC, Meijboom WB, Mollet NR et al. (2007) Reliable high-speed coronary computed tomography in symptomatic patients. J Am Coll Cardiol 50:786–794

Yates SJ, Pike LC, Goldstone KE (2004) Effect of multislice scanners on patient dose from routine CT examinations in East Anglia. Br J Radiol 77:472–478

Zanzonico P, Rothenberg LN, Strauss HW (2006) Radiation exposure of computed tomography and direct intracoronary angiography: risk has its reward. J Am Coll Cardiol 47:1846–1849

3.4 MDCT in Acute Coronary Syndrome

Hatem Alkadhi, Riksta Dikkers, Cristoph R. Becker, Charles White, and Udo Hoffman

CONTENTS

H. Alkadhi, MD
Institute of Diagnostic Radiology, University Hospital Zurich, Raemisstrasse 100, 8091 Zurich, Switzerland
R. Dikkers, MD, PhD
Department of Radiology, University Medical Center Groningen, University Groningen, Hanzeplein 1, PO Box 30.001, 9700 RB Groningen, the Netherlands
C. Becker, MD
Department of Clinical Radiology, Klinikum Grosshadern, University of Munich, Marchioninistrasse 15, 81377 Munich, Germany
C. White, MD
Professor of Radiology and Medicine, Department of Diagnostic Radiology, University of Maryland Medical Center, 22 S. Greene Street, Baltimore, MD 21201, USA
U. Hoffman, MD
Department of Radiology, Massachusetts General Hospital, 55 Fruit Street, Boston, MA 02114, USA
and
Harvard School of Public Health, 677 Huntington Avenue, Boston, MA 02115, USA

3.4.1 Introduction

Acute coronary syndrome (ACS) is a clinical syndrome that presents as chest pain or its angina equivalent (e.g. dyspnea, jaw or arm pain) as the manifestation of decreased coronary blood flow to the myocardium. The clinical symptoms depend on the severity of coronary blood flow reduction which determines the severity of ischemia and the amount of myocardial necrosis. Thus, the spectrum of ACS ranges from unstable angina with ischemia, but without detectable myocardial necrosis, to ACS with variable degrees of myocardial necrosis, i.e., myocardial infarction. The latter encompasses ST-elevated myocardial infarction (STEMI) and non-ST-elevated myocardial infarction (NSTEMI) (Fig. 3.4.1).

The clinical diagnosis of patients with ACS remains a considerable challenge. In the US alone, approximately 6 million patients with acute chest pain present to the emergency department (ED) each year. Because of the potentially serious consequences of an inappropriate discharge, ED patients with suspected ACS are usually admitted to the hospital with admission rates between 30% and 72%. This leads to the high annual healthcare costs that are estimated to be in the range of $8 billion (Hoffmann et al. 2006a). Ultimately, only 15%–25% of patients presenting with acute chest pain are diagnosed as having an ACS as underlying cause. Despite the high admission rates, between 2% and 8% of patients with ACS who present to the ED are inappropriately sent home (Pope et al. 2000), resulting in a mortality rate that is twice as high in the discharged patients compared to those who are admitted to hospital (Lee et al. 1987). Failure to diagnose ACS has shown to be strongly related to young age, female gender, non-white race, absence of typical symptoms, and no prior acute myocardial infarction or angina (Pope et al. 2000; Lee et al. 1987).

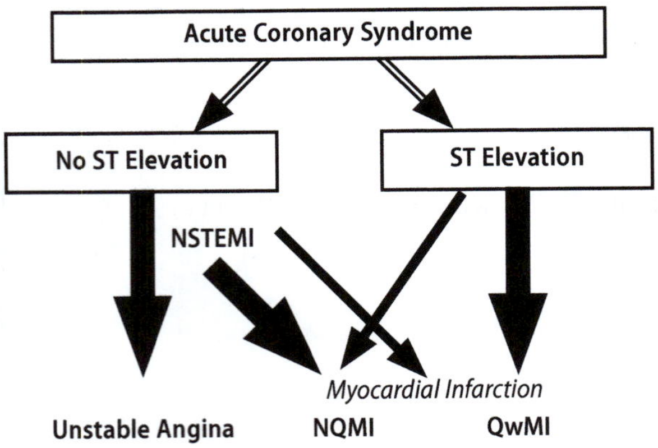

Fig. 3.4.1. Nomenclature of ACSs. Patients with ischemic discomfort may present with or without ST-segment elevation on the ECG. The majority of patients with ST-segment elevation (*large arrows*) ultimately develop a Q-wave AMI (*QwMI*), whereas a minority (small arrow) develop a non–Q-wave AMI (*NQMI*). Patients who present without ST-segment elevation are experiencing either UA or an NSTEMI. The distinction between these 2 diagnoses is ultimately made based on the presence or absence of a cardiac marker detected in the blood. Most patients with NSTEMI do not evolve a Q wave on the 12-lead ECG and are subsequently referred to as having sustained a non–Q-wave MI (*NQMI*); only a minority of NSTEMI patients develop a Q wave and are later diagnosed as having Q-wave MI. Not shown is Prinzmetal's angina, which presents with transient chest pain and ST-segment elevation but rarely MI. The spectrum of clinical conditions that range from US to non–Q-wave AMI and Q-wave AMI is referred to as ACSs. Braunwald E, et al. ACC/AHA guidelines for the management of patients with unstable angina and non-ST-segment elevation myocardial infarction. A report of the American College of Cardiology/American Heart Association Task Force on Practice Guidelines (Committee on the Management of Patients With Unstable Angina). J Am Coll Cardiol. 2000;36(3):970-1062.

In the emergency setting, the symptoms, the ECG, and the serum cardiac enzyme levels guide the triage of patients suspected of having an ACS. However, frequently patients with ACS may also present with atypical features depending on the time point of onset or release of symptoms. Cardiac enzymes may be in the normal range early after onset of a myocardial event, and conversely, elevated cardiac enzymes require also the consideration of a number of other differential diagnoses. In the event of an ACS with normal ECG and cardiac enzymes, the blood testing needs to be repeated within 6–8 h to check for a delayed increase of myocardium infarction markers. Patients with previous coronary artery disease may further complicate the situation by their baseline abnormal ECG.

This scenario points to the need for a fast and widely available, non-invasive diagnostic filter test that may either confirm the final diagnosis of ACS or may present findings related to other differential diagnoses. A reliable negative test would allow discharging patients immediately after relieving of symptoms, with major impact of health care costs. A number of different imaging modalities such as trans-thoracic echocardiography, acute radioisotope perfusion scanning, magnetic resonance imaging, coronary artery calcium (CAC) screening and CT angiography (CTA) have already been discussed for this purpose (Barnett et al. 2005). All of the listed modalities may serve for the purpose of diagnosing ACS to a certain degree.

The current chapter will focus on the review of studies describing the role of CAC and CTA in patients with ACS.

3.4.2 Pathogenesis

It was previously believed that the gradual progression of coronary artery stenosis was the cause of acute cardiac events. However, pathologic and angiographic studies have shown that an ACS often is caused by the disruption of a non-severely stenosing atherosclerotic lesion (Martinez-Rumayor and Januzzi 2006). Many patients with ACS have only mild to moderate disease before plaque rupture, with the culprit lesion in up to 80% of patients being less than 70% of the lumen diameter (Roe et al. 2000). Plaque components might therefore be more likely to predict the risk for rupture instead of the pure severity of luminal stenosis.

Vulnerable or 'soft plaques' are defined by a large lipid pool containing a high percentage of inflammatory cells, as well as a thin fibrous cap separating the lipid core from the blood pool. Especially when the fibrous cap is less than 65 µm, it may be vulnerable to rupture and thus exposing the highly thrombogenic core to the blood pool. This results in acute intra-coronary thrombosis obstructing the blood flow to the myocardium (Schroeder and Falk 1995). In contrast collagen-rich 'hard plaques may progress with regard to stenosis severity and result may in stable angina pectoris.

After rupture of a coronary plaque, a rapid sequence of intense platelet-mediated activity occurs ultimately leading to an intra-luminal thrombus partially or completely obstructing the coronary artery. This process can be followed by embolization of fragments of thrombus into the distal coronary circulation which cause micro-infarctions (Martinez-Rumayor and Januzzi 2006). This embolization process might explain why between 60% to 85% of patients with a NSTEMI show a patent infarct-related artery, but do develop symptoms of myocardial ischemia and signs of myocardial necrosis. Micro-infarction in these cases have shown an independent effect on outcome, regardless of the flow in the epicardial artery (Wong et al. 2002).

The current resolution of MDCT scanners does not permit an accurate visualisation of the initial phases of coronary plaque formation and cannot distinguish the subtle features of plaque, such as fibrous cap thickness or signs of inflammation. MDCT is able to classify the obstruction caused by different plaques into obstructive or non-obstructive stenosis. However, to date, precise quantification of the size of plaques is not possible due to the tendency to overestimate high density or calcified plaques and due to the underestimation of low-density plaques. Low density plaques can be either soft plaques with lipid core, fibrous tissue, necrotic tissue or thrombus. Since attenuation of these plaque components are in close range of each other and tend to overlap, it is difficult to distinguish them with a high accuracy using MDCT (Stillman et al. 2007; Pohle et al. 2007).

3.4.3 Risk Stratification

Treatment of ACS patients should in general be directed at stabilizing the hemodynamic situation, relieving ischemic pain, and reducing the risk for recurrent ischemia. It has been estimated that 80% of ACS patients can be stabilized within 48 h after being started on an intensive medical program for ischemia, while the rest require urgent catheterization and revascularization (Yeghiazarians et al. 2000). Risk stratification should therefore be utilized to identify these patients for which medical therapy will not suffice and who are in need for revascularization.

Patient presenting with acute chest pain are typically risk stratified based on the history, physical examination, ECG, chest X-ray, and laboratory studies including cardiac biomarkers. ECG is important to identify the small subset of patients with an ST-elevated myocardial infarction (STEMI) who will benefit from a coronary revascularization. Furthermore, baseline ECG has important prognostic value for ACS, as the risk of new or reversible ST segment depression greater or equal to 0.5 mm has comparable risks to transient ST elevation or new left bundle branch block. It nearly doubles the risk for death (from 8.2% to 15.8%) and it increases the risk for myocardial infarction or recurrent rest ischemia, as well as failure of medical therapy from three to six-fold (Martinez-Rumayor and Januzzi 2006). ECG is, however, less sensitive and has poor negative predictive value; thus a negative ECG does not offer reassurance (Martinez-Rumayor and Januzzi 2006).

Treatment of STEMI patients is directed towards early revascularization as recommended in the ACC/AHA guidelines (Smith et al. 2001). Clinical trials and large scale registry programmes have shown that the outcome for NSTEMI patients is not benign with a death rate of 12%–13% at 6 months in GRACE (global registry of acute coronary events) and PRAIS-UK (prospective registry of acute ischemic syndromes in the UK) which is similar to the 6-month survival of patients with STEMI who reach the hospital alive (Collinson et al. 2000; Fox et al. 2002). Also patients with unstable angina pectoris do not have a benign prognosis when the diagnosis is supported by evidence of underlying ischemic heart disease (5% death at 6 months) (Collinson et al. 2000; Fox et al. 2002). However, the time course and nature of the cardiac consequences differ substantially. Therefore, patients with NSTEMI and unstable angina pectoris at higher risk may benefit from acute interventional strategies and certain pharmacological treatment (glycoprotein IIb/IIIa inhibitors, low molecular weight heparin) compared with patients who do not have an increased risk.

Patients suspected of ACS can be stratified into STEMI, NSTEMI, and unstable angina pectoris with high or low risk for adverse cardiac events and into non-cardiac chest pain. A number of clinical decision tools are available to stratify patients into one of the above categories, but none have a high sensitivity and specificity, and some have an accuracy that is no better than the clinical impression alone (Stillman et al. 2007).

A widely used stratification tool is the Thrombosis In Myocardial Infarction (TIMI) risk score

(Table 3.4.1) (Antman et al. 2000). This seven-point risk score predicts the risk of death, development of new or recurrent infarction, or need for urgent vessel revascularization at 14 days after presentation. The low-risk group is defined by a score of 0 or 1 and a < 5% likelihood of requiring intervention. The high-risk group is defined by a score of 6 or 7 and a 40% likelihood of requiring intervention. This approach has been validated and can easily be used to supplement other ED risk stratification approaches (Manoharan and Adgey 2007; Mega et al. 2005). The TIMI risk score may be useful not only for identifying those patients at risk for ischemic complications from their ACS, such as progression to myocardial infarction or death, but also offers useful information regarding the benefit from specific interventions for ACS management ((Martinez-Rumayor and Januzzi 2006; Pollack et al. 2003).

Despite of the strength of the TIMI risk score, risk stratification for acute chest pain patients in the ED in the absence of diagnostic ECG findings remains an inexact science. Clinical acumen, ECG results, and biomarker assays are largely reliable but still miss 2%–8% of patients with myocardial infarction (Pollack et al. 2003). Quick and accurate risk stratification of patients with acute chest pain in the ED is essential for early and aggressive medical and interventional management of ACS patients. If it were possible to accurately predict high risk in patients with potential NSTEMI or, conversely, to accurately exclude ACS during the early observation period, the number of patients admitted for evaluation of chest pain could be significantly reduced with a commensurate reduction in cost of care. In addition, the earlier identification of high-risk ACS patients could lead to earlier treatment initiated in the ED with the possibility of improved patient outcomes.

Tabel 3.4.1. Thrombosis in myocardial infarction (TIMI) risk score for unstable angina and non-ST-elevated myocardial infarction (NSTEMI)

Age ≥ 65 years
History of known coronary artery disease (documented prior coronary artery stenosis > 50%)
≥ 3 Conventional cardiac risk factors (age, male sex, family history, hyperlipidemia, diabetes mellitus, smoking, obesity)
Use of aspirin in the past 7 days
ST-segment deviation (persistent depression or transient elevation)
Increased cardiac biomarkers (troponins)
≥ 2 Anginal events in the preceding 24 h

Score = sum of number of above characteristics.
Low-risk group is defined by a score of 0 or 1 and a < 5% likelihood of requiring intervention. The high-risk group is defined by a score of 6 or 7 and a 40% likelihood of requiring intervention.

3.4.4 Calcium Scoring in Patients with ACS

Quantification of coronary calcium by CT is a fast and simple procedure that allows determining the amount of calcified plaques in the coronary arteries and by that, estimation of the extent of the patient's atherosclerotic plaque burden. Coronary calcium scoring has been introduced more than a decade ago with the use of electron beam CT. Electron beam CT is a dedicated cardiac CT systems without any moving parts and by that allowing very short exposure times when scanning the heart. The design of this machine made it well suitable for low dose cross-sectional scanning of the heart to detect coronary calcium.

Primarily, coronary calcium scanning was intended as a screening tool for coronary atherosclerosis in asymptomatic persons to determine the risk of acute coronary events. However, in the late nineties some authors reported the use of coronary calcium screening also for patients with angina-like symptoms and negative cardiac enzymes. In two independent studies which both included more than 100 patients presenting with acute chest pain to the ED, electron beam CT was used as a triage tool (Laudon et al. 1999; McLaughlin et al. 1999). An Agatston score of 0 resulted in a negative predictive value of 100% and 98% in these studies (Laudon et al. 1999; McLaughlin et al. 1999). Another study followed almost 200 patients with acute chest pain in the ED for 50 months and found that coronary calcium in this cohort was a strong predictor for future cardiac events with an annual event rate of 0.6% for patients having an Agatston score of 0 (Georgiou et al. 2001). The conclusions from these studies were that patients with a negative coronary calcium scan may be safely discharged home from the ED. A problem with EBT calcium scoring is, however, its high costs and limited availability. Therefore EBT has never been widely used as a stand-alone tool to triage patients with acute chest pain.

Coronary calcium scoring may also be performed with MDCT systems. Depending on the number and width of the detector elements, the spiral scan can be performed within 6–20 s. To improve the reproducibility of the measurements, overlapping slice reconstruction on the basis of retrospective ECG-gating were recommended (Ohnesorge et al. 2000). However, this approach results in a higher radiation dose as compared to the prospective or sequential triggering approach.

It is important to note that the results from calcium scoring do not translate to a diseased coronary segment with regard to a stenosis, but to a diseased patient with atherosclerosis of the coronary arteries. A recent study has shown, that 7% of the patients having a negative calcium score suffer from obstructive CAD, and additional 13% with a zero Agatston score have non-obstructive coronary atheroma (Rubinshtein et al. 2007a). Nevertheless, the patient population of this study was relatively young and included 45% women for which CT calcium scoring in the triage of ED patients has proven to be less reliable. We should be aware that most studies assessing the predictive value of calcium scoring had been performed on electron beam CT, and we do not know yet if these results can be extrapolated to MDCT without adjustments. Guidelines are now being developed to address the use of MDCT calcium scoring in more detail.

3.4.5 CTA for the Diagnosis of ACS

Advanced MDCT technology allows not only assessment of the calcified atherosclerotic plaque burden but also enables the visualization of the lumen of the coronary arteries by the use of contrast material. A typical CT angiography (CTA) investigation of the heart with most modern CT scanners usually does not take longer than a breath-hold period of 10 s and 60–80 ml of contrast media. MDCT scanners with the option to scan the heart and the coronary arteries are in the meanwhile widely available.

Coronary artery plaques are of particular interest in patients with high risk for cardiac events. Although these lesions may not be flow limiting or causing stenosis at the time of detection because of positive remodeling of the artery, they may under certain circumstances rupture and cause acute occlusion of the vessel lumen with consecutive infarction.

Exceeding a certain size, CTA may, similar to intravascular ultrasound, demonstrate plaques and giving hereby a guess of their composition (Leber et al. 2005). Plaque assessment tools are implemented in cardiac software packages for evaluation of CTA data and help to quantify the volume and density of different coronary artery plaques. Ex-vivo studies have shown that plaques with a high lipid composition tend to have lower CT numbers than those presenting with fibrous tissue (Becker et al. 2003). CTA appears to be a well suited tool to image lesions in the coronary arteries that appear near normal in cardiac catheter and are only seen by intravascular ultrasound. The remodeling of coronary arteries with underlying atherosclerotic disease can be determined with MDCT in a similar fashion as with intravascular ultrasound (Imazeki et al. 2004). CTA provides information about the extent and density of culprit lesions in patients after myocardial infarction, whereas in patients with myocarditis these lesions are absent (Caussin et al. 2003). Studies reported that non-calcified plaques are seen more frequently in patients with acute myocardial infarction and calcified lesions were more common in patients with stable angina (Hoffmann et al. 2006b; Leber et al. 2003). Furthermore, plaques in the remote arteries of patients with ACS more frequently present with low CT densities as compared to patients with stable angina and therefore should intent a systemic rather then a local therapy (Kunimasa et al. 2005). In patients with ACS, plaques in the culprit vessel had a lower CT number as compared to those in non-culprit arteries, concluding that CTA by that is able to discriminate between stable and unstable plaques within the different coronary arteries of the same patient (Inoue et al. 2004).

Sato et al. (2005) investigated in a four-slice CT study 31 patients with ACS. By taking a 75% diameter stenosis and plaque densities with less than 50 HU as a positive finding at CT, the authors report for catheter coronary angiography or troponin I as the study endpoint a sensitivity and specificity for CT of 95.5% and 88.9%, respectively.

Dorgelo et al. (2005) reported in 22 patients undergoing 16-slice CT about the possibility to triage patients with ACS for conservative treatment, PCI, or CABG. The authors followed a simplified stratification scheme taking the number of coronary vessels into account that were affected by stenoses (defined as ≥ 50% luminal reduction). An excellent agreement for decision making using MDCT and catheter coronary angiography for triaging patients with ACS could be demonstrated.

Tsai et al. (2007) have evaluated the ability of 40-slice CT to triage 78 patients into early conservative or early invasive therapy. Early invasive therapy was assigned for the patients if there was significant stenosis (defined as ≥ 50% diameter reduction) in any coronary segment. The authors reported an overall agreement of 92.3% with a kappa value of 0.82 between MDCT and catheter coronary angiography.

Gallagher and colleagues (2007) have shown in a 64-slice CT study in 92 patients that the accuracy of CT is comparable to that of stress nuclear imaging for the detection of ACS in low-risk patients with negative serial ECG and cardiac biomarker results.

Hoffmann and coworkers (2006a) have demonstrated in a 64-slice CT study in 103 patients that CT has good performance characteristics for ruling out ACS in patients presenting to the emergency department with acute chest pain. The authors demonstrated in ACS patients in whom initial triage was inconclusive, that the absence of coronary artery plaque or significant stenosis (defined as diameter reduction ≥ 50%) on CT coronary angiography had an excellent negative predictive value for the subsequent diagnosis of ACS. Furthermore, in those patients with CAD at CT, the extent of coronary atherosclerotic plaque burden provided incremental information to standard baseline patient variables and standard clinical risk assessment.

Rubinshtein et al. (2007b) have shown in 58 patients that 64-slice CT allows for the diagnosis of acute coronary syndrome with a sensitivity of 100%, specificity of 92%, positive predictive value of 87%, and negative predictive value of 100%. In addition, during a 15-month follow-up period, no deaths or myocardial infarctions occurred in the 35 patients discharged from the ED after initial triage and CT findings. Overall, CT sensitivity for predicting major adverse cardiovascular events (death, myocardial infarction, or revascularization) during hospitalization and follow-up was 92%, specificity was 76%, positive predictive value was 52%, and negative predictive value was 97%.

Goldstein and colleagues (2007) have shown in a randomized study of 197 patients that 64-slice CT coronary angiography is able to definitely establish or exclude CAD as the cause of acute chest pain. The high negative predictive value of all these studies suggests that CT coronary angiography is useful for facilitating and optimizing triage of patients with acute chest pain and inconclusive initial clinical emergency department evaluation (Hoffmann et al. 2006a; Goldstein et al. 2007).

Currently, for a cardiac CTA examination, scanning for several heartbeats is necessary to acquire the entire heart volume. CTA therefore offers not only information about the amount of coronary calcium, degree of coronary artery stenosis, density and thereby composition of atherosclerotic plaques with the underlying remodeling but also information about the left ventricular function and regional wall motion. So far, authors using MDCT for diagnosing ACS always used only one or few of these different aspects. According to Dirksen et al. (2005), assessing left ventricular function in patients with unstable angina by cardiac CTA helps to specify the diagnosis of coronary artery disease over the assessment of the coronary arteries alone. In particular, the combination of normal left ventricular function and normal coronary arteries showed a very high negative predictive value for ruling out CAD as compared to cardiac catheter and echocardiography (Dirksen et al. 2005).

3.4.6 CTA for the Differential Diagnosis in ACS

Most modern MDCT scanners are now able to acquire not only selectively the heart but also the entire chest with ECG gating within one breath-hold period. Together with an adjusted contrast media administration protocol, this, at some institutions called "chest pain" or "triple rule out" protocol, allows for investigating the pulmonary arteries, the aorta and the coronary arteries at the same time. Furthermore, this protocol may allow investigation of the chest wall, pleura, lung, mediastinum, and osseous thoracic cage.

The scanning protocol for global assessment differs from dedicated coronary CTA in several important respects. First, the entire z-length of the thorax must be imaged in order to assess the pulmonary vasculature to a subsegmental level, as well as the thoracic aorta. Such imaging requires a longer data acquisition time of up to 15 s, depending on the type of the detector width and the pitch of the examination. This longer scan time goes along with increasing motion artifacts due to breathing. Because the pulmonary vessels are less susceptible to motion artifacts than are coronary arteries, it is advisable to start image acquisition below the cardiac apex and to scan in a caudo-cranial direction, in contrast to the typical cranio-caudal direction that usually is used for a cardiac CTA examination alone. This approach permits imaging of coronary arteries during the first part of the scan, when breath-holding is presumably better. A second important difference is the protocol for contrast media administration. Unlike coronary CTA, when partial washout of contrast in the right heart is desirable, a triple rule-out protocol must provide optimal enhancement of both the right and left heart for simultaneous visualization of the pulmonary arteries, the aorta, and the coronary arteries. Thus, a larger total amount of contrast media along with a longer contrast media administration period is recommended (Schertler et al. 2007; Johnson et al. 2008; Vrachliotis et al. 2007).

White et al. (2005) investigated with 16-slice CT 69 patients with acute chest pain using an ECG-gated protocol of the entire chest. The amount of coronary calcium, the degree of stenosis, the left ventricular ejection fraction, the wall motion, and perfusion lesions in the myocardium as well as non-cardiac causes of chest pain such as pulmonary embolism or pneumonia was assessed. The final diagnosis was derived from clinical examination or one month follow-up. The CT was normal, showed coronary artery disease, non-cardiac related or non-concordant findings in 75%, 14%, 4%, 7% of the patients, respectively. For the diagnosis of ACS the authors reported a sensitivity and specificity of 87% and 96%, respectively. In addition, non-cardiac findings including the lung, mediastinum and the bones were found.

Schertler et al. (2007) investigated 60 patients with acute chest pain with an ECG-gated whole chest dual-source CT protocol. The authors have found such a protocol to provide diagnostic information about the aorta, the pulmonary and the coronary arteries without foregoing heart rate control, and found various cardiac and non-cardiac causes for acute chest pain.

Despite these studies, however, there are still no large prospective studies evaluating the accuracy of an ECG-gated MDCT protocol of the entire chest (i.e., triple-rule-out protocol), and further research is needed to better define its role in ED patient care.

3.4.7 Current Recommendations and Guidelines

The North American Society of Cardiac Imaging and the European Society of Cardiac Radiology have recently published a consensus statement about the use of CT for the assessment of patients with acute chest pain. In consensus, the writing group states that CT provides – beyond the evaluation of aortic dissection and pulmonary embolism – novel and accurate information on the presence of coronary artery disease in this patient population. Nevertheless, large blinded clinical trials are still needed to determine the accuracy and precision of CT for the triage of these patients with acute chest pain. Randomized trials should be performed to evaluate the degree to which CT enhances patient risk stratification, the consequences of a universally standardized as opposed to a targeted protocol, patient outcomes, and cost-effectiveness as compared with the current clinical standard of care. Staffing issues also need to be addressed since sufficient numbers of CT trained physicians and technologists will be needed in order to offer ECG-gated chest CT examinations fully around the clock, including 7 days per week.

Whereas the initial literature evidence for performing a cardiac CT in patients with suspicion of ACS is encouraging, there is until now no agreement on the use and application of an extended ECG-gated CT examination covering the entire chest (i.e., triple rule-out protocol). The question for the need of such a protocol certainly must be answered from the clinical point of view. Emergency department physicians usually feel that it is relatively uncommon that they are uncertain of all three diagnostic considerations (i.e., aorta, pulmonary or coronary arteries). Thus, a single or dual rule-out CT examination most often will be sufficient. Until now, there is a lack on large prospective studies where triple rule-out CT has been used and further research is desirable to better define the role and indication of such a protocol.

3.4.8 Conclusion

Modern MDCT systems are capable of a comprehensive assessment of the cardiovascular system that includes the noninvasive assessment of coronary artery disease. Despite of the increasing role of MDCT in the noninvasive imaging for the coronary arteries, however, the clinical experience in ACS patients is still limited. Clinical guidelines are necessary to establish appropriate clinical indications for coronary CTA in the emergency department. Further evaluation of this evolving technology will benefit from cooperation between different medical specialties supporting multidisciplinary teams that are focused on the diagnosis and treatment of this acute and life-threatening disease. It appears undoubtedly that CT has a considerable potential for improving the management of selected patients with ACP, and that the necessary clinical research trials to clarify and establish its role in the emergency department should proceed with urgency.

References

Agatston AS, Janowitz WR, Hildner FJ, Zusmer NR, Viamonte M, Jr., Detrano R (1990) Quantification of coronary artery calcium using ultrafast computed tomography. J Am Coll Cardiol 15:827–832

Antman EM, Cohen M, Bernink PJ, McCabe CH, Horacek T, Papuchis G et al. (2000) The TIMI risk score for unstable angina/non-ST elevation MI: a method for prognostication and therapeutic decision making. JAMA 284:835–842

Barnett K, Feldman JA (2005) Noninvasive imaging techniques to aid in the triage of patients with suspected acute coronary syndrome: a review. Emerg Med Clin North Am 23:977–998

Becker CR, Nikolaou K, Muders M, Babaryka G, Crispin A, Schoepf UJ et al. (2003) Ex vivo coronary atherosclerotic plaque characterization with multi-detector-row CT. Eur Radiol 13:2094–2098

Braunwald E, Antman EM, Beasley JW et al. (2000) ACC/AHA guidelines for the management of patients with unstable angina and non-ST-segment elevation myocardial infarction. A report of the American College of Cardiology/American Heart Association Task Force on Practice Guidelines (Committee on the Management of Patients With Unstable Angina). J Am Coll Cardiol 36:970–1062

Caussin C, Ohanessian A, Lancelin B, Rahal S, Hennequin R, Dambrin G et al. (2003) Coronary plaque burden detected by multislice computed tomography after acute myocardial infarction with near-normal coronary arteries by angiography. Am J Cardiol 92:849–852

Collinson J, Flather MD, Fox KA, Findlay I, Rodrigues E, Dooley P et al. (2000) Clinical outcomes, risk stratification and practice patterns of unstable angina and myocardial infarction without ST elevation: Prospective Registry of Acute Ischaemic Syndromes in the UK (PRAIS-UK). Eur Heart J 21:1450–1457

Dirksen MS, Jukema JW, Bax JJ, Lamb HJ, Boersma E, Tuinenburg JC et al. (2005) Cardiac multidetector-row computed tomography in patients with unstable angina. Am J Cardiol 95:457–461

Dorgelo J, Willems TP, Geluk CA, van Ooijen PM, Zijlstra F, Oudkerk M (2005) Multidetector computed tomography-guided treatment strategy in patients with non-ST elevation acute coronary syndromes: a pilot study. Eur Radiol 15:708–713

Fox KA, Goodman SG, Klein W, Brieger D, Steg PG, Dabbous O et al. (2002) Management of acute coronary syndromes. Variations in practice and outcome; findings from the Global Registry of Acute Coronary Events (GRACE). Eur Heart J 23(15):1177–1189

Gallagher MJ, Ross MA, Raff GL et al. (2007) The diagnostic accuracy of 64-slice computed tomography coronary angiography compared with stress nuclear imaging in emergency department low-risk chest pain patients. Ann Emerg Med 49:125–136

Gallagher MJ, Ross MA, Raff GL, Goldstein JA, O'Neill WW, O'Neil B (2007) The diagnostic accuracy of 64-slice computed tomography coronary angiography compared with stress nuclear imaging in emergency department low-risk chest pain patients. Ann Emerg Med 49:125–136

Georgiou D, Budoff MJ, Kaufer E, Kennedy JM, Lu B, Brundage BH (2001) Screening patients with chest pain in the emergency department using electron beam tomography: a follow-up study. J Am Coll Cardiol 38:105–110

Goldstein JA, Gallagher MJ, O'Neill WW et al. (2007) A randomized controlled trial of multi-slice coronary computed tomography for evaluation of acute chest pain. J Am Coll Cardiol 49:863–871

Hoffmann U, Nagurney JT, Moselewski F et al. (2006a) Coronary multidetector computed tomography in the assessment of patients with acute chest pain. Circulation 114:2251–2260

Hoffmann U, Moselewski F, Nieman K, Jang IK, Ferencik M, Rahman AM et al. (2006b) Noninvasive assessment of plaque morphology and composition in culprit and stable lesions in acute coronary syndrome and stable lesions in stable angina by multidetector computed tomography. J Am Coll Cardiol 47:1655–1662

Imazeki T, Sato Y, Inoue F, Anazawa T, Tani S, Matsumoto N et al. (2004) Evaluation of coronary artery remodeling in patients with acute coronary syndrome and stable angina by multislice computed tomography. Circ J 68:1045–1050

Inoue F, Sato Y, Matsumoto N, Tani S, Uchiyama T (2004) Evaluation of plaque texture by means of multislice computed tomography in patients with acute coronary syndrome and stable angina. Circ J 68:840–844

Johnson TR, Nikolaou K, Becker A, Leber AW, Rist C, Wintersperger BJ, Reiser MF, Becker CR (2008) Dual-source CT in chest pain assessment. Eur Radiol Apr; 18(4):773–80

Kunimasa T, Sato Y, Sugi K, Moroi M (2005) Evaluation by multislice computed tomography of atherosclerotic coronary artery plaques in non-culprit, remote coronary arteries of patients with acute coronary syndrome. Circ J 69:1346–1351

Laudon DA, Vukov LF, Breen JF, Rumberger JA, Wollan PC, Sheedy PF (1999) Use of electron-beam computed tomography in the evaluation of chest pain patients in the emergency department. Ann Emerg Med 33:15–21

Leber AW, Knez A, White CW, Becker A, von ZF, Muehling O et al. (2003) Composition of coronary atherosclerotic plaques in patients with acute myocardial infarction and stable angina pectoris determined by contrast-en-

hanced multislice computed tomography. Am J Cardiol 91:714–718
Leber AW, Knez A, von Ziegler F, Becker A, Nikolaou K, Paul S et al. (2005) Quantification of obstructive and nonobstructive coronary lesions by 64-slice computed tomography: a comparative study with quantitative coronary angiography and intravascular ultrasound. J Am Coll Cardiol 46:147–154
Lee TH, Rouan GW, Weisberg MC, Brand DA, Acampora D, Stasiulewicz C et al. (1987) Clinical characteristics and natural history of patients with acute myocardial infarction sent home from the emergency room. Am J Cardiol 60:219–224
Manoharan G, Adgey AA (2002) Current management of unstable angina: lessons from the TACTICS-TIMI 18 trial. Am J Cardiovasc Drugs 2:237–243
Martinez-Rumayor A, Januzzi JL, Jr (2006) Non-ST segment elevation acute coronary syndromes: A comprehensive review. South Med J 99:1103–1110
McLaughlin VV, Balogh T, Rich S (1999) Utility of electron beam computed tomography to stratify patients presenting to the emergency room with chest pain. Am J Cardiol 84:327–328, A8
Mega JL, Morrow DA, Sabatine MS, Zhao XQ, Snapinn SM, DiBattiste PM et al. (2005) Correlation between the TIMI risk score and high-risk angiographic findings in non-ST-elevation acute coronary syndromes: observations from the Platelet Receptor Inhibition in Ischemic Syndrome Management in Patients Limited by Unstable Signs and Symptoms (PRISM-PLUS) trial. Am Heart J 149:846–850
Ohnesorge B, Flohr T, Becker C, Kopp AF, Schoepf UJ, Baum U et al. (2000) Cardiac imaging by means of electrocardiographically gated multisection spiral CT: initial experience. Radiology 217:564–571
Pohle K, Achenbach S, MacNeill B, Ropers D, Ferencik M, Moselewski F et al. (2007) Characterization of non-calcified coronary atherosclerotic plaque by multi-detector row CT: comparison to IVUS. Atherosclerosis 190:174–180
Pollack CV, Jr., Roe MT, Peterson ED (2003) 2002 update to the ACC/AHA guidelines for the management of patients with unstable angina and non-ST-segment elevation myocardial infarction: implications for emergency department practice. Ann Emerg Med 41:355–369
Pope JH, Aufderheide TP, Ruthazer R, Woolard RH, Feldman JA, Beshansky JR et al. (2000) Missed diagnoses of acute cardiac ischemia in the emergency department. N Engl J Med 342:1163–1170
Roe MT, Harrington RA, Prosper DM, Pieper KS, Bhatt DL, Lincoff AM et al. (2000) Clinical and therapeutic profile of patients presenting with acute coronary syndromes who do not have significant coronary artery disease. The Platelet Glycoprotein IIb/IIIa in Unstable Angina: Receptor Suppression Using Integrilin Therapy (PURSUIT) Trial Investigators. Circulation 102:1101–1106
Rubinshtein R, Gaspar T, Halon DA, Goldstein J, Peled N, Lewis BS (2007a) Prevalence and extent of obstructive coronary artery disease in patients with zero or low calcium score undergoing 64-slice cardiac multidetector computed tomography for evaluation of a chest pain syndrome. Am J Cardiol 99:472–475
Rubinshtein R, Halon DA, Gaspar T et al. (2007b) Usefulness of 64-slice cardiac computed tomographic angiography for diagnosing acute coronary syndromes and predicting clinical outcome in emergency department patients with chest pain of uncertain origin. Circulation 115:1762–1768
Sato Y, Matsumoto N, Ichikawa M, Kunimasa T, Iida K, Yoda S et al. (2005) Efficacy of multislice computed tomography for the detection of acute coronary syndrome in the emergency department. Circ J 69:1047–1051
Schertler T, Scheffel H, Frauenfelder T et al. (2007) Dual-source computed tomography in patients with acute chest pain: feasibility and image quality. Eur Radiol 17:3179–3188
Schroeder AP, Falk E (1995) Vulnerable and dangerous coronary plaques. Atherosclerosis 118[Suppl]:S141–S149
Smith SC, Jr., Dove JT, Jacobs AK, Kennedy JW, Kereiakes D, Kern MJ et al. (2001) ACC/AHA guidelines for percutaneous coronary intervention (revision of the 1993 PTCA guidelines)-executive summary: a report of the American College of Cardiology/American Heart Association task force on practice guidelines (Committee to revise the 1993 guidelines for percutaneous transluminal coronary angioplasty) endorsed by the Society for Cardiac Angiography and Interventions. Circulation 103:3019–3041
Stillman AE, Oudkerk M, Ackerman M, Becker CR, Buszman PE, de Feyter PJ et al. (2007) Use of multidetector computed tomography for the assessment of acute chest pain: a consensus statement of the North American Society of Cardiac Imaging and the European Society of Cardiac Radiology. Int J Cardiovasc Imaging 23:415–427
Tsai IC, Lee T, Lee WL, Tsao CR, Tsai WL, Chen MC et al. (2007) Use of 40-detector row computed tomography before catheter coronary angiography to select early conservative versus early invasive treatment for patients with low-risk acute coronary syndrome. J Comput Assist Tomogr 31:258–264
Vrachliotis TG, Bis KG, Haidary A et al. (2007) Atypical chest pain: coronary, aortic, and pulmonary vasculature enhancement at biphasic single-injection 64-section CT angiography. Radiology 243:368–376
White CS, Kuo D, Kelemen M, Jain V, Musk A, Zaidi E et al. (2005) Chest pain evaluation in the emergency department: can MDCT provide a comprehensive evaluation? AJR Am J Roentgenol 185:533–540
Wong GC, Morrow DA, Murphy S, Kraimer N, Pai R, James D et al. (2002) Elevations in troponin T and I are associated with abnormal tissue level perfusion: a TACTICS-TIMI 18 substudy. Treat Angina with Aggrastat and Determine Cost of Therapy with an Invasive or Conservative Strategy-Thrombolysis in Myocardial Infarction. Circulation 106:202–207
Yeghiazarians Y, Braunstein JB, Askari A, Stone PH (2000) Unstable angina pectoris. N Engl J Med 342:101–114

Non-Invasive Coronary Imaging

3

3.5 Coronary CT Angiography Guidance for Percutaneous Transluminal Angioplasty

Jean-Louis Sablayrolles and Philippe Guyon

CONTENTS

J.-L. Sablayrolles, MD
P. Guyon, MD
Centre Cardiologique du Nord, 32-36 Avenue des Moulins Gémeaux, 93200 Saint Denis, France

The angiographic "gold standard" for coronary stenosis is "luminography", whereby the interventional cardiologist does not see the disease being diagnosed or treated. This disease comes from the arterial wall. Invasive cardiology only treats the consequences of a pathology on the arterial lumen and the drop in local flow.

The rapid evolution of coronary computed tomographic angiography (CTA) and the accuracy of 64-slice scanners has resulted in the development of applications deemed highly improbable just a few years ago. The aim of this chapter is to demonstrate that coronary CTA can be a guide to percutaneous coronary interventions (PCI), particularly for complex coronary stenosis.

3.5.1 General Principles

Slice imaging [CT, intravascular ultrasound (IVUS), and optical coherence tomography (OCT)] has the major advantage of being able to visualize the lumen of the coronary arteries as well as their wall, therefore providing the ability to define the atheromatous plaques. Cardiac CT is the only non-invasive, but irradiating, imaging modality for plaques and atheromatous disease of the coronary arteries.

Coronary CTA has become a medium and an aid to the interventional cardiologist. CTA will be able to analyze the plaque that needs to be treated, perhaps less in terms of its composition (the resolution is somewhat low) than its location, especially its distribution around the coronary arteries bifurcations.

The appeal of this imaging technique in interventional cardiology is illustrated by the growing number of examinations requested directly by the catheterizing physician (Table 3.5.1).

Table 3.5.1. Change in the number of coronary CT scans performed at the request of the interventional cardiology department over 5 years

Year	2003	2004	2005	2006	2007
Scheduled ATCs	338	271	214	175	143
Total ATCs	1457	1483	1375	1308	1247
MSCT	10	20	71	124	215

ATC, MSCT, multi-slice computed tomography.

Increasing numbers of examinations are being requested directly by the catheterization lab, while the total number of coronary angioplasties, and especially the number of scheduled coronary angioplasties, has been dropping consistently for 5 years (Fig. 3.5.1). This drop reflects the maturity of patient care prior to a coronary angiography, which has become less a diagnostic examination for coronary lesions and more an anatomical check-up prior to a revascularization procedure either by coronary angioplasty or bypass surgery.

The resolution of the 0.4-mm multi-row CT scanner is probably still inadequate for a reliable assessment of atheromatous plaque. Still, its potential is unequaled for a non-invasive examination: analysis of the lesion topography, extent of lesions, their distribution in relation to the coronary arterial tree, particularly arterial bifurcations, and especially the composition and topography of the atheromatous plaque.

Technical limits of coronary angiography (CAG) and PCI:

- Left main trunk (LMT) and right coronary artery (RCA) ostium
- Bifurcation lesion
- Total chronic occlusion
- Highly calcified lesion
- Plaque characterization
- Plaque volume vs. stenosis

The advantages of coronary CTA include the ability to:

- Detect stenosis
- Specify the topography and volume of the plaque vs. stenosis
- Provide information for revascularization PCI or coronary artery bypass grafting (CABG)
- Optimize procedures: PCI guidance

CAG performs a perfect analysis of the lumen while cardiac CT scan provides plaque visualization. Is a fusion of the images with their analysis possible? This is the concept of multi-slice CT (MSCT) guidance prior to coronary angioplasty (Fig. 3.5.2).

In our institution, we use coronary CTA as PCI guidance for complex coronary lesions (ostial or bifurcation lesions) and for chronic total occlusion.

The rate of adverse events associated with CAG and PCI is 1%–2%, with a 0.05%–0.1% mortality rate. Events which may occur during procedures include:

- Plaque shifting
- Dissection
- Occlusion
- Emboli (gas, thrombus, ca++)
- Spasm
- Rupture
- Left ventricle (LV) perforation
- The aim is to choose the optimal procedure to:
- Cover the lumen stenosis and the whole plaque
- Prevent events during the procedure such as plaque shifting (Fig. 3.5.3)
- Reduce various risk factors for restenosis after coronary PCI

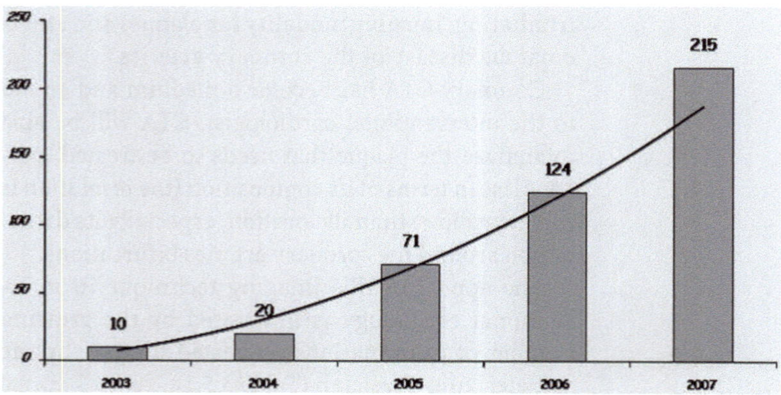

Fig. 3.5.1. Rapid exponential increase in the number of cardiac CT scans requested by the interventional cardiology department

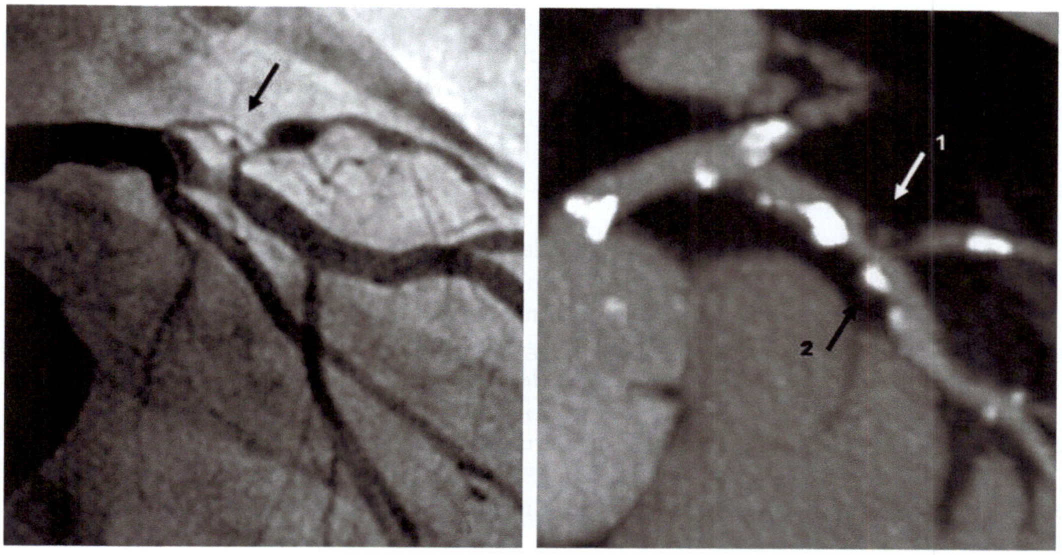

a b

Fig. 3.5.2a,b. Left anterior descending artery/diagonal artery stenosis. **a** Coronary angiography = "luminography". **b** Coronary CT angiography = lumen + soft plaque (*1*) and calcified plaque (*2*)

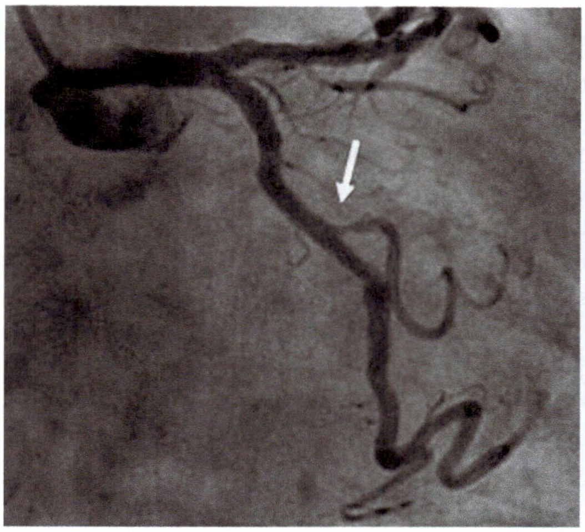

a

Fig. 3.5.3. **a** Ostial stenosis of a left main bronchus (LMB). **b** Balloon inflated in the LMB (*1*), evidence of a snowplow effect, shifting of the plaque toward the left circumflex artery segment II (*2*)

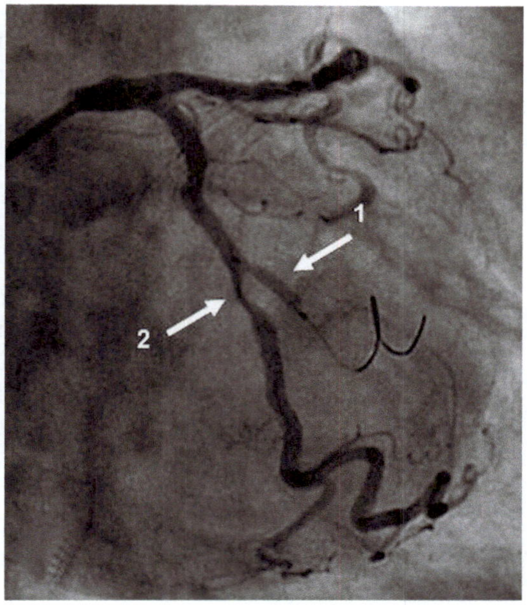

b

3.5.2 CTA Protocol for PCI Guidance of Complex CA Lesions

1. CAG in Cath Lab
2. Low dose CTA
3. Post processing: lesion classification and plaque study
4. Integration CAG and CT data in Cath Lab

3.5.2.1 Coronary Angiography

Following CAG, if there is a complex lesion of the coronary artery, we decide to perform a coronary CTA prior to angioplasty to identify these lesions (Fig. 3.5.4).

In CAG, the radiation dose is 1.10±0.42 mSv (0.42–5.47).

The contrast volume is 35–40 ml for standard CAG and 20–25 ml for rotational acquisition.

3.5.2.2 Protocol of Coronary CTA

In order to reliably assess coronary arteries and cardiac structures, it is essential to use optimal techniques in terms of patient preparation, scan parameters, and injection protocol. To reduce the radiation dose, we use the SnapShot Pulse acquisition (GE Lightspeed VCT XT). The SnapShot Pulse mode, which was installed at the CCN in September 2006, is an advanced axial step-and-shoot mode with prospective ECG synchronization developed by the engineers at General Electric. Using the axial mode instead of the helical mode already reduces the radiation dose, since the overlap related to the very principle of a tight-pitch helix (0.16–0.24) is eliminated. Lastly, in contrast to the helical mode, the X-ray tube does not emit continuously, but only during the window of the heart cycle chosen by the user (Fig. 3.5.5).

SnapShot Pulse thus makes it possible to drastically reduce the radiation dose while maintaining image quality. The dose is reduced by 70%–80% compared to the helical mode. Indeed, with this technique, it is now possible to perform a cardiac examination with an average of 5 mSv or even less (1–6 mSv). The acquisition parameters (kVp and mAS) are adjusted to the patient's BMI (height and weight).

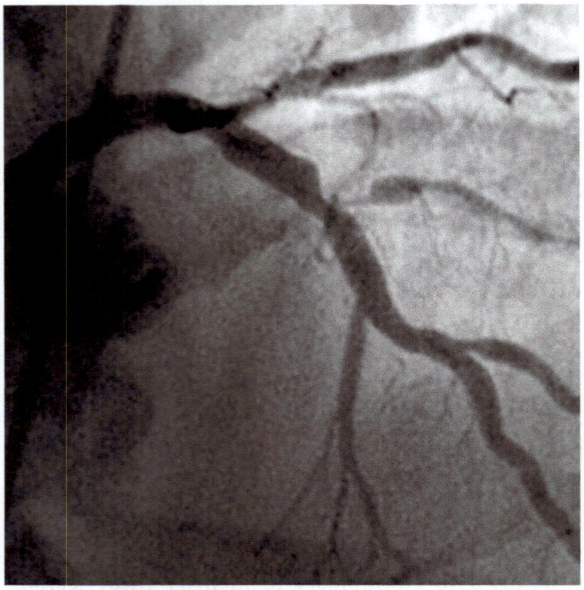

Fig. 3.5.4. Rotational coronary angiography; complex lesion of the left anterior descending artery/diagonal artery bifurcation

For an example of a male patient, 69 years old, 170 cm, 75 kg – BMI=22 kg/m^2, HR=55 bpm, see Table 3.5.2.

In the case given in Table 3.5.2, the radiation dose is only 3 mSv (DLP=176 mGy.cm) with equivalent image quality than spiral acquisition.

Heart scans are routinely performed with an intravenous injection of iodinated contrast medium. Image acquisition must be synchronized to the ECG, but also to the arrival of contrast medium in the chambers of the heart and the coronary artery. To achieve this ideal vascular enhancement, we use:

- A contrast volume of 60–80 ml depending on the patient's weight and the acquisition time.
- An iodine concentration of 300–350 mg I/ml.
- An automatic injector for proper control of the injection parameters, preferably with two syringes and a contrast medium dilution program.
- A triphasic injection:
  - The first phase consists of injecting 50 ml of contrast medium at a flow rate of 5 cc/s.
  - During the second phase, a mix of contrast medium and isotonic solution is injected (20 ml+20 ml) at a slower flow rate (2 ml/s).
  - In the third phase, 20 ml of isotonic solution is injected at 2 ml/s to flush the arm veins.
- A system for automatically detecting the arrival of contrast medium in the ascending aorta, such as SmartPrep.

3.5.2.3 Post Processing

Image processing is indispensable to extract information such as lesion classification and plaque study. Fast and reliable dedicated reconstruction software programs have been developed for the purpose of extracting this information. Thanks to volume acquisition of the multi-detector CT (MDCT) and an isotropic voxel, it is possible to reconstruct 3D or 2D images regardless of the plane in space, with a spatial resolution identical to that of basic axial cross sections.

When studying the coronary arteries, the first stage is to select the best phase in which the coro-

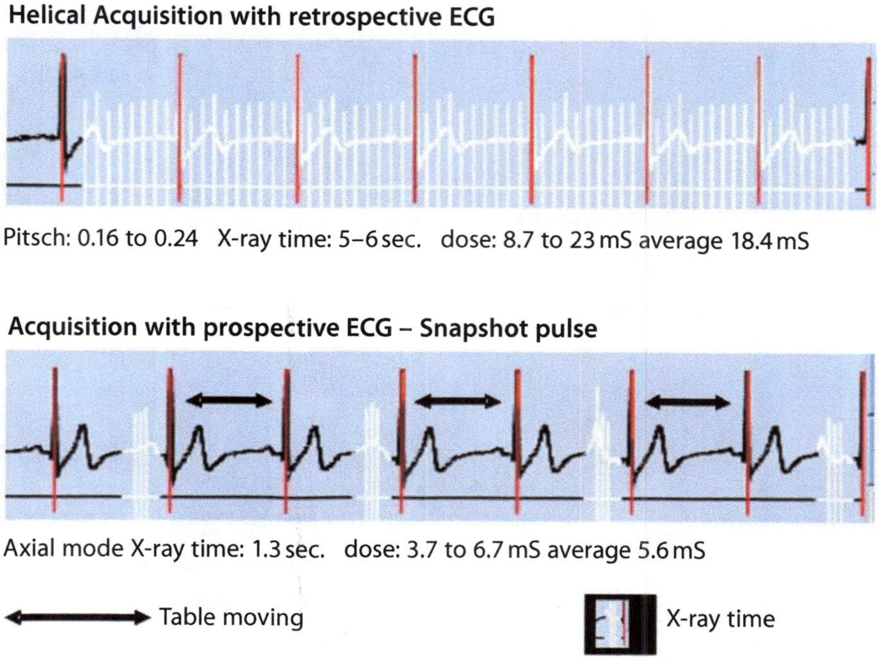

Fig. 3.5.5. Helical mode vs. SnapShot Pulse mode

Table 3.5.2. An example of reduced radiation dose using SnapShot Pulse mode in a 69-year-old male patient, 170 cm, 75 kg – BMI=22 kg/m², HR=55 bpm

Acquisition parameters	
Anatomical coverage	140 mm
Scan direction	Craniocaudal
Acquisition time X ray time	5–7 s 1.7 s
mA	650
kVp	120
Scan rotation	0.35 s
Temporal resolution Padding	227 m 1 Phase: 75%
FOV	200 mm
Slice thickness/increment Data filter	0.6 mm/0.6 mm Standard

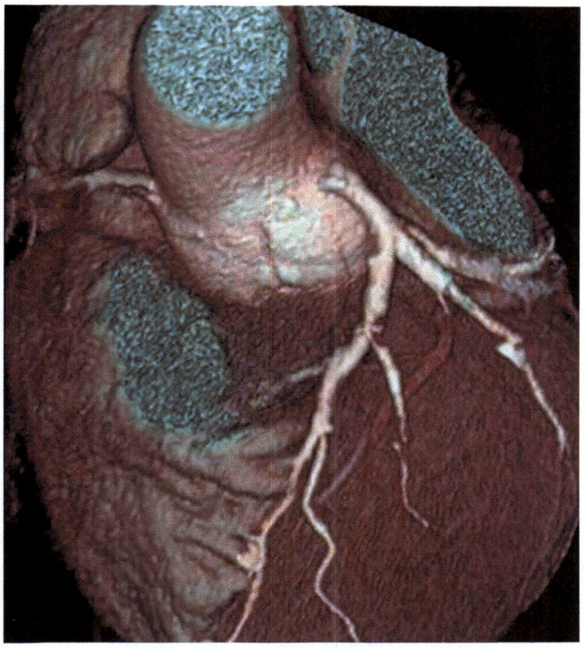

Fig. 3.5.6. Same patient as in Fig. 3.5.5. 3D Computed-assisted reconstruction

nary arteries are displayed optimally without kinetic artefacts. Once this first phase is selected, 3D imaging such as volume rendering or maximum intensity projection (MIP) identifies the right and left coronary arteries and their collateral branches (Fig. 3.5.6). The study of the lumen and vessel wall is then done with curved 2D after automatic tracking of each branch of the coronary arteries (Figs. 3.5.7 and 3.5.8). This 2D imaging not only assesses the lumen but also performs a plaque study: topography, volume and type (soft, calcified or mixed).

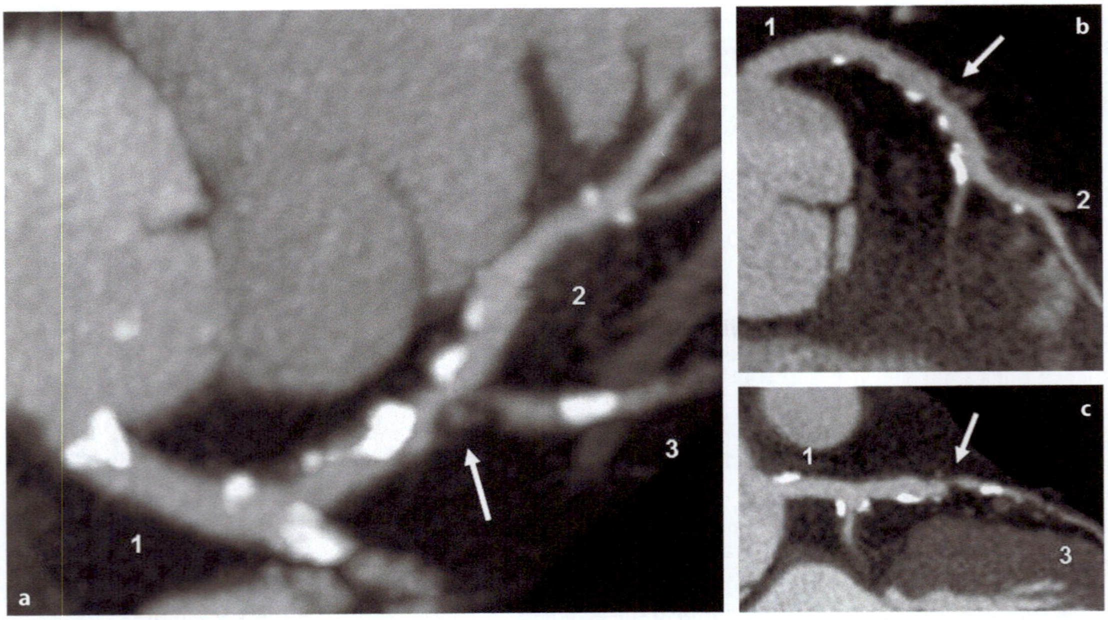

Fig. 3.5.7a–c. Left anterior descending artery (LAD)/diagonal artery stenosis. **a** Maximum intensity projection. **b** LAD 2D curved (*long axis*). **c** Diagonal 2D curved (*long axis*). *1*, Left main trunk; *2*, LAD; *3*, diagonal artery

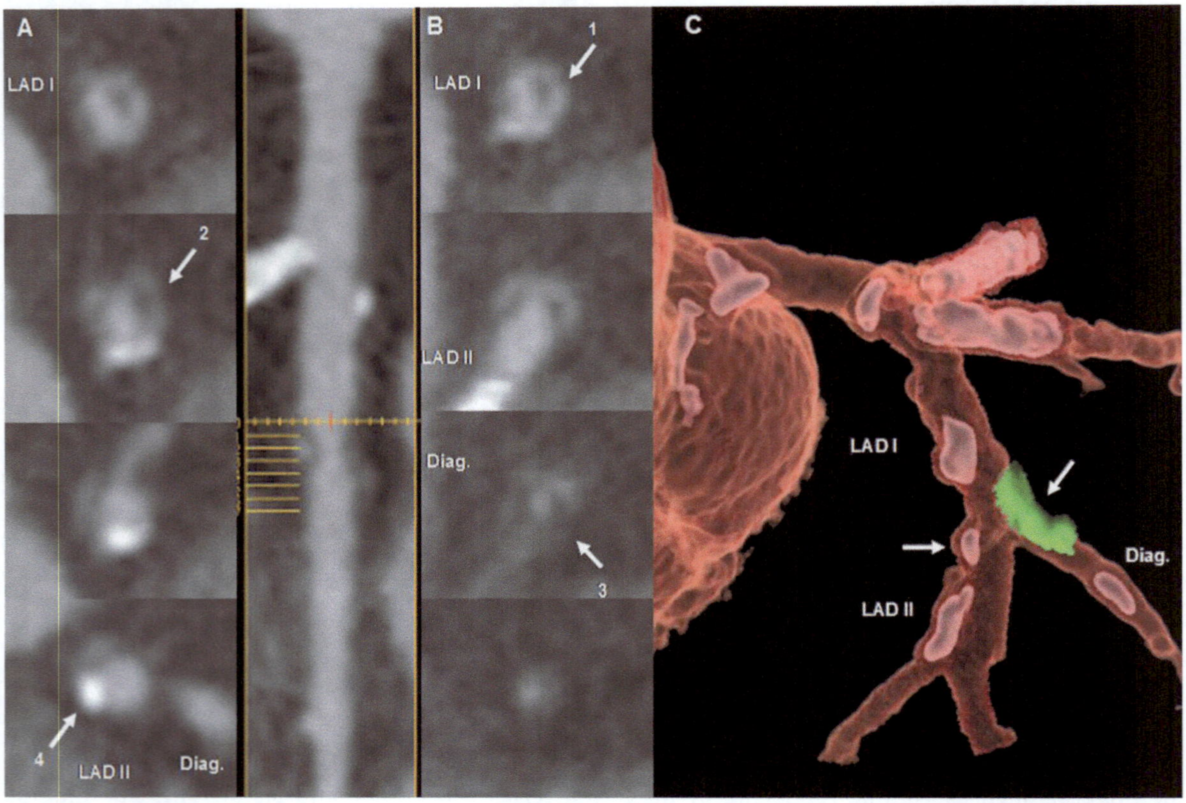

Fig. 3.5.8. Same lesion as in Fig. 3.5.7. Left anterior descending artery (LAD) (**A**) and diagonal artery. **B** 2D Curved in short axis. **C** Volume rendering. Plaque study: *1*, mixed plaque (LAD I); *2*, soft plaque (LAD I and diagonal artery); *3*, calcified plaque (LAD II)

3.5.2.4
Integration of CAG and CT Data in the Cath Lab

With new post-processing software (AngioCT of Shina systems), we integrate angiography and CT data during the catheterization procedure to optimize PCI planning and performance.

It presents a 3D reconstruction of coronary vessels as well as CT cross-sectional information, and recommends the optimal C-arm orientation for viewing an area of stenosis. AngioCT thus makes it possible to view and evaluate previously acquired cardiac CT images and register them with respect to fluoroscopic images that are being acquired during a cardiac catheterization procedure. This enables the user to visualize real-time CT image data that is associated with specific points in the fluoroscopic images (Fig. 3.5.9).

In real time, we have gained significant information for our PCI procedure:

- Optimal C-arm orientation
- Plaque location, length and type (calcified, mixed or soft)
- Real length of the stenosis or chronic total occlusion (CTO)
- Suggested stent size and positioning

3.5.3
CT Guidance of Chronic Total Occlusion

This is one of the major challenges of intravascular coronary procedures. This type of coronary lesion is characterized by a complete obstruction of the coronary artery over a segment of some length. An analysis of the plaque and occlusion in the CT scan images anticipates the pitfalls of these angioplasties, which are always difficult, by visualizing the presence of thrombi, the location of arterial calcifications, the virtual lumen, and the path of the artery's journey through the plaque (Fig. 3.5.10).

The fusion of images gained from techniques as diverse as CT and CAG is an unequalled opportunity. The "road mapping" of the artery to be unclogged as

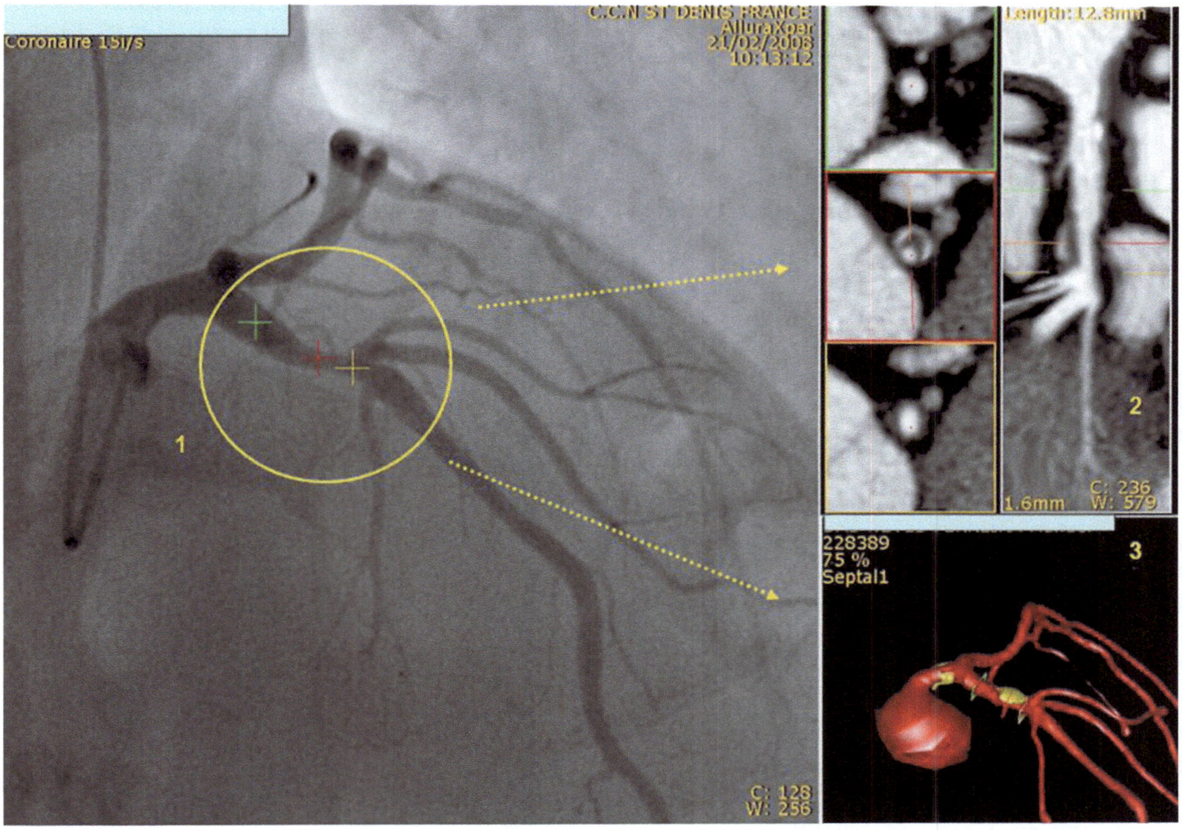

Fig. 3.5.9. Integration coronary angiography (CAG) and CT data in the Cath Lab. In real time, for specific points in GAG: *1*, visualization of 2D; *2*, and 3D; *3*, CT imaging (lumen and mixed plaque)

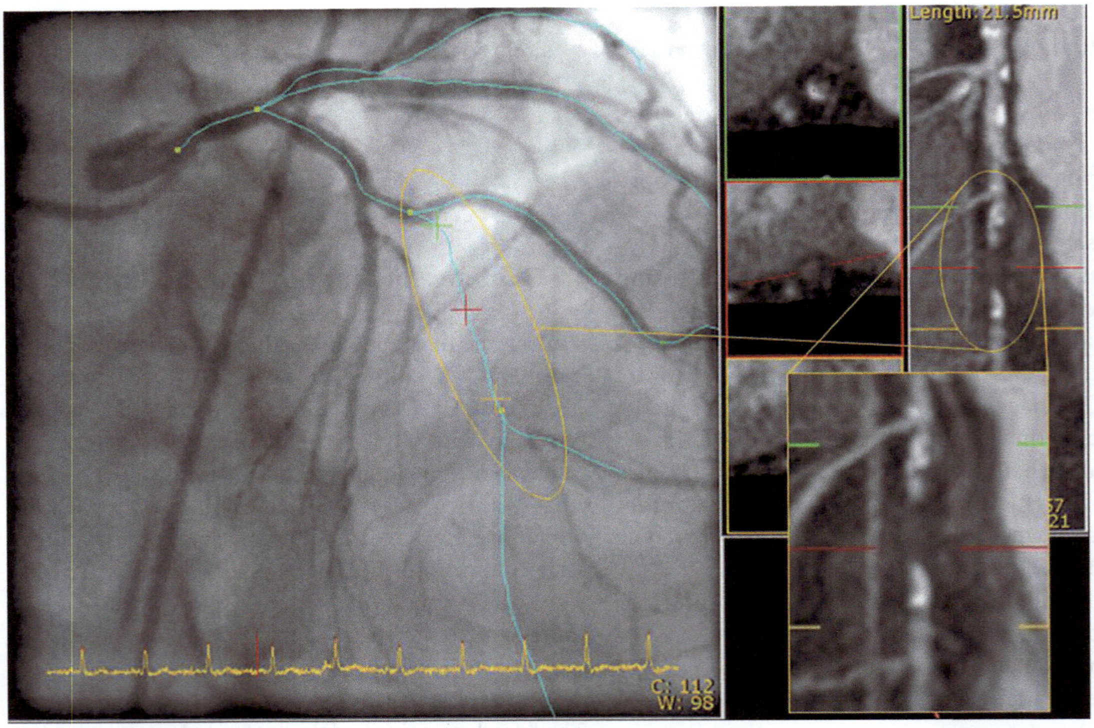

Fig. 3.5.10. Superimposition of the CT scan and coronary angiography images obtained with the same incidence on the registration of the coronary arteries. The CT scan shows the virtual lumen and the path of the epicardial vessel. This assists in the manipulation of the unclogging guide and steers it to the true arterial lumen

seen on the fluoroscopy must facilitate and steer the path of the guide. Synchronization of a Cath Lab C-arm to the projections of the images coming from a CT scanner is reality.

3.5.4 CT Guidance of Coronary Ostia

This concept of virtual reality also assumes an important role in the treatment of coronary ostia by means of transluminal angioplasty, in which the positioning of the stent is particularly challenging. The implantation of a medical spring must cover the entire initial path of the coronary artery with its radial force; however, the extreme proximal portion of the coronary artery has a wall in common with that of the aorta. The result is that, in order to be effective, the prosthesis must cover the coronary ostium and even protrude slightly, although not significantly, into the lumen of the ascending aorta. The superimposing of the anatomy of the aorta and the arterial tree obtained by the CT scanner on the angiography image (fluoroscopy and X-ray) provides an aid for stent positioning (Figs. 3.5.11, 3.5.12). Convergence of the types of imaging should

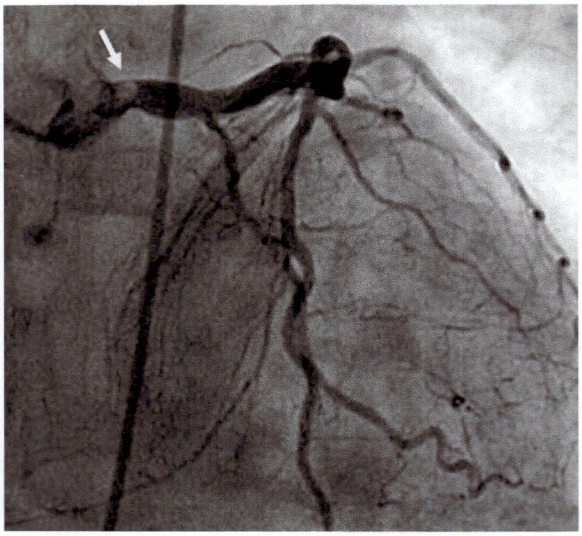

Fig. 3.5.11. Coronary angiography of left main trunk ostium stenosis

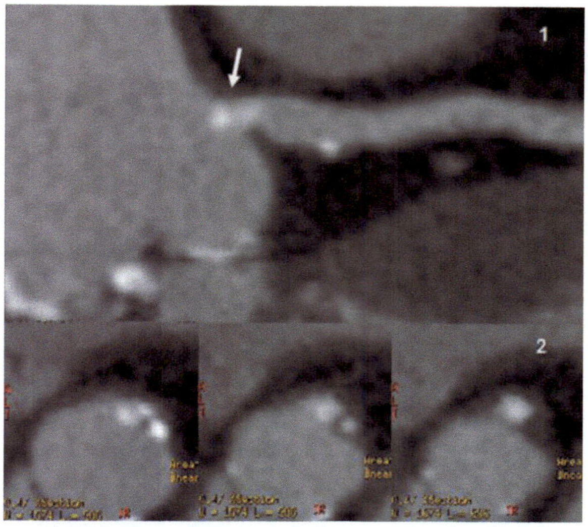

Fig. 3.5.12. CT 2D curved. Long axis (*1*) and short axis (*2*). Calcified plaque of aortic wall and left main trunk ostium

allow for perfectly adequate stent implantation with complete coverage of the coronary ostium without significant protrusion of the proximal portion of the stent into the aorta. The check-up scan performed after implantation of the endoprosthesis documents the position of the stent after the fact and will obviously determine a portion of the secondary and future evolution (Fig. 3.5.13).

3.5.5 CT Guidance of Bifurcation Lesions

Any analysis of the lumen and consequently the coronary stenosis during a coronary angiography is incomplete and is often even completely erroneous. Before an atheromatous plaque develops in the lumen, it develops toward its wall. The iceberg image is used to characterize this phenomenon. Narrowing of the arterial lumen is only one of the consequences of the development of the atheromatous plaque. It does not account for its extent or its surrounding distribution in the wall of the artery. This is particularly significant in bifurcation lesions where the so-called risk of plaque shifting and therefore occlusion of an artery during coronary angioplasty is very high. It is essential to know the distribution of the atheromatous plaque around the coronary bifurcation and its extension along the coronary arterial tree during coronary angioplasty.

3.5.5.1 The Limits of Coronary Angiography

Here, types of coronary lesion are illustrated by a comparative analysis of CT and CAG for coronary artery imaging.

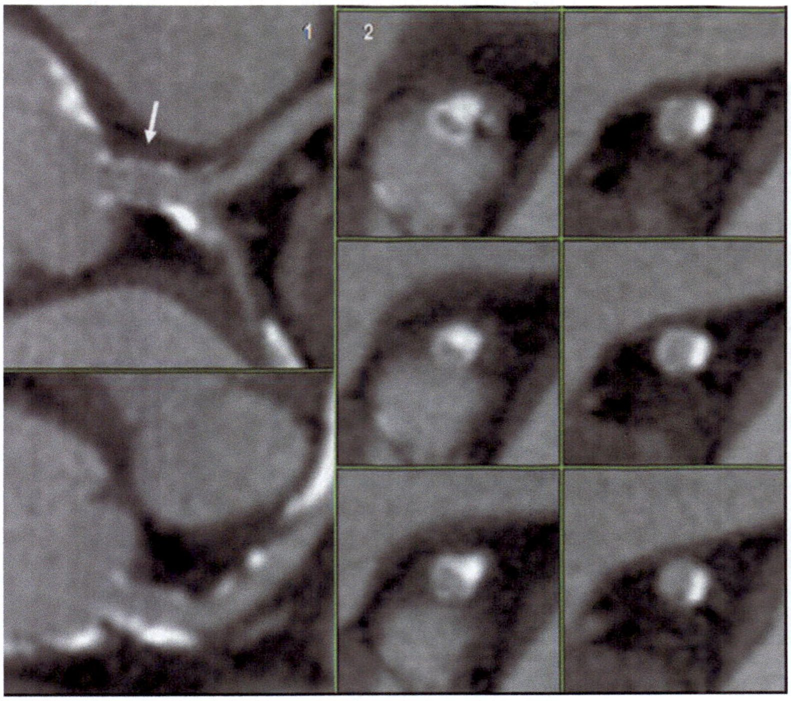

Fig. 3.5.13. Same patient as in Fig. 3.5.12. Normal stent follow-up (Taxus, 3.5 mm)

Of 81 bifurcation lesions, 26 lesions involved the main branch of the left coronary artery, 33 bifurcations were located on the left anterior descending artery and diagonal artery, 13 on the left circumflex and marginal artery, and nine on the right coronary artery in its distal bifurcation (tripod) (Table 3.5.3).

These patients all had at least one bifurcation lesion either on the main branch or on one of the three primary epicardial vessels. CT and CAG are interpreted blindly and independently by two different operators. The analysis targets the pathological arterial bifurcation area and 10 mm upstream and downstream when possible.

The bifurcation area was divided into three segments for the purpose of this analysis: proximal and distal on the main vessel and on the ostium of the collateral vessel (classification by Dr. Medina) (Fig. 3.5.14). The topography of the plaque was taken into account in its entirety on the CT scan, whereas the CAG analysis was performed using the arterial stenoses and their repercussions on the arterial lumen. A semi-quantitative analysis of the composition of the plaque (calcified, mixed or soft plaque), other upstream and/or downstream lesions and thrombi were also reported

Table 3.5.3. Classification of 81 bifurcation lesions in patients included in a comparative study of CT and CAG

Distal LMT	26
LAD/Diag.	33
LCx/LMB	13
RCA III	9

3.5.5.2 Results

In 70% of the cases, CAG did not clearly analyze the plaque volume distribution around the bifurcation lesion.

These results show that CAG does not correctly analyze the topography of the bifurcation lesion in

Table 3.5.4. Distribution of coronary bifurcation lesions according to the Medina classification depending on the imaging mode

Bifurcation site	1,1,1	1,1,0	1,0,0	0,1,1
CAG	41 (50%)	21 (25%)	7 (10%)	12 (15%)
CTA	70 (85%)	7 (10%)	4 (5%)	0

CAG, coronary angiography; CTA, multi-detector CT angiography

Table 3.5.5. Quantitative analysis of coronary bifurcation lesions according to imaging mode

Plaque Composition	Calcifications	Soft plaque	Thrombus	Other plaques
CAG	43 (54%)	NA	0	0
CTA	73 (86%)	24 (30%)	8 (10%)	73 (95%)

CAG, coronary angiography; CTA, multi-detector CT angiography; NA, not applicable.

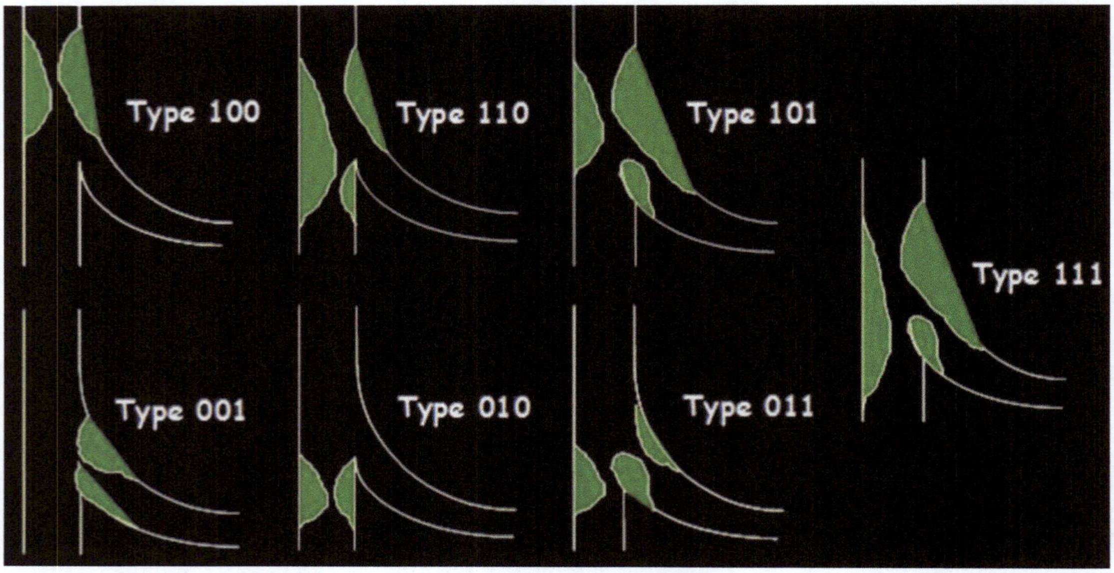

Fig. 3.5.14. Definition, classification, and distribution of bifurcation lesions according to the Medina classification

more than two thirds of cases. However, the CT scan, by correctly visualizing the atheromatous plaque, is capable of properly showing its distribution in three dimensions around the coronary branch divisions (Figs. 3.5.15–3.5.17). The decision of whether, and how ,to revascularize (CABG or CAG) or not is made according to the complexity of the lesion to be treated. If an indication for CAG is given, the prior analysis of the plaque and other lesions will guide the intervention in its implementation, e.g. whether or not to use of a protective guide in the collateral artery, installation of one or two stents.

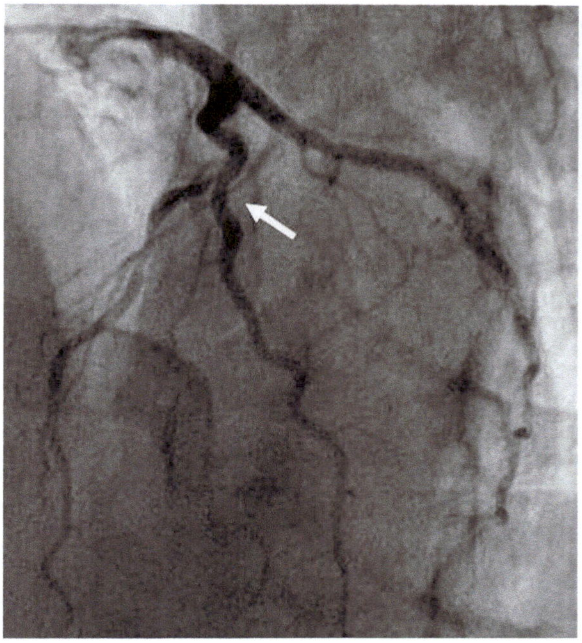

Fig. 3.5.15. Coronary angiography. Stenosis of left anterior descending artery segment II. The stenosis is located in a bifurcation area (ostial branch lesion) of the type 0,1,0 according to the Medina classification

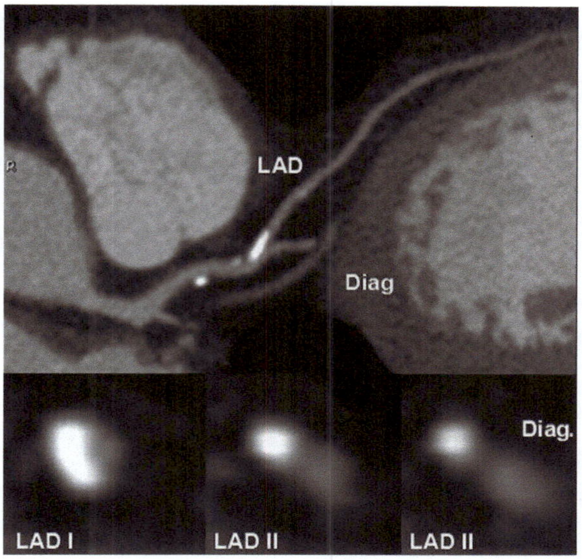

Fig. 3.5.16. CT 2D curved (long and short axis). The bifurcation lesion with calcified plaque is more complex than in coronary angiography (1,1,0 according to the Medina classification)

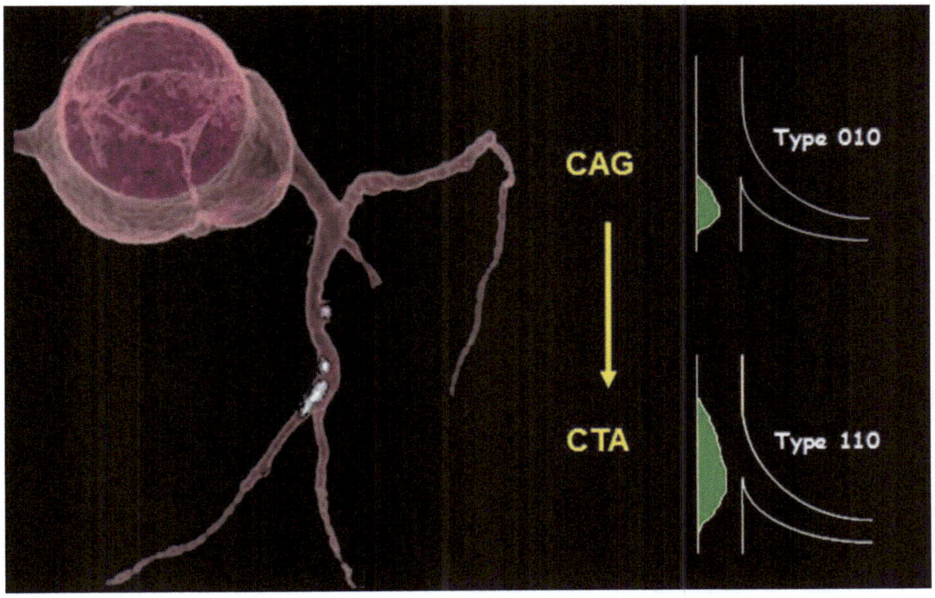

Fig. 3.5.17. The CT scan modifies the classification of this left anterior descending artery/diagonal artery bifurcation lesion by visualizing the plaque in reformatted 2D

3.5.5.2
Example of a Lesion on the Main Branch and the LAD/LCX Bifurcation

3.5.5.2.1
CAG and CTA Assessment Prior to the Procedure

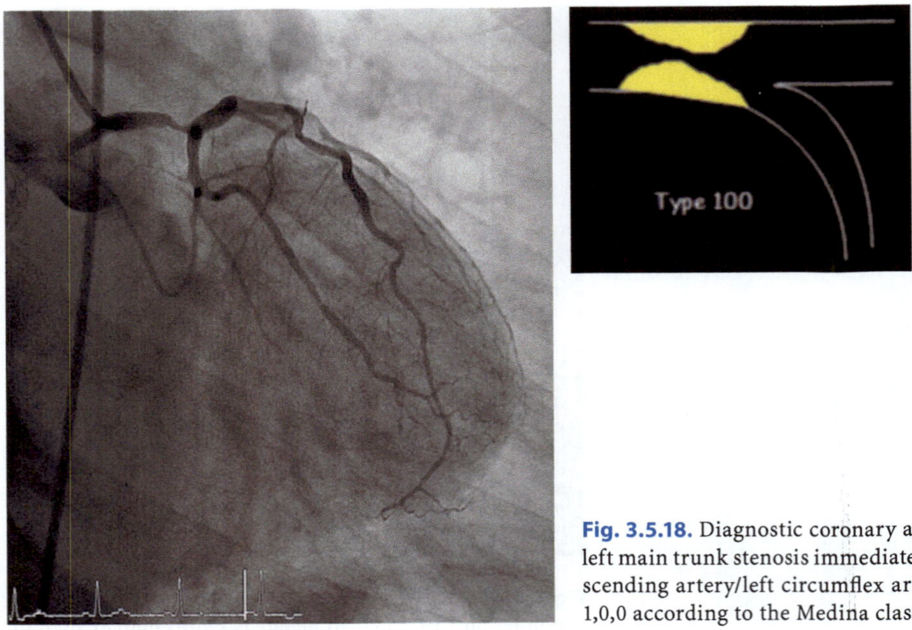

Fig. 3.5.18. Diagnostic coronary angiography showing a distal left main trunk stenosis immediately before the left anterior descending artery/left circumflex artery bifurcation (lesion type 1,0,0 according to the Medina classification)

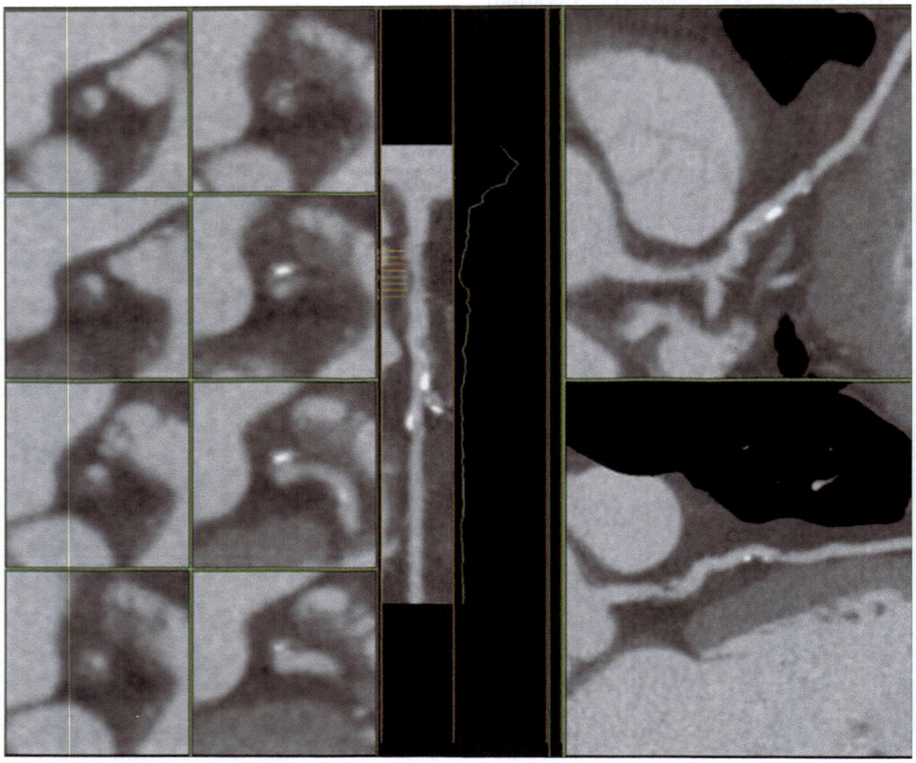

Fig. 3.5.19. Left main trunk and left anterior descending artery (LAD). Reformatted 2D CT (long and short axis). The distal lesion of the distal main branch very broadly includes the proximal portion of the LAD while leaving the circumflex ostium intact (lesion type 1,1,0 according to the Medina classification)

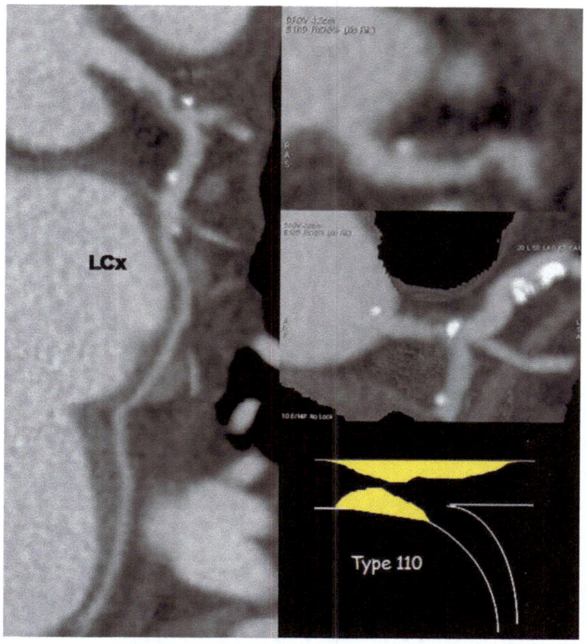

Fig. 3.5.20. Left main trunk and left circumflex artery on reformatted 2D CT. The plaque is located in phase opposition at the root of the circumflex artery, indicating a bifurcation lesion with a very low risk of plaque shifting. Note the presence of moderate calcifications, particularly at the medial left anterior descending artery. Lesion type 1,1,0 according to the Medina classification

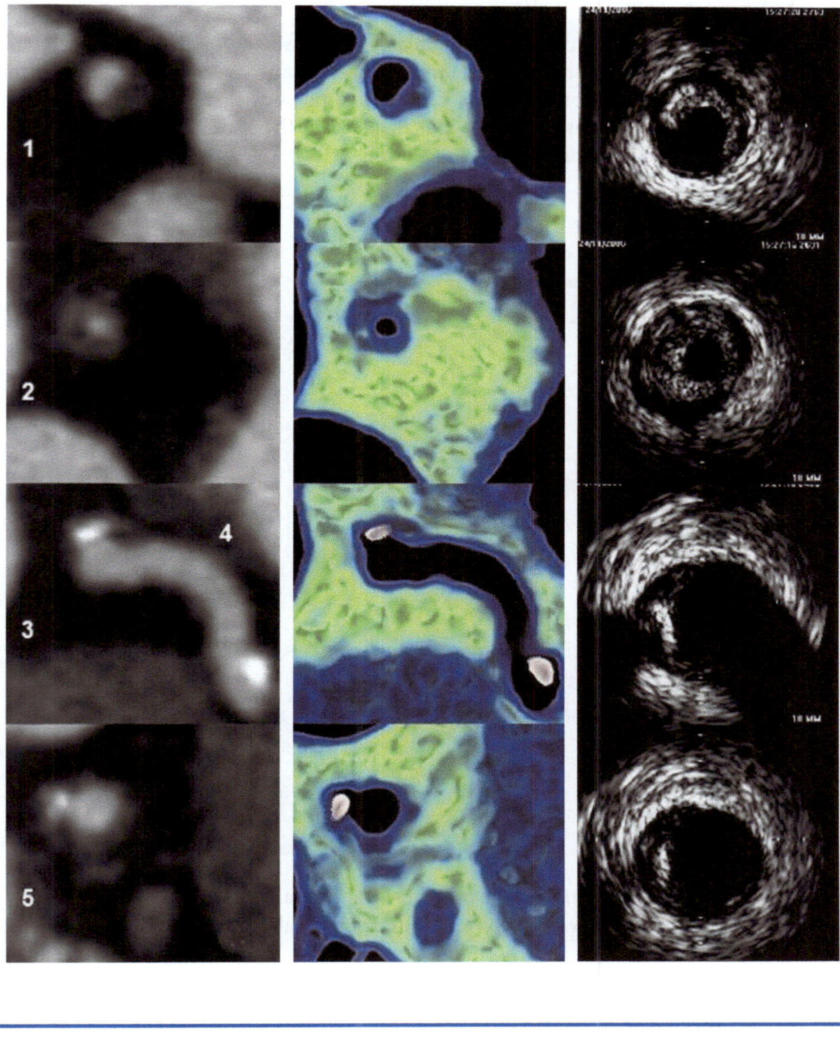

Fig. 3.5.21a–c. Stenosis of the distal main branch and the left anterior descending artery (LAD)/left circumflex artery (LCX) bifurcation. 2D Short axis correlation (**A**), CT IVUS (**B**), and IVUS (**C**). *1*, Medial left main trunk (LMT) with soft plaque; *2*, distal LMT with severe stenosis with soft plaque; 3, LAD ostium with calcified plaque; *4*, normal LCX ostium; *5*, juxta ostial LAD with calcified plaque

3.5.5.2.2
Performance of the Procedure

3.5.5.2.3
Results

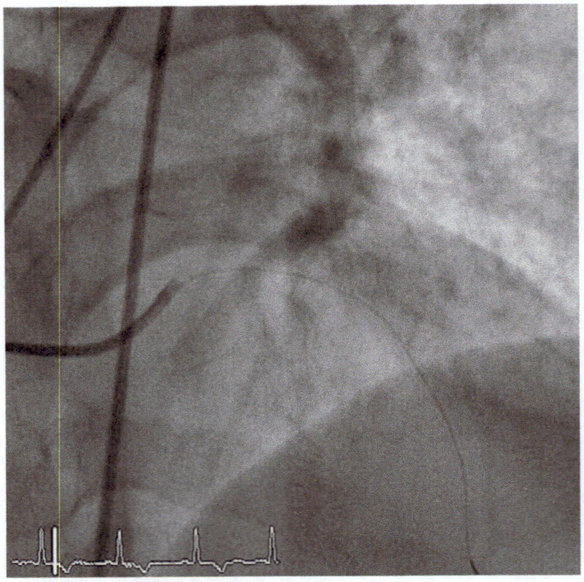

Fig. 3.5.22. Transluminal coronary angioplasty of a main branch of the unprotected coronary artery, guided by cardiac CT scan: the bifurcation lesion has a low risk of plaque shifting. A single angioplasty guide is put in place in the main branch line and the left anterior descending artery

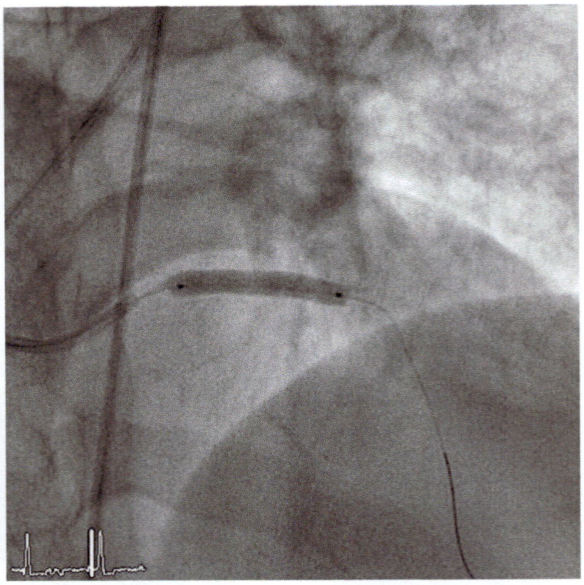

Fig. 3.5.23. Direct stenting of the main branch of the left coronary artery and the proximal left anterior descending artery. Significant indentation during inflation of the endoprosthesis was absent

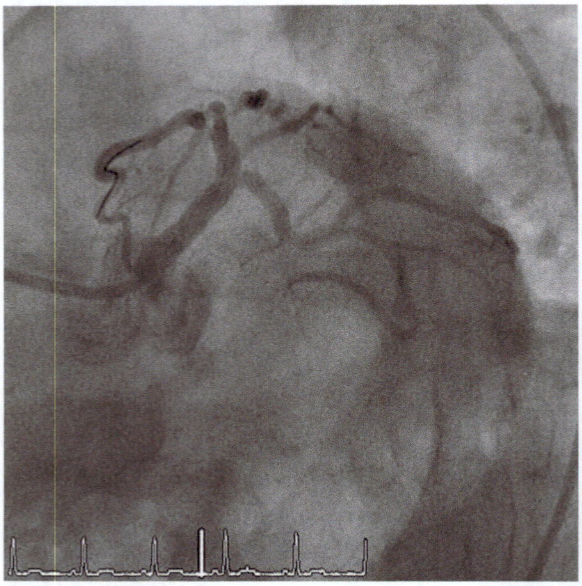

Fig. 3.5.24. After implantation of the prosthesis in the main branch, plaque shifting toward the circumflex artery is absent

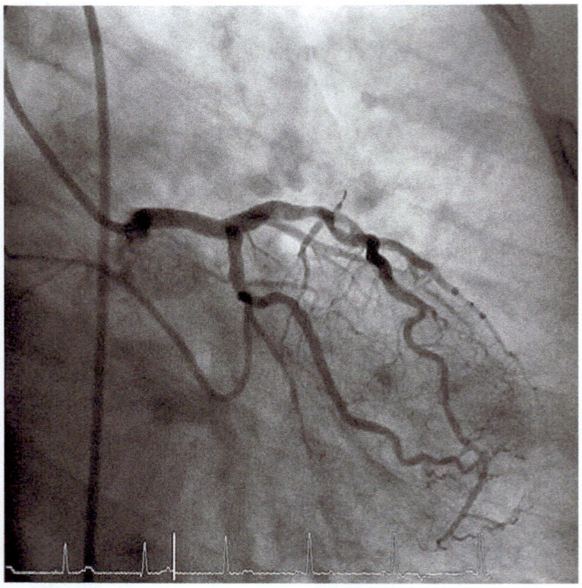

Fig. 3.5.25. End result of the coronary angioplasty of the main branch of the left coronary artery after performing the kissing balloon technique

3.5.6 Conclusion

Coronary CTA as a guide for PCI helps choose the optimal procedure, prevents events during procedures, such as plaque shifting, and increases the immediate and long-term results. The cumulative equivalent dose combining low dose CTA and CAG is now less than 10 mSV, permitting these two imaging modalities to be performed on the same day. By resolving patient radiation dose in particular, MDCT has become a fantastic tool for guiding percutaneous transluminal coronary angiography in complex lesions, as well as for daily practice.

References

Abdulla J, Abildstrom SZ, Gotzsche O, Christensen E, Kober L, Torp-Pedersen C (2007) 64-Multislice detector computed tomography coronary angiography as potential alternative to conventional coronary angiography: a systematic review and meta-analysis. Eur Heart J 28:3042–3050

Achenbach S, Giesler T, Ropers D, Ulzheimer S, Derlien H, Schulte C, Wenkel E, Moshage W, Bautz W, G. Daniel WG, Kalender WA, Baum U (2001) Detection of coronary artery stenoses by contrast-enhanced, retrospectively electrocardiographically-gated, multislice spiral computed tomography Circulation 103:2535–2538

Budoff MJ, Achenbach S, Blumenthal RS, Carr JJ, Goldin JG, Greenland P, Guerci AD, Lima JAC, Rader DJ, Rubin GD et al. (2006) Assessment of coronary artery disease by cardiac computed tomography: a scientific statement from the American Heart Association Committee on Cardiovascular Imaging and Intervention, Council on Cardiovascular Radiology and Intervention, and Committee on Cardiac Imaging, Council on Clinical Cardiology. Circulation 114:1761–1791

Cordeiro MAS, Lima JAC (2006) Atherosclerotic plaque characterization by multidetector row computed tomography angiography. J Am Coll Cardiol 47[8 Suppl]:C40–C47

Fuster, Fayad ZA, Moreno PR, Poon M, Corti R, Badimon JJ (2005) Atherothrombosis and high-risk plaque: part II: approaches by noninvasive computed tomographic/magnetic resonance imaging. J Am Coll Cardiol 46:1209–1218

Gaspar T, Halon DA, Lewis BS, Adawi S, Schliamser JE, Rubinshtein R, Flugelman MY, Peled N (2005) Diagnosis of coronary in-stent restenosis with multidetector row spiral computed tomography. J Am Coll Cardiol 46:1573–1579

Hoffmann U, Moselewski F, Cury RC, Ferencik M, Jang I-K, Diaz LJ, Abbara S, Brady TJ, Achenbach S (2004) Predictive value of 16-slice multidetector spiral computed tomography to detect significant obstructive coronary artery disease in patients at high risk for coronary artery disease: patient- versus segment-based analysis. Circulation 110:2638–2643

Louvard Y, Thomas M, Dzavik V, Hildick-Smith D, Galassi AR, Pan M, Burzotta F, Zelizko M, Dudek D, Ludman P, Sheiban I, Lassen JF, Darremont O, Kastrati A, Ludwig J, Iakovou I, Brunel P, Lansky A, Meerkin D, Legrand V, Medina A, Lefèvre T (2008) Classification of coronary artery bifurcation lesions and treatments: time for a consensus! Catheter Cardiovasc Interv 71:175–183

Medina A, Suárez de Lezo J, Pan M (2006) A new classification of coronary bifurcation lesions. Rev Esp Cardiol 59:183

Mollet NR, Cademartiri F, van Mieghem CAG, Runza G, McFadden EP, Baks T, Serruys PW, Krestin GP, de Feyter PJ (2005a) High-resolution spiral computed tomography coronary angiography in patients referred for diagnostic conventional coronary angiography. Circulation 112:2318–2323

Mollet NR, Cademartiri F, Krestin GP, McFadden EP, Arampatzis CA, Serruys PW, de Feyter PJ (2005b) Improved diagnostic accuracy with 16-row multi-slice computed tomography coronary angiography. J Am Coll Cardiol 45:128–132

Schroeder S, Achenbach S, Bengel F, Burgstahler C, Cademartiri F, de Feyter P, George R, Kaufmann P, Kopp AF, Knuuti J et al. (2007) Cardiac computed tomography: indications, applications, limitations, and training requirements: report of a Writing Group deployed by the Working Group Nuclear Cardiology and Cardiac CT of the European Society of Cardiology and the European Council of Nuclear Cardiology. Eur Heart J 29:531–556

Van Mieghem CAG, Cademartiri F, Mollet NR, Malagutti P, Valgimigli M, Meijboom WB, Pugliese F, McFadden EP, Ligthart J, Runza G, Bruining N, C. PC, Regar E, van der Giessen WJ, Sianos G, van Domburg R, de Jaegere P, Krestin GP, Serruys PW, de Feyter PJ (2006) Multislice spiral computed tomography for the evaluation of stent patency after left main coronary artery stenting: a comparison with conventional coronary angiography and intravascular ultrasound Circulation 114:645–653

Van Mieghem CA, Thury A, Meijboom WB, Cademartiri F, Mollet NR, Weustink AC, Sianos G, de Jaegere PP, Serruys PW, de Feyter P (2007) Detection and characterization of coronary bifurcation lesions with 64-slice computed tomography coronary angiography. Eur Heart J 28:1968–1976

Wilson GT, Gopalakrishnan P, Tak T (2007) Noninvasive cardiac imaging with computed tomography. Clin Med Res 5:165–171

3.6 Use of Multidetector Computed Tomography for the Assessment of Acute Chest Pain: Guidelines of the North American Society of Cardiac Imaging and the European Society of Cardiac Radiology

Arthur E. Stillman, Matthijs Oudkerk, Margaret Ackerman, Christoph R. Becker, Pawel E. Buszman, Pim J. de Feyter, Udo Hoffman, Matthew T. Keadey, Riccardo Marano, Martin J. Lipton, Gilbert L. Raff, Gautham P. Reddy, Michael R. Rees, Geoffrey D. Rubin, U. Joseph Schoepf, Giuseppe Tarulli, Edwin J. R. van Beek, Lewis Wexler, and Charles S. White*

CONTENTS

This contribution has already been published in *The International Journal of Cardiovascular Imaging* (2007) 23:415–427, as well as in *European Radiology* (2007) 17:2196–2207

A. E. Stillman, MD, PhD, FAHA
Department of Radiology, Emory University Hospital, 1365 Clifton Rd NE, Suite AT 506, Atlanta GA 30322, USA
M. Oudkerk, MD, PhD
Department of Radiology, University Medical Center Groningen, University of Groningen, Hanzeplein 1, 9700 RB Groningen, The Netherlands
M. Ackerman, MD, PhD
Division of Emergency Medicine, Department of Medicine, McMaster University, 1280 Main Street West, Hamilton, Ontario, Canada
**complete authors' adresses see List of Contributors*

3.6.1 Preamble

The diagnosis of patients with acute chest pain remains a challenging problem. There are approximately 6 million chest pain related emergency department (ED) visits annually in the US alone (Selker et al. 1997). Approximately 5.3% of all ED patients are seen because of chest pain and reported admission rates are between 30% and 72% for these patients (Graff et al. 1997).

Only 15%–25% of patients presenting with acute chest pain are ultimately diagnosed as having an acute coronary syndrome (ACS). Of those patients who were admitted to the chest pain unit, 44% ultimately had significant pathology ruled-out in one series (Pozen et al. 1984). The cost of chest pain triage and management has been estimated to be as high as $8 billion dollars annually with most of those patients ultimately not having ACS (Fineberg et al. 1984). Moreover, 2%–8% of patients are discharged from the ED and later diagnosed as having ACS (Goldman et al. 1996; Lee and Goldman 2000; Lee et al. 1987; Pope et al. 2000). The mortality rate for these patients is approximately 25%, which is twice as high as those who are admitted (Lee et al. 1987). Malpractice litigation over missed myocardial infarction (MI) represents the largest proportion of ED lawsuits in the US (Rusnak et al. 1989). There is thus great desire to find new tests to safely and expeditiously discharge low risk patients.

Recent technical advances in cardiovascular CT angiography (CCTA) have shown great promise for improving our diagnostic capabilities through non-invasive imaging. There are several articles showing excellent accuracy for diagnosing coronary heart disease with the latest 64-slice multi-detector CT (MDCT) scanner (Leber et al. 2005; Pugliese et al. 2006; Raff et al. 2005). Newer technology has arrived with dual-source 64-slice MDCT (Scheffel et al. 2006) and the imminent introduction of 256-slice MDCT that are expected to further improve on this diagnostic accuracy. Scanners that can perform cardiovascular CT are becoming more widely available. As has been the case for many rapid developments in medicine, in concert with this diffusion of technology there is the risk of application for clinical patient care without the scientific, rigorous study required. The concept of evaluating patients with acute chest pain with ECG-gated CT in the ED is but one such example, where, based on rapidly evolving technology, tests are being pushed to clinical application faster than our ability to scientifically evaluate their benefit. This is in part driven by industry, which wishes to sell more scanners, pioneering entrepreneurs, and by the ED in the setting of acute chest pain, which increasingly relies on imaging to enable faster risk stratification of patients and thereby minimize patient stay and costs. While there is a consensus that CT may indeed improve disposition of patients with acute chest pain, at this point, there is little data demonstrating typical coronary CT findings in patients with and without ACS among patients with chest pain. Thus, there is the potential of inappropriate use of new technology leading to additional testing rather than saving admissions or cost. Data from observational trials are needed to demonstrate the safety and feasibility of CT in the setting of acute chest pain, to identify the target population in whom admissions could be reduced, the relation of CT findings on plaque and stenosis to MI and unstable angina pectoris. Eventually randomized diagnostic trials are essential to prove the incremental value of cardiac CT to current standard of care, including stress testing similar to the evaluation of SPECT a decade ago (Udelson et al. 2002).

Currently there are no guidelines that have been published for the use of CT for acute chest pain. Appropriateness criteria have recently been published (Hendel et al. 2006). More general guidelines are currently under development. However, because of the great interest and pressure from a variety of groups to utilize this technology, there is value in providing interim guidance. For this reason, the North American Society for Cardiac Imaging (NASCI) and the European Society of Cardiac Radiology (ESCR) assembled a group of expert radiologists, cardiologists and emergency physicians representing the collective experience from the United States, Canada and Europe to review the literature, indicate areas in need of more research and provide a basis in the future for the development of comprehensive guidelines.

Co-endorsed White Papers and guidelines by various societies have been written before on various topics. We believe however that this is the first attempt to bring together the different experiences from different countries and continents whose medical systems are significantly different. We believe that this combined experience has the advantage that underlying biases from local practice becomes less relevant and that the underlying fundamental truths become relatively more important. The ESCR and NASCI are planning to work together in the future to bring together experts to discuss available evidence, to provide guidance to the practitioner and to further advance the field of cardiovascular imaging and provide a basis for practice with evolving technologies.

3.6.2 How to Manage Chest Pain: The Emergency Department Perspective

In the ED setting, the symptoms and clinical signs of patients with chest pain are variable but it is important to distinguish life threatening causes that need rapid or immediate intervention from those that are less likely to be fatal but still need in-patient treatment and those that can be managed supportively on an out-patient basis (Table 3.6.1) (Jeudy et al. 2006).

Table 3.6.1. Common potential causes of non-traumatic chest pain

Life threatening	Non-life threatening
Acute coronary syndrome	Pneumonia/pulmonary parenchymal disease
Pulmonary embolism	Pulmonary, mediastinal, or pleural neoplasm
Aortic dissection	Musculoskeletal injury or inflammation
Intramural hematoma	Cholecystitis
Penetrating aortic ulcer	Pancreatitis
Aortic aneurysm/rupture	Herpes zoster
Esophageal rupture	Hiatus hernia/GERD/esophageal spasm
Pericardial tamponade	Pericarditis/myocarditis
Tension pneumothorax	Simple pneumothorax

3.6.2.1
Acute Coronary Syndrome

In the United States more than 335,000 people die of heart disease in an ED or before reaching a hospital every year. Of patients who die suddenly because of coronary heart disease, 50% of men and 64% of women have no previous symptoms. When a patient presents with chest pain, they are typically risk stratified with an appropriate history and physical, and electrocardiogram (ECG), chest X-ray and laboratory studies including cardiac biomarkers. Obtaining a timely ECG is important to identify the small subset of patients with an ST elevation myocardial infarction (STEMI) who will benefit from a coronary intervention (PCI or thrombolysis). The majority of patients without a STEMI are further risk stratified into one of three categories: (1) high risk for acute coronary syndrome (ACS) or non ST elevation MI (NSTEMI), (2) low risk for ACS, or (3) noncardiac chest pain. A number of clinical decision rules tools are available to risk stratify patients into one of the above three categories, but none have a high sensitivity and specificity with some no better than clinical impression.

One risk stratification tool that is widely used in EDs is the thrombosis in myocardial infarction (TIMI) risk score that predicts the triple endpoint of death, new or recurrent myocardial infarction, or need for urgent target vessel revascularization within 2 weeks of presentation (Table 3.6.2) (Antman et al. 2000).

Table 3.6.2. Thrombosis in myocardial infarction (TIMI) risk score for unstable angina and non-ST-elevated myocardial infarction (NSTEMI)

•	Age ≥65 years
•	History of known coronary artery disease (documented prior coronary artery stenosis >50%)
•	≥3 Conventional cardiac risk factors (age, male sex, family history, hyperlipidemia, diabetes mellitus, smoking, obesity)
•	Use of aspirin in the past 7 days
•	ST-segment deviation (persistent depression or transient elevation)
•	Increased cardiac biomarkers (troponins)
•	≥2 Anginal events in the preceding 24 h
•	Score = sum of number of above characteristics

The low risk group is defined by a score of 0 or 1 and a <5% likelihood of requiring intervention. The high risk group is defined by a score of 6 or 7 and a 40% likelihood of requiring intervention. This approach has been validated in a number of additional trials (Cohen et al. 1998; Manoharan and Adgey 2002; Mega et al. 2005).

A computerized system for risk assessment is in use in some EDs to aid in diagnosis (Selker et al. 1998). A risk score for patients with normal troponin concentrations has recently been proposed (Sanchis et al. 2005a,b). Specific recommendations for an early invasive strategy in patients with NSTEMI include any of the following high-risk indicators (Braunwald et al. 2002):

- Recurrent angina/ischemia at rest or with low-level activities despite intensive anti-ischemic therapy.
- Elevated cardiac specific biomarkers, TnT or Tnl
- New or presumably new ST-segment depression
- Recurrent angina/ischemia with congestive heart failure symptoms, an S_3 gallop, pulmonary edema, worsening râles, new or worsening mitral valve regurgitation
- High-risk findings on noninvasive stress testing
- Depressed left ventricular systolic function (e.g., ejection fraction < 40% on noninvasive study)
- Hemodynamic instability
- Sustained ventricular tachycardia
- Percutaneous coronary intervention (PCI) within 6 months
- Prior coronary artery bypass graft (CABG)

Treatment and disposition is based on the level of risk assigned to the patient. Patients with a NSTEMI or who are deemed at high risk for ACS are typically admitted to the hospital. Patients with non-cardiac and non-life threatening chest pain are typically discharged home with outpatient follow-up. Low-risk ACS patients usually present a quandary. These patients usually require a period of observation with serial enzymes and then a determination is made whether provocative stress testing is required. In some facilities, observation units tailored toward the evaluation of chest pain have made prolonged evaluations in the ED possible. Patients receive serial biomarkers, observation in a telemetry setting, and most receive some form of cardiac stress testing. Cardiac stress testing ranges from simple treadmill tests to the newer cardiac PET scans. None of these tests is perfect and most if not all are not available 24 h/day/7 days a week. If the patient has rising cardiac biomarkers or has a positive cardiac stress test, they are usually admitted for cardiac catheterization and further management.

In spite of this aggressive approach to chest pain in the ED, even in the population at low risk for ACS, between 2%–8% of patients are inappropriately discharged and later found to have an ACS (GOLDMAN et al. 1996; LEE and GOLDMAN 2000; LEE et al. 1987; POPE et al. 2000). These discharged patients have a significantly increased morbidity and mortality. If it were possible to accurately predict high risk in patients with potential NSTEMI or, conversely, to accurately exclude ACS during the early observation period, the number of patients admitted for evaluation of chest pain could be significantly reduced with a commensurate reduction in cost of care. In addition, the earlier identification of high risk ACS patients could lead to earlier treatment initiated in the ED with the possibility of improved patient outcomes.

CCTA may be used in order to visualize the coronary arteries and to determine whether there are plaques or thrombi narrowing or occluding the vessel. If CCTA could be performed immediately or during the observation period for ACS at a cost that is less than that required for outpatient monitoring, there would be a significant saving to the health care system. Because of medical malpractice issues in the US (KATZ et al. 2005) and the high likelihood of a poor outcome if a patient with ACS is discharged, the test must have a high negative predictive value minimizing missed ACS. Ideally, the true positives would all undergo coronary artery revascularization and the number of indeterminate cases that require further observation would be reduced. A model cardiac chest pain pathway that incorporates CCTA is shown in Figure 3.6.1. Early supporting data for the use of CCTA for acute chest pain is now appearing in the literature (HOFFMANN et al. 2006a,b; WHITE et al. 2005).

Although this pathway represents one possible concept, further work is necessary to clarify the role of stenosis and plaque assessment for risk assessment of patients with acute chest pain. This relates both to the concept of mild to moderate stenosis as detected by CCTA and the necessity of stress testing or coronary angiography (CAG) in these patients, as well as the concept of plaque burden in CCTA as a tool for risk stratification. Both concepts have been recently addressed (HOFFMANN et al. 2006a).

Very important for the success of cardiac CT in this application will be our ability to exactly determine the target patient population. While the broader population of all comers with undifferentiated chest pain has a very low incidence of ACS, pulmonary embolism (PE), or aortic dissection, patients with inconclusive initial ED evaluation admitted to the hospital to rule out MI may benefit the most as 10%–15% of those patients will develop an ACS. Besides the detection of stenosis and plaque it may prove useful to evaluate the additional benefit from the assessment of global and regional LV function, which may identify stunned myocardium.

3.6.2.2 Pulmonary Embolism

Patients who present to the ED with a suspected PE can be risk stratified using the Wells' clinical decision rule (Table 3.6.3). The likelihood of a PE is low if the score is four or less and the D-dimer is negative. If the patient has a score greater than 4 then further investigations are required to exclude the diagnosis of PE. The most commonly used imaging techniques are a nuclear ventilation/perfusion scan or chest CT depending on institution and availability. A negative CT study is associated with a low risk for subsequent fatal and nonfatal venous thromboembolism (VTE) (WHITE et al. 2005). Therefore, in the patient with undifferentiated chest pain and a moderate to high probability of PE, a CT is indicated. If the patient is high risk for PE but has a negative CT scan, further testing may be indicated. A normal D-dimer or a negative evaluation of the lower extremity venous system with a contrast CT or US makes the diagnosis of PE unlikely. When the clinical probability is low, a normal D-dimer test excludes the diagnosis of PE and a CT is typically not performed.

Clinical probability of pulmonary embolism unlikely: 4 or less points; clinical probability of pulmonary embolism likely: more than 4 points.

3.6.2.3 Acute Aortic Syndromes

The clinical presentation of patients with acute aortic syndromes typically present with ripping or tearing chest discomfort that is sudden in onset, severe, substernal and may radiate to arms or back. The most common predisposing factors are hypertension, increasing age and pregnancy, while less common syndromes include Marfan's syndrome and Be-

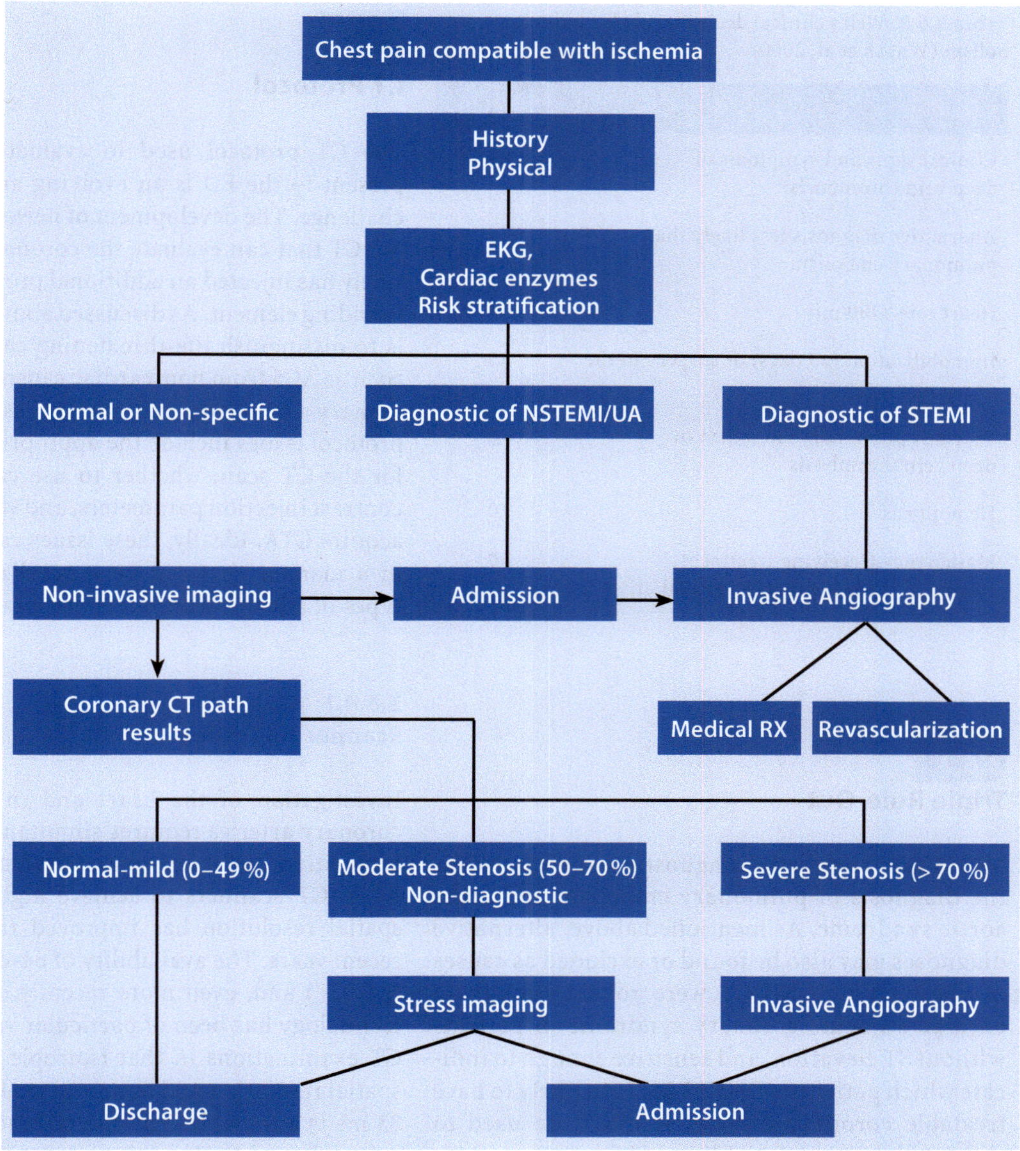

Fig. 3.6.1. A model cardiac chest pain pathway incorporating cardiovascular CT angiography

hçet's disease. The pain may start in the epigastrium or abdomen and radiate to the back. Hypotension, unequal pulses, acute aortic regurgitation or suggestive electrocardiographic changes may be features as well. Aortic disease includes entities such as acute aortic dissection, dissecting intramural hematoma, aortic penetrating ulcer, mycotic aneurysm, and atherosclerotic aneurysm with and without rupture. Because these may be fatal, rapid diagnosis and institution of therapy is desirable. MDCT is the diagnostic test most often used to make the diagnosis because it can distinguish among the various etiologies of the acute aortic syndrome and define the extent of the disease process (Khan and Nair 2002).

3.6.2.4
Alternative Diagnoses

MDCT is capable of detecting a multitude of alternative causes of acute chest pain. These include hiatus hernia, pneumonia, intrathoracic mass, pericardial effusion and pericarditis, esophageal mass or rupture, pleural effusion, pancreatitis, spontaneous fracture (spine, sternum, cough fracture of rib). Many patients with ill-defined symptoms or uncharacteristic presentations may be initially considered to have an acute coronary syndrome but may have a pulmonary embolism or another disease. Some patients have more than one disease process causing their symptoms (Thoongsuwan and Stern 2002).

Table 3.6.3. Well's clinical decision rule for pulmonary embolism (Wells et al. 2000)

Variable	Points
Clinical signs and symptoms of deep vein thrombosis	3.0
Alternative diagnosis less likely than pulmonary embolism	3.0
Heart rate >100/min	1.5
Immobilization (>3 days) or surgery in the previous 4 weeks	1.5
Previous pulmonary embolism or deep vein thrombosis	1.5
Hemoptysis	1.0
Malignancy (receiving treatment, treated in the last 6 months or palliative)	1.0

3.6.3 Triple Rule-Out

MDCT is currently the diagnostic test of choice for the diagnosis of pulmonary embolism and acute aortic syndrome. As mentioned above, alternative diagnoses may also be found or excluded as causes of chest pain. If MDCT were robust enough to exclude an acute coronary syndrome in patients without ST elevation, and sensitive enough to indicate which patients with NSTEMI are likely to have treatable coronary disease, it might be used to shorten the observational period for patients with suspected ACS to either rule-out cardiac causes for chest pain or ensure timely institution of specific therapy. Ultimately, we must ask: Is there a single MDCT study that can be performed that can accurately, expeditiously and cost-effectively diagnose coronary, pulmonary and aortic disease in the ED, the so-called "triple rule-out?" The question may also be asked, is there a clinical need for such a test? ED physicians usually feel that it is relatively uncommon that they are uncertain of all three diagnostic considerations, thus, single or dual rule out may be sufficient. As of this writing, there are no large prospective studies where MDCT has been used for this purpose and further research is desirable to better define the role for triple rule-out.

3.6.4 CT Protocol

The CT protocol used to evaluate patients who present to the ED is an evolving and multifaceted challenge. The development of newer generations of MDCT that can evaluate the coronary arteries routinely has injected an additional promising but confounding element. As discussed above, the challenge is to distinguish life-threatening cardiac etiologies such as ACS from non-cardiac causes including pulmonary embolism, and aortic dissection. Specific protocol issues include the appropriate preparation for the CT scan, whether to use calcium scoring, contrast injection parameters, and strategies used to acquire CTA. Ideally, these issues can be addressed in a manner that can be generalized to different types of advanced scanners and practice settings.

3.6.4.1 Scanner Technology

Investigation of the heart and in particular the coronary arteries requires simultaneous fast image acquisition and high spatial resolution. The ability of CT scanners to achieve high temporal and spatial resolution has improved tremendously in recent years. The availability of 64-detector-row CT (64DCT) and, even more recently, dual-source CT technology has been of particular value for cardiac CT examinations in that isotropic half-millimeter spatial resolution and temporal resolution as fast as 83 ms is attainable. The spatial resolution of CT is now only two to three times lower than that of the most optimal conventional coronary angiography (CAG), which is sufficient to visualize small segments of the coronary artery tree down to the third generation vessels (Wintersperger et al. 2006).

3.6.4.2 Preparation for the CT Scan

In patients with heart rates above 65 bpm, patient preparation with beta-blockers is necessary to achieve sufficiently low heart rates with ≤ 64-slice technology (Pannu et al. 2006). This typically involves administration of 50–100 mg Metoprolol 1 h prior to the CT scan, followed by 5–20 mg Metoprolol intravenously to patients in whom the heart rate is still above 65 bpm once in the CT scanner. In patients in whom the scan must be obtained with a heart rate of 80 bpm and above, image reconstruction in the systolic phase of the cardiac cycle often results in superior image quality (Wintersperger et al. 2006). Nitroglycerin (0.5 µg sublingual) is given to dilate the coronary arteries if the patient's blood pressure will tolerate it. With further improvement of technology, beta-blockers may no longer be indicated.

3.6.4.3 Calcium Scoring

Screening for coronary calcium by CT is a fast and simple procedure that allows determination of the amount of calcified plaques in the coronary arteries and estimation of the extent of the entire atherosclerotic plaque burden. Screening for coronary calcium was introduced more than a decade ago with the use of electron beam CT (EBT). EBT is a dedicated cardiac CT system without moving parts and permits very short exposure times when scanning the heart. The design of this machine made it suitable for low dose cross sectional scanning of the heart to detect coronary calcium.

Coronary calcium screening by EBT is performed with 3-mm consecutive slices through the range of the entire heart. No administration of contrast media is required. Every scan is triggered prospectively by the ECG signal to the mid diastole interval. Usually 40 heartbeats are necessary to acquire the entire volume resulting in a breath-hold time of approximately 30 s. Coronary calcium is identified as lesions in the coronary arteries with a density of 130 HU and above. A score value is calculated by a dedicated algorithm, which takes the peak density and the area of any individual lesion into account (Agatston et al. 19990). The total score corresponds to the sum of all lesions in all three coronary arteries, and is commonly provided in percentile for age and gender.

Coronary calcium screening may also be performed with MDCT systems. Four slices are minimally required to perform coronary calcium scanning with a MDCT. Depending on the number of slices available, the spiral scan can be performed within 10–20 s (Becker et al. 2001). To improve reproducibility of the measurement, overlapping slice reconstruction is recommended (Ohnesorge et al. 2002). However, this results in a relatively high dose of radiation so that a prospectively triggered sequential imaging approach analogous to EBT is commonly used. Images are evaluated according to the procedure suggested for coronary calcium screening with the EBT. To improve the reproducibility and comparability of coronary calcium screening with different CT scanners an international consortium has been founded with the aim to standardize the measurement. The consortium proposed to use the quantification of the absolute mass in mg calcium-hydroxyapatite rather than assessing the calcium score. For the standardized measurement frequent calibration of the CT scanner is required with dedicated phantoms. The foremost issue with coronary calcium screening for patients with acute coronary syndrome is to detect coronary calcium with a sensitivity that is as high as possible.

Initially, scanning for coronary calcium with EBT was intended to screen for coronary atherosclerosis in asymptomatic persons to determine the risk of acute coronary events. However, in the late nineties some authors reported the use of coronary calcium screening for patients with angina-like symptoms and negative cardiac enzymes. Laudon et al. (1999) described the use of CAC scanning in the ED in more than 100 patients, pointing out a negative predictive value of 100%. McLaughlin et al. (1999) reported a negative predictive value of 98% in 134 patients presenting with chest pain to the ED. Georgiou et al. (2001) followed almost 200 patients with chest pain in the ED and found that the presence of coronary artery calcium in this cohort is a strong predictor for future cardiac events and conversely patients with a negative coronary calcium scan may safely be discharged immediately from the ED. A problem with these studies is that the negative predictive value is not as great in younger patients. Thus coronary calcium may not be widely applicable in this patient population. In addition, because of its high costs and limited availability, EBT has never been widely used as a stand-alone tool to triage patients with chest pain.

Coronary artery calcium scoring by MDCT may be useful in the ED setting prior to CTA in that the quality of the CTA is likely to be impaired or non-diagnostic if large quantities of coronary calcium are found. A decision to proceed with CTA must then be made. Moreover, the calcium score can be compared to existing age and gender benchmarks to guide primary prevention as an outpatient if the patient is not admitted (Hoff et al. 2001; Naghavi et al. 2006). CAC is relatively common in this patient population even in patients with non-cardiac causes of chest pain. Thus CTA may still be of value to evaluate for stenoses. Clearly, there is a need for more research to define the relative roles of both CAC and CTA for acute chest pain patients. Calcium screening will be addressed in more detail in a future ESCR-NASCI Consensus Statement.

3.6.4.4 CTA Protocol

More advanced MDCT technology allows not only assessment of the calcified atherosclerotic plaque burden but also visualization of the lumen and wall of the coronary arteries using contrast material. In addition, other causes of chest pain such as pulmonary embolism, aortic dissection, and pneumonia can be evaluated using CTA. Provided that optimized images of the entire cardiac cycle are not required, dose modulation or ECG-pulsing can be used to reduce redundant radiation during the systolic phase while preserving coronary artery images of good quality (Poll et al. 2002). Specific ED chest pain protocols in which the differential diagnosis includes a coronary artery etiology can be divided into two groups. If the patient is stable and primary clinical suspicion is angina, a dedicated cardiac CTA may be sufficient. Alternatively, if the clinical evaluation is less specific and differential considerations include angina and other serious causes of acute chest pain, a comprehensive or global evaluation may be deemed appropriate. The latter protocol is also termed the triple threat or triple rule-out protocol. Each of these protocols is discussed in turn.

3.6.4.5 Dedicated CTA

A typical CT angiography (CTA) investigation of the heart with most modern CT scanners usually requires a breath-hold time of 10 s or less and 60–80 ml of contrast media. The regimen for intravenous contrast medium administration has changed with newer scanners. Formerly, with slower scanning the priority was to extend the contrast bolus in order to maintain homogenous enhancement during the entire scanning period. Now that the scan time with 64-DCT is typically no more than 10 s for the entire heart, high contrast enhancement must be achieved during the comparatively short scanning period. One method is to calculate the amount of contrast medium based on the bodyweight of the patient; for every kilogram of bodyweight administering 0.5 g of iodine. For a cardiac CT study the bodyweight-adapted amount of contrast medium is administered within 20 s. Highly concentrated contrast media is well suited to this approach, in order to keep the intravenous flow rate within a reasonable order of magnitude, particularly in obese patients. To lower the viscosity and to improve administration the contrast medium should be warmed to body temperature. In order to achieve correct timing, either a test injection or automated threshold-based bolus timing may be used. The threshold with automated bolus timing is often set at 150 HU.

In principle it is advisable to have some contrast in the right ventricle in order to identify the septum and the right ventricular myocardium. However, any CTA study should be performed in mid-inspiration in order to avoid the "Valsalva maneuver". This effect occurs during deep inspiration when an influx of contrast medium into the right atrium is impeded resulting in non-homogenous enhancement of the cardiac structures. A saline flush should always be performed immediately after the administration of contrast medium in order to flush the veins of remaining contrast medium and to maintain a tight contrast bolus, while it aids in the assessment of the right coronary artery and posterior descending artery. The scanning range extends from the level of the carina inferiorly to below the cardiac apex.

A number of studies have compared 64DCT and CAG on a segment-by-segment basis for the detection of coronary artery stenoses in the non-emergent setting (Pugliese et al. 2006; Raff et al. 2005; Leschka et al. 2005; Mollet et al. 2005). Although 10%–20% of coronary artery segments cannot be assessed by CTA because of motion artifacts or severe calcifications, the negative predictive value of this technique is close to 100%, rendering CT a reliable method to rule out coronary artery disease if the study can be performed successfully. Unfortunately, the positive predictive value is only around 75%, revealing a tendency of CTA to overestimate the degree of coronary artery stenoses. One of the reasons for overestimation may be the presence of plaques which appear to narrow the lumen, if adjacent widening of the outer lumen (positive remodeling) is not taken into account. Underestimation of the degree of stenosis by CAG due to eccentric stenosis and suboptimal angulation is presumably another cause. The largest cohort reported so far with CCTA in the ED comprised 103 patients with acute chest pain. By using ≥ 50%

coronary artery stenosis as detected by MDCT as a threshold with clinical follow-up as the reference standard, Hoffmann et al. (2006a) reported a positive and negative predictive value of 47% and 100% for ACS, respectively.

In a pilot study of 22 patients, Dorgelo et al. (2005) reported on the potential use of MDCT to triage patients with ACS among conservative treatment, percutaneous intervention or bypass grafting. They followed a simplified stratification scheme taking the number of coronary vessels into account affected by coronary artery disease with stenosis ≥ 50%. According to this scheme, the absence of coronary artery disease, single- or two-vessel disease, and left main or three-vessel disease initiated conservative, interventional and surgical therapy, respectively. They reported excellent agreement for decisions made by MDCT and CAG for triaging these patients with ACS. Interestingly, in some patients MDCT more often showed the tendency to triage for coronary intervention whereas after cardiac catheterization these few patients were treated conservatively. This presumably resulted from lack of adequate clinical information such as co-morbidity risk at MDCT that was available and influenced the final decision after cardiac catheterization (Dorgelo et al. 2005).

3.6.4.6 Global Assessment (Triple Rule-Out)

The protocol for global assessment differs from dedicated coronary CTA in several important respects. First, a large field of view is used to encompass the entire chest. Second, the entire length of thorax must be imaged in order to assess the pulmonary vasculature to a subsegmental level, as well as the thoracic aorta. Such imaging requires a longer acquisition of 15 s or more with 64-DCT with more opportunity for motion artifact due to breathing. It is therefore advisable to begin image acquisition below the cardiac apex and scan superiorly, in contrast to the cephalocaudal direction typically used for dedicated CCTA. This approach permits imaging of the coronary arteries during the first part of the scan, when breath-holding is presumably better.

A third important difference is the protocol for contrast administration. Unlike dedicated coronary CTA, where partial or complete washout of contrast in the right heart is desirable, a triple rule-out protocol must provide optimal enhancement of both the right and left heart for simultaneous visualization of the pulmonary arteries, the aorta and the coronary arteries. Thus, a small amount of additional contrast may be necessary and contrast bolus administration may need to be lengthened.

Using the global assessment chest pain protocol, White et al. (2005) investigated 69 patients with chest pain in whom they assessed the amount of calcium, the degree of stenosis, ejection fraction, wall motion abnormalities, and perfusion defects in the myocardium. The final diagnosis was derived from clinical exam or follow up for 1 month. The CT was normal, showed coronary artery disease, non-cardiac related or non-concordant findings in 75%, 14%, 4%, 7% of patients, respectively. For the diagnosis of acute coronary syndrome they reported a sensitivity and specificity of 87% and 96%, respectively. In addition White et al. (2005) reported findings in other areas such as the lung, mediastinum and the bones. In this study there were too few patients with aortic dissection or pulmonary embolism to adequately establish the diagnostic accuracy of this protocol for non-coronary causes of acute chest pain.

3.6.5 Imaging Evaluation and Post Processing

Within the context of an urgent clinical presentation, the initial assessment of the CT scan must be rapid and accurate for effective risk assessment of the patient. In the broadest sense this means determining if the patient is suffering from a life threatening condition necessitating urgent therapy, such as an acute coronary syndrome, an acute aortic syndrome, or venous thromboembolism. This assessment rarely requires visualization techniques beyond appropriately windowed transverse reconstructions. Although transverse sections represent the most basic output of the CT scanner, attention must be focused on proper assessment, as lesions can be missed or mischaracterized. In particular if the window center is too low or narrow, an intimal flap within the aorta or a pulmonary embolism can disappear within the contrast-enhanced lumen or a coronary occlusion associated with calcific plaque could be mistaken for a patent artery. As a general rule of thumb, proper window width and center settings require that the arterial lumen be not rendered as white, but an intermediate gray level. Moreover, the size of mural calcium will be overestimated (blooming) if it is not rendered with an opacity level below white. As was previously discussed, a thin-section acquisition, preferably with overlapping reconstructions is critical to fully assessing vascular abnormalities. With a thoracic CT angiogram comprising 400–4000 transverse reconstructions, it is impractical to effectively track the structures of interest across multiple sheets of film and spatial relationships will be difficult to ascertain.

If one of the aforementioned acute vascular abnormalities is excluded based upon transverse section review, then post processing will not be necessary. While this should almost always be the case when diagnosing an acute aortic syndrome or pulmonary embolism, the confident exclusion of an acute coronary syndrome may require a post-processing workstation, particularly if there are motion-related artifacts or calcified plaque.

A post-processing workstation is required if an acute aortic or an acute coronary syndrome is diagnosed or if an acute coronary syndrome cannot be excluded. With an acute aortic syndrome, planning of definitive therapy or triage to a period of monitoring necessitates characterization of the aortic lumen, wall, branches, and adjacent structures. A detailed description of the full scope of evaluations necessary to fully characterize an acute aortic syndrome is beyond the scope of this manuscript, but the use of multiplanar reformations (MPRs), curved planar reformations (CPRs), maximum intensity projections (MIP), and volume renderings are key to enabling complete characterization and documentation of the abnormality to facilitate communication with the treating physicians. Moreover, a post-processing workstation is necessary to measure important distances along axes and curved paths that are aligned with aortic landmarks and not the CT table, as is the case with the primary transverse reconstructions.

When characterizing or excluding acute coronary syndromes or acute aortic syndromes assessed with ECG gated CT acquisitions, the post-processing workstation must also be capable of managing multiphasic or four-dimensional data to allow seamless volumetric exploration and analysis across the temporal phases. While the tools of MPR, CPR, MIP and volume rendering frequently are all necessary for a complete assessment, the workstation must be capable of managing up to 3–4000 images simultaneously to allow seamless exploration of the 4D data. In the case of an acute coronary syndrome, the primary goal of the analysis should be the identification of the location and extent of the coronary artery occlusion. While, as mentioned above, primary transverse section review can allow exclusion of the diagnosis, full characterization of the extent of the abnormality, particularly in association with chronic atherosclerotic coronary occlusive disease, requires MPRs oriented perpendicular to median axis of the artery and/or CPRs. Volume rendering can provide an exquisite display of the relationships of the coronary arteries relative to the myocardium, but this is rarely necessary for urgent risk assessment.

When all phases are reconstructed across the cardiac cycle, then MPRs oriented along the standard cardiac axes can be viewed to assess for wall motion abnormalities and perfusion deficits.

3.6.6 Physician Requirements

In the US there are competency guidelines that provide minimum training requirements for radiologists, cardiologists, and nuclear medicine physicians for the interpretation of CTA (Budoff et al. 2005; Jacobs et al. 2006). In both Europe and Canada, government regulations largely limit interpretation to radiologists. Like all of imaging, there is a learning curve and some training is desirable in order to achieve a measure of competence. The extra-cardiac portion of the examination must be thoroughly evaluated as it has been shown that there may be significant non-cardiac abnormalities in the population of interest (Onuma et al. 2006; Rumberger 2006). Generally, this will require a radiologist over-read if the radiologist is not the primary reader. The American College of Radiology cautions against the practice of split-reads, and legal consultation is advisable in the US (ACR 2006).

3.6.7 Future Directions

Ongoing research in CT technology suggests that the evaluation of coronary arteries with MDCT will improve substantially in the coming years. Software improvements in post-processing will permit rapid reconstruction of the coronary arteries with automated selection of the optimal cardiac phase. Hardware improvements include better z-axis coverage generating a larger number of slices as well as better temporal resolution through the use of multiple tube technology or faster gantry rotation. Such advances in technology can be expected to improve the quality of coronary artery imaging, particularly for the large coverage required for the global assessment and will undoubtedly stimulate further modifications in the CT imaging protocols for ED patients with chest pain.

3.6.8 Summary

The major diagnostic concerns for acute chest pain are acute myocardial infarction and acute coronary syndrome. However, since enzyme blood levels may be normal for many hours following an event, and because ECG findings are often non-diagnostic, 2.8 million patients with acute chest pain in the US are admitted to hospital for evaluation and management of chest pain. This patient subgroup has a low risk for ACS yet undergo expensive investigations since the likelihood of bad outcome is extremely high with a missed diagnosis.

In patients with chest pain whose history, clinical findings and/or predisposing conditions suggest other life threatening diseases, specifically acute aortic syndromes or pulmonary embolism, MDCT is proven to be the diagnostic study of choice (Hayter et al. 2006; Stein et al. 2006). The CT protocol used should be optimized to evaluate each of these specific diagnoses, as completely as possible; this implies that no single protocol is ideal for all chest pain disease.

Regarding myocardial ischemia, numerous studies have established that 16 and 64 slice MDCT has high diagnostic accuracy for detecting significant coronary artery stenosis in stable patients with a high prevalence of coronary artery disease. Furthermore, preliminary studies indicate that MDCT can also detect and characterize atherosclerotic plaque, and these findings are in good agreement with intravascular ultrasound (IVUS). It is therefore tempting to believe that MDCT could identify patients with chest pain of uncertain cause in the ED, many of whom could then be safely discharged. Published pilot studies in which MDCT was used to evaluate patients in the ED for this purpose look promising, but have only involved small patient numbers, and cannot be regarded as definitive (Hoffmann et al. 2006a,b; White et al. 2005). The Writing Group feels that MDCT may provide novel and accurate information on the presence of CAD, and can also evaluate aortic dissection and pulmonary embolism. However, large blinded clinical trials are needed to determine the accuracy and precision of MDCT for triage of patients with acute chest pain. Randomized trials should be performed to evaluate the degree to which MDCT enhances patient risk stratification, the consequences of a universally standardized as opposed to a targeted protocol, patient outcomes, and cost-effectiveness compared with the current standard of care. Staffing issues also need to be addressed since sufficient numbers of CT trained physicians and technologists will be needed; ideally, facilities should offer ECG gated MDCT service 24 h/day and 7 days per week.

Finally, the Writing Group was unanimous in its belief that minimally invasive MDCT has indeed considerable potential for improving the management of selected patients with acute chest pain, and that the necessary clinical research trials to clarify and establish its role in the ED should proceed with urgency.

References

ACR (2006) White Paper on Split Interpretations. American College of Radiology, Reston, VA. Available from: http://www.acr.org/s_acr/doc.asp?CID=2600&DID=24277

Agatston AS, Janowitz WR, Hildner FJ, Zusmer NR, Viamonte M, Jr., Detrano R (1990) Quantification of coronary artery calcium using ultrafast computed tomography. J Am Coll Cardiol 15:827–832

Antman EM, Cohen M, Bernink PJ et al. (2000) The TIMI risk score for unstable angina/non-ST elevation MI: a method for prognostication and therapeutic decision making. Jama 284:835–842

Becker CR, Kleffel T, Crispin A et al. (2001) Coronary artery calcium measurement: agreement of multirow detector and electron beam CT. AJR Am J Roentgenol 176:1295–1298

Braunwald E, Antman EM, Beasley JW et al. (2002) ACC/AHA 2002 guideline update for the management of patients with unstable angina and non-ST-segment elevation myocardial infarction – summary article: a report of the American College of Cardiology/American Heart Association task force on practice guidelines (Committee on the Management of Patients With Unstable Angina). J Am Coll Cardiol 40:1366–1374

Budoff MJ, Cohen MC, Garcia MJ et al. (2005) ACCF/AHA clinical competence statement on cardiac imaging with computed tomography and magnetic resonance: a report of the American College of Cardiology Foundation/American Heart Association/American College of Physicians Task Force on Clinical Competence and Training. J Am Coll Cardiol 46:383–402

Cohen M, Demers C, Gurfinkel EP et al. (1998) Low-molecular-weight heparins in non-ST-segment elevation ischemia: the ESSENCE trial. Efficacy and Safety of Subcutaneous Enoxaparin versus intravenous unfractionated heparin, in non-Q-wave Coronary Events. Am J Cardiol 82:19L–24L

Dorgelo J, Willems TP, Geluk CA, van Ooijen PM, Zijlstra F, Oudkerk M (2005) Multidetector computed tomography-guided treatment strategy in patients with non-ST elevation acute coronary syndromes: a pilot study. Eur Radiol 15:708–713

Fineberg HV, Scadden D, Goldman L (1984) Care of patients with a low probability of acute myocardial infarction. Cost effectiveness of alternatives to coronary-care-unit admission. N Engl J Med 310:1301–1307

Georgiou D, Budoff MJ, Kaufer E, Kennedy JM, Lu B, Brundage BH (2001) Screening patients with chest pain in the emergency department using electron beam tomography: a follow-up study. J Am Coll Cardiol 38:105–110

Goldman L, Cook EF, Johnson PA, Brand DA, Rouan GW, Lee TH (1996) Prediction of the need for intensive care in patients who come to the emergency departments with acute chest pain. N Engl J Med 334:1498–1504

Graff LG, Dallara J, Ross MA et al. (1997) Impact on the care of the emergency department chest pain patient from the chest pain evaluation registry (CHEPER) study. Am J Cardiol 80:563–568

Hayter RG, Rhea JT, Small A, Tafazoli FS, Novelline RA (2006) Suspected aortic dissection and other aortic disorders: multi-detector row CT in 373 cases in the emergency setting. Radiology 238:841–852

Hendel RC, Patel MR, Kramer CM et al. (2006) ACCF/ACR/SCCT/SCMR/ASNC/NASCI/SCAI/SIR 2006 appropriateness criteria for cardiac computed tomography and cardiac magnetic resonance imaging: a report of the American College of Cardiology Foundation Quality Strategic Directions Committee Appropriateness Criteria Working Group, American College of Radiology, Society of Cardiovascular Computed Tomography, Society for Cardiovascular Magnetic Resonance, American Society of Nuclear Cardiology, North American Society for Cardiac Imaging, Society for Cardiovascular Angiography and Interventions, and Society of Interventional Radiology. J Am Coll Cardiol 48:1475–1497

Hoff JA, Chomka EV, Krainik AJ, Daviglus M, Rich S, Kondos GT (2001) Age and gender distributions of coronary artery calcium detected by electron beam tomography in 35,246 adults. Am J Cardiol 87:1335–1339

Hoffmann U, Nagurney JT, Moselewski F et al. (2006a) Coronary multidetector computed tomography in the assessment of patients with acute chest pain. Circulation 114:2251–2260

Hoffmann U, Pena AJ, Moselewski F et al. (2006b) MDCT in early triage of patients with acute chest pain. AJR Am J Roentgenol 187:1240–1247

Jacobs JE, Boxt LM, Desjardins B, Fishman EK, Larson PA, Schoepf UJ (2006) ACR Practice Guideline for the Performance and Interpretation of Cardiac Computed Tomography (CT). J Am Coll Radiol 3:677–685

Jeudy J, Waite S, White CS (2006) Nontraumatic thoracic emergencies. Radiol Clin North Am 44:273–293, ix

Katz DA, Williams GC, Brown RL et al. (2005) Emergency physicians‘ fear of malpractice in evaluating patients with possible acute cardiac ischemia. Ann Emerg Med 46:525–533

Khan IA, Nair CK (2002) Clinical, diagnostic, and management perspectives of aortic dissection. Chest 122:311–328

Laudon DA, Vukov LF, Breen JF, Rumberger JA, Wollan PC, Sheedy PF, 2nd. (1999) Use of electron-beam computed tomography in the evaluation of chest pain patients in the emergency department. Ann Emerg Med 33:15–21

Leber AW, Knez A, von Ziegler F et al. (2005) Quantification of obstructive and nonobstructive coronary lesions by 64-slice computed tomography: a comparative study with quantitative coronary angiography and intravascular ultrasound. J Am Coll Cardiol 46:147–154

Lee TH, Goldman L (2000) Evaluation of the patient with acute chest pain. N Engl J Med 342:1187–1195

Lee TH, Rouan GW, Weisberg MC et al. (1987) Clinical characteristics and natural history of patients with acute myocardial infarction sent home from the emergency room. Am J Cardiol 60:219–224

Leschka S, Alkadhi H, Plass A et al. (2005) Accuracy of MSCT coronary angiography with 64-slice technology: first experience. Eur Heart J 26:1482–1487

Manoharan G, Adgey AA (2002) Current management of unstable angina: lessons from the TACTICS-TIMI 18 trial. Am J Cardiovasc Drugs 2:237–243

McLaughlin VV, Balogh T, Rich S (1999) Utility of electron beam computed tomography to stratify patients presenting to the emergency room with chest pain. Am J Cardiol 84:327–328, A328

Mega JL, Morrow DA, Sabatine MS et al. (2005) Correlation between the TIMI risk score and high-risk angiographic findings in non-ST-elevation acute coronary syndromes: observations from the Platelet Receptor Inhibition in Ischemic Syndrome Management in Patients Limited by Unstable Signs and Symptoms (PRISM-PLUS) trial. Am Heart J 149:846–850

Mollet NR, Cademartiri F, van Mieghem CA et al. (2005) High-resolution spiral computed tomography coronary angiography in patients referred for diagnostic conventional coronary angiography. Circulation 112:2318–2323

Naghavi M, Falk E, Hecht HS et al. (2006) From vulnerable plaque to vulnerable patient – Part III: Executive summary of the Screening for Heart Attack Prevention and Education (SHAPE) Task Force report. Am J Cardiol 98:2H–15H

Ohnesorge B, Flohr T, Fischbach R et al. (2002) Reproducibility of coronary calcium quantification in repeat examinations with retrospectively ECG-gated multisection spiral CT. Eur Radiol 12:1532–1540

Onuma Y, Tanabe K, Nakazawa G et al. (2006) Noncardiac findings in cardiac imaging with multidetector computed tomography. J Am Coll Cardiol 48:402–406

Pannu HK, Alvarez W, Jr., Fishman EK (2006) Beta-blockers for cardiac CT: a primer for the radiologist. AJR Am J Roentgenol 186[6 Suppl 2]:S341–345

Poll LW, Cohnen M, Brachten S, Ewen K, Modder U (2002) Dose reduction in multi-slice CT of the heart by use of ECG-controlled tube current modulation («ECG pulsing»): phantom measurements. Rofo 174:1500–1505

Pope JH, Aufderheide TP, Ruthazer R et al. (2000) Missed diagnoses of acute cardiac ischemia in the emergency department. N Engl J Med 342:1163–1170

Pozen MW, D'Agostino RB, Selker HP, Sytkowski PA, Hood WB, Jr (1984) A predictive instrument to improve coronary-care-unit admission practices in acute ischemic heart disease. A prospective multicenter clinical trial. N Engl J Med 310:1273–1278

Pugliese F, Mollet NR, Runza G et al. (2006) Diagnostic accuracy of non-invasive 64-slice CT coronary angiography in patients with stable angina pectoris. Eur Radiol 16:575–582

Raff GL, Gallagher MJ, O'Neill WW, Goldstein JA (2005) Diagnostic accuracy of noninvasive coronary angiography using 64-slice spiral computed tomography. J Am Coll Cardiol 46:552–557

Rumberger JA (2006) Noncardiac abnormalities in diagnostic cardiac computed tomography: within normal limits or we never looked! J Am Coll Cardiol 48:407–408

Rusnak RA, Stair TO, Hansen K, Fastow JS (1989) Litigation against the emergency physician: common features in cases of missed myocardial infarction. Ann Emerg Med 18:1029–1034

Sanchis J, Bodi V, Llacer A et al. (2005a) Risk stratification of patients with acute chest pain and normal troponin concentrations. Heart 91:1013–1018

Sanchis J, Bodi V, Nunez J et al. (2005b) New risk score for patients with acute chest pain, non-ST-segment deviation, and normal troponin concentrations: a comparison with the TIMI risk score. J Am Coll Cardiol 46:443–449

Scheffel H, Alkadhi H, Plass A et al. (2006) Accuracy of dual-source CT coronary angiography: first experience in a high pre-test probability population without heart rate control. Eur Radiol 16:2739–2747

Selker HP, Zalenski RJ, Antman EM et al. (1997) An evaluation of technologies for identifying acute cardiac ischemia in the emergency department: a report from a National Heart Attack Alert Program Working Group. Ann Emerg Med 29:13–87

Selker HP, Beshansky JR, Griffith JL et al. (1998) Use of the acute cardiac ischemia time-insensitive predictive instrument (ACI-TIPI) to assist with triage of patients with chest pain or other symptoms suggestive of acute cardiac ischemia. A multicenter, controlled clinical trial. Ann Intern Med 129:845–855

Stein PD, Fowler SE, Goodman LR et al. (2006) Multidetector computed tomography for acute pulmonary embolism. N Engl J Med 354:2317–2327

Thoongsuwan N, Stern EJ (2002) Chest CT scanning for clinical suspected thoracic aortic dissection: beware the alternate diagnosis. Emerg Radiol 9:257–261

Udelson JE, Beshansky JR, Ballin DS et al. (2002) Myocardial perfusion imaging for evaluation and triage of patients with suspected acute cardiac ischemia: a randomized controlled trial. Jama 288:2693–2700

Wells PS, Anderson DR, Rodger M et al. (2000) Derivation of a simple clinical model to categorize patients probability of pulmonary embolism: increasing the models utility with the SimpliRED D-dimer. Thromb Haemost 83:416–420

White CS, Kuo D, Kelemen M et al. (2005) Chest pain evaluation in the emergency department: can MDCT provide a comprehensive evaluation? AJR Am J Roentgenol 185:533–540

Wintersperger BJ, Nikolaou K, von Ziegler F et al. (2006) Image quality, motion artifacts, and reconstruction timing of 64-slice coronary computed tomography angiography with 0.33-second rotation speed. Invest Radiol 41:436–442

Non-Invasive Measurement of Coronary Atherosclerosis

4

4.1 Pathophysiology of Coronary Atherosclerosis and Calcification

WILFRED F. A. DEN DUNNEN and ALBERT J. H. SUURMEIJER

CONTENTS

4.1.1 Normal Artery Histology and Cell Function

In order to understand plaque formation and plaque composition it is necessary to have a knowledge of the normal histology. In general, arteries contain three concentric layers: the intima, media and adventitia (Fig. 4.1.1). The intima consists of a single layer of endothelial cells with only a small amount of underlying connective tissue. The intima is separated from the media by a thick layer of elastic fibers called the intern elastic lamina. The media is mostly composed of smooth muscle cells. Approximately the inner half of the smooth muscle cell layer receives its nutrients from the lumen via diffusion. The outer half, however, needs nourishment from blood vessels themselves, called the vasa vasorum, which course into the media from the adventitia. Between the media and the adventitia lies the external elastic lamina. The adventitia consists of connective tissue, nerve fibers and the vasa vasorum.

W. F. A. DEN DUNNEN, MD, PhD
A. J. H. SUURMEIJER, MD, PhD
Department of Pathology and Laboratory Medicine, University Medical Center Groningen, University of Groningen, Hanzeplein 1, P.O. Box 30.001, 9700 RB Groningen, The Netherlands

Based upon their location in the circulatory system, size, and functional microscopic anatomy, arteries can be divided into: large or elastic arteries (such as the aorta), medium sized or muscular arteries (such as the coronary arteries), small arteries with a diameter smaller than 2 mm, and arterioles. The thickness of the arterial wall gradually diminishes as the vessel becomes smaller, but its ratio to the lumen diameter becomes proportionally greater. Depending on their position and function in the arterial system, the basic configuration of the arterial walls, as described above, may vary, especially in the media and the extracellular matrix. For instance, the aorta needs to be able to expand during the systole. Therefore, the media is rich in elastic fibers and arranged in functional lamellae of smooth muscle cells and elastic fibers. In contrast, muscular arteries and arterioles regulate regional blood flow and blood pressure by changing luminal size by contraction or relaxation of the smooth muscle cells. In this part of the arterial system, the media contains cir-

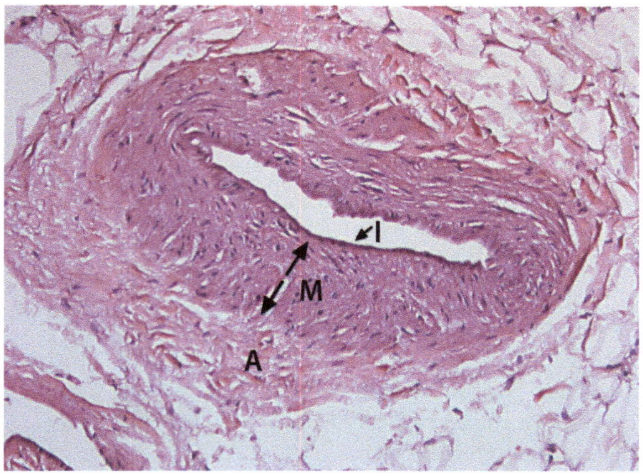

Fig. 4.1.1. Micrograph showing a normal muscular artery with a single layer thick intima (*I*), the media (*M*, *arrows* mark the borders) and adventitia (*A*)

cularly and spirally arranged smooth muscle cells, and the elastic fibers are limited to the internal and external elastic laminas.

The main cellular components of arteries are endothelial cells and smooth muscle cells. Endothelial cells form a continuous lining called the endothelium. The integrity of this single cell-thick layer is essential for the maintenance of vessel wall homeostasis and normal circulatory function. Endothelial cells have many different properties and functions, including: (1) permeability barrier function, (2) anticoagulant, antithrombotic and fibrinolytic effects, (3) extracellular matrix production, (4) oxidation of LDL, (5) regulation of inflammation and (6) regulation of cell growth. In addition to their contractile and relaxing properties, smooth muscle cells are able to synthesize collagen, elastin and proteoglycans and change (the function of) growth factors and cytokines.

4.1.2 Endothelial Dysfunction and the Pathogenesis of Atherosclerotic Plaques

Endothelial cells can respond to several stimuli by adjusting their normal physiological functions and by inducing new properties. This so-called endothelial activation can cause an increase in the expression of adhesion molecules and an increased production of growth factors and coagulation proteins. Endothelial dysfunction, however, can be responsible for the initiation of thrombus formation and atherosclerosis. Certain forms of endothelial dysfunction may develop within minutes and can be reversible, whereas others may require alterations in gene expression and protein synthesis, which may take days to develop.

Concerning the etiology of atherosclerosis, several major and minor clinical risk factors have been recognized. Well-established or major risk factors of atherosclerosis are cigarette smoking, hypertension, hypercholesterolemia, and diabetes mellitus. In addition to these clinical risk factors, hemodynamic factors, in particular disturbed arterial flow and increased arterial pulsatile shear stress, also contribute to endothelial dysfunction. Moreover, patients with more than one risk factor will more often experience complications of atherosclerosis at a younger age than patients with only one risk factor. Hemodynamically disturbed arterial flow and pulsatile shear stress provide us with an explanation why atherosclerosis mainly arises at the level of bifurcations of the larger elastic arteries. Sites of predilection of atherosclerosis, in addition to coronary arteries, are the aorta, the carotid arteries and the femoral and popliteal arteries. According to the response to injury theory, endothelial dysfunction is thought to play a key role in the development of atherosclerosis. In dysfunctional endothelial cells increased abluminal transport of serum proteins occurs, in particular LDL-cholesterol. Upon oxidation in the intima of the arterial wall, LDL-cholesterol is phagocytosed by macrophages, which enter the intima as monocytes from peripheral blood. The initial stage of atherosclerosis, which may be observed already at young

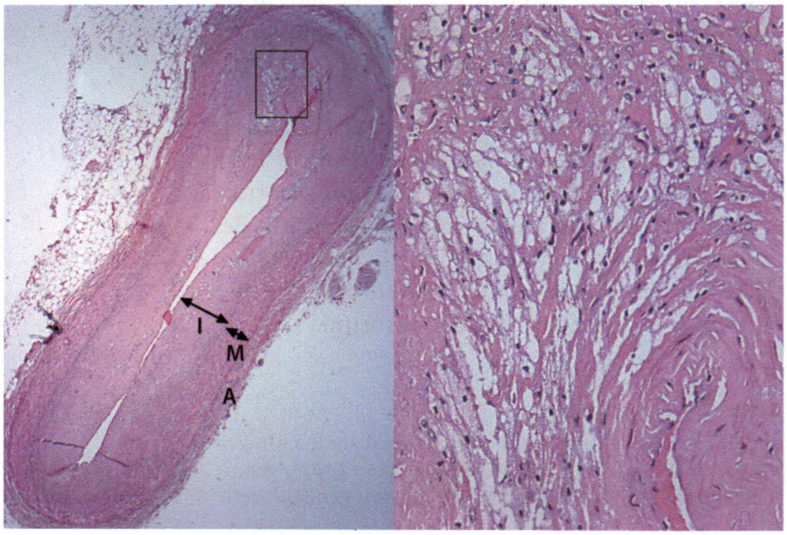

Fig. 4.1.2. The micrograph on the *left* shows a coronary artery with a thick intima (*I*) with fibrosis. The *box* indicates the detailed micrograph shown on the *right*, containing a large number of foamy macrophages

age is called fatty streak (Fig. 4.1.2). Histologically, the fatty streak consists almost only of foamy macrophages which have ingested LDL-cholesterol and other serum proteins. After this initial stage, atherosclerosis may develop over decades to become a fibrofatty atherosclerotic plaque. In its typical presentation the fibrofatty plaque is an eccentric plaque in the intima of an elastic or larger muscular artery (Fig. 4.1.3). In textbooks of pathology, the atherosclerotic plaque is usually depicted as an advanced fibrofatty plaque. The advanced fibrofatty plaque contains a large lipid core containing cell debris, cholesterol crystals, foamy macrophages, and calcifications (Fig. 4.1.4). The lipid core is separated from the vascular lumen by a fibrous cap, a band of collagen synthesized by myofibroblasts, often called smooth muscle cells. Inflammatory cells are also found in an advanced atherosclerotic plaque, indicating that immune reactions have occurred. In addition, in most advanced fibrofatty plaques ingrowth of small capillaries is observed (Fig. 4.1.5). The eccentric plaque bulges into the narrowed arterial lumen. The adaptation of the vessel wall, by which lumen diameter may increase to a certain extent, is called positive arterial remodeling. However, progression of the atherosclerotic plaque will finally result in severe narrowing of the vessel lumen and this will give rise to clinical symptoms, e.g. angina pectoris due to severe narrowing of a coronary artery. The more life threatening acute coronary syndromes such as unstable angina pectoris and myocardial infarct are nearly always caused by atherothrombosis with partial or complete lumen stenosis. The morphology of atherosclerotic plaques complicated by atherothrombosis is heterogeneous. About 60% of complicated plaques are due to plaque rupture, by which the highly thrombogenic plaque core is exposed to the luminal surface. Another 30% of cases of atherothrombosis are due to plaque erosion. In these cases the eroded surface usually contains smooth muscle cells embedded in myxoid stroma rich in small capillaries, quite different from the fibrous cap observed in most fibrofatty plaques. The final 10% of cases of atherothrombosis are related to a plaque bleeding or a large calcified nodule exposed to the surface. Interestingly, in patients presenting with an acute coronary syndrome, the culprit fibrofatty plaque lesion with atherothrombosis is more often seen in segments with less than 70% stenosis also showing positive arterial remodeling in stead of segments with severe stenosis.

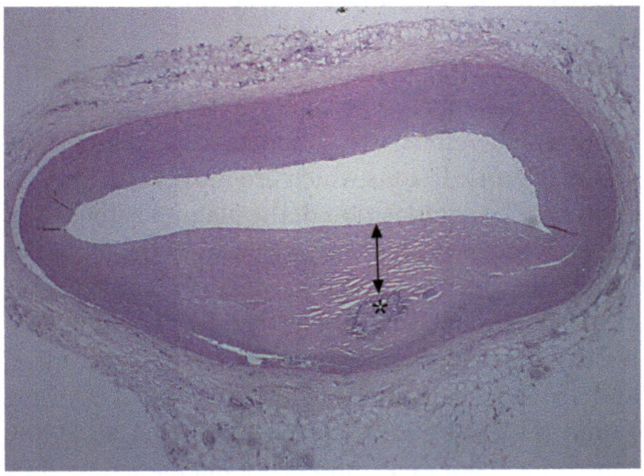

Fig. 4.1.3. Coronary artery with an eccentric plaque with a small calcification (*asterisk*) and a thick fibrous cap (*double arrow*)

4.1.3 Calcification of Plaques

From the radiologist's point of view the calcification process in atherosclerosis is interesting, because of the possibility to visualize calcium deposits and the fact that the calcification process parallels the formation of the atherosclerotic plaque. In this context it is important to note that calcification is usually much less prominent in complicated plaques due to erosion of a myxoid and cellular intima when compared to complicated plaques with rupture of a lipid rich core. Thus, it is important to be aware of the fact that calcification is present in a subset of morphologically heterogeneous atherosclerotic plaques. In the early stage of the prototypical atherosclerotic plaque called fatty streak no calcium can be detected. On the other hand, in nearly all advanced classical fibrofatty plaques a certain amount of calcification may be observed. Calcification in advanced fibrofatty atherosclerotic lesions may already present in relatively young people (Stary 1990). With increasing age, calcium granules grow in size, form lumps and sometimes plates. The lumps and plates tend to be in the periphery of the lipid core, especially in the base. In type VII ('calcific lesion') and type VIII ('fibrocalcific lesion') lesions, the necrotic core has become much smaller and is predominantly replaced by calcium and fibrotic tissue, respectively (Stary 1995, 2000).

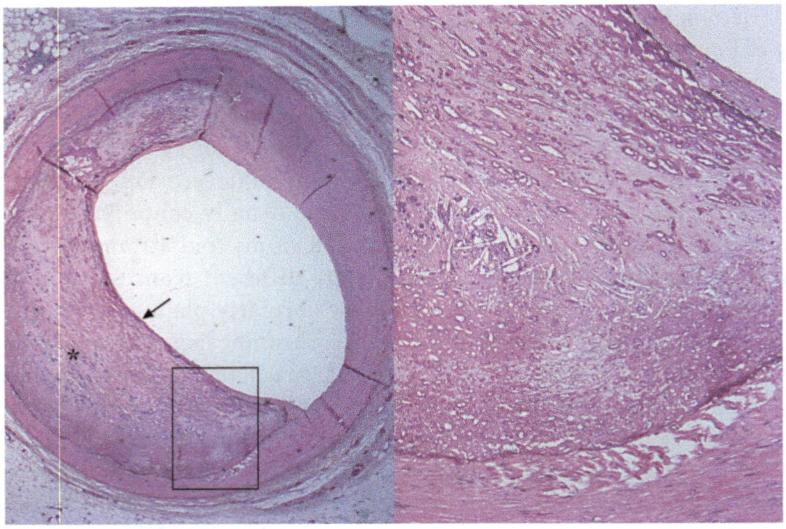

Fig. 4.1.4. Eccentric plaque with a necrotic core, calcification (*asterisk*) and a very thin fibrous cap (*arrow*). On the *right hand side* a detail showing cholesterol needles (*white spikes*) surrounded by deposited calcium (*purple material*)

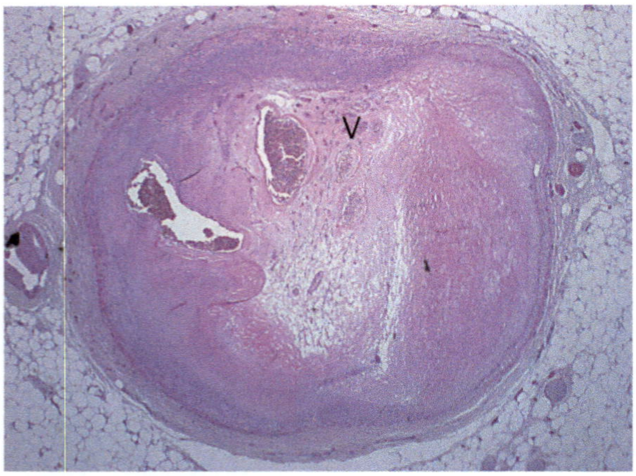

Fig. 4.1.5. A coronary artery with a very narrow lumen, as well as newly formed vessels (*V*) inside the plaque

As calcium deposition parallels the progression of atherosclerotic lesions, it is conceivable that the amount of calcification is associated with the atherosclerotic plaque burden (Detrano et al. 2008). However, atherosclerotic lesion types in coronary arteries of older adults can be quite heterogeneous, including early and advanced stages. In morphometric analysis of the composition of plaques in coronary events, the overall plaque area and the area of calcification were linearly associated (Kragel et al. 1989). The coronary calcium area of hearts as a whole, of individual coronary arteries and of individual coronary segments was highly correlated with the histologically quantified coronary plaque area (Rumberger et al. 1995). The detected amount of coronary calcification was about one fifth of the measured atherosclerotic plaque burden in corresponding segments. Further analyses showed that the increase in amount of coronary calcification with advancing age was similar to the increase in coronary atherosclerosis (Sangiorgi et al. 1998). Although the absence of calcification did not exclude the presence of possibly unstable plaque, there was a low plaque burden on average. Nevertheless, despite significant correlations between calcification area and plaque area, the individual variability in calcification was large.

4.1.4 Calcification and Plaque Rupture

Most myocardial infarctions are caused by thrombotic occlusion of a coronary artery after plaque rupture. Therefore, it is important to identify the atherosclerotic lesions which are most vulnerable to rupture. The composition of the plaques rather than lumen stenosis is presently regarded as the main determinant of acute coronary events (Van der Wal et al. 1994). Evidence on the composition of vulnerable lesions comes predominantly from autopsy studies, and from investigations with intravascular ultrasound (IVUS) or MRI (Briley-Saebo et al. 2007). The three major determinants of plaque vulnerability are the size and structure of the lipid core, the thickness of the fibrous cap covering the core, and inflammation in and near the cap (Virmani et al.

2000). If the lipid core of a lesion is large and soft, the plaque is at higher risk of rupture. Thinning of the fibrous cap and reduction of the collagen content of the cap also increase rupture risk. Part of this increased risk may be due to break-down of matrix proteins by proteases, released by activated macrophages, and a reduction in synthesis of matrix proteins by smooth muscle cells (Davies et al. 1993). If cap thickness is low, circumferential stress at the luminal border of the plaque shows a critical increase (Loree et al. 1994). It has been demonstrated that local variations in stress, possibly due to variations in plaque composition, may contribute to rupture of plaques (Cheng et al. 1993). Furthermore, heavy infiltration of macrophages in the cap and at the shoulder region is associated with plaque rupture. The role of calcification in the pathogenesis of coronary events is unclear. As mentioned before, the amount of calcium is related to the total amount of plaque, including unstable plaque sections. Since the plaque burden is related to myocardial infarction and sudden cardiac death, the quantity of calcification can possibly identify the persons at highest risk of coronary events (Schenker et al. 2008). A histopathological comparison of coronary arteries of subjects dying from sudden cardiac death (cases) and subjects dying from noncardiac causes (controls) showed that the plaque area, lipid core size and calcified area were larger in cases than in controls (Schmermund et al. 2001). In an analysis restricted to narrowed coronary sections from cases, ruptured plaques had an increased plaque area, lipid core size, calcified area, and percentage of segments with calcification, compared to stable plaques. It was stated that the surplus of calcium in ruptured plaques could simply reflect the larger plaque burden of ruptured plaques, and not a causal relationship between calcium and rupture. Using electron-beam CT (EBT) to compare infarct-related and non-infarct-related arteries in subjects with myocardial infarction, the amount of calcium, calcified areas and number of calcifications were higher for culprit arteries than for non-culprit arteries (Mascola et al. 2000). Clearly, a relation exists between coronary calcification and severity of coronary disease (Finn et al. 2007). However, whether calcification itself is a harmful or protective process, is a matter of debate. One necropsy study found that plaques in severely narrowed vessel segments contained less calcium in subjects with fatal myocardial infarction than in subjects with sudden cardiac death. It was therefore suggested that calcified deposits may impart stability and tend to reduce vulnerability for plaque rupture. Observations in a helical CT study corroborate this view (Shemesh et al. 1998). In this study myocardial infarction was prone to originate from non- or mildly calcified culprit arteries, while in subjects with stable angina pectoris coronary arteries were generally extensively calcified. Thus, increasing calcification of individual atherosclerotic lesions may decrease the risk of thrombotic obstruction at the lesion site and therefore of a coronary event. Biomechanical results are ambiguous. Calcification of individual plaques was found to make plaques stiffer and induce resistance to fibrous cap rupture, and extensive calcification may reduce stress in the fibrous cap (Lee 2000; Lee et al. 1991). However, focal calcification may increase stress at the shoulder regions and in the cap (Veress et al. 2000). This leads to the conclusion that coronary calcification may have a different significance in the context of individual plaques and of the total plaque burden. Further research is needed to elucidate the precise role of coronary calcification in plaque formation and stabilization.

References

Briley-Saebo KC, Mulder WJM, Mani V et al (2007) Magnetic resonance imaging of vulnerable atherosclerotic plaques: current imaging strategies and molecular imaging probes. J Magn Reson Imaging 26:460–479

Cheng GC, Loree HM, Kamm RD et al (1993) Distribution of circumferential stress in ruptured and stable atherosclerotic lesions. A structural analysis with histopathological correlation. Circulation 87:1179–1187

Davies MJ, Richardson PD, Woolf N et al (1993) Risk of thrombosis in human atherosclerotic plaques: role of extracellular lipid, macrophage, and smooth muscle cell content. Br Heart J 69:377–381

Detrano R, Guerci AD, Carr JJ et al (2008) Coronary calcium as a predictor of coronary events in four racial or ethnic groups. N Engl J Med 358:1336–1345

Finn AV, Nakazawa G, Narula J, Virmani R (2007) Culprit plaque in myocardial infarction; going beyond angiography. J Am Coll Cardiol 50:2204–2206

Kragel AH, Reddy SG, Wittes JT et al (1989) Morphometric analysis of the composition of atherosclerotic plaques in the four major epicardial coronary arteries in acute myocardial infarction and in sudden coronary death. Circulation 80:1747–1756

Lee RT (2000) Atherosclerotic lesion mechanics versus biology. Z Kardiol 89[Suppl 2]:80–84

Lee RT, Grodzinsky AJ, Frank EH et al (1991) Structure-dependent dynamic mechanical behavior of fibrous caps from human atherosclerotic plaques. Circulation 83:1764–1770

Loree HM, Tobias BJ, Gibson LJ et al (1994) Mechanical properties of model atherosclerotic lesion lipid pools. Arterioscler Thromb 14:230–234
Mascola A, Ko J, Bakhsheshi H et al (2000) Electron beam tomography comparison of culprit and non-culprit coronary arteries in patients with acute myocardial infarction. Am J Cardiol 85:1357–1359
Rumberger JA, Simons DB, Fitzpatrick LA et al (1995) Coronary artery calcium area by electron-beam computed tomography and coronary atherosclerotic plaque area. A histopathologic correlative study. Circulation 92:2157–2162
Sangiorgi G, Rumberger JA, Severson A et al (1998) Arterial calcification and not lumen stenosis is highly correlated with atherosclerotic plaque burden in humans: a histologic study of 723 coronary artery segments using nondecalcifying methodology. J Am Coll Cardiol 31:126–133
Schenker MP, Dorbala S, Cho Tek Hong E et al (2008) Interrelation of coronary calcification, myocardial ischemia and outcomes in patients with intermediate likelihood of coronary artery disease. A combined positron emission tomography/computed tomography study. Circulation 117:1693–1700
Schmermund A, Schwartz RS, Adamzik M et al (2001) Coronary atherosclerosis in unheralded sudden coronary death under age 50: histo-pathologic comparison with 'healthy' subjects dying out of hospital. Atherosclerosis 155:499–508
Shemesh J, Stroh CI, Tenenbaum A et al (1998) Comparison of coronary calcium in stable angina pectoris and in first acute myocardial infarction utilizing double helical computerized tomography. Am J Cardiol 81:271–275
Stary HC (1990) The sequence of cell and matrix changes in atherosclerotic lesions of coronary arteries in the first forty years of life. Eur Heart J 11 [Suppl E]:3–19
Stary HC (1995) The histological classification of atherosclerotic lesions in human coronary arteries. In: Fuster V, Ross R, Topol E (eds) Atherosclerosis and coronary artery disease. Lippincott-Raven Publishers, Philadelphia
Stary HC (2000) Natural history and histological classification of atherosclerotic lesions: an update. Arterioscler Thromb Vasc Biol 20:1177–1178
Van der Wal AC, Becker AE, van der Loos CM et al (1994) Site of intimal rupture or erosion of thrombosed coronary atherosclerotic plaques is characterized by an inflammatory process irrespective of the dominant plaque morphology. Circulation 89:36–44
Veress AI, Vince DG, Anderson PM et al (2000) Vascular mechanics of the coronary artery. Z Kardiol 89[Suppl 2]:92–100
Virmani R, Kolodgie FD, Burke AP et al (2000) Lessons from sudden coronary death: a comprehensive morphological classification scheme for atherosclerotic lesions. Arterioscler Thromb Vasc Biol 20:1262–1275

Non-Invasive Measurement of Coronary Atherosclerosis

4

4.2 Detection and Quantification of Coronary Calcification

Rozemarijn Vliegenthart Proença and Christopher Herzog

CONTENTS

R. Vliegenthart Proença, MD, PhD
Department of Radiology, University Medical Center Groningen, University of Groningen, Hanzeplein 1, P.O. Box 30.001, 9700 RB Groningen, The Netherlands
C. Herzog, MD, PhD
Department of Radiology, Rotkreuzklinikum Munich, Winthirstrasse 9, 80639 Munich, Germany

4.2.1 Introduction

A number of radiological techniques have the potential to detect calcification of the coronary arteries, namely plain chest radiography, fluoroscopy, conventional computed tomography, electron-beam computed tomography, multidetector-row computed tomography, intravascular ultrasound, magnetic resonance imaging, and transthoracic and transesophageal echocardiography. In the following, the methods that are most commonly used for visualization of coronary calcification are discussed.

Coronary calcification has been demonstrated incidentally with plain chest radiography. However, most patients with coronary artery disease have no visible calcifications in the coronary arteries on chest radiographs. This is mainly due to distinct cardiac moving artefacts masking the commonly rather discrete coronary calcifications. The accuracy of chest radiography thus was only 42% compared to fluoroscopy, which is also a rather insensitive technique (see below) (Souza et al. 1978).

4.2.2 Fluoroscopy

Already in 1968, coronary calcification seen fluoroscopically was found to be related to the presence of symptomatic heart disease (McGuire et al. 1968). In the 1970s, cardiologists reported the detection of coronary calcification by fluoroscopy as a potential aid in the diagnosis of coronary artery disease (CAD) (Bartel et al. 1974; Aldrich et al. 1979). Until then, the only noninvasive method for detecting CAD was exercise testing. There are, however, a number of limitations to exercise testing: it can only detect plaque constricting the lumen severely enough to compromise blood flow, it may cause a coronary event in high-risk subjects, and the possibility to perform the test depends on the exercise capacity of the patient. In contrast to exercise testing, cardiac fluoroscopy was a rapid, inexpensive and widely available procedure. With different projections, the presence of calcification in the individual coronary arteries could be assessed. A number of studies since then have been performed that integrated fluoroscopy in the precatheterization evaluation of patients undergoing selective coronary angiography (Hamby et al. 1974; Bierner et al. 1978; Aldrich et al. 1979; Detrano et al. 1985; Uretsky et al. 1988). After fluoroscopic images were relayed to a TV monitor or recorded on cinefilm, observers rated each coronary artery as to the presence or absence of calcification. Table 4.2.1 shows the results of eight studies comparing fluoroscopic detection of coronary calcification with angiographically detected disease (at least 50% luminal narrowing). Because it is difficult to justify an invasive procedure like coronary angiography without suspicion of CAD, these studies were all conducted in patients with symptomatic CAD. Aldrich et al. (1979) found that the diagnostic accuracy of fluoroscopy approached that of exercise testing. The accuracy of a positive test result was 86% for fluoroscopy but 69% for exercise testing. In the published studies, the sensitivities for detecting any angiographic disease ranged from 40% to 79%, while the specificities varied from 52% to 93%. The large variability in test parameter values can partly be explained by differences in threshold for significant coronary obstruction, differences in disease prevalence in the different populations, and bias caused by evaluation of angiographic or fluoroscopic images without blinding to the result of the other test. A meta-analytic review on the value of cardiac fluoroscopy reported a weighted mean sensitivity of 59% and a weighted mean specificity of 82% (Gianrossi et al. 1990). It can be concluded that the sensitivity of fluoroscopy for detection of CAD is quite low, so many patients with significant luminal narrowing do not have a positive fluoroscopic test result. The low sensitivity is partially due to image quantum noise and to interfering background structures like ribs, spine and great vessels that obscure calcification during the fluoroscopic examination. Notwithstanding the low sensitivity, Margolis et al. (1980) found that coronary calcification detected by fluoroscopy has prognostic significance: in a population of patients undergoing selective angiography because of suspected CAD, the 5-year survival rate was 58% in subjects with calcification while survival was 87% in subjects without calcification. However, the low sensitivity limits the use of fluoroscopy as a screening test for latent CAD. In addition, there are some technical difficulties in detecting small calcified lesions by fluoroscopy that prohibit its use for mass screening: a high kilovoltage is needed to penetrate subjects with large body habitus, and only trained radiologists can reliably evaluate the presence of coronary calcification.

Table 4.2.1. Studies on the comparison of coronary calcification detected by fluoroscopy with angiographically detected coronary artery disease

Study	Patients (n)	Sensitivity (%)	Specificity (%)
Hamby et al. (1974)	500	76	78
Bierner et al. (1978)	436	57	92
Aldrich et al. (1979)	181	66	52
Margolis et al. (1980)	800	40	93
Hung et al. (1984)	92	79	83
Detrano et al. (1986)	297	66	81
Uretsky et al. (1988)	600	76	79
de Korte et al. (1995)	778	52	91

To improve the sensitivity of conventional fluoroscopy, Detrano et al. (1985) employed a temporal blurred mask subtraction technique after digitalization of the fluoroscopic images. With this technique, interfering background structures are subtracted from the image, while moving cardiac structures partly escape from elimination. Furthermore, image averaging over part of the cardiac cycle results in blurring of the subtracted mask and at the same time in enhancement of radiodense objects like calcifications within a less radiodense field. This method was tested in 191 patients referred for coronary angiography. The sensitivity of digital subtraction fluoroscopy for significant luminal narrowing was superior to that of conventional fluoroscopy (92% versus 63%). Despite a decrease in specificity (65% versus 81%), the diagnostic accuracy of digital subtraction fluoroscopy was higher. Reading of coronary arteries on digital subtraction fluoroscopic images, scored as having heavy, mild or no calcification, was found to be highly reproducible (Tang et al. 1994). A study of 1461 asymptomatic, high-risk subjects voluntarily undergoing digital subtraction fluoroscopy had some important findings (Detrano et al. 1994). Firstly, coronary calcification was detectable in the majority of asymptomatic subjects. Secondly, coronary calcification showed the strongest association with age. Since coronary calcification is increasingly common with age, the authors concluded that detection of coronary calcification alone may be inadequate for screening. They proposed that the severity of coronary calcification should be assessed in a quantitative manner, to determine thresholds for different age categories. Two radiological techniques were suggested to quantify coronary calcification: dual energy digital subtraction fluoroscopy (Molloi et al. 1991) and ultrafast computed tomography (see Sect. 4.2.4).

Dual energy fluoroscopy exploits the energy dependence of tissue attenuation coefficients. Images are obtained by switching a high- and a low-energy beam at a high frequency. After correction for scatter and veiling glare (for the purpose of calcium quantification), weighted logarithmically transformed high-energy images are subtracted from low-energy images. From the resulting dual energy images, the absolute calcium mass can be quantified. Molloi et al. (1991) reported that calcium masses estimated from dual energy images correlated well with true calcium masses in a calcium phantom and in calcified arteries. However, the distribution of calcifications within the coronary arteries has not been determined by this method, and will probably heavily depend on the projection. No in vivo reports have been published using dual energy digital subtraction fluoroscopy to quantitate coronary calcification.

4.2.3 Conventional Computed Tomography

Because calcium attenuates the X-ray beam, and because computed tomography (CT) provides excellent contrast resolution, CT can easily detect coronary calcifications. Calcification of the coronary arteries is often noted on chest scans performed for non-cardiac indications (Stanford and Thompson 1999). Rienmüller and Lipton (1987) compared CT, fluoroscopy and coronary angiography in 47 patients (mean age 57 years). In vessels with significant CAD, calcification was visible on 62% of the CT scans, but only on 35% of the fluoroscopic images. CT detected calcification in all patients with angiographic coronary stenosis and in all patients with fluoroscopic calcification. Another study of patients referred for coronary angiography evaluated the sensitivity and specificity for significant stenosis in the different coronary arteries (Timins et al. 1991). Sensitivity of coronary calcification ranged from 16% for the right coronary artery (RCA) to 78% for the left anterior descending coronary artery (LAD), while the specificities ranged from 78% for LAD to 100% for RCA. The high positive predictive values (between 83% and 100%) suggested that significant CAD is very likely when coronary calcification is present. In a Japanese study 90% of patients with coronary calcification detected by CT had significant angiographic stenosis, while 80% of patients with stenosis showed calcification on the CT scan (Masuda et al. 1990). On an individual artery basis, sensitivity of calcification for stenosis in a coronary artery was 65%, while the specificity was found to be 87%. All three studies recorded calcification in the individual coronary arteries as present or absent. However, more sophisticated determination of the degree of calcification is necessary to predict coronary disease in older subjects, because of the increasing prevalence of coronary calcification with age. Moore et al. (1989) attempted to devise a scoring system to assess the amount of coronary calcification. The length of a calcification at the level of the aortic root (in centimeters), the number of slices with calcification, and the maximum width of calcification (in millimeters) were added. Thus, a score was yielded per vessel. Severe calcification was highly predictive of significant CAD. However, many vessels with significant stenosis did not show calcification. In a sub-study of patients undergoing thoracotomy, the presence of coronary calcification increased the risk of cardiac complications. The authors concluded that CT was not sensitive enough to be used for cardiac screening, but recommended it to report the presence of calcification on chest CT scans to alert cardiac surgeons. In general conventional CT suffers from slow scan times, resulting in considerable motion artifacts, partial volume effects, breathing misregistration, low sensitivity for small calcified lesions, and inability to quantify calcification accurately.

4.2.4 Electron-Beam Computed Tomography

Electron-beam computed tomography (EBCT) has resolved many of the problems of conventional CT, owing to an acquisition time of 100 ms or less (therefore formerly called 'ultrafast'). The very short acquisition time freezes cardiac motion, and greatly improves image quality. The scan commonly consists of 20 or 40 adjacent 3 mm images obtained by incremental table feed. The images are usually acquired during one or two breath-holds and are scanned at the moment of lowest cardiac motion usually the mid-diastole (diastasis) or end-systole. This approach is enabled by ECG-synchronized image acquisition also known as prospective ECG-triggering. Usually image acquisition is done within the mid-diastole (diastasis), which commonly represents the longest and calmest period in the cardiac cycle (Herzog et al. 2006). This period is commonly located at approximately 70% of the cardiac cycle. However, at elevated heart rates the length of the diastase gradually diminishes to a point (approximately 95 bpm) where the total duration of the diastole merely matches the length of the phase of rapid inflow (Herzog et al. 2006). According to cardiomechanics it is the transition between the end-systole and early-diastole that in fact displays the phase of least cardiac motion. Thus in the presence of elevated heart rates less motion artefacts and therefore improved image quality is observed if images are acquired at approximately 30% of the cardiac cycle (end-systole). This observation is reinforced by other investigators who earlier demonstrated that lowest velocity of coronary arterial movement is observed during the end-systole (Achenbach et al. 2000).

Tanenbaum et al. (1989) were the first to document the detection of coronary calcification by EBCT, and studied the correlation with angiographic findings. In 54 patients angiographic results were compared with the presence of calcified deposits on 50 ms scans with 1.5 mm² pixel size. Significant stenosis was present in 43 patients. The sensitivity and specificity of coronary calcification for the presence of significant CAD were 88 and 100%, respectively. Agatston et al. (1990) reported the first large study of 584 subjects using EBCT for the detection of coronary calcification. Of the subjects, 475 had no history of coronary disease. The scoring protocol consisted of 20 adjacent 3-mm slices with an acquisition time of 100 ms. EBCT identified calcification in 90% of subjects, while fluoroscopy detected calcium in only 52% of subjects. Figure 4.2.1 shows an image obtained with EBCT, with identification of several structures.

Investigators soon realized the potential of EBCT to perform quantitative measurements of coronary calcification. In an attempt to determine the amount of coronary calcification, Agatston et al. (1990) devised an arbitrary scoring algorithm. This method has become the standard for the quantification of calcium in the coronary arteries. On each image level, only pixels with a density over 130 Hounsfield Units (HU) are regarded as calcified. A value of 130 HU corresponds to a density which lies two standard deviations above the average density of blood in the aorta. The spatial threshold for a calcified lesion is set at ≥ 2 pixels. After placing a region of interest around all lesions found in a coronary artery, the lesion area and density are determined. The calcium score of the individual calcified lesions is calculated by multiplying the calcium area (in mm^2) and a factor based on the maximum density of the lesion. This factor ranges from 1 to 4 in the following manner: 1 = 130–199 HU, 2 = 200–299 HU, 3 = 300–399 HU, 4 = at least 400 HU. The total calcium score results from adding up the scores for all individual calcified lesions.

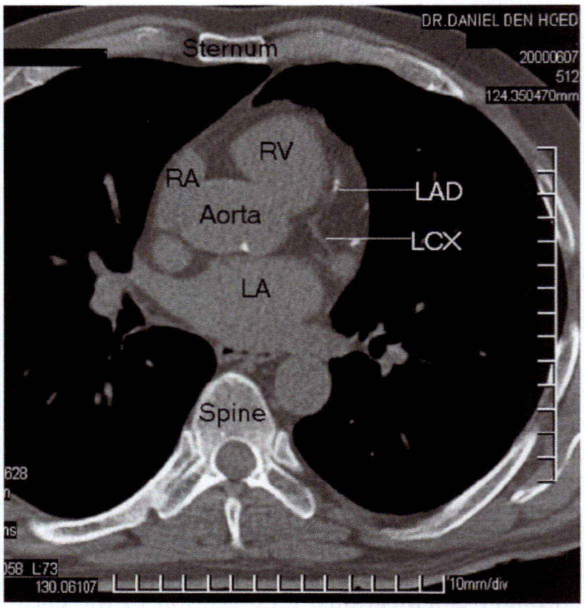

Fig. 4.2.1. Left circumflex coronary artery (*LCX*). *LA*, left atrium; *LAD*, left anterior descending artery; *RA*, right atrium; *RV*, right ventricle;

This calcium scoring protocol has been incorporated in a number of dedicated software programs. Figure 4.2.2 shows the interface of a calcium scoring software program, while examples of different amounts of coronary calcification are visible in Figure 4.2.3.

Agatston et al. (1990) found an increase in calcium score with age. Sensitivity, specificity and predictive values were calculated for different calcium scores in each decade. The negative predictive value of a calcium score of 0 for age groups 40–49, 50–59, and 60–69 years, was 98%, 94%, and 100%, respectively. Furthermore, the interobserver agreement for 88 scans scored by two independent readers was excellent. The authors put forward that the range of calcium scores allows the choice of threshold values tailored to the scan population. Rumberger et al. (1995) found that the amount of coronary calcification, expressed in the calcium score, was also strongly related to the total amount of plaque. In a study by Mautner et al. (1994) there was a close correlation between the calcium score and the histomorphometric calcium area in over 4000 segments from heart specimens.

Reliability of calcification measurements is of utmost importance if EBCT is to be a screening test for CAD. However, there is debate on the accuracy and reproducibility of calcium scores using EBCT. Unfortunately intra- and interobserver (Kaufmann et al. 1994; Hernigou et al. 1996) as well as interscan variability of calcification measurements is low, the latter ranging from 14% to 37% (Kajinami et al. 1993; Bielak et al. 1994; Shields et al. 1995; Wang et al. 1996; Callister et al. 1998a; Yoon et al. 2000; Achenbach et al. 2001a; Möhlenkamp et al. 2001). Part of the inter-scan variability can be attributed to the susceptibility of Agatston's scoring method to substantial change in calcium scores with minimal variation in plaque attenuation or area. Reproducibility found in different studies has been summarized in Table 4.2.2. Different scan protocols have been investigated that may help to increase the reproducibility of calcium scoring, such as use of thicker slice thickness (Wang et al. 1996; Callister et al. 2000), use of a calibration phantom (McCullough et al. 1995), heart rate dependent choice of the image acquisition window (see above) (Mao et al. 2001), use of higher section increment (Achenbach et al. 2001b) and new scoring methods (Detrano et al. 1995; Kaufmann et al. 1994; Callister et al. 1998b).

In a study by Wang et al. (1996), reproducibility increased when scan slices of 6 mm instead of 3 mm were obtained. Mao et al. (2001) showed that triggering at 40% of the R-R interval reduced the calcium score variability by 34% as compared

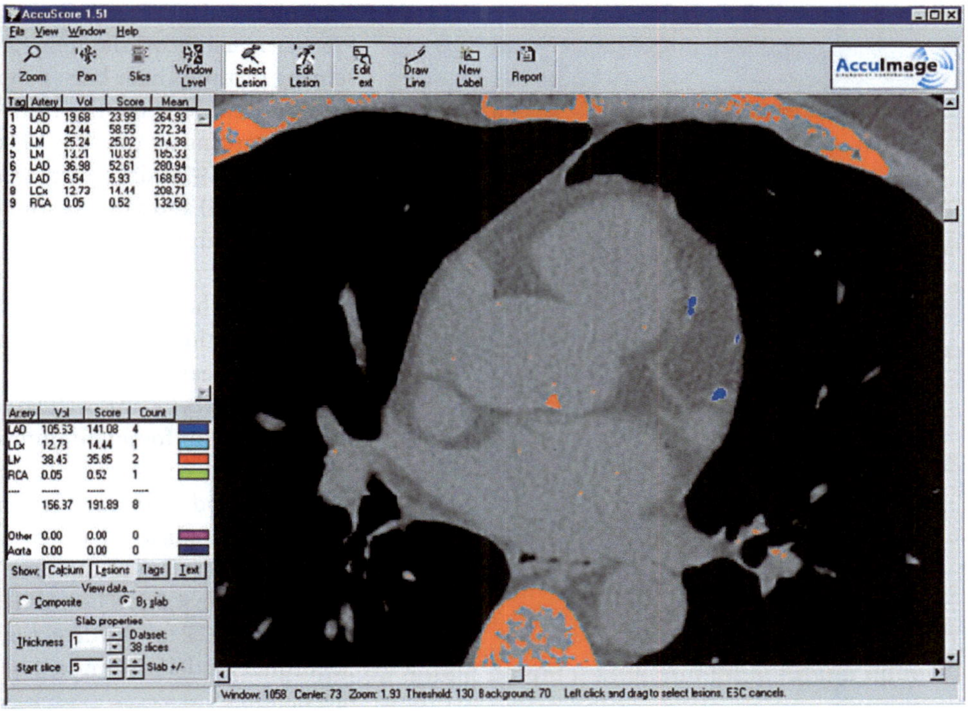

Fig. 4.2.2. Interface of calcium scoring program software

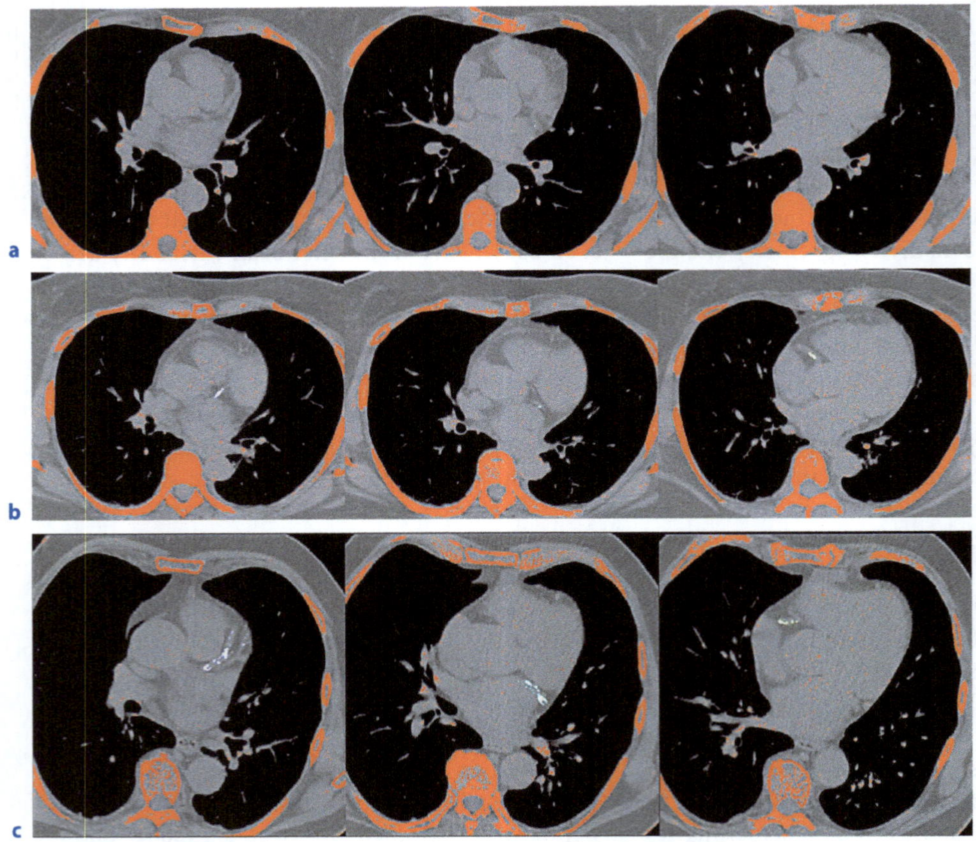

Fig. 4.2.3a–c. Examples of none to mild (**a**), moderate (**b**), and extensive (**c**) coronary calcification shown on EBCT

Table 4.2.2. Interscan variability of calcium scores in EBCT studies

Study	Patients (n)	Variability (%)
Kajinami et al. (1993)	75	34
Shields et al. (1995)	50	38
Wang et al. (1996)		
3-mm Slices	72	29
6-mm Slices	77	14
Callister et al. (1998b)		
Traditional calcium score	52	19
Volumetric score		13
Yoon et al. (2000)	1000	39
Achenbach et al. (2001b)		
Traditional calcium score	120	20
Volumetric score		16
Möhlenkamp et al. (2001)		
Traditional calcium score	50	19 (median)
Area score		13

to standard triggering at 80%. Achenbach et al. (2001b) found a decrease in variability from 23% to 9% when using overlapping cross-sections. Other scoring methods have been proposed which seem to be more reproducible than the traditional calcium score according to Agatston et al. (1990). Detrano et al. (1994, 1995) described an arterial summation method (1994) and a mass estimation method (1995). Although both the traditional scoring method and the alternative methods reflected the actual mass of calcium, the reproducibility was higher for the mass estimation method. Other methods such as summing areas or regions of interest have been proposed by Kaufmann (1994). Callister and coworkers (1998b) found an improved reproducibility when scoring coronary calcifications with a volumetric method, with a reduction in variability from 19% for the traditional score to 13% for the volume score. An overview of the scoring methods is provided in Table 4.2.3. The validation and validity of the use of EBCT for the detection and quantification of coronary calcification will be discussed in detail in Chap. 4.3.

Table 4.2.3. Different methods for quantification of coronary calcification, detected by EBCT

Traditional calcium score (Agatston et al. 1990):
Σ [area (≥ 130 HU) × 1 if (peak CT number 130–199 HU) 2 if (peak CT number 200–299 HU) 3 if (peak CT number 300–399 HU) 4 if (peak CT number ≥400 HU)]
Area score (Kaufmann et al. 1994): Σ [area (≥130 HU)]
Lesion score (Kaufmann et al. 1994): Σ [n (ROI { ≥130 HU})]
Arterial summation (Detrano et al. 1994):
A = {Σ [area (≥130 HU) × (mean of each calcified ROI – mean of ROI without Ca)]}
A / slope [a] × slice thickness = arterial summation
Mass estimation (Detrano et al. 1995):
Σ^{b} [proportion Ca × mass of voxel pure Ca]
Proportion Ca can be calculated:
1. CT number = (proportion soft tissue × CT soft tissue) + (proportion Ca × CT Ca)
2. In each voxel, proportion soft tissue + proportion Ca = 1
3. Proportion Ca = $\frac{\text{CT number} - \text{CT soft tissue}}{\text{CT Ca} - \text{CT soft tissue}}$
Volume score (Callister et al. 1998b):
Σ [area (≥130 HU) × slice thickness]
Or: Σ [volume (≥130 HU) using isotropic interpolation]

Σ, Sum of all slices, except for mass estimation method. Ca is calcium hydroxyapatite.

[a] Slope is regression line calculated from known calcium concentrations and the mean CT numbers in each slice of cylindrical inserts in a calcium phantom.

[b] For all voxels with CT number > 100 HU.

4.2.5 Multidetector Computed Tomography

Lastly, with the availability of sub-second slice acquisition times conventional sequential CT has been considered as a possible imaging modality for detection of coronary calcification. Becker et al. (1999) compared 50 patients using EBCT and conventional 500-ms partial scan CT. Conventional scans were acquired during two breath-holds and without ECG-triggering. Although a high correlation coefficient was found between calcium scores of both modalities, variability in calcium scores between both modalities was 42%. However, other study groups earlier were able to perform calcium scoring within a single breath-hold on a dual-slice spiral CT scanner with only 1-s rotation time (Shemesh et al. 1995; Broderick et al. 1996). Whereas sensitivity of calcified plaques regarding the detection of CAD was high, ranging from 81% to 92%, specificity (52% to 61%) and thus diagnostic accuracy was low (74%–84%). Although the test characteristics were comparable to those reported in EBCT studies, CT images were acquired without use of ECG-triggering. The problem with this approach was a distinct over- and underestimation of calcium scores respectively when compared to EBCT, primarily due to cardiac motion artifact (Baskin et al. 1995).

By applying retrospective ECG-gating to CT imaging Woodhouse et al. (1997) obtained CT images with distinctly less motion artifacts and thus a higher reproducibility than in the case of non-gated CT scans. Retrospective ECG-gating allows continuous image reconstruction from volume data sets during any phase of the cardiac cycle. Temporal resolution in this feasibility study amounted to 630 ms but came along with the trade-off of rather increased slice thickness.

In 1999, the market introduction of four-row multidetector CT (MDCT) with sub-second rotation and sub-millimeter collimation resolved this long-lasting trade-off between scan volume and section thickness, now allowing for acquisition of large scan volumes in sub-millimeter section thickness. Due to this innovation effective slice scan time could be decreased to 250 ms and slice thickness to 1.3 mm, respectively (Becker et al. 2000; Carr et al. 2000; McCullough et al. 2000; Becker et al. 2001; Budoff et al. 2001). Several studies compared MDCT and EBCT and demonstrated high correlation coefficients (Becker et al. 2000, 2001; Carr et al. 2000; McCullough et al. 2000; Budoff et al. 2001). Correlation coefficients ranged between 0.96 and 0.99, thus showing an excellent agreement (Table 4.2.4). Variability between both methods was 17% – comparable to variability in repeated ECBT examinations. Thus, mostly due to its wider availability nowadays, MDCT has largely replaced EBCT.

However, MDCT-based determination of coronary artery calcium bears fundamental problems such as a high variability, lack of standardization or insufficient quality assurance (Achenbach

Table 4.2.4. Coefficients of correlation for EBCT and MDCT regarding the detection and quantification of coronary artery calcifications

Author	Journal	Patients (n)	Modality	Ca++ score	r
Becker et al. (1999)	Eur Radiol	50	1-Slice CT triggered	983	0.98
Becker et al. (2000)	AJR Am J Roentgenol	160	1-Slice CT triggered	n.a.	0.98
Carr et al. (2000)	AJR Am J Roentgenol	36	1-Slice CT gated	432	0.98
Budoff et al. (2001)	Int J Cardiol	33	1-Slice CT un-triggered	52.1	0.68
Knez et al. (2002)	Int J Cardiac Imaging	99	4-Slice CT triggered	722	0.99
Stanford et al.	Radiology	78	4-Slice CT triggered	n.a.	0.96–0.99

n.a., Not available.

et al. 2001c; Ulzheimer et al. 2002; Becker et al. 2003). Particularly a high inter-scan, inter-observer, and intra-observer variability associated with this test have been recognized (Devries et al. 1995; Hernigou et al. 1996; Wang et al. 1996; Yoon et al. 2000; Achenbach et al. 2001c; Lu et al. 2002). The lowest inter-scan variability and highest reproducibility for coronary artery calcium measurements have been reported for mechanical spiral CT by use of narrow collimation and retrospective ECG-gating technique. More recent studies found inter-scan variability of about 10% or less for repeated four-detector row CT examinations (Detrano et al. 2002; Moser et al. 2002; Ohnesorge et al. 2002), which may be accurate enough to enable sensitive detection of changes in the total atherosclerotic disease burden in patients with and in those without specific therapy. In comparison to the prospectively ECG-triggered technique, however, CT acquisition with retrospective ECG gating is associated with a higher effective radiation dose (2.6–4.1 mSv) (Morin et al. 2003). With sophisticated technical devices, such as ECG-based tube current modulation, radiation exposure can be reduced to levels that are comparable to those of the prospectively ECG-triggered acquisition technique (Jakobs et al. 2002; Poll et al. 2002). At present, quantification of the actual amount of calcified plaques is still done semi-quantitatively and based on section-by-section analysis of CT images. This approach was first proposed by Agatston et al. (1990) and been used ever since (for details see Sect. 4.2.4). However, recent studies (Callister et al. 1998b; Kopp et al. 2002; Ohnesorge et al. 2002; Ulzheimer et al. 2003) reveal less variability and more accurate results when using quantitative measures (Ca^{++} volume, absolute Ca^{++} mass) as compared to the traditional scoring method according to Agatston. Nowadays results for all three measurement approaches are standardized and provided on most software platforms (Callister et al. 1998b; Kopp et al. 2002; Ohnesorge et al. 2002; Ulzheimer et al. 2003). Determination of the absolute Ca^{++} mass is based on a scanner-specific calibration and thus appears most promising not only in terms of accuracy, consistency, and reproducibility of coronary calcium assessment (Ulzheimer et al. 2003), but also regarding a future replacement of traditional scoring methods (Becker et al. 2003).

4.2.6 Intravascular Ultrasound

Intravascular ultrasound (IVUS) is the most sensitive in vivo imaging modality for the characterization of plaque components, including calcium (Mintz et al. 1992; Tuzcu et al. 1996). IVUS imaging makes use of a high-frequency ultrasound transducer, and can be performed during any coronary angiographic procedure. On IVUS images, calcified deposits appear as bright echoes casting acoustic shadows. Qualitative description of calcifications include location (lesion or reference) and distribution (superficial or deep). Furthermore, the arc of calcium in degrees and the length of calcific deposits can be measured. On sequential images, the arc and length of calcification can be used to calculate the percentage of plaque surface that is calcified (Scott et al. 2000). A comparison of IVUS imaging and histology of 54 atherosclerotic lesions showed that IVUS predicted the plaque composition correctly in 96% of cases (Potkin et al. 1990). All calcified plaque quadrants were identified by IVUS. FRIEDRICH et al. (1994) examined 50 atherosclerotic arteries by IVUS and histology. Three histological types of calcification were found: dense calcification, microcalcification (size, up to 0.5 mm^2) and a combination of the two. Sensitivity and specificity for densely calcified plaques was 90% and 100%, respectively. However, only two of the 12 micro-calcifications (17%) were detected by IVUS. In a study comparing IVUS and histologic findings, IVUS identified calcified lesions with a high sensitivity and specificity (89% and 97%, respectively), but underestimated the calcified plaque cross-sectional area by 39% (KOSTAMAA et al. 1999). Two evident factors may contribute to the underestimation of the calcified plaque cross-sectional area. The first is a limited depth of ultrasound penetration due to the high reflectivity of the acoustic signal by calcium. The second, a non-uniform rotation of the IVUS catheter drive shaft. In a clinical study by MINTZ et al. (1995) 1155 coronary lesions were evaluated by IVUS and coronary angiography. While IVUS detected calcium in 73% of lesions, angiography could only identify calcium in 38%. Compared to IVUS, angiography had a sensitivity of only 48%, and a specificity of 89%. This finding was confirmed by TUZCU et al. (1996): the presence of calcium was much higher by IVUS than by angiography. In patients with angiographically evident calcification, the mean arc of calcium on IVUS images was larger (175° vs. 108°). The distribution and amount of calcium within the vessel wall has a major significance in the diagnostic classification of lesion subsets (stable or unstable). Furthermore, the calcification pattern is regarded as a prognostic indicator for the outcome after coronary interventions, and thus influences the choice of treatment. The disadvantages of IVUS are its invasive nature and the limited portion of the coronary tree that can be visualized. Thus, currently IVUS has no important role in screening for sub-clinical CAD.

4.2.7 Magnetic Resonance Imaging

Magnetic resonance imaging (MRI) receives increasing attention for the characterization of atherosclerotic plaques. Noninvasive MRI has been shown as a highly potent modality to differ between fibrous and lipid components of coronary plaques (FAYAD et al. 2000; VILES-GONZALES et al. 2004). However, the ability of MRI to detect calcification is limited. The most common finding of calcification on T1- and T2-weighted spin-echo images is reduced signal intensity, primarily as a result of a low mobile proton density (HOLLAND et al. 1985). However, another study found extremely variable spin-echo findings for calcifications but demonstrated that gradient-echo images showed a marked (but non-specific) decrease in intensity in case of calcification, due to T2 shortening (ATLAS et al. 1988). Interestingly, concentrations of calcium particulate of up to 30% in weight seem to reduce T1 relaxation times, resulting in increased signal intensity (HENKELMAN et al. 1991). Thus currently an important role of MRI in the detection of coronary calcification is not expected.

References

Achenbach S, Ropers D, Holle J et al. (2000) In-plane coronary arterial motion velocity: measurement with electron-beam CT. Radiology 216:457–463

Achenbach S, Ropers D, Mohlenkamp S et al (2001a) Variability of repeated coronary artery calcium measurements by electron beam tomography. Am J Cardiol 87:210–213, A218

Achenbach S, Meissner F, Ropers D et al (2001b) Overlapping cross-sections significantly improve the reproducibility of coronary calcium measurements by electron beam tomography: a phantom study. J Comput Assist Tomogr 25:569–573

Achenbach S, Daniel W, Moshage W (2001c) Recommendations for standardization of EBT and MSCT scanning. Herz 26:273–277

Agatston AS, Janowitz WR, Hildner FJ et al (1990) Quantification of coronary artery calcium using ultrafast computed tomography. J Am Coll Cardiol 15:827–832

Aldrich RF, Brensike JF, Battaglini JW et al (1979) Coronary calcifications in the detection of coronary artery disease and comparison with electrocardiographic exercise testing. Results from the national heart, lung, and blood institute's type ii coronary intervention study. Circulation 59:1113–1124

Atlas SW, Grossman RI, Hackney DB et al (1988) Calcified intracranial lesions: detection with gradient-echo-acquisition rapid MR imaging. AJR Am J Roentgenol 150:1383–1389

Bartel AG, Chen JT, Peter RH et al (1974) The significance of coronary calcification detected by fluoroscopy. A report of 360 patients. Circulation 49:1247–1253

Baskin KM, Stanford W, Thompson BH et al (1995) Comparison of electron beam and helical computed tomography in assessment of coronary artery calcification. Circulation 92:I-651

Becker CR, Knez A, Jakobs TF et al (1999) Detection and

quantification of coronary artery calcification with electron-beam and conventional CT. Eur Radiol 9:620–624
Becker CR, Jakobs TF, Aydemir S et al (2000) Helical and single-slice conventional CT versus electron beam CT for the quantification of coronary artery calcification. AJR Am J Roentgenol 174:543–547
Becker CR, Kleffel T, Crispin A et al (2001) Coronary artery calcium measurement: agreement of multirow detector and electron beam CT. AJR Am J Roentgenol 176:1295–1298
Becker CR, Schoepf UJ, Reiser MF (2003) Coronary artery calcium scoring: medicine and politics. Eur Radiol 13:445–447
Bielak LF, Kaufmann RB, Moll PP et al (1994) Small lesions in the heart identified at electron-beam CT: calcification or noise? Radiology 192:631–636
Bierner M, Fleck E, Dirschinger J et al (1978) [Significance of coronary artery calcification: relationship to localization and severity of coronary artery stenosis (author's translation)]. Herz 3:336–343
Broderick LS, Shemesh J, Wilensky RL et al (1996) Measurement of coronary artery calcium with dual-slice helical CT compared with coronary angiography: evaluation of CT scoring methods, interobserver variations, and reproducibility. AJR Am J Roentgenol 167:439–444
Budoff MJ, Mao S, Zalace CP et al (2001) Comparison of spiral and electron beam tomography in the evaluation of coronary calcification in asymptomatic persons. Int J Cardiol 77:181–188
Callister TQ, Raggi P, Cooil B et al (1998a) Effect of HMG-CoA reductase inhibitors on coronary artery disease as assessed by electron-beam computed tomography. N Engl J Med 339:1972–1978
Callister TQ, Cooil B, Raya SP et al (1998b) Coronary artery disease: improved reproducibility of calcium scoring with an electron-beam CT volumetric method. Radiology 208:807–814
Callister T, Janowitz W, Raggi P (2000) Sensitivity of two electron beam tomography protocols for the detection and quantification of coronary artery calcium. AJR Am J Roentgenol 175:1743–1746
Carr JJ, Crouse JR III, Goff DC Jr et al (2000) Evaluation of subsecond gated helical CT for quantification of coronary artery calcium and comparison with electron-beam CT. AJR Am J Roentgenol 174:915–921
de Korte PJ, Kessels AG, van Engelshoven JM et al (1995) Comparison of the diagnostic value of cinefluoroscopy and simple fluoroscopy in the detection of calcification in coronary arteries. Eur J Radiol 19:194–197
Detrano R, Markovic D, Simpfendorfer C et al (1985) Digital subtraction fluoroscopy: a new method of detecting coronary calcifications with improved sensitivity for the prediction of coronary disease. Circulation 71:725–732
Detrano R, Salcedo EE, Hobbs RE et al (1986) Cardiac cinefluoroscopy as an inexpensive aid in the diagnosis of coronary artery disease. Am J Cardiol 57:1041–1046
Detrano R, Kang X, Mahaisavariya P et al (1994) Accuracy of quantifying coronary hydroxyapatite with electron beam tomography. Invest Radiol 29:733–738
Detrano R, Tang W, Kang X et al (1995) Accurate coronary calcium phosphate mass measurements from electron beam computed tomograms. Am J Card Imaging 9:167–173
Detrano R, Anderson M, Nelson J et al (2002) Effect of scanner type and calcium measure on the re-scan variability of calcium quantity by computed tomography. Circulation 106:II-479
Devries S, Wolfkiel C, Shah V et al (1995) Reproducibility of the measurement of coronary calcium with ultrafast computed tomography. Am J Cardiol 75:973–975
Fayad ZA, Fuster V, Fallon JT et al (2000) Noninvasive in vivo human coronary artery lumen and wall imaging using black-blood magnetic resonance imaging. Circulation 102:506–510
Friedrich GJ, Moes NY, Muhlberger VA et al (1994) Detection of intralesional calcium by intracoronary ultrasound depends on the histologic pattern. Am Heart J 128:435–441
Gianrossi R, Detrano R, Colombo A et al (1990) Cardiac fluoroscopy for the diagnosis of coronary artery disease: a meta analytic review. Am Heart J 120:1179–1188
Hamby RI, Tabrah F, Wisoff BG et al (1974) Coronary artery calcification: clinical implications and angiographic correlates. Am Heart J 87:565–570
Henkelman RM, Watts JF, Kucharczyk W (1991) High signal intensity in MR images of calcified brain tissue. Radiology 179:199–206
Hernigou A, Challande P, Boudeville JC et al (1996) Reproducibility of coronary calcification detection with electron-beam computed tomography. Eur Radiol 6:210–216
Herzog C, Arning-Erb M, Zangos S et al (2006) Multi-detector row CT coronary angiography. Influence of reconstruction technique and heart rate on image quality. Radiology 238:75–86
Holland BA, Kucharcyzk W, Brant-Zawadzki M et al (1985) MR imaging of calcified intracranial lesions. Radiology 157:353–356
Hung J, Chaitman BR, Lam J et al (1984) Noninvasive diagnostic test choices for the evaluation of coronary artery disease in women: a multivariate comparison of cardiac fluoroscopy, exercise electrocardiography and exercise thallium myocardial perfusion scintigraphy. J Am Coll Cardiol 4:8–16
Jakobs TF, Becker CR, Ohnesorge B et al (2002) Multislice helical CT of the heart with retrospective ECG gating: reduction of radiation exposure by ECG-controlled tube current modulation. Eur Radiol 12:1081–1086
Kajinami K, Seki H, Takekoshi N et al (1993) Quantification of coronary artery calcification using ultrafast computed tomography: reproducibility of measurements. Coron Artery Dis 4:1103–1108
Kaufmann RB, Sheedy PF, Breen JF et al (1994) Detection of heart calcification with electron-beam CT: interobserver and intraobserver reliability for scoring quantification. Radiology 190:347–352
Knez A, Becker C, Becker A et al (2002) Determination of coronary calcium with multi-slice spiral computed tomography: a comparative study with electron-beam CT. Internat J Cardiovasc Imaging 18:295–303
Kopp AF, Ohnesorge B, Becker C et al (2002) Reproducibility and accuracy of coronary calcium measurements with multi-detector row versus electron-beam CT. Radiology 225:113–119
Kostamaa H, Donovan J, Kasaoka S et al (1999) Calcified plaque cross-sectional area in human arteries: correlation between intravascular ultrasound and undecalcified histology. Am Heart J 137:482–488
Lu B, Budoff M, Zhuang N et al (2002) Causes of interscan

variability of coronary artery calcium measurements at electron-beam CT. Acad Radiol 9:654–661
Mao S, Bakhsheshi H, Lu B et al (2001) Effect of electrocardiogram triggering on reproducibility of coronary artery calcium scoring. Radiology 220:707–711
Margolis JR, Chen JT, Kong Y et al (1980) The diagnostic and prognostic significance of coronary artery calcification. A report of 800 cases. Radiology 137:609–616
Masuda Y, Naito S, Aoyagi Y et al (1990) Coronary artery calcification detected by CT: clinical significance and angiographic correlates. Angiology 41:1037–1047
Mautner GC, Mautner SL, Froehlich J et al (1994) Coronary artery calcification: assessment with electron-beam CT and histomorphometric correlation. Radiology 192:619–623
McCollough CH, Kaufmann RB, Cameron BM et al (1995) Electron-beam CT: use of a calibration phantom to reduce variability in calcium quantitation. Radiology 196:159–165
McCollough CH, Bruesewitz MR, Daly TR et al (2000) Motion artifacts in subsecond conventional CT and electron-beam CT: pictorial demonstration of temporal resolution. Radiographics 20:1675–1681
McGuire J, Schneider HJ, Chou TC (1968) Clinical significance of coronary artery calcification seen fluoroscopically with the image intensifier. Circulation 37:82–87
Mintz GS, Douek P, Pichard AD et al (1992) Target lesion calcification in coronary artery disease: an intravascular ultrasound study. J Am Coll Cardiol 20:1149–1155
Mintz GS, Popma JJ, Pichard AD et al (1995) Patterns of calcification in coronary artery disease. A statistical analysis of intravascular ultrasound and coronary angiography in 1,155 lesions. Circulation 91:1959–1965
Möhlenkamp S, Behrenbeck TR, Pump H et al (2001) Reproducibility of two coronary calcium quantification algorithms in patients with different degrees of calcification. Int J Cardiovasc Imaging 17:133–142; discussion 143
Molloi S, Detrano R, Ersahin A et al (1991) Quantification of coronary arterial calcium by dual energy digital subtraction fluoroscopy. Med Phys 18:295–298
Moore EH, Greenberg RW, Merrick SH et al (1989) Coronary artery calcifications: Significance of incidental detection on CT scans. Radiology 172:711–716
Morin R, Gerber T, McCullough C (2003) Radiation dose in computed tomography of the heart. Circulation 107:917–922
Moser K, Bateman T, Case J (2002) The influence of acquisition mode on the reproducibility of coronary artery calcium scores using multi-detector computed tomography. Circulation 106 (S):II–47
Ohnesorge B, Flohr T, Fischbach R et al. (2002) Reproducibility of coronary calcium quantification in repeat examinations with retrospectively ECG-gated multisection spiral CT. Eur Radiol 12:1532–1540
Poll LW, Cohnen M, Brachten S et al (2002) Dose reduction in multi-slice CT of the heart by use of ECG controlled tube current modulation ("ECG pulsing"): phantom measurements. Fortschr Rontgenstr 174:1500–1505
Potkin BN, Bartorelli AL, Gessert JM et al (1990) Coronary artery imaging with intravascular high-frequency ultrasound. Circulation 81:1575–1585
Rienmueller R, Lipton MJ (1987) Detection of coronary artery calcification by computed tomography. Dynam Cardiovasc Imaging 1:139–145
Rumberger JA, Simons DB, Fitzpatrick LA et al (1995) Coronary artery calcium area by electron-beam computed tomography and coronary atherosclerotic plaque area. A histopathologic correlative study. Circulation 92:2157–2162
Scott DS, Arora UK, Farb A et al (2000) Pathologic validation of a new method to quantify coronary calcific deposits in vivo using intravascular ultrasound. Am J Cardiol 85:37–40
Shemesh J, Apter S, Rozenman J et al (1995) Calcification of coronary arteries: detection and quantification with double-helix CT. Radiology 197:779–783
Shields JP, Mielke CH Jr, Rockwood TH et al (1995) Reliability of electron beam computed tomography to detect coronary artery calcification. Am J Card Imaging 9:62–66
Souza AS, Bream PR, Elliott LP (1978) Chest film detection of coronary artery calcification. The value of the CAC triangle. Radiology 129:7–10
Stanford W, Thompson BH (1999) Imaging of coronary artery calcification. Its importance in assessing atherosclerotic disease. Radiol Clin North Am 37:257–272, v
Stanford W, Thompson BH, Burns TL, Heery SD, Burr MC (2004) Coronary artery calcium quantification at multidetector row helical CT versus electron-beam CT. Radiology 230:397–402
Tanenbaum SR, Kondos GT, Veselik KE et al (1989) Detection of calcific deposits in coronary arteries by ultrafast computed tomography and correlation with angiography. Am J Cardiol 63:870–872
Tang W, Young E, Detrano R et al (1994) Reproducibility of digital subtraction fluoroscopic readings for coronary artery calcification. Invest Radiol 29:147–149
Timins ME, Pinsk R, Sider L et al (1991) The functional significance of calcification of coronary arteries as detected on CT. J Thorac Imaging 7:79–82
Tuzcu EM, Berkalp B, De Franco AC et al (1996) The dilemma of diagnosing coronary calcification: angiography versus intravascular ultrasound. J Am Coll Cardiol 27:832–838
Ulzheimer S, Kalender W (2003) Assessment of calcium scoring performance in cardiac computed tomography. Eur Radiol 13:484–497
Ulzheimer S, Halliburton S, McCollough C et al (2002) Quality assurance in cardiac computed tomography: latest initiatives and developments. Radiology 225:309
Uretsky BF, Rifkin RD, Sharma SC et al (1988) Value of fluoroscopy in the detection of coronary stenosis: influence of age, sex, and number of vessels calcified on diagnostic efficacy. Am Heart J 115:323–333
Viles-Gonzalez JF, Poon M, Sanz J et al (2004) In vivo 16-slice, multidetector-row computed tomography for the assessment of experimental atherosclerosis: comparison with magnetic resonance imaging and histopathology. Circulation 110:1467–1472
Wang S, Detrano RC, Secci A et al (1996) Detection of coronary calcification with electron-beam computed tomography: evaluation of interexamination reproducibility and comparison of three image-acquisition protocols. Am Heart J 132:550–558
Woodhouse CE, Janowitz WR, Viamonte M Jr (1997) Coronary arteries: retrospective cardiac gating technique to reduce cardiac motion artifact at spiral CT. Radiology 204:566–569
Yoon HC, Goldin JG, Greaser LE III et al (2000) Interscan variation in coronary artery calcium quantification in a large asymptomatic patient population. AJR Am J Roentgenol 174:803–809

Non-Invasive Measurement of Coronary Atherosclerosis

4

4.3 Measuring Coronary Calcium

Jaap M. Groen, Marcel J. W. Greuter, and Matthijs Oudkerk

CONTENTS

J. M. Groen, MSc, PhD
Department of Radiology, University Medical Center Groningen, University of Groningen, Hanzeplein 1, P. O. Box 30.001, 9700 RB Groningen, The Netherlands
M. J. W. Greuter, PhD
Departement of Radiology, University Medical Center Groningen, University of Groningen, Hanzeplein 1, P. O. Box 30.001, 9700 RB Groningen, The Netherlands
M. Oudkerk, MD, PhD
Professor of Radiology, University Medical Center Groningen, University of Groningen, Hanzeplein 1, P. O. Box 30.001, 9700 RB Groningen, The Netherlands

4.3.1 Introduction

The amount of calcium present in coronary arteries is related to the risk of coronary artery disease such as myocardial infarction and sudden death (Arad et al. 2000; Raggi et al. 2000; O'Rourke et al. 2000). Furthermore, the absence of calcium in the coronary arteries is believed to indicate the absence of coronary artery disease (Wexler et al. 1996). Due to the high density of calcium X-ray tomographic techniques are very suitable for imaging calcium, which is presented by bright spots in tomographic images. Electron-beam tomography (EBT) is established as the gold standard for determining the amount of coronary calcium and assessing the extent and progression of calcified plaques (Arad et al. 2000; Wong et al. 2000). However, EBT is becoming obsolete. Multi-detector computed tomography (MDCT), has become a commonly used alternative to determine the amount of coronary calcium, due to the general availability of this modality. Using the image data obtained from EBT or MDCT, the amount of calcium can be quantified. The amount of coronary calcium is reflected by a calcium score.

4.3.2 Scoring Algorithms

At present, three different algorithms exist to determine the calcium score from CT images. The first algorithm is the Agatston score, proposed in 1990 by Agatston et al. (1990). Originally, the Agatston score (AS) was determined from 20 contiguous EBT slices of the heart with a thickness of 3 mm for each slice. Nowadays the amount of slices is adjusted to the size of the heart. To calculate the Agatston score of an individual calcification, the area of that calcification is determined by selecting pixels above a threshold of 130 HU and ignoring structures smaller than 1 mm^2. The area is then multiplied by a weighting factor (w) which depends on the maximum HU number (HU_{max}) inside the calcification. This procedure is performed per slice.

$$AS_i = area_i \cdot w_i \tag{4.3.1}$$

where

$$w_i = \begin{cases} 1 \text{ if } 130\,HU \le HU_{\max} \le 200\,HU \\ 1 \text{ if } 200\,HU \le HU_{\max} \le 300\,HU \\ 1 \text{ if } 300\,HU \le HU_{\max} \le 400\,HU \\ 1 \text{ if } 400\,HU \le HU_{\max} \end{cases}$$

The total Agatston score is calculated by summing up the scores of the individual calcifications in all slices.

$$AS_{total} = \sum_i AS_i \tag{4.3.2}$$

The second algorithm is the Volume score (VS), proposed several years after the Agatston score to reduce variability of calcium scoring (Callister et al. 1998). The Volume score of a calcification is defined by the number of interconnected voxels (N) in that calcification which is above a threshold of 130 HU multiplied by the volume of one voxel (V).

$$VS_i = N_i \cdot V_i \tag{4.3.3}$$

The total Volume score is calculated by summing up the scores of all individual calcifications and reflects the total volume of the calcifications present in the coronary arteries given in mm^3.

$$VS_{total} = \sum_i VS_i \tag{4.3.4}$$

The third algorithm is the Equivalent Mass or Mass score (Yoon et al. 1997). The Mass score (MS) of a calcification is defined by the number of interconnected voxels (N) in that calcification which is above a threshold of 130 HU multiplied by the volume of one voxel (V), the averaged HU number (HU_{mean}) of that calcification and a calibration factor (c).

$$MS_i = N_i \cdot V_i \cdot HU_{mean,i} \cdot c \tag{4.3.5}$$

The calibration factor (c) relates a CT density (HU value) to a calcium density (mg/cc). The calibration factor is scanner-specific and defined by:

$$c = \frac{\rho_{HA}}{CT_{HA} - CT_{water}} \tag{4.3.6}$$

The calibration factor can be obtained by scanning a calcified object with a known density of calcium hydroxy apatite (ρ_{HA}), determining the mean CT number (CT_{HA}) of that calcification, and correcting for the mean CT number of water (CT_{water}) (McCollough et al. 1995, 2007). A per-patient calibration of the scanner is not useful, because the determined calibration factor will only be influenced by the table height (Deurholt et al. 2008, unpublished results). Correction of the determined calibration factor according to the table height yields a consistent calibration factor. Therefore, in accordance with guidelines a monthly calibration seems sufficient (Oudkerk et al. 2008). The total Mass score is calculated by summing up the scores of all individual calcifications and reflects the total mass of the calcifications present in the coronary arteries given in milligrams (mg).

$$MS_{total} = \sum_i MS_i \tag{4.3.7}$$

Equation 4.3.1 shows that the Agatston score depends on the area of the calcification, Eqs. 4.3.3 and 4.3.5 show that the Volume score and Mass score both depend on the volume of the calcification. Thus all three scoring algorithms depend on the size of the calcification.

Apart from the size of the calcification, both the Agatston score and the Mass score depend on the density of the calcification. For the Agatston score this is reflected by the weighting factor w, for the Mass score this is reflected by the HU_{mean} (Eqs. 4.3.1 and 4.3.5).

So, based upon the volume and the density, all three scoring algorithms quantify the amount of calcium in the coronary arteries, although the clinical standard is still the Agatston score. Agatston scores range from 0 for patients without coronary calcium, up to more than 3000 for patients with severely calcified arteries.

4.3.3 Calcium Scoring In Vivo

Calcium scoring has been investigated in numerous patient studies with large patient cohorts (Arad et al. 2000; Budoff et al. 1996; Hoff et al. 2003; Wong et al. 2000). The majority of these studies was performed using EBT combined with Agatston scoring since the original calcium scoring algorithm was developed for this technique and multi-slice MDCT was not yet available. In these studies an association between conventional risk factors for coronary artery disease and calcium in the coronary arteries was reported. Monitoring coronary calcium is suggested to assess the progression and regression of coronary calcium. For reliable detection of changes in calcium score in patient monitoring programs, a coronary calcium measurement is mandatory. Furthermore, the accuracy of the measurement should be lower than the normal progression of calcium scores. Study results showed that the normal progression of calcium scores varies between 14%–27% (Maher et al. 1999). In patients with significant coronary artery disease the progression is increased up to 33%–48% (Janowitz et al. 1991). Sevrukov et al. (2005) analyzed 2217 pairs of repeated calcium scans using EBT. They found that the smallest significant interval change was 4.930 × square root of the baseline Agatston score and 3.445 × square root of the baseline Volume score. In addition, it was shown that the square root of the Volume score stabilized interscan variability. A change in Volume score was defined as greater than or equal to 2.5 mm^3 of the difference in the square root-transformed Volume score (Hokanson et al. 2004).

The accuracy of calcium scoring is usually determined by the variability of the measurement. Using two consecutive scans, with or without repositioning the patient, the majority of the studies assessing the variability of calcium scoring defines the variability as

$$Var = \frac{|scan_A - scan_B|}{\frac{1}{2} \times (scan_A - scan_B)} \times 100\% \qquad (4.3.8)$$

Different variabilities have been reported in recent years. For EBT these reported variabilities ranged from 9% up to 37% (Budoff et al. 2008; Callister et al. 1998; Horiguchi et al. 2005a; Yoon et al. 1997; Lu et al. 2002). The difference in study outcome can partly be explained by different patient populations. For example, Yoon et al. (1997) selected patients with calcium scores between 2 and 100. Because the variability of low scores is higher, Yoon et al. (1997) reported higher variabilities than other studies (Stanford et al. 2004). Table 3.4.1 shows the results of several studies assessing the variability of EBT-based calcium scoring.

In recent years the variability of calcium scoring in MDCT has also been investigated. Reported variabilities ranged from 11% up to 41% (Hoffmann et al. 2006; Hong et al. 2003a; Horiguchi et al. 2005a, 2006; Mahnken et al. 2002; Ohnesorge et al. 2002). As with the studies performed with EBT, differences in study outcome can be explained by differences in

Table 4.3.1. Reported variabilities of electron-beam tomography (EBT) and multi-detector CT (MDCT) in patient studies (64-MDCT data has not yet been reported)

Author	Agatston	Volume	Mass	Modality	No. of patients
Yoon et al. (1997)	37.2	28.2	28.4	EBT	50
Callister et al. (1998)	15	9	-	EBT	79
Mahnken et al (2002)	24.1	20.0	-	4-MDCT	75
Ohnesorge et al. (2002)	12	7.5	7.5	4-MDCT	50
Lu et al. (2002)	21.6	17.8	-	EBT	298
Hong et al. (2003)	23.9	15.7	10.4	4-MDCT	37
Horiguchi et al. (2005)	25	20	21	EBT	61
	13–22	13–18	15–18	16-MDCT	
Hoffmann et al. (2006)	41	34	26	8-MDCT	69
Horiguchi et al. (2006)	12	11	-	16-MDCT	105
Budoff et al. (2008)	11.8	10.3	-	EBT	463

study population. In Table 4.3.1 results of different calcium scoring studies are given.

Apart from the variability of two consecutive scans, the variability between two imaging modalities can also be calculated. This can be of interest when different imaging modalities are being used in a patient monitoring program or when interpreting calcium scoring data between two modalities. Daniell et al. (2005) reported a variability of 27% for Agatston scoring and 16% for Volume scoring comparing EBT to MDCT. Similar variabilities were reported by other studies: 26.5% for Agatston scoring and 17% for Volume scoring (Knez et al. 2002; Horiguchi et al. 2004). These results show that intermodality variabilities are similar to interscan variabilities of EBT and MDCT individually.

Furthermore, these results show that there are also differences in variability for the three scoring algorithms. The reason for introducing the Volume score was a reduced variability compared to the Agatston score (Callister et al. 1998). This is illustrated in Table 4.3.1, where Volume scoring shows a smaller variability as compared to Agatston scoring for all imaging techniques. For the same reason, reduced variability, the Mass score was introduced (Yoon et al. 1997). Again, the studies mentioned in Table 4.3.1 show a reduced variability for Mass scoring compared to Agatston scoring. But also a reduced variability for Mass scoring is observed when compared to Volume scoring, although the differences are smaller. Thus, Mass scoring shows the smallest variability of all three scoring algorithms in these in vivo studies. Based on this smallest variability for Mass scoring, this scoring algorithm is advocated for quantifying the amount of calcium in the coronary arteries. However, the current standard for calcium scoring is still the Agatston score, so a transition from Agatston score to Mass score is needed to decrease the variability and thus increase the accuracy of calcium scoring.

In addition to an accurate calcium score with a low variability, the absolute score is also important. Because the association between calcium scores and conventional risk factors for coronary artery disease are mostly related to EBT-based calcium scores, MDCT-based calcium scores should be equivalent.

The correlation between EBT and single-slice CT is excellent according to Carr et al. (2000), with a correlation coefficient of 0.98 for Agatston scoring, 0.97 for Volume scoring and 0.98 for Mass scoring. The same excellent correlation was shown in another study, although the mean calcium score was significantly greater with EBT than with single-slice CT (Goldin et al. 2001). Going from single- to multislice CT, the results are equivalent. Again an excellent correlation between EBT and four-slice MDCT was found. Based on the results of 51 patients, a very strong linear association between EBT and four-slice MDCT was found by Stanford et al. (2004) with a correlation coefficient of 0.99. Although the results for EBT and four-slice MDCT appeared comparable, this was only true with an equivalence limit of 20%. Based on the results of 100 patients Becker et al. (2001) found correlation coefficients of 0.987 for Agatston scoring and 0.986 for Volume scoring, although the need for larger cohort studies was indicated, particularly in younger subjects. In addition, both studies showed that calcium scores using EBT were higher than calcium scores using four-slice MDCT. Excellent correlations were also found by Horiguchi et al. (2004) in a study comparing EBT to 16-slice MDCT. For Agatston scoring the correlation coefficients were 0.952, 0.955 and 0.977 for Agatston, Volume and Mass scoring, respectively (Table 4.3.2).

4.3.4 Calcium Scoring In Vitro

Because calcium scoring is hampered by large variabilities it has been the subject of many in vitro studies. Phantom studies are particularly useful for calcium scoring investigations because they offer the possibility of systematic analysis of the influence of different parameters without the problem of patient dose. Furthermore, the Volume score and Mass score are both suitable for comparison to actual known phantom values, in contrast to Agatston scoring which has no physical equivalent. This offers the possibility of a quantitative analysis of calcium scoring in addition to a qualitative analysis in terms of variability and absolute scores compared to EBT. The two measurable quantities, volume and mass, of an individual calcification depend on the measured HU values, as explained in Sect. 4.3.2.

The major problem in calcium scoring is the partial volume effect (PVE), which is related to the point spread function (PSF) of the scanner. The PVE is the effect wherein the HU value of a voxel is determined by a mixing of different tissues within that voxel. The PVE is related to the spatial resolution of the

Table 4.3.2. Reported correlations between electron-beam tomography (EBT) and multi-detector (MDCT) in patient studies (64-MDCT data has not been reported yet)

Author	Agatston	Volume	Mass	Modalities
Carr et al. (2000)	0.98	0.97	0.98	EBT vs. 1SCT
Goldin et al. (2001)	0.99	-	-	EBT vs. 1SCT
Becker et al. (2001)	0.987	0.986	-	EBT vs. 4-MDCT
Stanford et al. (2004)	0.99	-	-	EBT vs. 4-MDCT
Horiguchi et al. (2004)	0.955	0.952	0.977	EBT vs. 16-MDCT

1SCT, single-slice CT

scanner. An increase in spatial resolution leads to a decrease in PVE and visa versa. The problems arising from the PVE in calcium scoring are reflected by under- or overestimation of the volume and/or mass of the calcification as compared to the actual volume and or mass. For calcifications with a high density the voxels at the edges of the calcification are exaggerated due to the PVE. Combined with the standard threshold of 130 HU this leads to an overestimation of the volume of the calcification. For calcifications with a low density the reverse effect is observed. The voxels at the edges of the calcification are undervalued. Combined with the standard threshold of 130 HU this leads to an underestimation of the volume of the calcification. The described phenomenon can be observed when the Volume scores of equally sized calcifications with different densities are compared (Fig. 4.3.1) (Groen et al. 2007a,b).

The incorrect volume of a calcification influences the measured mass of the calcification. In Figure 4.3.2 the true and measured masses of the same equally sized calcifications with different densities are shown.

Although the volume of the calcifications with higher densities is exaggerated the measured mass is underestimated. This can be explained by the fact that the measured mass does not solely depend on the volume but also on the HU_{mean} (Eq. 4.3.5). Due to the PVE the HU_{mean} within the calcification is underestimated. For example, a phantom calcification with a density of 800 HU will have a HU_{mean} of approximately 400 HU when measured, when a standard acquisition protocol is used with a voxel size of 0.6 × 0.6 × 3.0 mm.

Different in vitro studies confirm these results. Mühlenbruch et al. (2007) investigated calcium scoring using a phantom containing different kinds of calcifications. The volumes of calcifications with a relatively high density were highly exaggerated, whereas the volumes of relatively low densities calcifications were underestimated. The Mass scores of the calcifications showed that the masses of the calcifications were underestimated for all densities. Underestimated masses were also reported by Mao et al. (2003) in a study investigating calcifications with a relatively low density. Although both studies

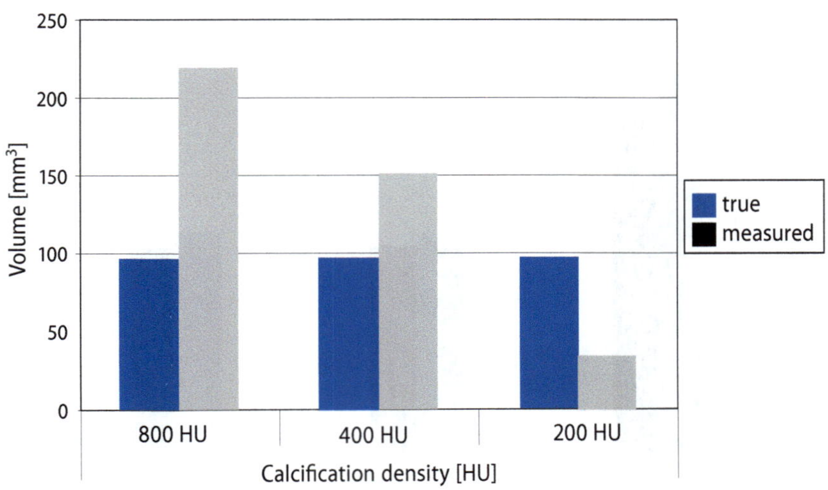

Fig. 4.3.1. True and measured volume of three equally sized calcifications with different densities. Measurements were performed with a 64-slice MDCT with a slice thickness of 3.0 mm (Groen et al. 2007a,b)

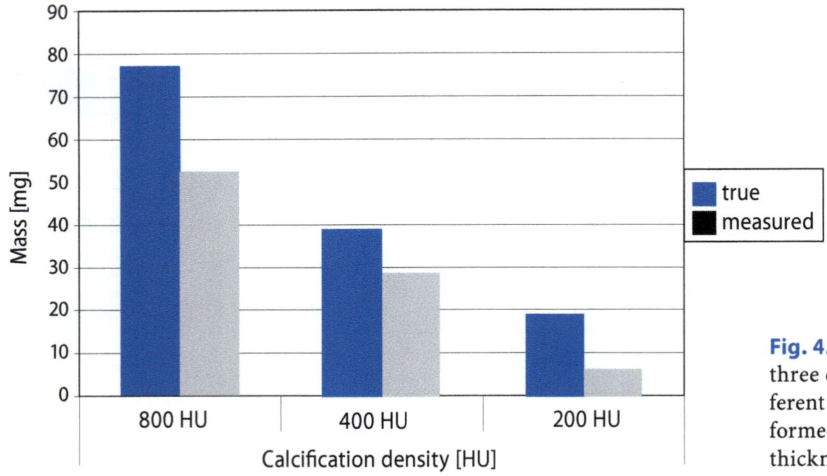

Fig. 4.3.2. True and measured mass of three equally sized calcifications with different densities. Measurements were performed with a 64-slice MDCT with a slice thickness of 3.0 mm (Groen et al. 2007a,b)

are in concordance to the results in Figures 4.3.1 and 4.3.2, the measured masses did not deviate severely from the true masses. This can be explained by the fact that the overestimation of the volume cancels out the underestimation of the HU_{mean}, resulting in measured masses comparable to the true masses in spite of the PVE. However, both factors, the volume and HU_{mean}, are incorrect. Both studies used the same phantom. Larger discrepancies between measured and true mass can be expected when analyzing different kinds of calcifications.

To reduce the PVE CT modalities with higher spatial resolutions are required. Another partial solution is the use of thinner collimations. The original protocol utilizes relative thick slices of 3.0 mm, but modern MDCT offers sub-millimeter scanning. Apart from a reduction in the PVE this will increase the detectability of smaller calcifications and increase noise levels in the image data (Groen et al. 2007b; Mao et al. 2003; Mühlenbruch et al. 2007). Due to this increased detectability of smaller calcifications and increased noise levels the calcium score will increase for thinner slices. In Figure 4.3.3 Agatston scores of three different calcifications at different slice thicknesses are shown. The figure shows increased Agatston scores for thinner slices.

Another approach to overcome the over- and underestimated volumes might be the use of a segmentation threshold adapted to the calcification (Hong et al. 2003b; Raggi et al. 2002). The segmentation threshold should be increased for high density calcifications, whereas the threshold should be decreased for low density calcifications.

A second problem in calcium scoring is cardiac motion. Cardiac motion influences the HU values of the calcification and thus the volume and the HU_{mean}. Depending on the density of the calcification, the volume of the calcification will increase or

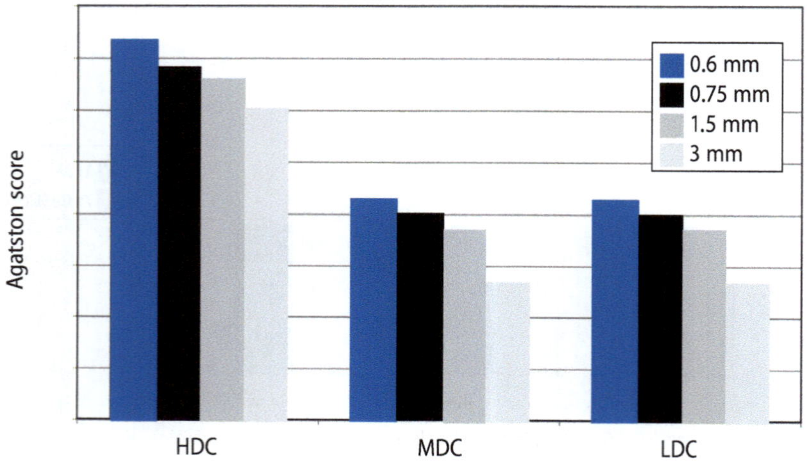

Fig. 4.3.3. Agatston scores of three calcifications with different densities. The scans were performed with a 64-slice MDCT at four different slice thicknesses (Groen et al. 2007b). *HDC*, high density calcification; *MDC*, medium density calcification; *LDC*, low density calcification

decrease with increasing motion, shown by volume scores of the different calcifications in an in vitro study (Fig. 4.3.4) (Groen et al. 2007b). With increased heart rate the volume score of the high density calcification is increased whereas the volume score of the low density calcification is decreased.

A theoretical explanation for this phenomenon is given in Figure 4.3.5. Two calcifications of identical size are shown by black lines, one with a relatively high density (X) and one with a relatively low density (Y). The corresponding reconstructed blurred CT images at a relatively low velocity are represented by the solid grey line. The corresponding reconstructed blurred CT images at a relatively high velocity are represented by the dotted grey line. In addition, the default calcium scoring threshold of 130 HU is shown by the dotted black line. At the level of the threshold, the apparent width of the high density calcification (X) is larger at the high velocity than at the low velocity. The low density calcification shows the opposite behaviour as a function of velocity. Because the calcium score is proportional to the volume of the calcification (Eqs. 4.3.1, 4.3.3 and 4.3.5), high density calcifications show an increased calcium score at increased velocity, whereas low density calcifications show a decreased calcium score at increased velocity.

To reduce the influence of cardiac motion a high temporal resolution is required (Mühlenbruch et al. 2007). Comparing 64-slice MDCT with a temporal resolution of 165 ms, dual source CT (DSCT) with a temporal resolution of 83 ms and EBT with a temporal resolution of 50 ms, the latter was shown to be the least influenced by cardiac motion in a phantom study (Groen et al. 2007a). Furthermore, DSCT was shown to be 50% less influenced by cardiac motion compared to 64-slice MDCT (Groen et al. 2007a). In addition, Brown et al. (2007) showed that increased

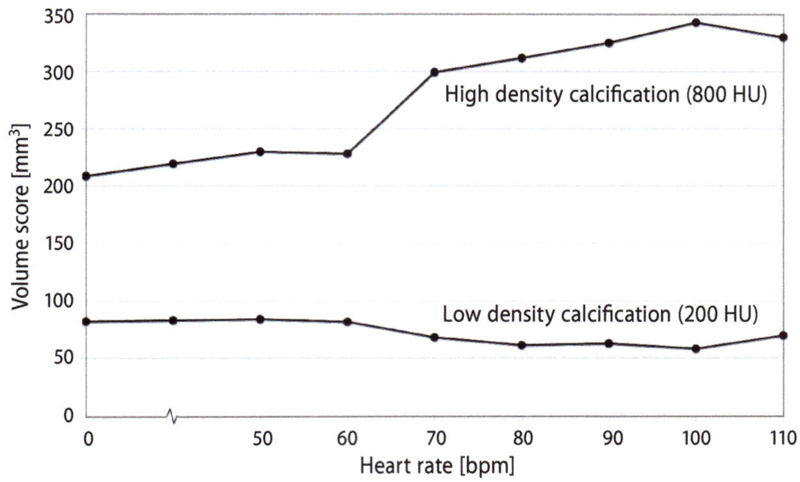

Fig. 4.3.4. Volume scores as a function of cardiac motion of two equally sized calcifications. Scans were performed with a 64-slice MDCT at 0.6-mm slice thickness (Groen et al. 2007b)

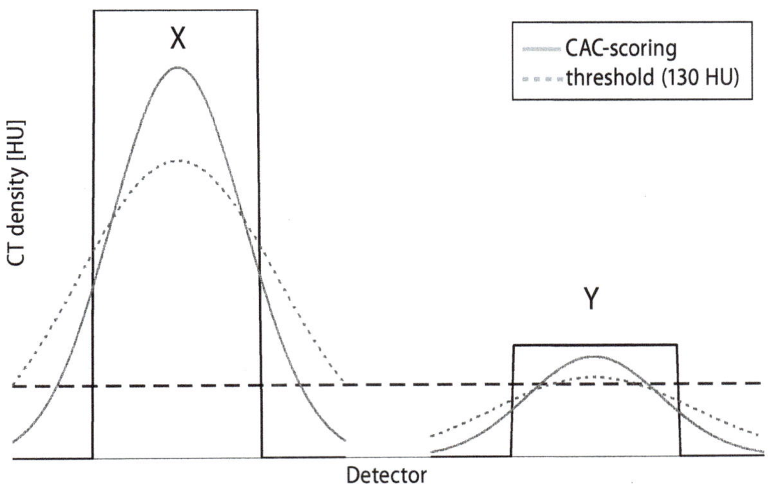

Fig. 4.3.5. Theoretical CT profile of two objects (*black*) with a relatively high (*X*) and low (*Y*) density which exhibit a relatively low (*solid grey*) and high (*dotted grey*) movement. The *dotted line* represents the calcium scoring threshold of 130 HU (Groen et al. 2007a,b)

motion during scanning resulted in an apparent increase in the Agatston score. A second advantage of less motion during the calcium scoring scan is a reduced variability. Comparing calcium scoring scans at 60 bpm and 85 bpm, the variability was less at 60 bpm for EBT and 16-slice MDCT (Horiguchi et al. 2005b). Similar results were found for 64-slice MDCT; the variability increased with increasing heart rate (Groen et al. 2007b).

In conclusion, calcium scoring in vitro showed that calcium scoring can be improved in terms of variability and absolute score by a reduction of the PVE with higher spatial resolutions and a reduction of cardiac motion with higher temporal resolutions.

4.3.5 Combining In Vivo and In Vitro

Research on calcium scoring in vitro can be translated to calcium scoring in vivo and vice versa. Different phantom studies supported the underestimation of the calcium score with MDCT compared to EBT (Groen et al. 2007a; Ulzheimer and Kalender 2003). In a study comparing two different 64-slice MDCT systems to EBT, the Agatston and Volume scores obtained with 64-slice MDCT were highly correlated with EBT-obtained (Fig. 4.3.6). However, the MDCT systems both significantly underestimated the calcium scores compared to the EBT-based scores (–10% to –2%, mean –8%) (Greuter et al. 2007). This suggests that as a consequence MDCT-based calcium scores should be increased by approximately 8% to acquire MDCT-based calcium scores similar to EBT-based calcium scores. This might enable the use of the EBT-based cut-points for MDCT-based calcium scores. A second serious consequence of the underestimation of the calcium score on MDCT is that when the outcome of the calcium scan is zero, this does not mean that there is no calcium present in the coronary arteries. Due to the large variabilities and underestimation, smaller calcifications might be missed by MDCT.

In addition to systematic comparisons between EBT and MDCT, calcium scoring in vitro showed that a reduced spatial and temporal resolution is required to enhance calcium scoring in vivo.

An increased spatial resolution in calcium scoring in vivo can be achieved by the use of smaller slice thicknesses, although this will also increase the patient dose. Calcium scoring in vitro already showed that smaller slice thicknesses increased the calcium score (Groen et al. 2007b; Mao et al. 2003; Mühlenbruch et al. 2007). This result was confirmed in different patient studies. Vliegenthart et al. (2003) showed that the median Volume score was increased by 44% comparing 1.5-mm slices to 3.0-mm slices in 1302 patients using EBT. Increased Agatston, Volume and Mass scores were also reported for 16-slice MDCT (Sabour et al. 2007) and 64-slice MDCT (Schlosser et al. 2007). In addition, Schlosser et al. (2007) also showed a reduced variability for thinner slices.

A second approach to reduce the PVE is the use of overlapping slices. Different patient studies con-

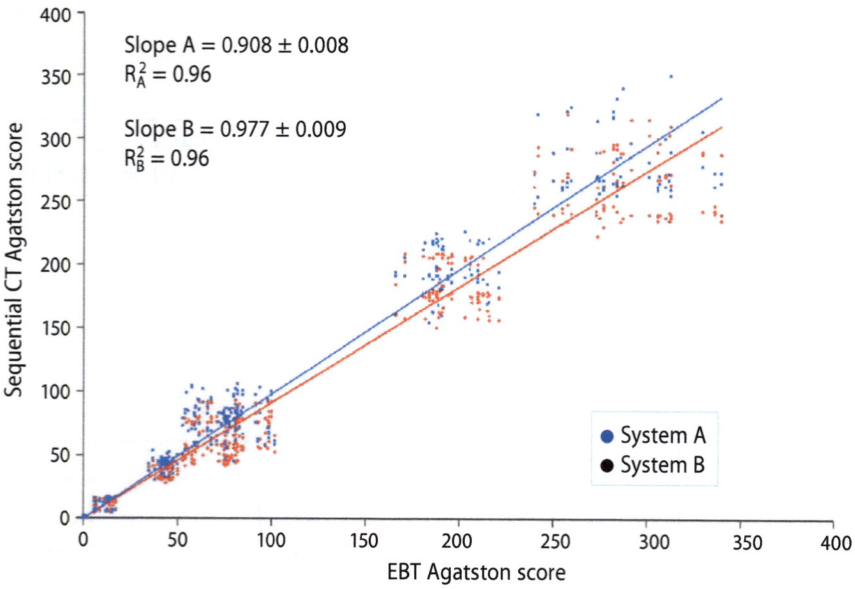

Fig. 4.3.6. Comparison of two different 64-slice MDCT to EBT with respect to Agatston scores of a phantom (Greuter et al. 2007). Scans were performed with a sequential scanning protocol at 3.0-mm slice thickness

firmed the use of overlapping slices to be beneficial for calcium scoring. A reduced variability was observed for 16-slice MDCT (Horiguchi et al. 2005a) and 64-slice MDCT (Schlosser et al. 2007).

An increased temporal resolution in calcium scoring in vivo can only be achieved by the use of scanners with faster rotation times (Flohr et al. 2006). However, an alternative approach is to reduce the amount of motion during scanning. In MDCT scanning this can be achieved by the use of ECG-gating or β-blockers. ECG-gating ensures that the scan is performed during a period of reduced movement of the heart, therefore reducing the amount of cardiac motion during the scan. The use of this technique to reduce the amount of motion reduces the variability (Horiguchi et al. 2007; Mao et al. 2001; Rutten et al. 2008). Absolute scoring results have not been reported.

4.3.6 Implications

The presented research results show that MDCT could function as an alternative to EBT for quantifying the amount of calcium in the coronary arteries. However, the obtained calcium score does come with a few pitfalls. First of all, calcium scoring is hampered by large variabilities, thus the obtained score has relatively large margins of error. Furthermore, if the score is zero, there might still be calcium present in the coronary arteries, due to the underestimation inherent to MDCT. This underestimation also hampers the use of the calcium score as a risk factor for coronary artery disease, especially for low calcium scores. A simple one-to-one translation from EBT to MDCT might underestimate the patients risk for coronary artery disease. And finally, different parameters of the scan protocol have an impact on the outcome of the calcium score. Therefore, these parameters should be taken into account when interpreting the obtained score.

4.3.7 Conclusion

MDCT can be used to quantify the amount of coronary calcium and shows equal or improved variabilities as compared to EBT. Furthermore, research shows that calcium scoring using the Mass score is advocated due to a lower variability compared to the other calcium scoring algorithms. The variability can be further reduced by the use of appropriate scan protocols using thinner slices combined with techniques to reduce the amount of motion. Although the accuracies of EBT and MDCT are similar and different scanning techniques of MDCT are useful in the reduction of variability, the absolute scoring results of MDCT may not be equivalent to the scoring results of EBT. MDCT underestimates the total amount of calcium in the coronary arteries compared to EBT. Therefore, one should be cautious when using a calcium score obtained with MDCT for risk assessment, since this risk assessment is based upon EBT-data.

Although standardized protocols and calibrations are helpful in obtaining standardized calcium scores, a thorough understanding of the underlying principles involved in calcium scoring is essential. A proper analysis of algorithms and measurements will benefit the calcium score in terms of variability, absolute score and equality of MDCT and EBT.

For now, MDCT and EBT calcium scores may not be equivalent. Knowledge of the system and scan protocol remain important and are therefore needed for every calcium score procedure to ensure a correct clinical interpretation of the obtained calcium score results.

References

Agatston AS, Janowitz WR, Hildner FJ et al (1990) Quantification of coronary artery calcium using ultrafast computed tomography. J Am Coll Cardiol 15:827–832

Arad Y, Spadaro LA, Goodman K et al (2000) Prediction of coronary events with electron beam computed tomography. J Am Coll Cardiol 36:1253–1260

Becker CR, Kleffel T, Crispin A et al (2001) Coronary artery calcium measurement: agreement of multirow detector and electron beam CT. AJR Am J Roentgenol 176:1295–1298

Brown SJ, Hayball MP, Coulden RA (2007) Impact of motion artefact on the measurement of coronary calcium score. Br J Radiol 73:956–962

Budoff MJ, Georgiou D, Brody A et al (1996) Ultrafast computed tomography as a diagnostic modality in the detection of coronary artery disease: a multicenter study. Circulation 93:898–904

Budoff MJ, Kessler P, Gao YL et al (2008) The interscan variation of CT coronary artery calcification score: analysis of the Calcium Acetate Renagel Comparison (CARE)-2 study. Acad Radiol 15:58–61

Callister TQ, Cooil B, Raya SP et al (1998) Coronary artery disease: improved reproducibility of calcium scoring with an electron-beam CT volumetric method. Radiology 208:807–814

Carr JJ, Crouse JR III, Goff DC Jr et al (2000) Evaluation of subsecond gated helical CT for quantification of coronary artery calcium and comparison with electron beam CT. AJR Am J Roentgenol 174:915–921

Daniell AL, Wong ND, Friedman JD et al (2005) Concordance of coronary artery calcium estimates between MDCT and electron beam tomography. AJR Am J Roentgenol 185:1542–1545

Deurholt WY, Groen JM, Visser R et al (2008) Per-patient calibration in calcium mass scoring on DSCT and EBT. Per-patient calibration in calcium mass scoring on DSCT and EBT 2008 (unpublished results)

Flohr TG, McCollough CH, Bruder H et al (2006) First performance evaluation of a dual-source CT (DSCT) system. Eur Radiol 16:256–268

Goldin JG, Yoon HC, Greaser LE III et al (2001) Spiral versus electron-beam CT for coronary artery calcium scoring. Radiology 221:213–221

Greuter MJ, Dijkstra H, Groen JM et al (2007) 64 Slice MDCT generally underestimates coronary calcium scores as compared to EBT: a phantom study. Med Phys 34:3510–3519

Groen JM, Greuter MJ, Vliegenthart R et al (2007a) Calcium scoring using 64-slice MDCT, dual source CT and EBT: a comparative phantom study. Int J Cardiovasc Imaging 24:547–556

Groen, JM, Greuter, MJ, Schmidt, B et al (2007b) The influence of heart rate, slice thickness, and calcification density on calcium scores using 64-slice multidetector computed tomography: a systematic phantom study. Invest Radiol 42:848–855

Hoff JA, Daviglus ML, Chomka EV et al (2003) Conventional coronary artery disease risk factors and coronary artery calcium detected by electron beam tomography in 30,908 healthy individuals. Ann Epidemiol 13:163–169

Hoffmann U, Siebert U, Bull-Stewart A et al (2006) Evidence for lower variability of coronary artery calcium mineral mass measurements by multi-detector computed tomography in a community-based cohort – consequences for progression studies. Eur J Radiol 57:396–402

Hokanson JE, MacKenzie T, Kinney G et al (2004) Evaluating changes in coronary artery calcium: an analytic method that accounts for interscan variability. AJR Am J Roentgenol 182:1327–1332

Hong C, Bae KT, Pilgram TK et al (2003a) Coronary artery calcium quantification at multi-detector row CT: influence of heart rate and measurement methods on interacquisition variability initial experience. Radiology 228:95–100

Hong C, Pilgram TK, Zhu F et al (2003b) Improving mass measurement of coronary artery calcification using threshold correction and thin collimation in multi-detector row computed tomography: in vitro experiment. Acad Radiol 10:969–977

Horiguchi J, Yamamoto H, Akiyama Y et al (2004) Coronary artery calcium scoring using 16-MDCT and a retrospective ECG-gating reconstruction algorithm. AJR Am J Roentgenol 183:103–108

Horiguchi J, Yamamoto H, Akiyama Y et al (2005a) Variability of repeated coronary artery calcium measurements by 16-MDCT with retrospective reconstruction. AJR Am J Roentgenol 184:1917–1923

Horiguchi J, Shen Y, Akiyama Y et al (2005b) Electron beam CT versus 16-MDCT on the variability of repeated coronary artery calcium measurements in a variable heart rate phantom. AJR Am J Roentgenol 185:995–1000

Horiguchi J, Yamamoto H, Hirai N et al (2006) Variability of repeated coronary artery calcium measurements on low-dose ECG-gated 16-MDCT. AJR Am J Roentgenol 187:W1–W6

Horiguchi J, Fukuda H, Yamamoto H et al (2007) The impact of motion artifacts on the reproducibility of repeated coronary artery calcium measurements. Eur Radiol 17:81–86

Janowitz WR, Agatston AS, Viamonte M Jr (1991) Comparison of serial quantitative evaluation of calcified coronary artery plaque by ultrafast computed tomography in persons with and without obstructive coronary artery disease. Am J Cardiol 68:1–6

Knez A, Becker C, Becker A et al (2002) Determination of coronary calcium with multi-slice spiral computed tomography: a comparative study with electron-beam CT. Int J Cardiovasc Imaging 18:295–303

Lu B, Budoff MJ, Zhuang N et al (2002) Causes of interscan variability of coronary artery calcium measurements at electron-beam CT. Acad Radiol 9:654–661

Maher, JE, Bielak, LF, Raz, JA et al (1999) Progression of coronary artery calcification: a pilot study. Mayo Clin Proc 74:347–355

Mahnken AH, Wildberger JE, Sinha AM et al (2002) Variation of the coronary calcium score depending on image reconstruction interval and scoring algorithm. Invest Radiol 37:496–502

Mao S, Bakhsheshi H, Lu B et al (2001) Effect of electrocardiogram triggering on reproducibility of coronary artery calcium scoring. Radiology 220:707–711

Mao S, Child J, Carson S et al (2003) Sensitivity to detect small coronary artery calcium lesions with varying slice thickness using electron beam tomography. Invest Radiol 38:183–187

McCollough CH, Kaufmann RB, Cameron BM et al (1995) Electron-beam CT: use of a calibration phantom to reduce variability in calcium quantitation. Radiology 196:159–165

McCollough CH, Ulzheimer S, Halliburton SS et al (2007) Coronary artery calcium: a multi-institutional, multimanufacturer international standard for quantification at cardiac CT. Radiology 243:527–538

Mühlenbruch G, Klotz E, Wildberger JE et al (2007) The accuracy of 1- and 3-mm slices in coronary calcium scoring using multi-slice CT in vitro and in vivo. Eur Radiol 17:321–329

Ohnesorge B, Flohr T, Fischbach R et al (2002) Reproducibility of coronary calcium quantification in repeat examinations with retrospectively ECG-gated multisection spiral CT. Eur Radiol 12:1532–1540

O'Rourke RA, Brundage BH, Froelicher VF et al (2000) American College of Cardiology/American Heart Association Expert Consensus document on electron-beam computed tomography for the diagnosis and prognosis of coronary artery disease. Circulation 102:126–140

Oudkerk M, Stillman AE, Halliburton SS et al (2008) Coronary artery calcium screening: current status and recommendations from the European Society of Cardiac Radiology and North American Society for Cardiovascular Imaging. Int J Cardiovasc Imaging 24:645- 671
Raggi P, Callister TQ, Cooil B et al (2000) Identification of patients at increased risk of first unheralded acute myocardial infarction by electron-beam computed tomography. Circulation 101:850–855
Raggi P, Callister TQ, Cooil B (2002) Calcium scoring of the coronary artery by electron beam CT: how to apply an individual attenuation threshold. AJR Am J Roentgenol 178:497–502
Rutten A, Krul SP, Meijs MF et al (2008) Variability of coronary calcium scores throughout the cardiac cycle: implications for the appropriate use of electrocardiogram-dose modulation with retrospectively gated computed tomography. Invest Radiol 43:187–194
Sabour S, Rutten A, van der Schouw YT et al (2007) Inter-scan reproducibility of coronary calcium measurement using multi detector-row computed tomography (MDCT). Eur J Epidemiol 22:235–243
Schlosser T, Hunold P, Voigtlander T et al (2007) Coronary artery calcium scoring: influence of reconstruction interval and reconstruction increment using 64-MDCT. AJR Am J Roentgenol 188:1063–1068
Sevrukov AB, Bland JM, Kondos GT (2005) Serial electron beam CT measurements of coronary artery calcium: has your patient‘s calcium score actually changed? AJR Am J Roentgenol 185:1546–1553
Stanford W, Thompson BH, Burns TL et al (2004) Coronary artery calcium quantification at multi-detector row helical CT versus electron-beam CT. Radiology 230:397–402
Ulzheimer S, Kalender WA (2003) Assessment of calcium scoring performance in cardiac computed tomography. Eur Radiol 13:484–497
Vliegenthart R, Song B, Hofman A et al (2003) Coronary calcification at electron-beam CT: effect of section thickness on calcium scoring in vitro and in vivo. Radiology 229:520–525
Wexler L, Brundage B, Crouse J et al (1996) Coronary artery calcification: pathophysiology, epidemiology, imaging methods, and clinical implications. A statement for health professionals from the American Heart Association. Writing Group. Circulation 94:1175–1192
Wong ND, Hsu JC, Detrano RC et al (2000) Coronary artery calcium evaluation by electron beam computed tomography and its relation to new cardiovascular events. Am J Cardiol 86:495–498
Yoon HC, Greaser LE III, Mather R et al (1997) Coronary artery calcium: alternate methods for accurate and reproducible quantitation. Acad Radiol 4:666–673

Non-Invasive Measurement of Coronary Atherosclerosis

4

4.4 Coronary Calcium as an Indicator of Coronary Artery Disease

AXEL SCHMERMUND, STEFAN MÖHLENKAMP, and RAIMUND ERBEL

CONTENTS

4.4.1 Coronary Calcium as an Indicator of Atherosclerosis

Non contrast-enhanced cardiac CT imaging allows for direct, noninvasive visualization of calcified coronary plaques. The primary aim is not to diagnose coronary stenoses, but rather to detect and quantify coronary plaque burden. Coronary plaques, usually not highly stenotic, are the underlying substrate of the acute coronary syndromes (SCHMERMUND and ERBEL 2001). Coronary calcium is a specific expression of coronary atherosclerotic plaque disease (BUDOFF et al. 2006; DEBACKER et al. 2003). There is a relationship between the extent of calcified plaque burden and that of total plaque burden (BUDOFF et al. 2006; DEBACKER et al. 2003; RUMBERGER et al. 1995; SCHMERMUND et al. 1999). Total plaque burden is one of the most important predictors of coronary risk (EMOND et al. 1994; PROUDFIT et al. 1980). The more calcium is detected, the more plaque there is (Fig. 4.4.1). This carries direct implications for an individual's coronary risk (BUDOFF et al. 2006; DEBACKER et al. 2003; SCHMERMUND and ERBEL 2001).

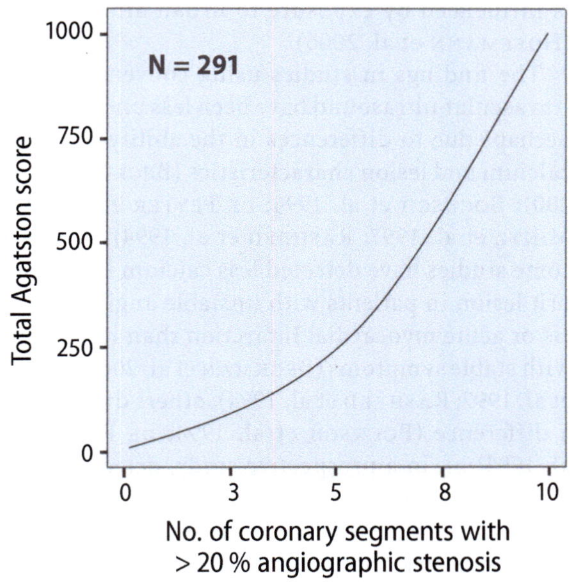

Fig. 4.4.1. Extent of coronary calcium (*Total Agatston score*) in relation to the number of coronary segments with angiographic stenoses > 20% diameter narrowing. *10*, ≥ 10 Segments. A curvilinear fit of the total Agatston calcium score median values is shown. On the basis of data presented in SCHMERMUND et al. (1999)

A. SCHMERMUND, MD, FESC
Associate Professor of Internal Medicine and Cardiology, Cardioangiologisches Centrum Bethanien, Im Prüfling 23, 60389 Frankfurt/Main, Germany
S. MÖHLENKAMP, MD
West German Heart Center Essen, Department of Cardiology, University Duisberg-Essen, Hufelandstrasse 55, 45122 Essen, Germany
R. ERBEL, MD
Professor, West German Heart Center Essen, Department of Cardiology, University Duisberg-Essen, Hufelandstrasse 55, 45122 Essen, Germany

It may be argued that calcium is associated with an overall increased activity of coronary atherosclerotic disease. Histo-pathologic studies have demonstrated that coronary calcium is a frequent feature of plaque rupture (Burke et al. 2000; Farb et al. 1996; Schmermund et al. 2001a) and is found even in subjects who die of sudden coronary death as the first manifestation of ischemic heart disease under the age of 50 years (Schmermund et al. 2001a). Among all types of histologically defined types of plaques detected in young victims of sudden coronary death, acute ruptures contain calcium most frequently (80%), while healed ruptures contain the greatest amount of calcium (Burke et al. 2000, 2001). Plaque erosions, on the other hand, are associated with little calcium (Farb et al. 1996; Burke et al. 2000). Calcium is found preferentially in plaques with expansive ("positive") arterial remodeling (Burke et al. 2002). The mechanisms leading to expansive arterial remodeling appear to share common aspects with those ultimately leading to plaque rupture, and plaques displaying positive remodeling of the arterial segment are prone to rupture (Ward et al. 2000). Further evidence supporting the active role of coronary calcium in coronary atherosclerosis stems is, among others, derived from the observation that the extent of coronary artery calcium is influenced by exposure to urban air pollution (Hoffmann et al. 2006).

The findings in studies using conventional intravascular ultrasound have been less unequivocal, perhaps due to differences in the ability to define calcium and lesion characteristics (Beckman et al. 2001; Bocksch et al. 1994; de Feyter et al. 1995; Mintz et al. 1997; Rasheed et al. 1994). Whereas some studies have detected less calcium in the culprit lesion in patients with unstable angina pectoris or acute myocardial infarction than in patients with stable symptoms (Beckman et al. 2001; Mintz et al. 1997; Rasheed et al. 1994), others did not find a difference (Bocksch et al. 1994; de Feyter et al. 1995) or, in a prospective study, detected more calcium in patients who later sustained an event (Abizaid et al. 1999). In summary, coronary calcium indicates the presence and extent of coronary atherosclerotic plaque disease. The weight of evidence suggests that coronary calcium indicates atherosclerotic disease activity and is associated with healed or acute plaque rupture and positive arterial remodeling.

4.4.2 Coronary Calcium – Prediction of Coronary Heart Disease Events

In symptomatic patients presenting to the emergency room with chest pain and no initial objective signs of myocardial ischemia, a negative coronary calcium scan indicated an excellent prognosis with regard to major cardiac events over the subsequent 1–4 months (Georgiou et al. 2001; Laudon et al. 1999; McLaughlin et al. 1999). Coronary calcium scans yielded negative predictive values in the range of 98%–100%. In symptomatic patients undergoing coronary angiography, increased amounts of coronary calcium detected by electron-beam computed tomography (EBCT) were highly predictive of subsequent events over 30 months (Detrano et al. 1996). In direct comparison, the coronary calcium scan performed better than coronary angiography (that is, number of stenotic major coronary arteries) in this respect.

Möhlenkamp et al. (2003) evaluated the prognostic value of high coronary calcium scores in symptomatic males undergoing coronary angiography. In these selected patients, clinical cardiac events occurred earlier and more frequently in patients with scores > 1000. Left main coronary artery disease and elevated calcium scores were the only independent predictors of hard events. Accordingly, even in symptomatic patients with an a priori high cardiovascular risk, extensive coronary calcium provided complementary prognostic information concerning future cardiovascular events.

The morphological information on the extent of coronary atherosclerosis provided by the coronary calcium score may complement the functional information obtained by exercise stress testing and, in particular, myocardial perfusion studies (Berman et al. 2004; Greenland et al. 2007; He et al. 2000; Schmermund et al. 1999). High coronary calcium scores are associated with a high rate of positive myocardial perfusion studies, demonstrating comparatively extensive perfusion abnormalities (Berman et al. 2004; He et al. 2000). On the other hand, myocardial perfusion defects are almost never observed in the absence of coronary calcium. In a middle-aged patient group with an intermediate coronary heart disease (CHD) risk, myocardial perfusion defects are detected in < 2% of all patients with a coronary calcium score < 100 (Berman et al. 2004).

Data are accumulating regarding the prognostic ability of calcium scanning in asymptomatic subjects. In 2004, PLETCHER et al. systematically analyzed the published evidence available on the prognostic value of measuring coronary calcium. All studies available for the analysis had been performed by using EBCT. These studies included > 13,000 person-years of observation time after the EBCT scan. To provide for a common standard, PLETCHER et al. (2004) analyzed four calcium score categories (0, 1–100, 101–400, and > 400). After adjusting for the established cardiovascular risk factors, they calculated the relative risk of a CHD event associated with each of the higher calcium score categories compared to a calcium score of 0. Figure 4.4.2 shows that the relative risk estimates increased progressively for each calcium score category. Accordingly, coronary calcium was associated with an increased risk of CHD events, even when established risk factors for CHD were taken into account.

A number of studies provided a detailed analysis of the potential of the calcium score to add prognostic information to the traditional risk factors. GREENLAND et al. (2004) analyzed data from the South Bay Heart Watch study, which had in part be included in the above named meta-analysis by PLETCHER et al. (2004) (GREENLAND et al. 2004). Risk factors were determined with state-of-the art methods and were used to compute the Framingham risk score, employing the algorithm provided by the National Cholesterol Education Program Adult Treatment Panel III report. The rate of cardiovascular death or myocardial infarction ("hard events") over 7.0 years was assessed in subgroups of patients classified according to the Framingham risk score or the calcium score. Across all Framingham risk score strata, a calcium score ≥ 301 (observed in 17%) predicted an increased hard event rate compared with a calcium score of 0 (observed in 24%). In the Framingham risk score strata ≥ 10%, a calcium score ≥ 301 predicted an increased hard event rate compared with all categories of lower calcium scores, thus suggesting useful additional prognostic information in "intermediate risk" subjects. Along these lines, receiver-operating characteristic (ROC) curve analysis demonstrated that the addition of the calcium score to the Framingham risk score provided for a significant improvement in the prediction of hard cardiac events (GREENLAND et al. 2004).

Table 4.4.1 gives an overview of the studies not included in the meta-analysis by PLETCHER et al. (2004), usually because they were published in the year 2004 or later. The endpoints of these studies vary, and most did not perform state-of-the-art measurements of the cardiovascular risk factors. Nevertheless, we are provided with large observational studies which demonstrate the ability of calcium scores to add independent and incremental information in addition to traditional risk factors in predicting important clinical events. Most of these studies included patients who had been referred for risk assessment or because of a presumed high-risk status, usually involving some selection of the study subjects. It has been questioned whether the results obtained in these populations also pertain to a more general population. In this respect, recent data from general, unselected populations are of great interest, as provided by the Rotterdam Calcification Study (VLIEGENTHART et al. 2005) and the St. Francis Heart Study (ARAD et al. 2005a).

The above named studies have established the prognostic ability of coronary calcium quantities determined by using cardiac CT. On the basis of these studies, coronary calcium scanning has been proposed as a means for risk stratification in certain subgroups of asymptomatic and symptomatic subjects by the major scientific societies in the USA and in Europe (BUDOFF et al. 2006; DEBACKER et al. 2003; GREENLAND et al. 2007). The clinical use of this method as detailed by the current scientific statements is outlined below (Sect. 4.4.4).

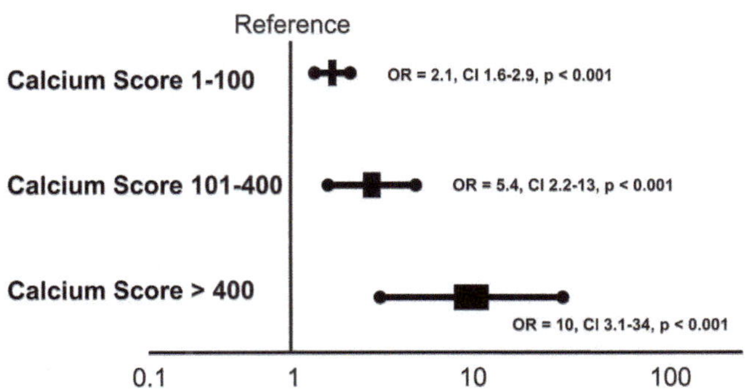

Fig. 4.4.2. Meta-analysis of prospective studies on the prognostic value of coronary calcium published between 1999 and 2001. Depending on the coronary calcium score, the odds ratio (*OR*) regarding cardiac events is shown after adjustment for the cardiovascular risk factors. The reference odds ratio equals 1 and pertains to the absence of detectable coronary calcium. On the basis of data presented in PLETCHER et al. (2004)

Table 4.4.1.
Prospective studies on the prognostic value of the coronary calcium score in asymptomatic subjects not included in the 2004 meta-analyses by Pletcher et al. (2004). CHD = coronary heart disease

First author	Number of study participants and mean duration of follow-up	Risk factor Assessment	Endpoint	Univariate relative risk	Multivariate relative risk	Comment
Kondos et al. (2003)	8,855 3.1 Years	Questionnaire	CHD events (a) "Hard events" = cardiac death and myocardial infarction (b) "All events" = also including revascularization	Analysis restricted to men: (a) Hard events: Presence of coronary calcium versus no calcium: 5.8 b) All events: Presence of coronary calcium versus no calcium: 16.7	Analysis restricted to men: (a) hard events: Presence of coronary calcium versus no calcium: 3.9 (b) all events: Presence of coronary calcium versus no calcium: 10.5	Too few women as participants and too few events to allow for a meaningful analysis in women
Shaw et al. (2003)	10,377 5.0 Years	Questionnaire/ interview	All-cause mortality	Calcium score ≤ 10: 1 Score 11–100: 2.5 Score 101–400: 3.6 Score 401–1,000: 6.2 Score > 1,000: 12.3	Calcium score ≤ 10: 1 Score 11–100: 1.6 Score 101–400: 1.7 Score 401–1,000: 2.5 Score > 1,000: 4.0	Overall mortality as the only clinical endpoint
LaMonte et al. (2005)	10,746 3.5 Years	Questionnaire	CHD events (a) "Hard events" = coronary death and myocardial infarction (b) "All events" = also including revascularization	Highest tertile of calcium score distribution versus no coronary calcium: Hard events: Men: 20.0 Women: 9.3 All events: Men: 67.0 Women: 9.3	Highest tertile of calcium score distribution versus no coronary calcium: Hard events: Men: 17.7 Women: 7.2 All events: Men: 61.7 Women: 6.2	Large, relatively healthy sample

4.4.3 Progression of Coronary Calcium

Coronary angiographic studies have established the prognostic importance of atherosclerosis progression (Kaski et al. 1995; Waters et al. 1993). Patients with increased progression of either the number of angiographic stenoses or worst stenosis degree have a several-fold increased risk of unstable angina and myocardial infarction. Importantly, it has been demonstrated that atherosclerosis progression does not occur in a graded, continuous fashion. Severe stenoses can appear in coronary segments showing no or minimal angiographic disease in the initial angiogram only weeks to months before the second examination, and lesions in the same patient do not necessarily develop in the same direction: some lesions progress whereas others remain stable or even regress (Ambrose 1988; Little 1988). Accordingly, it is usually impossible to predict the progression of coronary atherosclerosis in an individual patient.

Coronary calcium progression can be reliably determined in small groups of patients. Using up-to-date scanner technology, inter-scan variability is smaller than annual coronary artery calcification (CAC) progression in such groups, which is usually in the order of 20%–30% (Achenbach et al. 2002; Callister et al. 1998; Maher et al. 1999; Schmermund et al. 2001b; Yoon et al. 2002). In individual patients, only substantial CAC changes are beyond measurement variability (Bielak et al. 2001). In analogy with angiographic measures of coronary

First author	Number of study participants and mean duration of follow-up	Risk factor Assessment	Endpoint	Univariate relative risk	Multivariate relative risk	Comment
Taylor et al. (2005)	2,000 3.0 Years	Measurement	All CHD events	Not presented	Analysis restricted to men: Presence of coronary calcium versus no coronary calcium: 11.8 After further controlling for C-reactive protein: 10.8	Young, healthy population; few events; too few women as participants and too few events to allow for a meaningful analysis in women
Vliegenthart et al. (2005)	1,795 3.3 Years	Measurement	(a) Hard CHD events (only cardiac death and myocardial infarction) (b) All CHD events (also including revascularization) (In addition, also overall cardiovascular events and total mortality, not listed here)	Adjusted for age and sex (a) (Hard events) Score 0–100: 1 Score 101–400: 2.8 Score 401–1000: 3.9 Score > 1000: 7.5 (b) (All CHD events) Score 0–100: 1 Score 101–400: 3.2 Score 401–1000: 4.7 Score > 1000: 8.2	(a) (Hard events) Score 0–100: 1 Score 101–400: 2.7 Score 401–1000: 4.1 Score > 1000: 8.1 (b) (All CHD events) Score 0–100: 1 Score 101–400: 3.1 Score 401–1000: 4.6 Score > 1000: 8.3	Population-based study with no selection of the participants Higher age than in the other studies (mean age, 71 years)
Arad et al. (2005a)	4,613 4.3 Years	Measurement/questionnaire	All CHD events	Calcium score = 0: 1 Score 1–99: 1.9 Score 100–399: 10.2 Score ≥ 400: 26.2	Only available in a subgroup of subjects, not presented in detail, but coronary calcium adds significant information	Study participants were volunteers not selected on the basis of risk factors or clinical symptoms

atherosclerosis, increased CAC progression conveys an increased risk of suffering acute myocardial infarction and other cardiovascular events (Arad et al. 2005a; Raggi et al. 2003, 2004). Although this might have clinical consequences for selected patients, no factors have been reliably identified which modify coronary calcium progression.

In symptomatic patients who mostly underwent pharmacological treatment and who had a calcium score > 0, the mean annual progression of total calcium area was 42%, and the median 27% (Schmermund et al. 2001b). The baseline coronary calcium burden influenced the rate of progression (Fig. 4.4.3). This was later confirmed in other reports (Yoon et al. 2002). Patients with extensive coronary calcium had the greatest absolute rate of progression, whereas in patients with lower coronary calcium scores, absolute progression was much less. In the latter group (with lower coronary calcium scores), relative progression was significantly higher (Fig. 4.4.3). This reflects in part a mathematical phenomenon in that an increase in the coronary calcium score from 30 to 60 is an increase by 100%, whereas from 1030 to 1060, it is only an increase by 3%. Nevertheless, it appears clinically relevant that opposite trends in absolute and relative (percent) measures of progression can be seen.

It has been proposed that patients with increased coronary calcium progression (and normal renal function) have a higher rate of acute myocardial infarction, independent of statin treatment (Raggi et al. 2003, 2004). Raggi et al. (2004) conducted a retro-

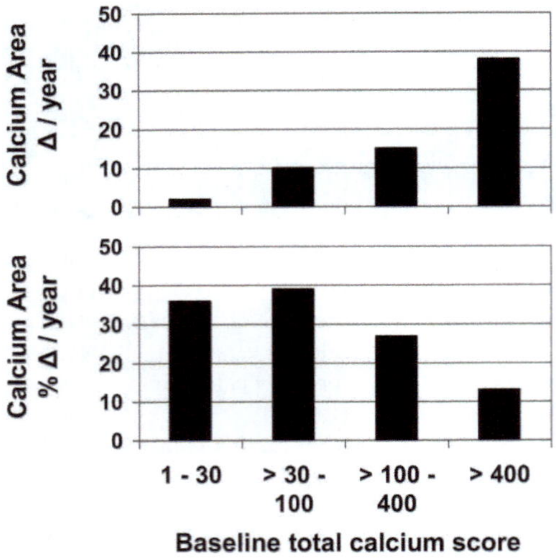

Fig. 4.4.3. The interpretation of the annualized progression of coronary calcium (median) depends on the baseline total calcium score. Patients are classified into four groups with different baseline scores. In the *top panel*, absolute changes (calcium score progression per year) are greater in patients with greater baseline scores. In the *bottom panel*, relative changes in percent of the baseline score are smaller in patients with greater baseline scores. On the basis of data presented in Schmermund et al. (2001b)

spective analysis in 495 patients who had no clinical coronary artery disease but were all treated with statins because of their coronary calcium burden. The mean follow-up time was 3.2 years. Although the baseline amount of coronary calcium was comparable, patients who later suffered an acute myocardial infarction had a mean coronary calcium progression of 42%, whereas it was 17% in the patients with no acute myocardial infarction ($p < 0.0001$). Patients with an annual coronary calcium progression ≥ 15% had a 17.2-fold increased risk of acute myocardial infarction. This risk appeared to be modified depending on the baseline coronary calcium score. In particular, patients with a high baseline score *and* an increased progression had an increased risk of acute myocardial infarction, underlining the importance of the relationship between the baseline amount of CAC and the rate of progression (Raggi et al. 2004).

Several randomized studies failed to detect an effect of lipid-lowering therapy on CAC progression, even though medications proven to reduce cardiovascular event rates were used (Arad et al. 2005b; Houslay et al. 2006; Raggi et al. 2005; Schmermund et al. 2006b). In a subgroup of participants in the St. Francis Heart Study who had increased coronary calcium scores, coronary calcium progression was examined over a mean duration of 4.3 years (Arad et al. 2005b). Apart from vitamin supplementation and aspirin, the treatment group received atorvastatin 20 mg/day, whereas the placebo group received only aspirin 81 mg/day. In the group treated with atorvastatin, the mean baseline LDL cholesterol value of 146 mg/dl was lowered by 47% over the course of the study. Despite the comparatively long treatment period and a trend for a lower event rate in the atorvastatin group, no difference in the progression of coronary calcium (Agatston method) was observed. Overall, the Agatston coronary calcium score increased by 331 in the atorvastatin group (+81%) and by 323 (+73%) in the control group treated with aspirin alone (Arad et al. 2005b).

In the Beyond Endorsed Lipid Lowering with EBT Scanning (BELLES) trial, EBCT scanning to track CAC progression was performed in hyperlipidemic postmenopausal women (Raggi et al. 2005). In a multicenter study, they were randomized to therapy with 80 mg/day atorvastatin or 40 mg/day pravastatin. Intensive statin therapy with 80 mg atorvastatin over 1 year lowered LDL cholesterol from 175 mg/dl to 92 mg/dl (–47%), whereas 40 mg pravastatin lowered LDL cholesterol from 174 mg/dl to 129 mg/dl (–25%). However, median coronary calcium progression (volume score) did not differ and was approximately 20% in both treatment groups. In another randomized multicenter study, patients who had no CHD but ≥ 2 cardiovascular risk factors and at least moderate coronary calcium scores were assigned to receive 80 mg or 10 mg atorvastatin per day over 12 months (Schmermund et al. 2006b). Mean coronary calcium progression was similar in both treatment groups. Corrected for the baseline calcium volume score, it was 27% in the 80 mg atorvastatin group and 25% in the 10 mg atorvastatin group ($p = 0.65$). There was no relationship of coronary calcium progression with on-treatment LDL cholesterol levels.

To explain these unexpected results, a recent analysis reevaluated intravascular ultrasound data from two large randomized trials examining coronary plaque progression in response to anti-atherosclerotic treatment (Nicholls et al. 2007). Whereas in general, coronary plaques with little or no calcification displayed measurable changes in volume (progression or even regression depending on the medical treatment regimen), calcified plaque volume appeared to be more resistant to such changes. This may imply that once calcified plaque formation has taken place, further changes are difficult to detect. In this respect, two more considerations deserve mention. Calcified plaque volume only represents a minor proportion of overall plaque volume, a proportion which may in part be too small to detect changes. Also, only a fraction of the extent of coronary calcium can be explained by cardiovascular risk factor variability (Schmermund et al. 1998). Accordingly, other factors apart from risk factors should also play a role in coronary calcium progression and were not accounted for in the randomized studies mentioned above.

Overall, accelerated coronary calcium progression signifies a significantly increased risk of adverse cardiac events. However, it remains open which determinants influence calcium progression over the course of 1–4 years, and likewise, potential therapeutic implications remain unclear. Apart from these issues, we do not know at which interval serial coronary calcium scanning might be considered and if the dynamic developments in scanner technology will influence serial measurements. Against this background, assessment of coronary calcium progression in clinical practice is currently discouraged (Greenland et al. 2007).

4.4.4 Guidelines for and Practical Use of Coronary Calcium Assessment

Assessment of coronary calcium provides for direct visualization of the coronary arteries and quantification of coronary artery calcium as a representation of coronary atherosclerosis. The extent of coronary calcium has unequivocally been demonstrated to predict clinical cardiovascular events. In appropriately selected patients, it provides additional and incremental prognostic information above that provided by clinical data and cardiovascular risk factor analysis alone. Assessment of coronary calcium should only be contemplated in patients who can potentially derive a benefit from this test. This will be the case in asymptomatic patients whose cardiovascular risk remains indeterminate despite thorough analysis of medical history, ECG data and other clinical information, and risk factor analysis. Depending on the definition of cardiovascular risk thresholds ("low versus intermediate versus high risk"), the proportion of the asymptomatic population with an indeterminate ("intermediate") risk may range between 5% and 40% (Greenland et al. 2001; Keevil et al. 2007).

For practical purposes, global cardiovascular risk assessment plays an important role in determining the a priori risk of an individual. This will usually involve one or more of the available risk scoring algorithms in Europe and in the USA such as the Framingham Risk Score (Greenland et al. 2001) or the European Score (deBacker et al. 2003). In addition, a family history of premature CHD certainly needs to be considered (Keevil et al. 2007; Nasir et al. 2004). In their most recent expert consensus statement, the leading American professional societies state: "The accumulating evidence suggests that asymptomatic individuals with an intermediate Framingham Risk Score may be reasonable candidates for CHD testing using coronary artery calcium as a potential means of modifying risk prediction and altering therapy" (Greenland et al. 2007). The statement published by the European societies reads: "The resulting calcium score is an important parameter to detect asymptomatic individuals at high risk for future cardiovascular disease events, independent of the traditional risk factors" (deBacker et al. 2003). In a large unselected European population in Germany, the Heinz Nixdorf Recall study demonstrated the impact of coronary calcium scoring on global risk assessment (Erbel et al. 2008). The majority of the subjects who had been classified as "intermediate risk" on the basis of the Framingham risk algorithm were reclassified on the basis o the coronary calcium score as having either a low risk (64%) or a high risk (32%).

Both the American and the European societies suggest that coronary calcium scanning in asymptomatic subjects with an indeterminate risk can be helpful for defining therapeutic aims and for guiding the intensity of medical therapy (deBacker et al. 2003; Greenland et al. 2007). Coronary calcium scanning does not appear to add useful prognostic information in subjects with a low cardiovascular risk on the basis of clinical data and the risk prediction algorithms. In high-risk subjects, coronary calcium scanning also appears unnecessary. The currently available data are insufficient to justify withholding therapy from high-risk patients who have no coronary calcium.

When defining a patient's individual risk, age and sex of the patient should be considered. Recent large population-based studies have provided "normograms" of calcium score distribution in the general population in the USA (Multi-Ethnic Study of Atherosclerosis) and in Europe (Heinz Nixdorf Recall Study) (McClelland et al. 2006, Schmermund et al. 2006a). These percentile values were calculated on the basis of EBCT studies. They appear to be very similar to values derived with four-slice spiral CT (Schmermund et al. 2002). However, with the ongoing scanner technology developments, there are dynamic changes in imaging parameters which need to be accounted for regarding the comparability and application of data from one system to another. Figures 4.4.4 and 4.4.5 show simple schemes for the indication and interpretation of coronary calcium scans in asymptomatic individuals.

In symptomatic individuals, coronary calcium scanning may be useful as a filter prior to invasive coronary angiography or stress nuclear imaging, because significant coronary stenoses are very unlikely in the absence of coronary calcium (Greenland et al. 2007). This also pertains to the examination of patients in the emergency room who have unexplained chest pain. However, the assessment of calcified plaques has clear limitations in a setting where it is the goal to rule out coronary stenoses. In rare instances, significant coronary stenoses can result from non-calcified plaque formation, being "silent" on a coronary calcium scan. Indeed, if coronary stenoses need to be ruled out with a high degree of certainty, CT coronary angiography may be preferable, as it also detects non-calcified plaque formation. Also, patients who are able to exercise should probably undergo exercise stress testing in the first line, because it provides inherently important prognostic information on cardiorespiratory fitness. Table 4.4.2 gives an overview of the current indications for coronary calcium scanning in asymptomatic and symptomatic patients.

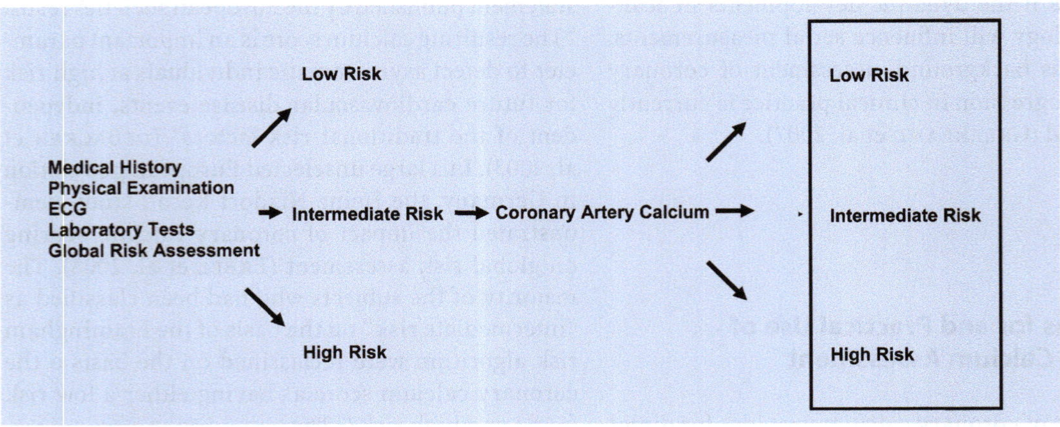

Fig. 4.4.4. Schematic representation of the indication for coronary calcium determination. The test can provide useful additional information in a subgroup of patients whose cardiovascular risk remains indeterminate after office-based risk assessment

Step I		Step II	
Coronary Calcium Score	Interpretation	Age- and sex-specific interpretation (Calcium Score percentiles)	Risk assessment
0 - 10	No/minimal plaque	0 - 25	Small risk
11 - 100	Some plaque present	26 - 50	Moderate risk
111 - 400	Moderate plaque burden	51 - 75	Moderately increased risk
401-1000	Extensive plaque burden	76 - 90	Increased risk
> 1000	Severe plaque burden	> 90	High risk

Fig. 4.4.5. The interpretation of the coronary artery calcium score can be carried out in two steps. In a first step, the overall amount of coronary calcium is assessed. In a second step, the percentile value of the calcium score is considered to put the amount of calcium in a perspective regarding other subjects of the same sex and age

Table 4.4.2. Indications for the use of CT coronary calcium scanning

Asymptomatic persons:	
1.	Specify cardiovascular risk in subjects with risk factors who cannot be determined by office-based risk assessment to have either a low or a high cardiovascular risk
2.	Specify cardiovascular risk in older subjects in whom the established risk factors lose some of their predictive value and whose risk remains indeterminate
3.	Identify subjects with an increased cardiovascular risk who might endanger others in the case of a clinical event (air travel, public traffic, high-risk environment)
4.	Subjects with markedly elevated levels of potential cardiovascular risk factors whose clinical impact remains uncertain such as lipoprotein(a), C-reactive protein, or homocysteine
Symptomatic persons:	
5.	Rule out calcified coronary atherosclerosis in patients with a low to intermediate likelihood of significant coronary stenoses to determine the necessity of further testing (myocardial perfusion study, coronary angiography)

References

Abizaid AS, Mintz GS, Abizaid A et al (1999) One-year follow-up after intravascular-ultrasound assessment of moderate left main coronary artery disease in patients with ambiguous angiograms. J Am Coll Cardiol 34:707–715

Achenbach S, Ropers D, Pohle K et al (2002) Influence of lipid-lowering therapy on the progression of coronary artery calcification: a prospective evaluation. Circulation 106:1077–1082

Ambrose JA, Tannenbaum MA, Alexopoulos D et al (1988) Angiographic progression of coronary artery disease and the development of myocardial infarction. J Am Coll Cardiol 12:56–62

Arad Y, Goodman KJ, Roth M, Newstein D, Guerci AD (2005a) Coronary calcification, coronary disease risk factors, C-reactive protein, and atherosclerotic cardiovascular disease events: the St. Francis Heart Study. J Am Coll Cardiol 46:158–165

Arad Y, Spadaro LA, Roth M et al (2005b) Treatment of asymptomatic adults with elevated coronary calcium scores with atorvastatin, vitamin C, and vitamin E. The St. Francis Heart Study randomized clinical trial. J Am Coll Cardiol 46:166–172

Beckman JA, Ganz J, Creager MA et al (2001) Relationship of clinical presentation and calcification of culprit coronary artery stenoses. Arterioscler Thromb Vasc Biol 21:1618–1622

Berman DS, Wong ND, Gransar H et al (2004) Relationship between stress-induced myocardial ischemia and atherosclerosis measured by coronary calcium tomography. J Am Coll Cardiol 44:923–30

Bielak LF, Sheedy PF II, Peyser PA (2001) Coronary artery calcification measured at electron-beam CT: agreement in dual scan runs and change over time. Radiology 218:224–229

Bocksch WG, Schartl M, Beckmann SH et al (1994) Intravascular ultrasound imaging in patients with acute myocardial infarction: comparison with chronic stable angina pectoris. Coron Artery Dis 5:727–735

Budoff MJ, Achenbach S, Blumenthal RS et al; American Heart Association Committee on Cardiovascular Imaging and Intervention; American Heart Association Council on Cardiovascular Radiology and Intervention; American Heart Association Committee on Cardiac Imaging, Council on Clinical Cardiology (2006) Assessment of coronary artery disease by cardiac computed tomography: a scientific statement from the American Heart Association Committee on Cardiovascular Imaging and Intervention, Council on Cardiovascular Radiology and Intervention, and Committee on Cardiac Imaging, Council on Clinical Cardiology. Circulation 114:1761–1791

Burke AP, Taylor A, Farb A et al (2000) Coronary calcification: insights from sudden coronary death victims. Z Kardiol 89:49–53

Burke AP, Kolodgie FD, Farb A et al (2001) Healed plaque ruptures and sudden coronary death: evidence that subclinical rupture has a role in plaque progression. Circulation 103:934–940

Burke AP, Kolodgie FD, Farb A et al (2002) Morphological predictors of arterial remodeling in coronary atherosclerosis. Circulation 105:297–303

Callister TQ, Raggi P, Cooil B et al (1998) Effect of HMG-CoA reductase inhibitors on coronary artery disease as assessed by electron-beam computed tomography. New Engl J Med 339:1972–1978

DeBacker G, Ambrosioni E, Borch-Johnsen K et al (2003) European guidelines on cardiovascular disease prevention in clinical practice. Third Joint Task Force of European and Other Societies on Cardiovascular Disease Prevention in Clinical Practice. Eur J Cardiovasc Prev Rehab 10:S1–S78

de Feyter PJ, Ozaki Y, Baptista J et al (1995) Ischemia-related lesion characteristics in patients with stable or unstable angina. A study with intracoronary angioscopy and ultrasound. Circulation 92:1408–1413

Detrano R, Hsiai T, Wang S et al (1996) Prognostic value of coronary calcification and angiographic stenoses in patients undergoing coronary angiography. J Am Coll Cardiol 27:285–290

Emond M, Mock MB, Davis KB et al (1994) Long-term survival of medically treated patients in the Coronary Artery Surgery Study (CASS) Registry. Circulation 90:2645–2657

Erbel R, Möhlenkamp S, Lehmann N et al; on behalf of the Heinz Nixdorf Recall Study Investigative Group (2008) Sex related cardiovascular risk stratification based on quantification of atherosclerosis and inflammation. Atherosclerosis 197:662–672

Farb A, Burke AP, Tang AL et al (1996) Coronary plaque erosion without rupture into a lipid core. A frequent cause of coronary thrombosis in sudden coronary death. Circulation 93:1354–1364

Georgiou D, Budoff MJ, Kaufer E et al (2001) Screening patients with chest pain in the emergency department using electron beam tomography: a follow-up study. J Am Coll Cardiol 38:105–110

Greenland P, Smith SC, Grundy SN (2001) Current perspective: improving coronary heart disease risk assessment in asymptomatic people. Role of traditional risk factors and noninvasive cardiovascular tests. Circulation 104:1863–1867

Greenland P, LaBree L, Azen SP et al (2004) Coronary artery calcium score combined with Framingham score for risk prediction in asymptomatic individuals. JAMA 291:210–215

Greenland P, Bonow RO, Brundage BH et al (2007) American College of Cardiology Foundation Clinical Expert Consensus Task Force (ACCF/AHA Writing Committee to Update the 2000 Expert Consensus Document on Electron Beam Computed Tomography); Society of Atherosclerosis Imaging and Prevention; Society of Cardiovascular Computed Tomography. ACCF/AHA 2007 clinical expert consensus document on coronary artery calcium scoring by computed tomography in global cardiovascular risk assessment and in evaluation of patients with chest pain: a report of the American College of Cardiology Foundation Clinical Expert Consensus Task Force (ACCF/AHA Writing Committee to Update the 2000 Expert Consensus Document on Electron Beam Computed Tomography). Circulation 115:402–426

He ZX, Hedrick TD, Pratt CM et al (2000) Severity of coronary artery calcification by electron beam computed tomography predicts silent myocardial ischemia. Circulation 101:244–251

Hoffmann B, Moebus S, Stang A et al; Heinz Nixdorf Recall Study Investigative Group (2006) Residence close to high traffic and prevalence of coronary heart disease. Eur Heart J 27:2696–2702

Houslay ES, Cowell SJ, Prescott RJ et al (2006) Progressive coronary calcification despite intensive lipid-lowering treatment: a randomised controlled trial. Heart 92:1207–1212

Kaski JC, Chester MR, Chen L et al (1995) Rapid angiographic progression of coronary artery disease in patients with angina pectoris. The role of complex stenosis morphology. Circulation 92:2058–2065

Keevil JG, Cullen MW, Gangnon R et al (2007) Implications of cardiac risk and low-density lipoprotein cholesterol distributions in the United States for the diagnosis and treatment of dyslipidemia. Data from National Health and Nutrition Examination Survey 1999 to 2002. Circulation 115:1363–1370

Kondos GT, Hoff JA, Sevrukov A et al (2003) Electron-beam tomography coronary artery calcium and cardiac events: a 37-month follow-up of 5635 initially asymptomatic low- to intermediate-risk adults. Circulation 107:2571–2576

LaMonte MJ, FitzGerald SJ, Church TS et al. (2005) Coronary artery calcium score and coronary heart disease events in a large cohort of asymptomatic men and women. Am J Epidemiol 162:421–429

Laudon DA, Vukov LF, Breen JF et al (1999) Use of electron-beam computed tomography in the evaluation of chest pain patients in the emergency department. Ann Emerg Med 33:15–21

Little WC, Constantinescu M, Applegate RJ et al (1988) Can coronary angiography predict the site of a subsequent myocardial infarction in patients with mild-to-moderate coronary artery disease? Circulation 78:1157–1166

Maher JE, Bielak LF, Raz JA et al (1999) Progression of coronary artery calcification: a pilot study. Mayo Clin Proc 74:347–355

McClelland RL, Chung H, Detrano R et al (2006) Distribution of coronary artery calcium by race, gender, and age: results from the Multi-Ethnic Study of Atherosclerosis (MESA). Circulation 113:30–37

McLaughlin VV, Balogh T, Rich S (1999) Utility of electron beam computed tomography to stratify patients presenting to the emergency room with chest pain. Am J Cardiol 84:327–328

Mintz GS, Pichard AD, Popma JJ et al (1997) Determinants and correlates of target lesion calcium in coronary artery disease: a clinical, angiographic and intravascular ultrasound study. J Am Coll Cardiol 29:268–274

Möhlenkamp S, Lehmann N, Schmermund A et al (2003) Prognostic value of extensive coronary calcium quantities in symptomatic males – a 5-year follow-up study. Eur Heart J 24:845–854

Nasir K, Michos ED, Rumberger JA et al (2004) Coronary artery calcification and family history of premature coronary heart disease: sibling history is more strongly associated than parental history. Circulation 110:2150–2156

Nicholls SJ, Tuzcu EM, Wolski K et al (2007) Coronary artery calcification and changes in atheroma burden in response to established medical therapies. J Am Coll Cardiol 49:263–270

Pletcher MJ, Tice JA, Pignone M et al (2004) Using the coronary artery calcium score to predict coronary heart disease events: a systematic review and meta-analysis. Arch Intern Med 164:1285–1292

Proudfit WL, Bruschke VG, Sones FM Jr (1980) Clinical course of patients with normal or slightly or moderately abnormal coronary arteriograms: 10-year follow-up of 521 patients. Circulation 62:712–717

Raggi P, Cooil B, Shaw LJ et al (2003) Progression of coronary calcium on serial electron beam tomographic scanning is greater in patients with future myocardial infarction. Am J Cardiol 92:827–829

Raggi P, Callister TQ, Shaw LJ (2004) Progression of coronary artery calcium and risk of first myocardial infarction in patients receiving cholesterol-lowering therapy. Arterioscler Thromb Vasc Biol 24:1272–1277

Raggi P, Davidson M, Callister TQ et al (2005). Aggressive versus moderate lipid-lowering therapy in hypercholesterolemic postmenopausal women: Beyond Endorsed Lipid Lowering with EBT Scanning (BELLES). Circulation 112:563–571

Rasheed Q, Nair R, Sheehan H et al (1994) Correlation of intracoronary ultrasound plaque characteristics in ath-

erosclerotic coronary artery disease patients with clinical variables. Am J Cardiol 73:753–758
Rumberger JA, Simons DB, Fitzpatrick LA et al (1995) Coronary artery calcium area by electron-beam computed tomography and coronary atherosclerotic plaque area. A histopathologic correlative study. Circulation 92:2157–2162
Schmermund A, Baumgart D, Görge G et al (1998) Measuring the effect of risk factors on coronary atherosclerosis: coronary calcium score vs. angiographic disease severity. J Am Coll Cardiol 31:1267–1273
Schmermund A, Denktas AE, Rumberger JA et al (1999) Independent and incremental value of coronary artery calcium for predicting the extent of angiographic coronary artery disease: comparison with cardiac risk factors and radionuclide perfusion imaging. J Am Coll Cardiol 34:777–786
Schmermund A, Erbel R (2001) Current perspective: unstable coronary plaque and its relation to coronary calcium. Circulation 104:1682–1687
Schmermund A, Schwartz RS, Adamzik M et al (2001a) Coronary atherosclerosis in unheralded sudden coronary death under age fifty: histo-pathologic comparison with "healthy" subjects dying out of hospital. Atherosclerosis 155:499–508
Schmermund A, Baumgart D, Möhlenkamp S et al (2001b) Natural history and topographic pattern of progression of coronary calcification in symptomatic patients: an electron-beam CT study. Arterioscler Thromb Vasc Biol 21:421–426
Schmermund A, Erbel R, Silber S (2002) Age and gender distribution of coronary artery calcium measured by four-slice computed tomography in 2,030 persons with no symptoms of coronary artery disease. Am J Cardiol 90:168–173
Schmermund A, Möhlenkamp S, Berenbein S et al (2006a) Population-based assessment of subclinical coronary atherosclerosis using electron-beam computed tomography. Atherosclerosis 185:177–182
Schmermund A, Achenbach S, Budde T et al (2006b) Effect of intensive versus standard lipid-lowering treatment with atorvastatin on the progression of calcified coronary atherosclerosis over 12 months: a multicenter, randomized, double-blind trial. Circulation 113:427–437
Shaw LJ, Raggi P, Schisterman E et al (2003) Prognostic value of cardiac risk factors and coronary artery calcium screening for all-cause mortality. Radiology 228:826–833
Taylor AJ, Bindeman J, Feuerstein I et al (2005) Coronary calcium independently predicts incident premature coronary heart disease over measured cardiovascular risk factors: mean three-year outcomes in the Prospective Army Coronary Calcium (PACC) project. J Am Coll Cardiol 46:807–814
Vliegenthart R, Oudkerk M, Hofman A et al (2005) Coronary calcification improves cardiovascular risk prediction in the elderly. Circulation 112:572–577
Ward MR, Pasterkamp G, Yeung AC et al (2000) Arterial remodeling. Mechanisms and clinical implications. Circulation 102:1186–1191
Waters D, Craven TE, Lespérance J (1993) Prognostic significance of progression of coronary atherosclerosis. Circulation 87:1067–1075
Yoon HC, Emerick AM, Hill JA et al (2002) Calcium begets calcium: progression of coronary artery calcification in asymptomatic subjects. Radiology 224:236–241

Non-Invasive Measurement of Coronary Atherosclerosis

4

4.5 Epidemiology of Coronary Calcification

Rozemarijn Vliegenthart Proença and Jacqueline C. M. Witteman

CONTENTS

R. Vliegenthart Proença, MD PhD
Department of Radiology, University Medical Center Groningen, University of Groningen, Hanzeplein 1, P. O. Box 30.001, 9700 RB Groningen, The Netherlands

J. C. M. Witteman, PhD
Associate Professor of Cardiovascular Epidemiology, Department of Epidemiology and Biostatistics, Erasmus MC, P. O. Box 1738, 3000 DR Rotterdam, The Netherlands

4.5.1 The Prevalence of Coronary Calcification

The amount of coronary calcification detected by electron-beam computed tomography (EBCT) depends on sex and age. Studies among populations of asymptomatic subjects have shown that men generally have higher calcium scores than women and that calcium scores increase with age (Hoff et al. 2001; Rumberger et al. 2003; Schmermund et al. 2006a; McClelland et al. 2006). Table 4.5.1 shows sex- and age-stratified calcium score nomogram of the largest study, which comprises 35,246 self-referred subjects (Hoff et al. 2001). Different studies have found that up to half of all men already have detectable coronary calcification before the age of 50. By the age of 65 years, almost all men have a positive calcium score. The median calcium score for men at the age of 65 years is at least 100, with a wide and skewed distribution. The prevalence of coronary calcium is much lower for relatively young women: only up to 25% of women have any coronary calcium before the age of 50. By the age of 75, coronary calcification is as ubiquitous for women as for men. However, at any age, the distribution of calcium scores is much lower for women than for men. Calcium scores in women are comparable to calcium scores in men who are 10–15 years younger. For example, the median calcium score for women aged 65 years is only 10–20. In Figure 4.5.1, median calcium score values from the different studies are depicted for men and women, per age category (Schmermund et al. 2006a). Depending on the specific characteristics of the study population, some median values differ. Compared to population-based studies, self-referred cohorts generally yield somewhat higher median calcium scores for men at higher ages and women at lower ages. Possible explanations for these differences include selection of study participants, geographic

Table 4.5.1. Electron-beam computed tomography calcium score percentiles for 25,251 men and 9995 women within age strata. [Reprinted from Hoff et al. (2001) with permission]

Calcium scores	Age (years)								
	<40	40–44	45–49	50–54	55–59	60–64	65–69	70–74	>74
Men (*n*)	3504	4238	4940	4825	3472	2288	1209	540	235
25th Percentile	0	0	0	1	4	13	32	64	166
50th Percentile	1	1	3	15	48	113	180	310	473
75th Percentile	3	9	36	103	215	410	566	892	1071
90th Percentile	14	59	154	332	554	994	1299	1774	1982
Women (*n*)	641	1024	1634	2184	1835	1334	731	438	174
25th Percentile	0	0	0	0	0	0	1	3	9
50th Percentile	0	0	0	0	1	3	24	52	75
75th Percentile	1	1	2	5	23	57	145	210	241
90th Percentile	3	4	22	55	121	193	410	631	709

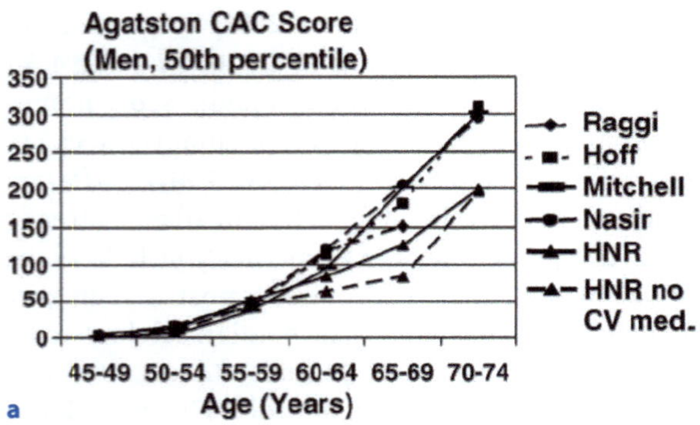

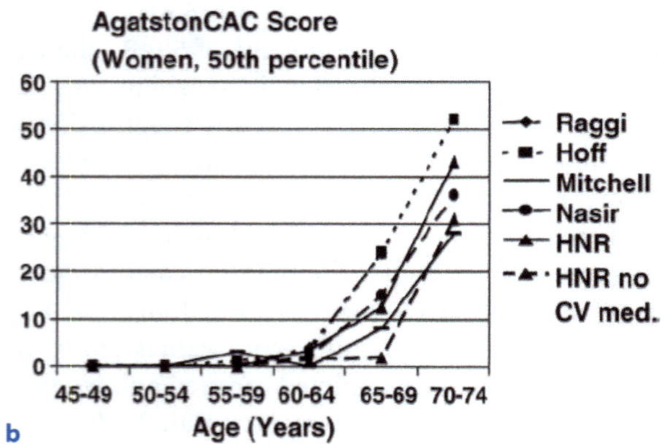

Fig. 4.5.1a,b. Median coronary calcium scores in men (**a**) and in women (**b**) in different cohort studies: Raggi et al. (2000), Hoff et al. (2001), Mitchell et al. (2001), Nasir et al. (2004a), HNR: Heinz Nixdorf Recall Study, HNR no CV med: Heinz Nixdorf Recall study population without cardiovascular medication (both from Schmermund et al. 2006a). [Reprinted from Schmermund et al. (2006a) with permission]

differences and differences in prescription of cardiovascular medication.

Although the amount of coronary calcification increases with age, age itself should not be considered as a risk factor for coronary calcification. Rather, the effect of age is to a great extent due to the cumulative measure of exposure to cardiovascular risk factors.

4.5.2 Cardiovascular Risk Factors and Coronary Calcification

It has been known for decades that cardiovascular risk factors like smoking, hypertension, hypercholesterolemia, obesity and diabetes increase the risk of coronary heart disease (CHD), mostly through initiating and accelerating the development of atherosclerosis. These risk factors are also called traditional risk factors. More recently, studies have identified new risk markers for cardiovascular disease like C-reactive protein (CRP), fibrinogen and homocysteine. There is clear evidence that conventional risk factors are associated with the presence and amount of coronary calcification. In a self-referred screening population of more than 30,000 subjects aged 30–90 years (mean age, 51 years), the mean calcium score increased with increasing number of conventional risk factors (Hoff et al. 2003). Significant associations were present with self-reported hypertension, smoking, hypercholesterolemia and diabetes. In the Rotterdam Coronary Calcification Study among elderly subjects (mean age, 71 years), risk factors assessed 7 years before scanning were strongly associated with coronary calcification (Oei et al. 2004). However, associations with blood pressure and cholesterol disappeared when measured concurrently to scanning, probably due to the decreasing predictive value of risk factors with increasing age. Remarkably, without risk factors, a high calcium score, above 400, was present in about 30% of men and 15% of women. In the following paragraphs, we will discuss the association between the separate conventional and newer risk factors and coronary calcification.

Pathology studies in the 1970s already showed that smoking increases the amount of coronary and aortic atherosclerosis (Strong and Richards 1976). The development of EBCT offered the opportunity to study the association of smoking and coronary atherosclerosis in vivo. In a population-based study among 740 adults between 20 and 59 years of age, Maher et al. (1996) showed that subjects with a history of smoking have higher calcium scores than subjects who never smoked. In a multivariate model a history of smoking was only in men associated with coronary calcification. In the study by Hoff et al. (2003), the percentage of ever smokers increased from 43% and 46% among men and women without coronary calcium to 65% and 59% in case of a high calcium score (2003). In elderly, smoking, expressed as the number of pack-years smoked, is still associated with coronary calcification (Newman et al. 2001; Oei et al. 2004). On the other hand, studies using intravascular ultrasound to detect coronary calcification in patients who underwent coronary angiography found a similar or even lower amount of calcification in smokers than in non-smokers (Tuzcu et al. 1996; Mintz et al. 1997; Kornowski 1999). This apparent contradiction is likely due to selection bias. Therefore, the results of the latter studies cannot be extrapolated to the general population.

Blood pressure is positively and linearly related to cardiovascular disease (Stokes et al. 1989). A net reduction of 5–6 mm Hg in diastolic blood pressure is associated with a 38% reduction in stroke risk and a 16% reduction in CHD risk (Stokes et al. 1989). Furthermore, hypertension is an important risk factor for atherosclerosis at extracoronary sites (Bots et al. 1992; O'Leary et al. 1992). Population-based studies have shown that systolic blood pressure and diastolic blood pressure are important risk factors for coronary calcification (Maher et al. 1996; Mahoney et al. 1996; Megnien et al. 1996; Arad et al. 2001; Bielak et al. 2004). Adults with coronary calcification have a higher systolic blood pressure and a higher diastolic blood pressure than adults without any coronary calcification. Adults above the 90th percentile of systolic blood pressure have been shown to be at least six times more likely to have coronary calcification, with corresponding relative risks for diastolic blood pressure of 4 for men and 3 for women (Mahoney et al. 1996). While coronary calcification is positively associated with both systolic and diastolic blood pressure below the age of 50 years, the positive association remains only for systolic blood pressure above 50 years, favoring pulse pressure as the best predictor of coronary calcium (Bielak et al. 2004). Analogous to the attenuation of the predictive value of hypertension for CHD in the very elderly, no association of hypertension and coronary calcification was found in subjects with a mean age of 80 years (Newman et al. 2001).

Compared to subjects who have cholesterol levels below 5.0 mmol/l, the risk of CHD is three-fold greater among subjects who have cholesterol levels between 6.5 mmol/l and 7.9 mmol/l and five-fold greater among subjects who have cholesterol levels >8.0 mmol/l (Jousilahti et al. 1998). In the study by Hoff et al. (2003), the percentage of hypercholesterolemia increased from 31% and 33% among men and women without coronary calcium to 42% and 52% in case of a high calcium score. Population-based studies with an age range of 20–74 years have shown that LDL cholesterol, triglycerides and cholesterol/HDL cholesterol ratio are positively associated with coronary calcification while HDL cholesterol is inversely associated with coronary calcification in both men and women (Maher et al. 1996; Arad et al. 2001; Allison et al. 2003; Allison and Wright 2004a). However, in the elderly an association between concurrently measured cholesterol and coronary calcification is lacking (Newman et al. 2001; Oei et al. 2004). In the MESA study, a multicenter study of 6814 participants, it was found that many drug-eligible persons with considerable coronary calcium are not treated with lipid-lowering therapy, while many persons who do not qualify for drug treatment have considerable coronary calcium (Goff et al. 2006). Thus, information on the severity of coronary calcification may improve the ability to predict who will benefit from lipid-lowering therapy.

Oxidation of LDL has been proposed as an intermediary step in the causal chain from risk factors to the development of subclinical cardiovascular disease. In the MESA study, persons with coronary calcification were found to have higher levels of oxidized LDL (Holvoet et al. 2006). Lipoprotein-associated phospholipase A2, a new predictor of cardiovascular disease, possibly exerts its effect through enhancement of the pro-inflammatory properties of oxidized LDL-cholesterol (Kardys et al. 2006). LDL-cholesterol to which a protein (a) is bound, also known as lipoprotein (a), has been established as an independent risk factor for coronary heart disease. Studies in which the relationship between lipoprotein (a) and coronary calcification was examined, generally showed no association between the two, suggesting that lipoprotein (a) influences lesion stability or susceptibility to thrombosis rather than the development of the atherosclerotic lesion (Nishino et al. 2000; Guerra et al. 2005).

Subjects with obesity have a relative risk of 2–2.5 for CHD as compared to subjects without obesity (Hubert et al. 1983). Studies in young to middle-aged populations have shown a strong relationship between measures of obesity and coronary calcification. Body mass index, waist to hip ratio, abdominal height and intra-abdominal fat are all associated with the amount of coronary calcification (Maher et al. 1996; Arad et al. 2001). In contrast, in elderly individuals body mass index shows a weak or no correlation with calcification (Newman et al. 2001; Oei et al. 2004). Whether the weaker association between obesity and coronary calcification in the elderly is caused by selection due to survival, by frailty due to underlying disease (e.g. cancer) or by another underlying mechanism is unclear.

There is a remarkable disparity between men and women with respect to measures of body morphology and coronary calcification (Allison and Michael Wright 2004b). The relationship between body mass index and the calcium score is much stronger for men than for women. Central adiposity was related to coronary calcification in men only, but not as strong as the body mass index. CT-based measures of abdominal fat do not seem to be superior to body mass index or waist circumference as risk factors to explain the presence of coronary calcium (Snell-Bergeon et al. 2004).

Studies on type II diabetes and coronary calcification consistently show that the prevalence and extent of coronary calcification is increased in diabetics (Schurgin et al. 2001; Mielke et al. 2001; Meigs et al. 2002; Hoff et al. 2003; Wong et al. 2003a). Table 4.5.2 shows calcium scores for diabetics and non-diabetics in different age-categories, by gender. Men with diabetes have higher calcium scores than men without diabetes. Similarly, women with diabetes have higher calcium scores than women without diabetes (Hoff et al. 2003). Compared to individuals without type II diabetes, patients are 70% more likely to have any coronary calcium (Wong et al. 2003a) and 70% more likely to have a calcium score in the highest age/gender quartile (Hoff et al. 2003). Whether the association between diabetes and coronary calcium persists at old age is unclear. While one population-based study (mean age, 71 years) showed a positive association between diabetes and the calcium score (Oei et al. 2004), another study in an even older population (mean age, 80 years) showed no association between diabetes mellitus and coronary calcification. Insulin resistance also shows an association with subclinical coronary atherosclerosis (Arad et al. 2001; Meigs et al. 2002). Insulin resistance is correlated with a constellation of abnormalities, including central adiposity, lipid abnormalities, hypertension and hypercoagulability – known together as the metabolic syndrome. In a population with a mean age of 53 years, the prevalence of coronary calcium increased with the number of risk factors for the metabolic syndrome, from 34% for 0 risk factors to 58% for five risk factors (Wong et al. 2003a).

The prevalence of coronary calcification is not only increased in patients with type II diabetes, but also in type I diabetics (Dabelea et al. 2003). In type I diabetes, coronary calcium is detected already in the third decade of life in a considerable proportion of patients. The gender difference in the presence of coronary calcium is smaller in case of type I diabetes than in the general population (Colhoun et al. 2000). Type I diabetes increases coronary calcification relatively more in women than in men, possibly related to gender differences in insulin resistance in these patients (Dabelea et al. 2003).

Population-based follow-up studies have shown that moderate alcohol consumption diminishes the risk of CHD (Hennekens et al. 1978; Klatsky et al. 1981; Suh et al. 1992; Camargo et al. 1997; Yang et al. 1999). Although it has been postulated that alcohol increases HDL cholesterol levels, the mechanism by which alcohol intake exerts this effect is not well understood. Conflicting results have been found in studies examining the relationship between alcohol consumption and coronary atherosclerosis. In

Table 4.5.2. Median coronary artery calcium (CAC) scores in men and women with and without diabetes. [Reprinted from HOFF et al. (2003) with permission]

	Diabetes		No Diabetes		
	Median CAC		Median CAC		
Men	**n**	**Score**	**n**	**Score**	**pValue**
Age group (years)					
<40	46	4	3,005	1	<0.001
40–44	63	13	3,653	1	<0.001
45–49	100	9.5	4,322	3	0.001
50–54	144	42	4,142	14	<0.001
60–64	117	192	1,860	105	<0.001
65–69	72	378	955	152	<0.001
≥70	45	343	592	301	0.77
Total	**747**	**63**	**21,441**	**6**	**<0.001**

	Diabetes		No Diabetes		
	Median CAC		Median CAC		
Women	**n**	**Score**	**n**	**Score**	**pValue**
Age group (years)					
<40	21	1	514	0	<0.001
40–44	32	0	846	0	0.14
45–49	32	1	1,398	0	0.01
50–54	74	8.5	1,826	0	<0.001
55–59	52	7.5	1,522	1	<0.001
60–64	47	21	1,105	2	0.003
65–69	34	104	712	5	0.006
≥70	36	114	465	52	0.54
Total	**328**	**5**	**8,388**	**1**	**<0.001**

The Mann-Whitney *U* test was used to compare coronary artery calcium (CAC) scores between diabetic and nondiabetic subjects within each five-year age group. the analyses were performed separately for men and women

the Rotterdam Coronary Calcification Study, a u-shaped association was reported, with the largest reduction in risk of extensive coronary calcification at a consumption level of one to two drinks per day (VLIEGENTHART et al. 2004). The protective effect was most prominent for wine types of alcoholic beverages. In contrast, two studies in younger populations found no inverse relation between alcohol intake and coronary calcification (TOFFERI et al. 2004; PLETCHER et al. 2005). In these studies, increasing number of drinks per day was associated with an increasing prevalence of coronary calcium. Also binge drinking (>five drinks on one day) increased the risk of coronary calcification (PLETCHER et al. 2005). In a large population-based study among white and African American subjects with a mean age of 56 years, no beneficial effect of alcohol on the extent of coronary calcification was found (ELLISON et al. 2006). Possibly different beverage preferences may have led to these contrasting results.

Inflammatory markers, like CRP and fibrinogen, are blood measurements that have recently gained interest as possible new variables for prediction of cardiovascular disease. The most studied inflammatory protein so far is CRP. CRP is a sensitive marker of inflammation that increases the risk of CHD in healthy subjects (Ridker et al. 1997, 1998a,b), in patients with stable and unstable angina pectoris (Liuzzo et al. 1994; Thompson et al. 1995; Haverkate et al. 1997), and in high-risk patients (Kuller et al. 1996). In addition, CRP has been related both cross-sectionally and prospectively to peripheral arterial disease (Ridker et al. 1998c; Erren et al. 1999). However, CRP is not associated with the amount of coronary calcification in most studies (Redberg et al. 2000; Bielak et al. 2000; Hunt et al. 2001; Newman et al. 2001; Reilly et al. 2003; Khera et al. 2006). Only one study found a modest correlation between high CRP levels and the calcium score (Wang et al. 2002). By far the largest study, among more than 3300 participants of the population-based Dallas Heart Study, found some increase in the extent of coronary calcification in subjects with higher CRP levels, but this association was explained by traditional cardiovascular risk factors (Khera et al. 2006). As a possible explanation for the lack of the association, it has been suggested that high-sensitivity CRP reflects an underlying propensity to plaque instability rather than overall atherosclerotic plaque burden (Khera et al. 2006).

Increased plasma fibrinogen concentration is related to an increased risk of cardiovascular disease (Danesh et al. 1998; Maresca et al. 1999). There are several mechanisms by which fibrinogen may increase the risk of cardiovascular disease. Fibrinogen is the main coagulation protein in plasma, is an important determinant of blood viscosity and can act as a cofactor for platelet aggregation (Meade et al. 1986; Maresca et al. 1999). Fibrinogen may also contribute to cardiovascular disease by other direct effects: it is a component of atherosclerotic plaques and stimulates smooth muscle cell migration and proliferation (Meade et al. 1986). Furthermore, the correlation with CRP suggests that fibrinogen reflects the inflammatory activity of progressing atherosclerosis (Folsom et al. 1997). Studies on the association of fibrinogen and coronary calcification have found conflicting results. A population-based study in 114 men and 114 women found that subjects who were selected on the basis of their high calcium score had higher fibrinogen than the control group (Bielak et al. 2000). In addition, a study in hypercholesterolemic patients found that fibrinogen was positively associated with coronary calcification (Levenson et al. 1997). However, other studies were not able to confirm these findings (Hunt et al. 2001; Newman et al. 2001). In conclusion, studies have suggested that fibrinogen may play a role in the process of atherosclerosis. Larger population-based studies have to be awaited before conclusions can be drawn on the association of fibrinogen and coronary calcification.

Although elevated serum homocysteine levels have been shown to correlate with CHD risk in cross-sectional studies, results from prospective studies are conflicting (Pearson 2002). A meta-analysis of 57 studies showed that homocysteine is only weakly related to CHD and somewhat more strongly related to cerebrovascular disease (Ford et al. 2002). Although recent experimental studies have shown that hyperhomocysteinemia is atherogenic, at least at early stages and in the presence of another potent risk factor (Hofmann et al. 2001; Zhou et al. 2001), most epidemiologic studies found no effect of serum homocysteine levels on coronary calcification (Mahoney et al. 1996; Superko and Hecht 2001; Taylor et al. 2001). However, in the largest study so far, including 1071 participants, homocysteine did show a correlation with the extent of coronary calcium (Kullo et al. 2006a), even after adjusting for conventional cardiovascular risk factors. Only in subjects at intermediate risk of coronary heart disease, based on risk factor levels, was an association present. In a study among patients with type II diabetes, a positive correlation between homocysteine and the calcium score was found, but the association disappeared after adjusting for risk factors (Godsland et al. 2006). The significance and clinical utility of homocysteine needs to be resolved.

Whether a family history of premature CHD is associated with coronary calcium is still unclear. The limited number of published studies showed differing results. A screening study showed a significant association between family history and the prevalence and extent of coronary calcification, stronger for a sibling history than for a parental history (Nasir et al. 2004b). Another study found a positive correlation for African-Americans, but not for Caucasians (Fornage et al. 2004). However, in a large predominantly Caucasian population, Hoff et al. (2003) found a positive, albeit moderate, association between family history and the extent of coronary calcium.

Various psychological and socio-economic factors are associated with coronary heart disease. One of the proposed pathways is increased atherogenesis. Studies examining the relationship of psychosocial risk factors to coronary calcium have yielded conflicting results. In a study of almost 800 individuals (mean age, 57 years), social network indices such as being single or widowed were associated with coronary calcification (Kop et al. 2005). The larger the social network, the lower the likelihood of coronary calcium being present. Socioeconomic status and depressive symptoms were not related to the presence of coronary calcification. In contrast, educational attainment, a correlate of socioeconomic status, was found to be inversely related to the prevalence of coronary calcium in two other studies among young adults and postmenopausal women (Gallo et al. 2001; Yan et al. 2006).

While single studies in different study populations showed a positive association of coronary calcium with hostility, depression and type A (coronary-prone) behaviour (Iribarren et al. 2000; Sparagon et al. 2001; Agatisa et al. 2005), the largest study so far found no correlation between the prevalence and extent of coronary calcification and depression, anxiety, hostility and stress (Diez Roux et al. 2006). Also a study among active army personnel found no associations (O'Malley et al. 2000). Thus, further research is needed to determine whether, and in which populations, psychosocial factors influence the development and progression of subclinical coronary atherosclerosis.

4.5.3 Ethnic Differences in Coronary Calcification

There are remarkable ethnic differences in the prevalence, progression, and risk of CHD. Pathological studies have found more extensive fatty streaks in the coronary arteries of African-American individuals than of Caucasians (McGill and Strong 1968; Freedman et al. 1988; Strong et al. 1999) but a similar amount of raised lesions (Strong et al. 1999), which are likely to contain calcium. In contrast, large US-based studies have shown that Caucasian men have the highest prevalence of coronary calcification compared to men from other ethnicities after controlling for risk factors (Bild et al. 2005; McClelland et al. 2006; Orakzai et al. 2006). Overall, compared to Caucasians, the prevalence and extent of coronary calcification is lowest for African-Americans, followed by Chinese and then by Hispanics. It is preferable to evaluate the amount of coronary calcification according to race-specific distributions of the calcium score. Tools are available on the internet to obtain a percentile of the calcium score for a specific combination of age, gender and race (McClelland et al. 2006). Among women from different ethnic groups, very little or no differences in coronary calcium are generally seen. Interestingly, African-American individuals have higher incidences of CHD, despite similar (women) or lower (men) calcium scores. The explanation for this difference is unclear. Possibly, ethnic differences in the process of calcifying plaques play a role (Doherty et al. 1999).

4.5.4 Coronary Calcification and Risk of Manifest Atherosclerotic Disease

The most important cause of morbidity and mortality in individuals with cardiovascular risk factors is coronary atherosclerosis. Atherosclerotic plaques in a coronary artery can rupture or erode, which can lead to thrombosis and partial or complete occlusion of the culprit artery. If occlusion of the coronary artery lasts for some time, ischemia and subsequently infarction of the cardiac tissue, which is normally nourished by the culprit artery, can occur – causing a coronary event. Most subjects at risk do not develop symptoms of coronary artery disease (CAD) until the occurrence of acute myocardial infarction or sudden cardiac death. The ability to predict and prevent the majority of coronary events is limited. Research has shown that asymptomatic individuals at risk benefit from aggressive risk factor modification or further testing (Grover et al. 1995). A commonly used method to assess cardiovascular risk is the Framingham risk score. This is an office-based scoring algorithm based on risk factors. According to the Framingham risk score, asymptomatic individuals are stratified into low, intermediate or high risk of CHD. However, risk factor assessment to identify high-risk subgroups is neither highly sensitive nor highly specific (Grover et al. 1995): many individuals, considered to be at high risk of a coronary event will not experience myocardial infarction or sudden cardiac death, while many other subjects, considered to be low-risk, will suffer a coronary event. Thus, there is a clear need for new strategies for the primary prevention of CAD. In recent years, an alternative approach to risk stratification has been proposed: noninvasive evaluation of coronary calcification by EBCT. This strategy is based on the close histopathological correlation between coronary calcium deposits and the total amount of coronary atherosclerosis (Rumberger et al. 1995).

To draw conclusions about the possible clinical use of the calcium score, prospective results from large follow-up studies in unselected populations are of utmost importance (Wexler et al. 1996). In recent years a number of studies have been published on the prognostic value of coronary calcification for coronary events in asymptomatic subjects – see the overview provided in Table 4.5.3.

In a study by Arad et al. (2000) 39 coronary events were observed in 1172 asymptomatic subjects (mean age 53 years) during an average follow-up of 3.6 years. The population consisted of subjects who were either referred by physicians or self-referred in response to advertisements. The 39 events included three sudden cardiac deaths, 15 (nonfatal) myocardial infarctions, and 21 revascularizations. The mean calcium score among subjects with events was much higher than the mean calcium score among subjects without events (764 ± 935 vs. 135 ± 432). A calcium score above 160 was associated with an odds ratio of all coronary events of 15.8 (CI, 7.4–33.9), while the odds ratio of only myocardial infarction and coronary death was 22.2 (CI, 6.4–77.4). Wong et al. (2000) observed in a study among 926 self-referred and GP-referred subjects a relative risk of cardiovascular events of 8.8 in the highest calcium score quartile compared to subjects without coronary calcification. However, of the 28 cardiovascular events that occurred during a mean of 3.3 years after scanning, 23 were revascularizations. Referral bias could have influenced the results since revascularizations may partially have taken place on the basis of a high calcium score. Raggi et al. (2000) reported a relative risk of 21.5 (95% CI, 2.8–162.4) for myocardial infarction or cardiac death in the fourth quartile of the calcium score when compared to the lowest quartile. The subjects in the study population were referred for scanning because of the presence of cardiovascular risk factors. The investigation was based on calcium scores of 632 subjects (mean age 52 years) and 27 coronary events in 32 months. In two large screening studies among 5635 and 10,746 subjects by Kondos et al. (2003) and LaMonte et al. (2005), respectively, 224 and 287 participants experienced an event during the follow-up period of 3–3.5 years. Strong associations between the calcium score and coronary events were found in men, with relative risks of the highest quartile and tertile, respectively, were 7.2 and 61.7 (versus a calcium score of 0). Interestingly, in a further analysis of the latter screening population (Church et al. 2007), a calcium score of zero was associated with a very low risk of coronary events, irrespective of the number of risk factors present. Statistical power enabled only LaMonte et al. (2005) to investigate relative risks in women. In gender-specific tertiles of non-zero calcium scores, lower relative risks were found for women than for men. However, the distribution of calcium scores for women was much lower than for men. In both screening studies, the majority of events concerned revascularizations, possibly due to referral bias. This limits the validity of the results.

Most of the aforementioned prospective studies were performed in populations of self-referred or physician-referred individuals. This is usually not a reflection of the general population, since referral for an EBCT examination may occur because of the presence of risk factors, or due to health-consciousness of asymptomatic persons. In these studies, risk factors were generally obtained by questionnaires or interviews, not by actual measurement. It is known that self-report may lead to misclassification of risk factors. Many individuals are unaware of the presence of risk factors like hypertension or hypercholesterolemia.

Recently, studies have been published in study populations that are more reflective of (a part of) the general population. In these studies, cardiovascular risk factors were measured [in the study by Arad (2005a) in part of the population]. In the South Bay Heart Watch Study, 1029 high-risk asymptomatic subjects without diabetes (mean age 66 years) were followed during more than 6 years (Greenland et al. 2004). The majority of the population was male. During the follow-up time, 84 myocardial infarctions and coronary deaths occurred. In this study, the predictive value of the calcium score was compared to that of the Framingham risk score. The calcium score was found to be an independent predictor of coronary events. Across categories of the Framingham risk score, the calcium score was predictive of risk among individuals with an intermediate and high Framingham risk score, but not in case of a low risk score. In the intermediate risk group, the extent of coronary calcification significantly modified the risk prediction, and allowed further categorization of these individuals into low or high

Table 4.5.3. Relative risks of coronary calcification for coronary heart disease in prospective electron-beam computed tomography studies

Study	Subjects (n)	Age (years, mean ± SD)	Population characteristics	Risk factors measured or reported	Mean follow-up (months); % compl.	Events (n); types (n)	Calcium score cut-off	Relative risk (95% CI)[b]
Arad et al. (2000)	1173 71% Male	53±11	Self-referred or referred by physician	Reported	43; 100	39; Nonfatal MI (15), CHD death (3), revascularization (21)	>80 (vs <80) >160 (vs <160) >600 (vs <600)	14.3 (4.9–42.3) 19.7 (6.9–56.4) 20.2 (7.3–55.8)
Wong et al. (2000)[a]	926 79% Male	54±10	Self-referred or referred by physician	Reported	40; 61	28; Nonfatal MI (6), revascularization (20), also included stroke (2)	0 Quartiles: Q1 (1–15) Q2 (16–80) Q3 (81–270) Q4 (>270)	1.0 (reference) 0.7 (0.1–6.6) 3.3 (0.9–12.8) 4.5 (1.2–16.8) 8.8 (2.2–35.1)
Raggi et al. (2000)	632 50% Male	52±9	Referred by physician because of risk factors	Reported	37; nr	27; Nonfatal MI (21), CHD death (8)	Quartiles: Q1 (nr) Q2 Q3 Q4	 1.0 (reference) 1.0 (0.1–16.1) 6.2 (0.7–52.1) 21.5 (2.8–162.4)
Kondos et al. (2003)	5635 74% Male	51±9	Self-referred	Reported	37; 64	224; Nonfatal MI (37), CHD death (21), revascularization (166)	In men:[c] 0 Quartiles: Q1 (1–4) Q2 (4–31) Q3 (31–169) Q4 (≥170)	 1.0 (reference) 1.8 (0.4–7.9) 2.8 (0.7–11.1) 5.6 (1.6–20.1) 7.2 (2.0–26.2)
LaMonte et al. (2005)	10746 64% Male	54±10	Preventive health examination, self-referred or referred by physician	Measured in 3619, in the others reported	42; 70	287; Nonfatal MI (62), CHD death (19), revascularization (206)	In men: 0 Tertiles: T1 (1–38) T2 (39–249) T3 (≥250) In women: 0 Tertiles: T1 (1–16) T2 (17–112) T3 (≥113)	1.0 (reference) 5.0 (1.8–13.8) 18.5 (7.3–46.6) 61.7 (24.7–153.7) 1.0 (reference) 1.8 (0.6–5.5) 3.7 (1.5–9.2) 6.2 (2.7–14.4)
Greenland et al. (2004)	1029 90% Male	66±8	South Bay Heart Watch Study, at least one risk factor, diabetics excluded	Measured	76; 88	84; Nonfatal MI and CHD death (84)	0 1–100 101–300 >300	1.0 (reference) 1.5 (0.7–2.9) 2.1 (1.0–4.3) 3.9 (2.1–7.3)
Arad et al. (2005b)	4613 65% Male	59±6	St Francis Heart Study, 50–70 years	Measured in random sample of 1293	52; 94	99; Nonfatal MI and CHD death (40), revascularization (59)	0 1–99 100–399 ≥400	1.0 (reference) 1.9 (0.8–4.2) 10.2 (4.8–21.6) 26.2 (12.6–53.7)
Vliegenthart et al. (2005)	1795 49% Male	71±6	Rotterdam Coronary Calcification Study, general population of elderly	Measured	40; 100	51; Nonfatal MI and CHD death (40), revascularization (11)	0–100 101–400 401–1000 >1000	1.0 (reference) 3.1 (1.2–7.9) 4.6 (1.8–11.8) 8.3 (3.3–21.1)
Taylor et al. (2005)	1983 82% Male	43±3	PACC Project, active-duty army personnel, 40–50 years	Measured	36; 99	9; Nonfatal MI, CHD death, and unstable angina (9)	In men:[c] > 0 (vs 0)	10.8 (2.2–51.8)

nr, Not reported. MI, myocardial infarction; CHD, coronary heart disease.
[a] Confidence intervals as reported by Pletcher et al. (2004). [b] Analyses adjusted for age, gender, and cardiovascular risk factors, except Greenland and Arad (2005): univariate analysis. [c] Relative risks not reported for women due to lack of power.

risk. Thus, it was concluded that calcium scoring can significantly alter clinical decision making. The authors refuted the notion that absence of coronary calcium precludes the risk of CHD, pointing to 14 coronary events in the group of 316 subjects with a calcium score of 0. However, in this study a scan protocol was used with a lower sensitivity for calcified plaques (6-mm slices instead of 3-mm slices). Thus, the amount of coronary calcification may have been underestimated, causing subjects to be falsely classified as having no calcium. The St Francis Heart Study is a study among 4903 asymptomatic individuals, aged 50–70 years. At 4.3 years, 119 of the 4613 subjects with complete follow-up suffered from CHD, stroke or peripheral vascular surgery (Arad et al. 2005a). The calcium score was a strong predictor of events, independent of traditional risk factors and CRP levels. Furthermore, the predictive power of the calcium score exceeded that of the Framingham risk score, and improved cardiovascular risk stratification of subjects falling into the intermediate or high risk category on the basis of risk factors. The table reports the main result for coronary events alone. So far the only truly population-based study with prospective results is the Rotterdam Coronary Calcification Study, a study among elderly taking part in the Rotterdam Study. In this study among 1795 asymptomatic elderly (mean age, 71 years) with a follow-up period of 3.3 years, a strong association was found between the calcium score and the risk of CHD, with relative risks up to 8.3 for a calcium score over 1000 compared to a calcium score between 0 and 100 (Vliegenthart et al. 2005). Risk prediction based on the Framingham risk score became more accurate when coronary calcification was added to risk assessment. The calcium score is not only predictive in older, but also in younger populations. In a study among mainly male army personnel, aged 40–50 years, nine coronary events occurred during 3 years of follow-up (Taylor et al. 2005). Compared to absence of coronary calcium, a calcium score above 0 increased the risk of CHD almost 11 times, independently of the Framingham risk score and a family history of CHD. The paucity of events diminished the ability to control for risk factors and diminished the precision of risk estimates. Finally, a large screening study among 10,377 individuals including 903 diabetics, showed that the calcium score also has predictive power in patients with diabetes, who are generally considered to be at high risk of CHD (Raggi et al. 2004a). In this study all-cause mortality was used as outcome measure. With increasing extent of coronary calcification, the risk of mortality increased more in diabetics compared to non-diabetics. Interestingly, in the case of a calcium score of 0, the short-term risk of death was similar for the two groups. Further studies should investigate whether the same is true in case of CHD events. Possibly, the notion of diabetes as a CAD equivalent may not apply in diabetic patients without coronary calcium.

Atherosclerosis is thought to be a generalized process. Manifestations of atherosclerosis not only occur in the coronary arteries but also at other sites of the vascular tree, such as the arteries in the leg (manifest as intermittent claudication), and the carotid or cerebral arteries (transient ischemic attack or stroke). Since calcification of the coronary arteries is also a marker of the amount of atherosclerosis elsewhere in the vessels, detection of the amount of coronary calcification could be related to manifestations of atherosclerosis distant from the heart. Vliegenthart et al. (2002) showed an association between the amount of coronary calcification and the presence of stroke in the Rotterdam Coronary Calcification Study. People whose calcium score was high (above 500) were three times more likely to have experienced stroke, compared to those with low calcium scores (0–100). Those with an intermediate score (101–500) were twice as likely to have had a stroke in comparison to the reference category. The results support the view that similar processes underlie CHD and stroke. More study is needed to determine if people with high levels of coronary calcification are at an increased risk of stroke.

It can be concluded that the amount of coronary calcification as assessed by CT is a strong predictor of coronary events, in younger and older populations. An analysis of the combined data of six prospective studies (Kondos et al. 2003; Greenland et al. 2004; Arad et al. 2005a; Taylor et al. 2005; Vliegenthart et al. 2005; LaMonte et al. 2005) in 27,622 individuals (395 coronary events) results in summary relative risks that can be appreciated in Figure 4.5.2, and have been reported in Greenland et al. (2007). Individuals without coronary calcium have a very low risk of CHD (0.4% over 3–5 years of observation), while the risk of CHD shows a steep increase with increasing amount of coronary calcification. The calcium score significantly improves CHD prediction compared to the assessment of risk factors. Recently, the long awaited update ACCF/AHA consensus document on calcium scoring was published. The document includes recommendations for

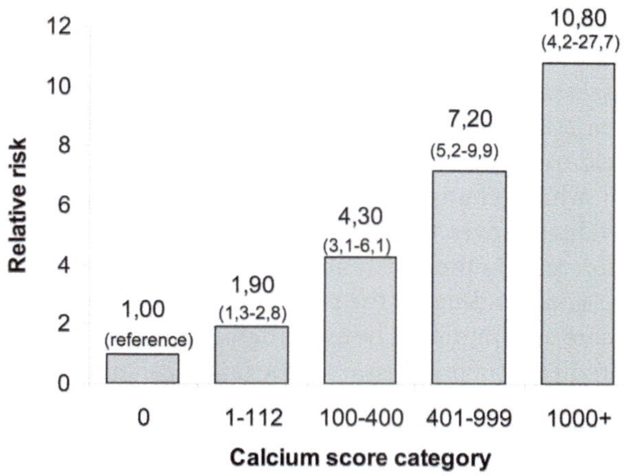

Fig. 4.5.2. Summary relative risks of myocardial infarction and coronary heart disease death, according to calcium score. [Modified from Greenland et al. (2007) with permission]

indications to perform calcium scoring and clinical implications (Greenland et al. 2007). With the evidence that has accrued in the last 6 years, the role of calcium scoring becomes more and more clear. According to the consensus document, calcium scoring is reasonable in asymptomatic individuals with intermediate CHD risk based on risk factors. These individuals may be reclassified to a higher risk status based on a high calcium score (Agatston score >400). In case of a high calcium score, individuals should be regarded as candidates for intensive risk factor modification. Use of calcium scoring in individuals at low or high CHD risk based on risk factors is not advised, since testing at this moment will have no consequences for the clinical strategy. An additional role of calcium scoring is noted in patients with atypical chest pain. The absence of coronary calcium basically rules out the presence of obstructive coronary disease.

4.5.5 Coronary Calcification and Measures of Extracoronary Atherosclerosis

Pathology studies in the 1960s already revealed that atherosclerosis is a generalized process that is not limited to the coronary arteries but is present in different vessel beds. With the development of EBCT, it became possible for the first time to directly evaluate the extent of coronary atherosclerosis in a non-invasive manner. This also created the possibility to study the association of extracoronary atherosclerosis and coronary atherosclerosis in the living. Since then several studies have examined to what extent measures of atherosclerosis in the extracoronary arteries reflect coronary atherosclerosis. Carotid atherosclerosis, most commonly examined by ultrasound, is assessed by the intima-media thickness and by the number of plaques. Both measures are associated with the amount of coronary calcification, carotid plaques more strongly than the intima-media thickness (Davis et al. 1999; Newman et al. 2002; Oei et al. 2002). The ankle-brachial blood pressure index, a measure of peripheral atherosclerosis, shows a moderate association with coronary atherosclerosis (Oei et al. 2002; McDermott et al. 2005). Calcific deposits in the abdominal aorta on lumbar radiographs (Kuller et al. 1999; Oei et al. 2002), CT-detected calcification of the thoracic aorta (Adler et al. 2004; Wong et al. 2003b) and of the aortic valve (Wong et al. 2003b) are closely related to the presence of coronary calcium.

The findings confirm the generalized nature of the development of atherosclerosis in vascular beds. However, atherosclerosis does not develop in all vascular beds concurrently: plaque formation in the aorta and peripheral arteries generally precede calcification of the coronary arteries.

Atherosclerosis induces macro- and microvascular changes, including stiffening of the arteries. Arterial stiffness leads to an increase in blood pressure and is predictive of cardiovascular events (Oliver and Webb. 2003; Mattace-Raso et al. 2006). Aortic pulse wave velocity and brachial artery distensibility – functional measures of arterial stiffness – have also been found to be related to coronary calcification (Budoff et al. 2003; Kullo et al. 2006b).

Measures of extracoronary atherosclerosis have been found to predict the risk of CHD (Witteman et al. 1986; Leng et al. 1996; Bots et al. 1997; Zheng et al. 1997; O'Leary et al. 1999; Wilson et al. 2001; Meer et al. 2004). Relative risks for an extensive level of atherosclerosis compared to a low level or absent atherosclerosis range between 1.7 and 4.5 for carotid intima-media thickness, between 1.7 and 6.4 for calcified plaques in the aorta, and between 1.4 and 3.3 for ankle-brachial blood pressure index. In an elderly population, the predictive value of the calcium score for CHD was compared with the predictive value of often used measures of extracoronary atherosclerosis (Vliegenthart et al. 2005).

The cut-off values for severe atherosclerosis versus mild or no atherosclerosis were chosen such that the percentages of individuals in the two categories were comparable. Relative risks of CHD for the most severe level of extracoronary atherosclerosis in comparison to the lowest level were 1.6 for carotid intima-media thickness, 2.7 for aortic calcification and 1.5 for ankle-brachial index. By far the strongest predictor of coronary events was the amount of coronary calcification, with a relative risk for a high calcium score versus a low calcium score of 8.2.

4.5.6 Progression and Regression of Coronary Calcification

A method to document the atherosclerotic process in the general population can be invaluable for the assessment of interventions or lifestyle modifications aimed at reducing cardiovascular risk. Accurate measurements of coronary calcification can be obtained by EBCT, with reasonable variability (down to about 10% with the new protocols). Since the amount of coronary calcium has been shown to be closely related to the total amount of coronary atherosclerosis (Rumberger et al. 1995), the assessment of coronary calcification may facilitate the study of the progression of coronary atherosclerosis. A number of studies has been conducted in which changes in coronary calcification were evaluated over time (Table 4.5.4). Annual progression rates in the different studies ranged from 0% to 52%, depending on the population and the calcium score distribution. The most important factor for the prediction of progression is the initial calcium score. Generally, the absolute increase in calcium score is largest in the case of a high baseline calcium score, and lower for lower baseline calcium scores. However, the relative increase (in percent) is largest for the lowest initial calcium scores, and decreases with the baseline calcium score. Interestingly, of subjects with no detectable coronary calcium on the baseline scan, the majority did not develop calcification in the next years (Gopal et al. 2006).

The associations between cardiovascular risk factors and progression of coronary calcification have not yet been completely elucidated. As stated, progression is most strongly related to the initial calcium score, while the relationship with cardiovascular risk factors is weaker and less consistent. Neither age nor sex was found to be a significant

Table 4.5.4. Annual progression of coronary calcification (in percent) in generally asymptomatic subjects, in observational electron-beam computed tomography studies

Study	Subjects (n)	Age (years, mean ± SD)	Follow-up (months)	Hypercholesterolemia[a] (%)	Annual progression (%)
Janowitz et al. (1991)	20	56 ± 9	13		
Asymptomatic					20
CAD					48
Callister et al. (1998b)	27	nr	12	nr	52
Maher et al. (1999)	82	46 ± 7	42	nr, 1% Medication	24
Pohle et al. (2001)	104	65 ± 8	15	nr, 52% Medication	27
Yoon et al. (2002)	217	57 ± 11	25	59	38
Hsia et al. (2004)	94	65 ± 9	40	21	14 (3rd Tertile) -33% (1st/ 2nd tertile)

CAD, coronary artery disease; nr, Not reported
[a]Either high LDL cholesterol level in blood or use of cholesterol-lowering medication

predictor of progression (Budoff et al. 2000; Yoon et al. 2002). Studies on different cardiovascular risk factors have shown that risk factors influence the progression of coronary calcification. In a study in 443 non-diabetic subjects (mean age, 51 years), subjects received a repeat scan after an average of 9 years (Cassidy et al. 2005). The Framingham risk score and measures of obesity were specifically studied in relation to progression of the calcium score. The mean 10-year CHD risk in this population was 7.5 ± 5.8%. Adjusted for the baseline calcium score, a higher Framingham risk score was associated with a greater increase in the calcium score: with a 1-unit increase in SD in the Framingham risk score, the annual change in coronary calcium area increased by 60%. In the group with a 10-year CHD risk <10%, age, male sex, hypertension, cholesterol level and measures of obesity were found to be associated with an increase in progression, but not in the higher risk group. In case of the presence of traditional cardiovascular risk factors, other factors for coronary calcium progression may be more difficult to identify. Hypertension and diabetes were also found to be independent predictors of progression of coronary atherosclerosis in a study by Yoon et al. (2002). The influence of lipid levels on progression of coronary calcium has been studied in a number of observational and interventional studies, to be discussed in a later paragraph. A study among asymptomatic post-menopausal women showed that the calcium progression for women without hormone therapy was similar to those taking hormone replacement therapy consisting of estrogen plus progestin (22% vs. 24%). The rate of progression was less in case of estrogen replacement only (9%). Whether combined hormone replacement therapy reduces cardiovascular risk is questionable (Staren and Omer 2004), probably due to the negative effect of progestin on the cardiovascular system.

The progression of coronary atherosclerosis may not only be evaluable by EBCT; multidetector computed tomography (MDCT) has also been proposed for this purpose. So far, one study, by Shemesh et al. (2000), examined the rate of calcium progression using dual-slice spiral CT in 246 hypertensive subjects, who underwent a second scan after 3 years. Of the patients with a baseline calcium score of 0 28% had calcium on the second scan, while of those with calcium on the first scan, 70% showed an increase in the extent of coronary calcium. The relative rate of calcium progression was found to be higher in hypertensive patients who had had a coronary event compared to those without an event (Shemesh et al. 2001).

The prognostic impact of coronary calcium progression was studied by one group. In a screening population (817 asymptomatic individuals) and subsets of this population, with an average follow-up period of 2.2–3.2 years, the rate of progression was found to be a significant predictor of the occurrence of myocardial infarction (Raggi et al. 2003, 2004b). Compared to subjects with stable calcium scores, individuals with significant increase of the calcium score had an increased risk of myocardial infarction (Raggi et al. 2003). Similar results were found in individuals receiving lipid-lowering therapy: even with similar LDL control, progression of coronary calcium was increased in MI patients compared to those without an event (Raggi et al. 2004b). The follow-up score and the score change were found to be independent predictors of events.

There is discussion on the calcium measure to be used for annual change, and the definition of a significant increase in coronary calcium. To accurately evaluate progression of coronary calcification over time, it is necessary to take into account the variability of calcium scores, which can occur in dual scan runs. Bielak et al. (2001) devised a regression method to evaluate the change in calcium scores over time, while accounting for disagreement in the quantity of calcium between dual scan runs. The regression method was then tested on 81 participants who were scanned after a mean interval of 3.5 years. No significant change in calcium quantity was present in 73% of participants, while 26% had a large increase. In all, 1% of the participants had a significant decrease in calcium score. Hokanson et al. (2003) performed dual EBCT scans 5 min apart in 1074 subjects, and calculated calcium volume scores. They assessed interscan variability, and found that use of the square root transformation of the volume score stabilized the variation the most. They then applied this transformation to data of baseline and follow-up scans from 109 diabetic patients. In their study, significant change in calcium volume score was defined as a difference between transformed scores of at least 2.5 mm^3 (>99th percentile of interscan variability). This analytic method may facilitate research on progression of coronary calcification.

Prospective trials to assess the effectiveness of an intervention on cardiovascular event rate require large numbers of subjects to be followed for many years, at high cost. As a means to obtain effect estimates for all participants in a clinical trial, and after a shorter period, the use of surrogate end-points was introduced. Surrogate end-points have the advantage that much smaller numbers of subjects can be studied for a shorter period of time, with sufficient statistical power. Before a marker can be used as a surrogate end-point, the validity of the marker should be established, i.e. whether the marker can be used to assess the risk of cardiovascular events. A number of potential end-points have been investigated, that are indeed able to predict cardiovascular events. Furthermore, most surrogate end-points, like lumen diameter by coronary angiography and carotid intima-media thickness, are continuous variables, which provide a much more precise measure of the effect of the studied intervention. In addition to the mentioned benefits, surrogate markers provide information on the natural history of and factors associated with progression. Coronary calcification by EBCT, which is non-invasive and a direct measure of coronary atherosclerosis, may be worthwhile as a surrogate end-point. The use of the development of coronary calcification through time as end-point in clinical studies is gaining interest. However, a number of studies has been published on the effect of control of lipid levels with or without lipid-lowering therapy on progression of coronary calcification. Two observational studies found that the progression of coronary calcification was lower under treatment with lipid-lowering drugs (Callister et al. 1998a; Achenbach et al. 2002).

In case of good control of lipid levels under lipid-lowering therapy, the progression decreased significantly compared to the untreated status, and even a net reduction in the calcium score was noted on the repeat scan after an average of 12–14 months of treatment.

A study in diabetic patients also showed a decrease in calcium score progression in case of lipid lowering (Budoff et al. 2005). These results suggest that treatment of hypercholesterolemia decreases the rate of calcium progression. However, conflicting results were found in clinical trials on different statin therapy strategies. Two study groups investigated the effect of standard versus intensive lipid-lowering therapy, and performed repeated EBCT scanning after an average of 12 months (Raggi et al. 2005; Schmermund et al. 2006b). One trial included 471 asymptomatic individuals with at least two cardiovascular risk factors (Schmermund et al. 2006b), while the other included 615 postmenopausal women with hypercholesterolemia. No statistically significant difference in progression of coronary calcium was found between the two drug regimes, despite a difference in reduction of LDL-cholesterol (decrease significantly larger in case of intensive treatment). As the authors suggest, possibly the follow-up period was too small to detect a significant difference in the rate of calcium progression. A trial in which 102 patients with calcific aortic stenosis, without indication for lipid-lowering, were assigned to either intensive lipid-lowering drugs or placebo, showed similar results: reduction of LDL-cholesterol levels in case of statins, but no major effect on the progression of coronary calcification (Houslay et al. 2006). However, this study used an outdated CT technique to detect and quantify coronary calcification, which limits the validity of the obtained calcium scores. Lastly, a trial was performed in 1005 asymptomatic individuals with a high calcium score percentile (Arad et al. 2005b). The individuals were randomized to a low-dose statin, vitamin C and vitamin E or to placebos, and followed for more than 4 years. Again, while LDL-cholesterol levels showed a reduction in treated individuals versus individuals taking placebos, no effect was found on the rate of progression of coronary calcium. However, a number of weaknesses, like a considerable number of low-risk individuals, affected the probability of finding a significant difference in progression of coronary calcification. Thus, no definitive answer is as yet available on the effect of statins on the rate of calcium progression. Results from a recent IVUS study suggest that calcified plaques are more resistant to the effect of medical therapy than non-calcified plaques (Nicholls et al. 2007). This indicates that changes in calcification may not give a clear indication of the effect on the plaque volume, including vulnerable plaque components.

More studies are needed to elucidate whether progression of coronary calcium is a useful tool in clinical practice.

In conclusion, the amount of EBCT-detected coronary calcification shows a steep increase with age, and is generally higher in men than in women. The coronary calcium score has been found to be related to many cardiovascular risk factors, and is considered to reflect the impact of known and unknown risk factors on the arterial wall. There are remarkable ethnic differences in coronary calcification. The calcium score is a very strong predictor of coronary heart disease, with higher relative risks than found for other non-invasive measures of atherosclerosis. Coronary calcification improves cardiovascular risk prediction based on conventional risk factors.

Evaluation of the calcium score may be valuable in cardiovascular risk stratification of asymptomatic individuals and in the clinical work-up of patients with atypical symptoms of chest pain. Future studies should investigate how the calcium score can be incorporated in clinical strategies for asymptomatic and symptomatic individuals. It is still uncertain whether repeated measurement of coronary calcium can be used to follow the progression of atherosclerosis.

References

Achenbach S, Ropers D, Pohle K et al (2002) Influence of lipid-lowering therapy on the progression of coronary artery calcification. A prospective evaluation. Circulation 106:1077–1082

Adler Y, Fisman EZ, Shemesh J et al (2004) Spiral computed tomography evidence of close correlation between coronary and thoracic aorta calcifications. Atherosclerosis 176:133–138

Agatisa PK, Matthews KA, Bromberger JT et al (2005) Coronary and aortic calcification in women with a history of major depression. Arch Intern Med 165:1229–1236

Allison MA, Wright CM (2004a) A comparison of HDL and LDL cholesterol for prevalent coronary calcification. Int J Cardiol 95:55–60.

Allison MA, Wright MC (2004b) Body morphology differentially predicts coronary calcium. Int J Obes 28:396–401

Allison MA, Wright M, Tiefenbrun J (2003) The predictive power of low-density lipoprotein cholesterol for coronary calcification. Int J Cardiol 90:281–289

Arad Y, Spadaro LA, Goodman K et al (2000) Prediction of coronary events with electron beam computed tomography. J Am Coll Cardiol 36:1253–1260

Arad Y, Newstein D, Cadet F et al (2001) Association of multiple risk factors and insulin resistance with increased prevalence of asymptomatic coronary artery disease by an electron-beam computed tomographic study. Arterioscler Thromb Vasc Biol 21:2051–2058

Arad Y, Goodman KJ, Roth M et al (2005a) Coronary calcification, coronary disease risk factors, C-reactive protein, and atherosclerotic cardiovascular disease events. J Am Coll Cardiol 46:158–165

Arad Y, Spadaro LA, Roth M et al (2005b) Treatment of asymptomatic adults with elevated coronary calcium scores with atorvastatin, vitamin C, and vitamin E. The St. Francis Heart study randomized clinical trial. J Am Coll Cardiol 46:166–172

Bielak LF, Klee GG, Sheedy PF et al (2000) Association of fibrinogen with quantity of coronary artery calcification measured by electron beam computed tomography. Arterioscler Thromb Vasc Biol 20:2167–2171

Bielak LF, Sheedy PF, Peyser PA (2001) Coronary artery calcification measured at electron-beam CT: agreement in dual scan runs and change over time. Radiology 218:224–229

Bielak LF, Turner ST, Franklin SS et al (2004) Age-dependent associations between blood pressure and coronary artery calcification in asymptomatic adults. J Hypert 22:719–725

Bild DE, Detrano R, Peterson D et al (2005) Ethnic differences in coronary calcification: the Multi-Ethnic Study of Atherosclerosis (MESA). Circulation 111:1313–1320

Bots ML, Breslau PJ, Briet E et al (1992) Cardiovascular determinants of carotid artery disease. The Rotterdam Elderly Study. Hypertension 19:717–720

Bots ML, Hoes AW, Koudstaal PJ et al (1997) Common carotid intima-media thickness and risk of stroke and myocardial infarction: the Rotterdam Study. Circulation 96:1432–1437

Budoff MJ, Lane KL, Bakhsheshi H et al (2000) Rates of progression of coronary calcium by electron beam tomography. Am J Cardiol 86:8–11

Budoff MJ, Flores F, Tsai J et al (2003) Measures of brachial artery distensibility in relation to coronary calcification. Am J Hypert 16:350–355

Budoff MJ, Yu D, Nasir K et al (2005) Diabetes and progression of coronary calcium under the influence of statin therapy. Am Heart J 149:695–700

Callister TQ, Raggi P, Cooil B et al (1998a) Effect of HMG-CoA reductase inhibitors on coronary artery disease as assessed by electron-beam computed tomography. N Engl J Med 339:1972–1978

Callister TQ, Cooil B, Raya SP et al (1998b) Coronary artery disease: improved reproducibility of calcium scoring with an electron-beam CT volumetric method. Radiology 208:807–814

Camargo CA Jr, Stampfer MJ, Glynn RJ et al (1997) Moderate alcohol consumption and risk for angina pectoris or myocardial infarction in U.S. male physicians. Ann Intern Med 126:372–375

Cassidy AE, Bielak LF, Zhou Y et al (2005) Progression of subclinical coronary atherosclerosis: does obesity make a difference? Circulation 111:1877–1882

Church TS, Levine BD, McGuire DK et al (2007) Coronary artery calcium score, risk factors, and incident coronary heart disease events. Atherosclerosis 190:224–231

Colhoun HM, Rubens MB, Underwood SR et al (2000) The effect of type 1 diabetes mellitus on the gender difference in coronary artery calcification. J Am Coll Cardiol 36:2160–2167

Dabelea D, Kinney G, Snell-Bergeon JK et al (2003) Effect of type I diabetes on the gender difference in coronary artery calcification: a role for insulin resistance? The coronary artery calcification in type I diabetes (CACTI) study. Diabetes 52:2833–2839

Danesh J, Collins R, Appleby P et al (1998) Association of fibrinogen, c-reactive protein, albumin, or leukocyte count with coronary heart disease: meta-analyses of prospective studies. JAMA 279:1477–1482

Davis PH, Dawson JD, Mahoney LT et al (1999) Increased carotid intimal-medial thickness and coronary calcification are related in young and middle-aged adults. The Muscatine Study. Circulation 100:838–842

Diez Roux AV, Ranjit N, Powell L et al (2006) Psychosocial factors and coronary calcium in adults without clinical cardiovascular disease. Ann Intern Med 144:822–831

Doherty TM, Tang W, Detrano RC (1999) Racial differences in the significance of coronary calcium in asymptomatic black and white subjects with coronary risk factors. J Am Coll Cardiol 34:787–794

Ellison RC, Zhang Y, Hopkins PN et al (2006) Is alcohol consumption associated with calcified atherosclerotic plaque in the coronary arteries and aorta? Am Heart J 152:177–182

Erren M, Reinecke H, Junker R et al (1999) Systemic inflammatory parameters in patients with atherosclerosis of the coronary and peripheral arteries. Arterioscler Thromb Vasc Biol 19:2355–2363

Folsom AR, Wu KK, Rosamond WD et al (1997) Prospective study of hemostatic factors and incidence of coronary heart disease: the atherosclerosis risk in communities (ARIC) study. Circulation 96:1102–1108

Ford ES, Smith SJ, Stroup DF et al (2002) Homocyst(e)ine and cardiovascular disease: a systematic review of the evidence with special emphasis on case-control studies and nested case-control studies. Int J Epidemiol 31:59–70

Fornage M, Lopez DS, Roseman JM et al (2004) Parental history of stroke and myocardial infarction predicts coronary artery calcification: the coronary artery risk development in young adults (CARDIA) study. Eur J Cardiovasc Prevention Rehab 11:421–426

Freedman DS, Newman WP 3rd, Tracy RE et al (1988) Black-white differences in aortic fatty streaks in adolescence and early adulthood: the Bogalusa Heart Study. Circulation 77:856–864

Gallo LC, Matthews KA, Kuller LH et al (2001) Educational attainment and coronary and aortic calcification in postmenopausal women. Psychosom Med 63:925–935

Godsland IF, Elkeles RS, Feher MD et al (2006) Coronary calcification, C-reactive protein and the metabolic syndrome in Type 2 diabetes: the Prospective Evaluation of Diabetic Ischaemic Heart Disease by Coronary Tomography (PREDICT) Study. Diab Med 23:1192–1200

Goff DC, Gertoni AG, Kramer H et al (2006) Dyslipidemia prevalence, treatment, and control in the Multi-Ethnic Study of Atherosclerosis (MESA). Circulation 113:647–656

Gopal A, Nasir K, Liu ST et al (2006) Coronary calcium progression rates with a zero initial score by electron beam tomography. Int J Cardiol doi:10.1016/j.ijcard.2006.04.081

Greenland P, LaBree L, Azen SP et al (2004) Coronary artery calcium score combined with Framingham score for risk prediction in asymptomatic individuals. JAMA 291:210–215

Greenland P, Bonow RO, Brundage BH et al (2007) ACCF/AHA 2007 clinical expert consensus document on coronary artery calcium scoring by computed tomography in global cardiovascular risk assessment and in evaluation of patients with chest pain. J Am Coll Cardiol 49:378–402

Grover SA, Coupal L, Hu XP (1995) Identifying adults at increased risk of coronary disease. How well do the current cholesterol guidelines work? JAMA 274:801–806

Guerra R, Yu Z, Marcovina S et al (2005) Lipoprotein(a) and apolipoprotein(a) isoforms: no association with coronary artery calcification in The Dallas Heart Study. Circulation 111:1471–1479

Haverkate F, Thompson SG, Pyke SD et al (1997) Production of c-reactive protein and risk of coronary events in stable and unstable angina. European concerted action on thrombosis and disabilities angina pectoris study group. Lancet 349:462–466

Hennekens CH, Rosner B, Cole DS (1978) Daily alcohol consumption and fatal coronary heart disease. Am J Epidemiol 107:196–200

Hoff JA, Chomka EV, Krainik AJ et al (2001) Age and gender distributions of coronary artery calcium detected by electron beam tomography in 35,246 adults. Am J Cardiol 87:1335–1339

Hoff JA, Guinn L, Sevrukov A et al (2003) The prevalence of coronary artery calcium among diabetic individuals without known coronary artery disease. J Am Coll Cardiol 41:1008–1012

Hofmann MA, Lalla E, Lu Y et al (2001) Hyperhomocysteinemia enhances vascular inflammation and accelerates atherosclerosis in a murine model. J Clin Invest 107:675–683

Hokanson JE, MacKenzie T, Kinney G et al (2003) Evaluating changes in coronary artery calcium: an analytic method that accounts for interscan variability. Am J Radiol 182:1327–1332

Holvoet P, Jenny NS, Schreiner PJ et al (2006) The relationship between oxidized LDL and other cardiovascular risk factors and subclinical CVD in different ethnic groups: the Multi-Ethnic Study of Atherosclerosis (MESA). Atherosclerosis doi: 10.1016/j.atherosclerosis.2006.08.002

Houslay ES, Cowell SJ, Prescott RJ et al (2006) Progressive coronary calcification despite intensive lipid-lowering treatment: a randomised controlled trial. Heart 92:1207–1212

Hsia J, Klouj A, Prasad A et al (2004) Progression of coronary calcification in healthy postmenopausal women. BMC Cardiovascular disorders 4:21

Hubert HB, Feinleib M, McNamara PM et al (1983) Obesity as an independent risk factor for cardiovascular disease: a 26-year follow-up of participants in the Framingham heart study. Circulation 67:968–977

Hunt ME, O'Malley PG, Vernalis MN et al (2001) C-reactive protein is not associated with the presence or extent of calcified subclinical atherosclerosis. Am Heart J 141:206–210

Iribarren C, Sidney S, Bild DE et al (2000) Association of hostility with coronary artery calcification in young adults: the CARDIA study. JAMA 283:2546–2551

Janowitz WR, Agatston AS, Viamonte M Jr (1991) Comparison of serial quantitative evaluation of calcified coronary artery plaque by ultrafast computed tomography in persons with and without obstructive coronary artery disease. Am J Cardiol 68:1–6

Jousilahti P, Vartiainen E, Pekkanen J et al (1998) Serum cholesterol distribution and coronary heart disease risk: observations and predictions among middle-aged population in eastern finland. Circulation 97:1087–1094

Kardys I, Oei HHS, Hofman A et al (2006) Lipoprotein-associated phospholipase A2 and coronary calcification: the Rotterdam Coronary Calcification Study. Atherosclerosis doi:10.1016/j.atherosclerosis.2006.04.004

Khera A, de Lemos JA, Peshock RM et al (2006) Relationship between C-reactive protein and subclinical atherosclerosis: the Dallas Heart Study. Circulation 113:38–43

Klatsky AL, Friedman GD, Siegelaub AB (1981) Alcohol and mortality. A ten-year kaiser-permanente experience. Ann Intern Med 95:139–145

Kondos GT, Hoff JA, Sevrukov A et al (2003) Electron-beam tomography coronary artery calcium and cardiac events: a 37-month follow-up of 5635 initially asymptomatic low-to intermediate-risk adults. Circulation 107:2571–2576

Kop WJ, Berman DS, Gransar H et al (2005) Social network and coronary artery calcification in asymptomatic individuals. Pscyhosom Med 67:343–352

Kornowski R (1999) Impact of smoking on coronary atherosclerosis and remodeling as determined by intravascular ultrasonic imaging. Am J Cardiol 83:443–445

Kuller LH, Tracy RP, Shaten J et al (1996) Relation of c-reactive protein and coronary heart disease in the mrfit nested case-control study. Multiple Risk Factor Intervention Trial. Am J Epidemiol 144:537–547

Kuller LH, Matthews KA, Sutton-Tyrrell K et al (1999) Coronary and aortic calcification among women 8 years after menopause and their premenopausal risk factors: the Healthy Women Study. Arterioscler Thromb Vasc Biol 19:2189–2198

Kullo IJ, Li G, Bielak LF et al (2006a) Association of plasma homocysteine with coronary artery calcification in different categories of coronary heart disease risk. Mayo Clin Proc 81:177–182

Kullo IJ, Bielak LF, Turner ST et al (2006b) Aortic pulse wave velocity is associated with the presence and quantity of coronary artery calcium: a community based study. Hypertension 47:1–6

LaMonte MJ, FitzGerald SJ, Church TS et al (2005) Coronary artery calcium score and coronary heart disease events in a large cohort of asymptomatic men and women. Am J Epidemiol 162:1–9

Leng GC, Fowkes FGR, Lee AJ et al (1996) Use of ankle brachial pressure index to predict cardiovascular events and death: a cohort study. BMJ 313:1440–1443

Levenson J, Giral P, Megnien JL et al (1997) Fibrinogen and its relations to subclinical extracoronary and coronary atherosclerosis in hypercholesterolemic men. Arterioscler Thromb Vasc Biol 17:45–50

Liuzzo G, Biasucci LM, Gallimore JR et al (1994) The prognostic value of c-reactive protein and serum amyloid a protein in severe unstable angina. N Engl J Med 331:417–424

Maher JE, Raz JA, Bielak LF et al (1996) Potential of quantity of coronary artery calcification to identify new risk factors for asymptomatic atherosclerosis. Am J Epidemiol 144:943–953

Maher JE, Bielak LF, Raz JA et al (1999) Progression of coronary artery calcification: a pilot study. Mayo Clin Proc 74:347–355

Mahoney LT, Burns TL et al (1996) Coronary risk factors measured in childhood and young adult life are associated with coronary artery calcification in young adults: the Muscatine Study. J Am Coll Cardiol 27:277–284

Maresca G, Di Blasio A, Marchioli R et al (1999) Measuring plasma fibrinogen to predict stroke and myocardial infarction: an update. Arterioscler Thromb Vasc Biol 19:1368–1377

Mattace-Raso FU, Van der Cammen TJ, Hofman A et al (2006) Arterial stiffness and risk of coronary heart disease and stroke: the Rotterdam Study. Circulation 113:657–663

McDermott MM, Liu K, Criqui MH et al (2005) Ankle-brachial index and subclinical cardiac and carotid disease: the Multi-Ethnic Study of Atherosclerosis. Am J Epidemiol 162:33–41

McGill HC Jr, Strong JP (1968) The geographic pathology of atherosclerosis. Ann N Y Acad Sci 149:923–927

McClelland RL, Chung H, Detrano R et al (2006) Distribution of coronary artery calcium by race, gender, and age: results from the Multi-Ethnic Study of Atherosclerosis (MESA). Circulation 113:30–37

Meade TW, Mellows S, Brozovic M et al (1986) Haemostatic function and ischaemic heart disease: principal results of the Northwick Park Heart Study. Lancet 2:533–537

Meer van der IM, Bots ML, Hofman A et al (2004) Predictive value of non-invasive measures of atherosclerosis for incident myocardial infarction: the Rotterdam Study. Circulation 109:1089–1094

Megnien JL, Simon A, Lemariey M et al (1996) Hypertension promotes coronary calcium deposit in asymptomatic men. Hypertension 27:949–954

Meigs JB, Larson MG, d'Agostino RB et al (2002) Coronary artery calcification in type II diabetes and insulin resistance: the Framingham Offspring study. Diab Care 25:1313–1319

Mielke CH, Shields JP, Broemeling LD (2001) Coronary artery calcium, coronary artery disease, and diabetes. Diabetes Res Clin Pract 53:55–61

Mintz GS, Pichard AD, Popma JJ et al (1997) Determinants and correlates of target lesion calcium in coronary artery disease: a clinical, angiographic and intravascular ultrasound study. J Am Coll Cardiol 29:268–274

Mitchell TL, Pippin JJ, Devers SM et al (2001) Age- and sex-based nomograms from coronary artery calcium scores as determined by electron beam computed tomography. Am J Cardiol 87:453–456

Nasir K, Raggi P, Rumberger JA et al (2004a) Coronary artery calcium volume scores on electron beam tomography in 12,936 asymptomatic adults. Am J Cardiol 93:1146–1149

Nasir K, Michos ED, Rumberger JA et al (2004b) Coronary artery calcification and family history of premature coronary heart disease: sibling history is more strongly associated than parental history. Circulation 110:2150–2156

Newman AB, Naydeck BL, Sutton-Tyrrell K et al (2001) Coronary artery calcification in older adults to age 99: prevalence and risk factors. Circulation 104:2679–2684

Newman AB, Naydeck BL, Sutton-Tyrrell K et al (2002) Relationship between coronary artery calcification and other measures of subclinical cardiovascular disease in older adults. Arterioscler Thromb Vasc Biol 22:1674–1679

Nicholls SJ, Tuzcu EB, Wolski K et al (2007) Coronary artery calcification and changes in atheroma burden in response to established medical therapies. J Am Coll Cardiol 49:263–70

Nishino M, Malloy MJ, Naya-Vigne J et al (2000) Lack of association of lipoprotein(a) levels with coronary calcium deposits in asymptomatic postmenopausal women. J Am Coll Cardiol 35:314–320

Oei HH, Vliegenthart R, Hak AE et al (2002) The association between coronary calcification assessed by electron beam computed tomography and measures of extracoronary atherosclerosis: the Rotterdam Coronary Calcification Study. J Am Coll Cardiol 39:1745–1751

Oei HHS, Vliegenthart R, Hofman A et al (2004) Risk factors for coronary calcification in older subjects: the Rotterdam Coronary Calcification Study. Eur Heart J 25:48–55

O'Leary DH, Polak JF, Kronmal RA et al (1992) Distribution and correlates of sonographically detected carotid artery disease in the cardiovascular health study. The chs collaborative research group. Stroke 23:1752–1760

O'Leary DH, Polak JF, Kronmal RA et al (1999) Carotid-artery intima and media thickness as a risk factor for myocardial infarction and stroke in older adults. Cardiovascular Health Study collaborative research group. N Engl J Med 340:14–22

Oliver JJ, Webb DJ (2003) Noninvasive assessment of arterial stiffness and risk of atherosclerotic events. Arterioscler Thromb Vasc Biol 23:554–566

O'Malley PG, Jones DL, Feuerstein IM et al (2000) Lack of correlation between psychological factors and subclinical coronary artery disease. N Engl J Med 343:1298–1304

Orakzai SH, Orakzai RH, Nasir K et al (2006) Subclinical coronary atherosclerosis: racial profiling is necessary! Am Heart J 152:819–827

Pearson TA (2002) New tools for coronary risk assessment: what are their advantages and limitations? Circulation 105:886–892

Pletcher MJ, Tice JA, Pignone M et al (2004) Using the coronary artery calcium score to predict coronary heart disease events: a systematic review and meta-analysis. Arch Intern Med 164:1285–1292

Pletcher MJ, Varosy P, Kiefe CI et al (2005) Alcohol consumption, binge drinking, and early coronary calcification: findings from the Coronary Artery Risk development in Young Adults (CARDIA) Study. Am J Epidemiol 161:423–433

Pohle K, Maffert R, Ropers D et al (2001) Progression of aortic valve calcification: association with coronary atherosclerosis and cardiovascular risk factors. Circulation 104:1927–1932

Raggi P, Callister TQ, Cooil B et al (2000) Identification of patients at increased risk of first unheralded acute myocardial infarction by electron-beam computed tomography. Circulation 101:850–855

Raggi P, Cooil B, Shaw LJ et al (2003) Progression of coronary calcium on serial electron beam tomographic scanning is greater in patients with future myocardial infarction. Am J Cardiol 92:827–829

Raggi P, Shaw LF, Berman DS et al (2004a) Prognostic value of coronary artery calcium screening in subjects with and without diabetes. J Am Coll Cardiol 43:1663–1669

Raggi P, Callister TG, Shaw LJ (2004b) Progression of coronary artery calcium and risk of first myocardial infarction in patients receiving cholesterol-lowering therapy. Arterioscler Thromb Vasc Biol 24:1–7

Raggi P, Davidson M, Callister TQ et al (2005) Aggressive versus moderate lipid-lowering therapy in hypercholesterolemic postmenopausal women. Beyond endorsed lipid lowering with EBT scanning (BELLES). Circulation 112:563–571

Redberg RF, Rifai N, Gee L et al (2000) Lack of association of c-reactive protein and coronary calcium by electron beam computed tomography in postmenopausal women: implications for coronary artery disease screening. J Am Coll Cardiol 36:39–43

Reilly MP, Wolfe ML, Localio AR et al (2003) C-reactive protein and coronary artery calcification: the Study of Inherited Risk of Coronary Atherosclerosis (SIRCA). Arterioscler Thromb Vasc Biol 23:1851–1856

Ridker PM, Cushman M, Stampfer MJ et al (1997) Inflammation, aspirin, and the risk of cardiovascular disease in apparently healthy men. N Engl J Med 336:973–979

Ridker PM, Glynn RJ, Hennekens CH (1998a) C-reactive protein adds to the predictive value of total and HDL cholesterol in determining risk of first myocardial infarction. Circulation 97:2007–2011

Ridker PM, Buring JE, Shih J et al (1998b) Prospective study of c-reactive protein and the risk of future cardiovascular events among apparently healthy women. Circulation 98:731–733

Ridker PM, Cushman M, Stampfer MJ et al (1998c) Plasma concentration of c-reactive protein and risk of developing peripheral vascular disease. Circulation 97:425–428

Rumberger JA, Simons DB, Fitzpatrick LA et al (1995) Coronary artery calcium area by electron-beam computed tomography and coronary atherosclerotic plaque area. A histopathologic correlative study. Circulation 92:2157–2162

Rumberger JA, Kaufman L (2003) A rosetta stone for coronary calcium risk stratification: Agatston, volume and mass scores in 11,490 individuals. AJR Am J Roentgenol 181:743–748

Schmermund A, Moehlenkamp S, Berenbein S et al (2006a) Population-based assessment of subclinical coronary atherosclerosis using electron-beam computed tomography. Atherosclerosis 185:177–182

Schmermund A, Achenbach S, Budde T et al (2006b) Effect of intensive versus standard lipid-lowering treatment with atorvastatin on the progression of calcified coronary atherosclerosis over 12 months. A multicenter, randomized, double-blind trial. Circulation 113:427–437

Schurgin S, Rich S, Mazzone T (2001) Increased prevalence of significant coronary artery calcification in patients with diabetes. Diabetes Care 24:335–338

Shemesh J, Apter S, Stroh CI et al (2000) Tracking coronary calcification by using dual-section spiral CT: a 3-year follow-up. Radiology 217:461–465

Shemesh J, Apter S, Stolero D et al (2001) Annual progression of coronary artery calcium by spiral computed tomography in hypertensive patients without myocardial ischemia but with prominent atherosclerotic risk factors, in patients with previous angina pectoris or healed acute myocardial infarction, and in patients with coronary events during follow-up. Am J Cardiol 87:1395–1397

Snell-Bergeon JK, Hokanson JE, Kinney GL et al (2004) Measurement of abdominal fat by CT compared to waist circumference and BMI in explaining the presence of coronary calcium. Int J Obes Relat Metab Disord 28:1594–1599

Sparagon B, Friedman M, Breall WS et al (2001) Type A behaviour and coronary atherosclerosis. Atherosclerosis 156:145–149

Staren ED, Omer S (2004) Hormone replacement therapy in postmenopausal women. Am J Surg 188:136

Stokes J 3rd, Kannel WB, Wolf PA et al (1989) Blood pressure as a risk factor for cardiovascular disease. The Framingham Study – 30 years of follow-up. Hypertension 13:I13–18

Strong JP, Richards ML (1976) Cigarette smoking and atherosclerosis in autopsied men. Atherosclerosis 23:451–476

Strong JP, Malcom GT, McMahan CA et al (1999) Prevalence and extent of atherosclerosis in adolescents and young adults: implications for prevention from the pathobiological determinants of atherosclerosis in youth study. JAMA 281:727–735

Suh I, Shaten BJ, Cutler JA et al (1992) Alcohol use and mortality from coronary heart disease: the role of high-density lipoprotein cholesterol. The Multiple Risk Factor Intervention Trial research group. Ann Intern Med 116:881–887

Superko HR, Hecht HS (2001) Metabolic disorders contribute

to subclinical coronary atherosclerosis in patients with coronary calcification. Am J Cardiol 88:260–264

Taylor AJ, Feuerstein I, Wong H et al (2001) Do conventional risk factors predict subclinical coronary artery disease? Results from the prospective army coronary calcium project. Am Heart J 141:463–468

Taylor AJ, Bindeman J, Feuerstein I et al (2005) Coronary calcium independently predicts incident premature coronary heart disease over measured cardiovascular risk factors: mean three-year outcomes in the Prospective Army Coronary Calcium (PACC) project. J Am Coll Cardiol 46:807–814

Thompson SG, Kienast J, Pyke SD et al (1995) Hemostatic factors and the risk of myocardial infarction or sudden death in patients with angina pectoris. European concerted action on thrombosis and disabilities angina pectoris study group. N Engl J Med 332:635–641

Tofferi JK, Taylor AJ, Feuerstein IM et al (2004) Alcohol intake is not associated with subclinical coronary atherosclerosis. Am Heart J 148:803–809

Tuzcu EM, Berkalp B, De Franco AC et al (1996) The dilemma of diagnosing coronary calcification: angiography versus intravascular ultrasound. J Am Coll Cardiol 27:832–838

Vliegenthart R, Hollander M, Breteler MM et al (2002) Stroke is associated with coronary calcification as detected by electron-beam CT: the Rotterdam Coronary Calcification Study. Stroke 33:462–465

Vliegenthart R, Oei HHS, Elzen van den APM et al (2004) Alcohol consumption and coronary calcification in a general population. Arch Intern Med 164:2355–2360

Vliegenthart R, Oudkerk M, Hofman A et al (2005) Coronary calcification improves cardiovascular risk prediction in the elderly. Circulation 112:572–577

Wang TJ, Larson MG, Levy D et al (2002) C-reactive protein is associated with subclinical epicardial coronary calcification in men and women: the Framingham Heart Study. Circulation 106:1189–1191

Wexler L, Brundage B, Crouse J et al (1996) Coronary artery calcification: pathophysiology, epidemiology, imaging methods, and clinical implications. A statement for health professionals from the American Heart Association. Writing group. Circulation 94:1175–1192

Wilson PW, Kauppila LI, O'Donnell CJ et al (2001) Abdominal aortic calcific deposits are an important predictor of vascular morbidity and mortality. Circulation 103:1529–1534

Witteman JCM, Kok FJ, van Saase JL et al (1986) Aortic calcification as a predictor of cardiovascular mortality. Lancet 2:1120–1122

Wong ND, Hsu JC, Detrano RC et al (2000) Coronary artery calcium evaluation by electron beam computed tomography and its relation to new cardiovascular events. Am J Cardiol 86:495–498

Wong ND, Sciammarella MG, Polk D et al (2003a) The metabolic syndrome, diabetes, and subclinical atherosclerosis assessed by coronary calcium. J Am Coll Cardiol 41:1547–1553

Wong ND, Sciammarella M, Arad Y et al (2003b) Relation of thoracic aortic and aortic valve calcium to coronary artery calcium and risk assessment. Am J Cardiol 92:951–955

Yan LL, Liu K, Daviglus ML et al (2006) Education, 15-year risk factor progression, and coronary artery calcium in young adulthood an dearly middle age. JAMA 295:1793–1800

Yang T, Doherty TM et al (1999) Alcohol consumption, coronary calcium, and coronary heart disease events. Am J Cardiol 84: 802–806

Yoon HC, Emerick AM, Hill JA et al (2002) Calcium begets calcium: progression of coronary artery calcification in asymptomatic subjects. Radiology 224:236–241

Zheng ZJ, Sharrett AR, Chambless LE et al (1997) Associations of ankle-brachial index with clinical coronary heart disease, stroke and preclinical carotid and popliteal atherosclerosis: the Atherosclerosis Risk in Communities (ARIC) Study. Atherosclerosis 131:115–125

Zhou J, Moller J, Danielsen CC et al (2001) Dietary supplementation with methionine and homocysteine promotes early atherosclerosis but not plaque rupture in apoE-deficient mice. Arterioscler Thromb Vasc Biol 21:1470–1476

Non-Invasive Measurement of Coronary Atherosclerosis

4

4.6 Coronary Artery Calcium Screening: Current Status and Recommendations from the European Society of Cardiac Radiology and North American Society for Cardiovascular Imaging

Matthijs Oudkerk, Arthur E. Stillman, Sandra S. Halliburton, Willi A. Kalender, Stefan Möhlenkamp, Cynthia H. McCollough, Rozemarijn Vliegenthart Proença, Leslee J. Shaw, William Stanford, Allen J. Taylor, Peter M. A. van Ooijen, Lewis Wexler, and Paolo Raggi *

CONTENTS

M. Oudkerk, MD, PhD, Professor
Department of Radiology, University Medical Center Groningen, University of Groningen, Hanzeplein 1, P.O. Box 30.001, 9700 RB Groningen, The Netherlands
A. E. Stillman, MD, PhD, FAAH, Professor
Director of the Division of Cardiothoracic Imaging
Department of Radiology, Emory University Hospital, 1365 Clifton Rd NE, Suite AT 506 Atlanta GA 30322, USA

* *complete authors' adresses see List of Contributors*

4.6.1 Introduction

In 1996 and 2000 the American Heart Association (AHA) issued statements on coronary artery calcium (CAC) quantification (O'Rourke et al. 2000; Wexler et al. 1996). In 2006 and 2007, several professional societies updated these statements describing new evidence related to CAC imaging (Budoff et al. 2006; Greenland et al. 2007; Hendel et al. 2006). The purpose of the present chapter is to summarize the rationale and content of those recommendations with regard to CAC quantification, to address differences among them and to point out controversial areas of CAC research of high clinical relevance among both asymptomatic and symptomatic persons.

Nearly all of the published clinical outcome data from CAC are based on results obtained with electron beam tomography (EBT) systems. However, these CT systems are largely no longer available and are being widely replaced with multi detector CT (MDCT) systems. EBT, produced by one manufacturer, provided much more standardization than exists for all the various generations of MDCT systems from different manufacturers. Standardization guidelines have been proposed for MDCT (McCollough et al. 2007), but are rarely used. Studies with earlier MDCT technology (four- to 16-slice) have demonstrated that similar mean CAC scores can be obtained with EBT and MDCT (Becker et al. 2001; Carr et al. 2000; Daniell et al. 2005; Detrano et al. 2005; Horiguchi et al. 2004; Knez et al. 2002). Nevertheless systematic differences exist which can likely affect serial measurements (McCollough et al. 2007; Greuter et al. 2007; Ulzheimer and Kalender 2003).

While large numbers of patients were included in the EBT outcome studies, most of these suffered from selection biases related to ethnicity, patient self-referral or referral by physicians concerned about subclinical coronary artery disease due to the presence of risk factors. The Dallas Heart Study (Jain et al. 2004), Multi-Ethnic Study of Atherosclerosis (Bild et al. 2005) and Rotterdam Study (Oei et al. 2004; Vliegenthart et al. 2005) have attempted to address some of these issues. The results from general populations cannot reliably be applied to special populations. Nevertheless it is clear from many studies that in all kinds of populations, even in high-risk populations such as diabetic patients, and in both symptomatic and asymptomatic patients, the absence of coronary artery calcium (zero calcium score) excludes most clinically relevant coronary artery disease. This information is highly relevant since many individuals of subjects among the general as well as special populations have a zero calcium score.

In this paper we review the evidence in support of the use of CAC for cardiac risk assessment in the general population as well as special populations with particular focus on the importance of a zero score. The need for standardization of CAC measurements with MDCT is also discussed.

4.6.2 Coronary Artery Calcium as a Predictor of Cardiac Events

Most published studies addressing the issue of coronary artery calcium as a predictor of cardiac events are based on EBT data. In the ACCF/AHA Consensus Document on Coronary Artery Calcium Scoring 6 such studies were selected for review because they fulfilled sufficient criteria for outcome analysis (Vliegenthart et al. 2005; Arad et al. 2000; Greenland et al. 2004; Kondos et al. 2003; LaMonte et al. 2005; Taylor et al. 2005a). From the data presented in these studies it was concluded that coronary artery calcium scores add incremental prognostic value in the evaluation of patients at intermediate risk for a coronary event. Other studies further support this conclusion. Raggi et al. (2000a) screened 632 asymptomatic patients with EBT and followed them for 32 months to determine the incidence of hard cardiac events (myocardial infarction and death). The majority of events occurred in individuals with high calcium scores and in individuals with scores > 75th percentile compared with age and sex matched controls. Arad et al. (2000) screened 1172 asymptomatic patients with EBT and followed them for a mean of 3.6 years to determine the incidence of cardiovascular end points (myocardial infarction, death and the need for revascularization). The authors concluded that in asymptomatic adults EBT calcium scores are highly predictive of events. Pletcher et al. (2004) conducted a meta-analysis of studies performed between 1980–2003 in ~13,000 asymptomatic patients screened with EBT and followed for 3.6 years or less to determine the odd ratios (OR) of hard coronary events. OR for Agatston CAC scores < 100, 100–400 and > 400 were 2.1, 4.2 and 7.2, respectively. The authors concluded that the EBT derived Agatston calcium score is an independent predictor of coronary events in asymptomatic subjects.

4.6.3 CAC as an Indicator of Coronary Artery Luminal Stenosis

Only studies based on EBT data have addressed the issue of CAC as an indicator of coronary artery luminal stenosis. HABERL et al. (2001) analyzed the value of EBT derived calcium CAC scores as an indicator of coronary luminal stenoses in 1764 patients undergoing conventional coronary angiography. The authors concluded that EBT CAC scores are highly sensitive but moderately specific determinants of stenosis. The ACC/AHA Expert Consensus document on electron-beam CT for the diagnosis and prognosis of coronary artery disease (2000) reported a pooled sensitivity of 91.8% and specificity of 55% for detection of a coronary artery stenosis >50% after reviewing 16 selected studies comparing CAC scores and invasive angiography. KNEZ et al. (2004) compared EBT derived Agatston CAC scores with calcium volume scores (CVS) as a predictor of coronary luminal stenoses in 2115 patients undergoing conventional coronary angiography. The authors reported overall results similar to those already reported by others, but also concluded that the CVS are as accurate as the Agatston score for stenosis prediction. Indeed, BUDOFF et al. (2002) utilized CVS obtained by EBT to predict the presence of coronary artery stenoses in 1851 patients undergoing conventional coronary angiography and concluded that CVS provide incremental value in predicting the severity and extent of angiographically significant coronary artery disease.

4.6.4 Clinical Comparison of MDCT and EBT for Coronary Artery Calcium Score Measurement

KNEZ et al. (2002) studied 99 symptomatic men (mean age: 60 years) with both MDCT (prospective triggering, Siemens Volume Zoom) and EBT imaging and found a correlation coefficient of 0.99 for CVS and 0.98 for the mass score (MS) with a mean overall variability of 17%. No significant differences for scores 1–100, 101–400, 401–1000, > 1000 were found. The authors concluded that MDCT is equivalent to EBT for CAC scoring. BECKER et al. (2001) compared a four-slice MDCT (Siemens Volume Zoom) with EBT (prospective triggering) in 100 patients and calculated the Agatston score, CVS and MS. The authors concluded that the score variability is highest for the Agatston score (32%) and the correlation between MSCT and EBT is excellent for CVS and MS. CARR et al. (2000) performed CT examinations with both GE Lightspeed LX/i four-slice MDCT (retrospective gating) and EBT in 36 patients and calculated the Agatston score in all of them. The authors reported excellent correlation between scores obtained on the two CT systems. HORIGUCHI et al. (2004) performed EBT and 16-MDCT with retrospective gating in 100 patients and reported a high degree of correlation between the two CT systems for the Agatston score ($r^2 = 0.955$), CVS ($r^2 = 0.952$) and MS ($r^2 = 0.977$). DANIELL et al. (2005) compared the results of EBT and four-slice MDCT (prospective triggering, Siemens Volume Zoom) in 68 patients. EBT and MDCT scores correlated well ($r = 0.98$–0.99) with a median variability between EBT and MDCT for the Agatston score of ~25% and ~16% for CVS. Scores were higher for EBT than MDCT in approximately half of the cases, with little systematic difference between the two (median EBT-MDCT difference: Agatston score, –0.55; volume score, 3.4 mm^3).

4.6.5 Review of Current Guidelines on Coronary Artery Calcification

4.6.5.1 Risk Assessment in Asymptomatic Persons

Risk stratification algorithms such as the Framingham risk score (FRS) (WILSON et al. 1998), the PROCAM score (ASSMANN et al. 2002) or the European SCORE-system (CONROY et al. 2003; GRAHAM et al. 2007) are used to assess an individual's global 10-year risk. Risk factors are measured and weighed and attributed to an empirically determined absolute risk of cardiovascular events, i.e. cardiac death and myocardial infarction (SMITH et al. 2000):

- Low risk = < 1% per year or < 10% in 10 years
- Intermediate risk = 1–2% per year or 10–20% in 10 years
- High risk = > 2% per year or > 20% in 10 years

This classification was slightly modified by the 2004 update of NCEP guidelines (Table 4.6.1) (Grundy et al. 2004).

It is argued that persons at high risk will most likely benefit from intensive risk modification, while persons at low risk are generally recommended to adhere to a healthy lifestyle and guideline based treatment of individual risk factors when present. In persons at intermediate risk, however, there remains a diagnostic gap and further tests, such as CAC scoring, measuring intima-media thickness (IMT), the ankle arm index, or exercise stress testing may be useful in distinguishing individuals who indeed have a high risk from those at low risk, leaving hopefully few that remain at intermediate risk (Smith et al. 2000). It should be recognized, though, that the Framingham score does not take into account life-style factors such as diet, exercise and body mass index. Neither does the score reflect a positive family history of cardiovascular disease. The extent of atherosclerotic disease burden, autonomic dysfunction, chronic inflammation, lipoprotein subfractions, blood thrombogenicity, the myocardial propensity to develop life-threatening arrhythmias, and immeasurable genetic factors are also not part of conventional risk assessment. Measuring the atherosclerotic sequelae of lifelong global exposure to all risk factors by virtue of measuring the extent of the disease in its early subclinical stages may overcome this limitation. The detection of calcified atherosclerosis is a general surrogate of total atheroma burden. It is noted however, that the extent of coronary calcification systematically differs among ethnic populations and by gender.

Table 4.6.1. Absolute risk categories "NCEP-Update 2004". [Modified from Grundy et al. (2004)]

10-Year risk categories	Definition of risk category
High risk	CAD[a], CAD-risk equivalents[b], ≥2 major risk factors[c], 10-year-risk >20%
Moderately high risk	≥2 Major risk factors but 10-year CAD risk 10%–20%
Moderate risk	≥2 Major risk factors but 10-year CAD risk <10%
Low risk	0–1 Major risk factor and 10-year CAD risk <10%

[a] History of myocardial infarction, coronary revascularisations or myocardial ischemia.

[b] Includes diabetes mellitus, stroke, TIA or carotid artery stenosis > 50%, symptomatic peripheral artery disease or abdominal aortic aneurysm.

[c] Smoking, hypertension, high LDL- cholesterol/low HDL-cholesterol, age (men > 45 years., women > 55 years.), and premature family history of coronary artery disease (1st grade family member, i.e. men < 55 years., women < 65 years). CAD, coronary artery disease.

4.6.5.2 The Focus of Current Guidelines on CAC Scoring

The AHA Scientific Statement on "Assessment of Coronary Artery Disease (CAD) by Cardiac Computed Tomography" (Budoff et al. 2006) reviewed scientific data for cardiac CT related to imaging of CAD and atherosclerosis in symptomatic and asymptomatic subjects, including a detailed description of technical aspects and radiation exposure of CAC CT and non-invasive CT angiography using electron beam CT (EBT) and multidetector CT (MDCT). According to AHA standards, recommendations were classified (Class I, IIa, IIb and III) and the level of evidence (A, B, or C) was provided (see http://circ.ahajournals.org/manual/ manual_IIstep6.shtml).

The ACC/AHA 2007 Clinical Expert Consensus Document (Greenland et al. 2007) discussed the role of CAC quantification with respect to: (1) identifying and modifying coronary event risk in asymptomatic subjects, (2) modifying clinical care and outcomes of symptomatic patients with suspected CAD and (3) understanding the role of CAC CT in selected patient sub-groups, including women, ethnic groups, and patients with renal disease or diabetes. (4) The clinical value of serial CAC CT, cost-effectiveness of CAC CT, and clinical implications of incidental findings were also addressed.

The purpose of the 2006 Appropriateness Criteria Statement (Hendel et al. 2006) was to create, review and categorize appropriateness criteria for cardiac CT and also cardiac magnetic resonance imaging (MRI) with regard to detection of CAD, cardiovascular risk stratification, as well as cardiac structure and function assessment. Members of the expert group assessed the risks and benefits of the imaging tests for several indications and clinical scenarios and scored them based on a scale of 1–9:

- 7–9 = Appropriate: the test is generally acceptable and is a reasonable approach
- 4–6 = Uncertain: uncertain indication or clinical setting
- 1–3 = Inappropriate: the test is generally not acceptable / is not a reasonable approach

Indications in the latter statement were derived from common applications or anticipated uses of cardiac CT and MRI. Working group panelists rated each indication based on the ACC methodology for valuating the appropriateness of cardiovascular imaging (Patel et al. 2005).

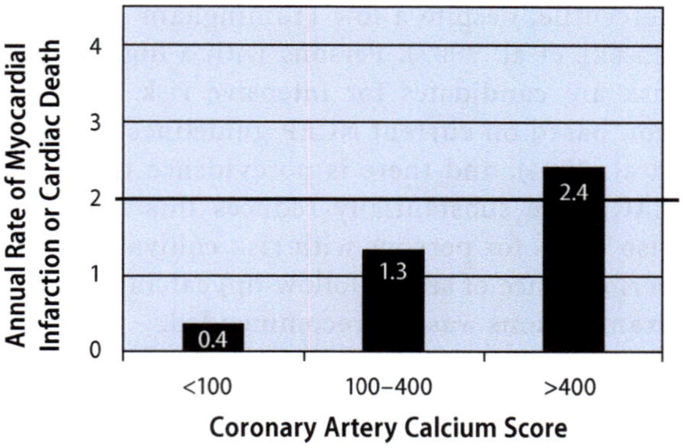

Fig. 4.6.2. Annual rate of myocardial infarction or cardiac death in categories of CAC burden in persons at intermediate risk based on convention risk factor assessment. In persons with a high CAC score (>400), the annual event rate exceeds the threshold for intensive risk factor modification, i.e. >2% per year (*black line*). A CAC score >400 in intermediate risk persons may therefore be considered as a risk equivalent. [Modified from Greuter et al. (2007)]

4.6.6 Indications for CAC Scoring in Asymptomatic Individuals

In the past several years, numerous publications have reported on the incremental prognostic value of CAC over measured conventional risk factors in large series of patients including asymptomatic population-based cohorts (Vliegenthart et al. 2005; Greenland et al. 2004; Kondos et al. 2003; LaMonte et al. 2005; Taylor et al. 2005a; Arad et al. 2005). The relative risk of coronary events increased with increasing CAC burden (Fig. 4.6.1). The majority of the expert writing committees agree that it may be reasonable to consider use of CAC measurement in asymptomatic intermediate risk patients, i.e. 10%–20% coronary events in 10 years. These patients might be reclassified to a higher risk status based on a high CAC score, and subsequent patient management may be modified (Fig. 4.6.2). In the ACC appropriateness criteria document, notably published prior to the most recent AHA and ACC statements and additional prospective CAC scoring studies, CAC scoring was considered appropriate only for very few indications. However, all of them were given a rating of "uncertain", most notably CAC scoring for risk assessment in the general population at moderate (score 6) or high (score 5) CAD Framingham risk. In patients with a low or a high 10-year risk of coronary events, i.e. <10% or >20% in 10 years, CAC quantification is not recommended: in low risk individuals, even a high CAC score does not generally elevate this person's risk above the threshold to initiate therapy (Greenland et al. 2007). Yet, lifetime risk may be elevated in 18% and 20% of asymptomatic men and women, respectively, who have a high CAC score, i.e. CAC >400 or >75th

Fig. 4.6.1. Increase in relative risk (*RR*) with increasing CAC scores in asymptomatic persons in comparison to asymptomatic persons without CAC. [Modified from Greuter et al. (2007)]

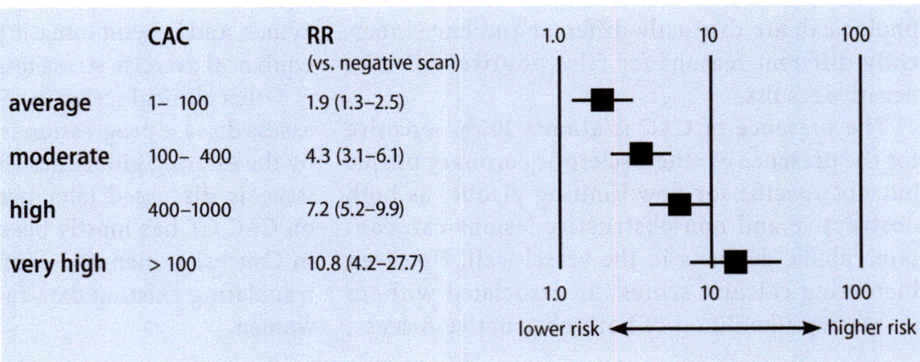

percentile, despite a low Framingham risk score (Erbel et al. 2007). Persons with a high 10-year risk are candidates for intensive risk modification based on current NCEP guidelines (Grundy et al. 2004), and there is no evidence that a low CAC score substantially reduces this risk. This also holds for persons with risk equivalents. The performance of serial (follow-up) calcium scoring examinations was not recommended.

4.6.7 Atherosclerotic Disease Quantification in Patients with Chest Pain

In symptomatic patients, diagnostic tests may be used for risk stratification, but the primary initial objective is to identify or rule out obstructive coronary artery disease. Especially in young persons with atypical chest pain, non-atherosclerotic non-obstructive coronary disease such as myocardial bridging, coronary anomalies, coronary vasospasm, intramyocardial small vessel disease, or non-coronary heart disease such as cardiomyopathy, valvular heart disease, pericardial disease, aortic disease, pulmonary disease, etc. must be considered as differential diagnoses. Persons with an intermediate pretest-likelihood of obstructive CAD, i.e. between 20%–80%, are most likely to benefit from additional testing (Gibbons et al. 2002).

Functional tests such as treadmill, exercise or pharmacological nuclear stress tests or stress-echocardiography are used to induce myocardial ischemia in patients with flow limiting coronary obstruction. In contrast, CAC CT is aimed at estimating coronary plaque severity and the associated likelihood of a flow-limiting lesion. These two approaches, the former functional and the latter morphological, are distinctly different and have inherently different reasons for false positive and false negative results.

The presence of CAC is almost 100% sensitive for the presence of atherosclerotic coronary plaque but not specific for flow limiting plaque, as both obstructive and non-obstructive lesions can contain calcific deposits in the vessel wall. However, increasing calcium scores are associated with an increasing likelihood of both obstructive disease, and an increased severity (number of vessels involved) of coronary artery disease. Moderately high coronary calcium scores (approximately 150) in symptomatic patients are associated with a roughly 80% sensitivity and specificity for the presence of an obstructive coronary artery lesion (among patients referred to coronary angiography) (Haberl et al. 2001; Budoff et al. 2002) an accuracy that is similar in magnitude to conventional stress tests (Gibbons et al. 2002; Fleischmann et al. 2002). Consistent with these data are findings from myocardial perfusion scintigraphy in which only 2% of patients with a CAC score <100 were shown to have a positive nuclear stress test (Berman et al. 2004). A clinical application of these relationships has been demonstrated among emergency department patients with chest pain, in whom a zero calcium score was associated with a very low risk of cardiovascular events (Georgiou et al. 2001). Caution in the interpretation of zero calcium scores is warranted among individuals with a high pretest probability for coronary artery disease (e.g., young smokers) in whom false negative studies may be observed (Shaw et al. 2006).

In summary, the majority of expert writing committee members agreed that patients at low risk of CAD by virtue of atypical cardiac symptoms may benefit from CAC testing to help exclude the presence of obstructive CAD. CAC scoring may be a useful filter prior to invasive angiography or further stress testing (Geluk et al. 2007; Raggi et al. 2000b). However, more data on direct comparisons with established forms of stress testing are needed. Currently, additional non-invasive testing in persons with a very high CAC score, e.g. >400 is not recommended as there is no evidence that such additional testing will improve appropriate selection of candidates for therapy. CAC CT was classified as "Class IIb, Level of Evidence: B" when used to rule out obstructive CAD in patients with chest pain with equivocal or normal ECGs and negative cardiac enzymes, and in symptomatic patients in the setting of equivocal exercise stress tests [3].

Other clinical scenarios: Serial imaging of CAC to assess disease progression is currently not indicated by the existing guidelines (Budoff et al. 2006); this issue is discussed later herein. Existing evidence on CAC CT has mostly been gathered from studies in Caucasian men and caution is warranted in extrapolating existing data to other ethnic groups or women.

4.6.7.1
Implications for Therapy

The NCEP/ATP III Guidelines have incorporated CAC CT as a complementary test to modify treatment intensity: Measurement of coronary calcium is an option for advanced risk assessment in appropriately selected persons. In persons with multiple risk factors, high coronary calcium scores (e.g., >75th percentile for age and sex) denote advanced coronary atherosclerosis and provide a rationale for intensified LDL-lowering therapy. Moreover, measurement of coronary calcium is promising for older persons in whom the traditional risk factors lose some of their predictive power (Grundy et al. 2004). The use of CAC percentile ranks, as advocated in the NCEP guidelines, is especially important in young individuals whose absolute scores may be low, yet "high-for-age", indicating a high life-long risk, even though short-term risk over the next 5–10 years may be low. As risk factor modification in high-risk subjects should be initiated as early as possible, such persons are likely appropriate candidates for intensive risk modification – a notion that needs to be further confirmed by prospectively collected outcome data.

4.6.7.2
Limitations

There is currently little evidence that CAC CT and knowledge of CAC score severity has an impact on the advice physicians give to patients or on patients' adherence to prescribed risk factor modification efforts (Kalia et al. 2006). Further, CAC CT may improve risk stratification in selected populations, but currently the data are limited that CAC CT improves outcome. Accordingly, current evidence does not support lowering treatment intensity in intermediate risk subjects even if the CAC score is zero (Greenland et al. 2007).

4.6.7.3
Summary

Current guidelines propose the use of CAC CT to improve risk stratification in subjects at intermediate 10-year risk of incident coronary events. The present writing committee agrees with this general recommendation.

4.6.8
Race and Calcium Score

There is still limited knowledge of the predictive value of CAC in non-Caucasians. It has been well documented that there is a notable difference in CAC accumulation not only between men and women, but also between subjects of different ethnicities and races. Doherty et al. (1999) using subtraction fluoroscopy first noted a significantly lower prevalence of CAC in Blacks than Whites (35.5% vs. 59.9%, $p=0.0001$) and warned of the different prognostic significance of CAC in these races. Indeed, during a follow up of 70 ± 13 months, 23.7% of the black and 14.8% of the white screened population suffered an incident cardiovascular event (odds ratio: 2.16, 95% CI 1.34–3.48). The significant difference in prevalence and distribution of CAC assessed by CT in four races in the US, was recently confirmed by the Multi-Ethnic Study of Atherosclerosis (MESA). Bild et al. (2005) showed that the prevalence of CAC on cardiac CT (score >0) was highest in Whites followed by Chinese, Hispanics and finally Blacks. Santos et al. (2006) showed that North American Caucasian subjects have more CAC than Caucasian subjects from Brazil and Portugal despite the higher prevalence of risk factors in the latter two ethnic groups. Interestingly, despite a substantial genetic similarity between Brazilian and Portuguese patients, and the presence of more smokers among the latter, Brazilians had a greater extent of coronary artery calcium than Portuguese subjects. These findings mirrored the national mortality and morbidity statistics indicating a greater cardiovascular event rate in the North American, followed by the Brazilian and finally the Portuguese population.

Despite the noted differences in CAC scores, there is currently limited evidence of the prognostic significance of CAC in different races. Detrano et al. (2008) showed that CAC is a strong predictor of cardiovascular death, non-fatal myocardial infarction, angina and revascularization (total events = 162) in all 6722 MESA patients independent of race. Furthermore, CAC added incremental prognostic value beyond traditional risk factors for the prediction of events.

Recently, Nasir et al. (2007) evaluated the use of CAC to predict all-cause mortality in 14,812 patients belonging to the same four races considered in MESA (505 deaths in 10 years of follow-up). Once again the prevalence of CAC was highest in Whites, although Blacks and Hispanics had a greater clustering of risk factors for CAD. Despite a lower prevalence of CAC and lower scores compared to the other races, black patients had the highest mortality rates even after multivariable adjustment for clinical risk factors and baseline CAC score ($p<0.0001$). Compared with Whites, the relative risk of death was 2.97 (CI:1.87–4.72) in Blacks, 1.58 (CI: 0.92–2.71) in Hispanics and 0.85 (CI: 0.47–1.54) in Chinese individuals. A 50-year-old black patient with a CAC score >400 had an estimated loss of 7 years of life, as opposed to 2.5 years of life for a white patient with the same score.

Therefore, it would appear appropriate to consider CAC a good marker of risk in all races so far investigated, although the prognostic significance of score categories varies between racial groups. This underscores the importance of racial specific risk categories defined according to CAC score thresholds. An attempt at defining such categories was recently published by Sirineni et al. (2008). In their publication the authors suggested substituting the chronological age of a patient undergoing CAC screening for his vascular age. The vascular age can be assessed according to the median CAC score for a subject of the same age, race and sex. For example a 50-year-old black man with a CAC score of 40 should be considered ~20 years older than his chronological age, since 40 is the median score of a 70 year old black man in MESA. On the other hand, a score of 40 adds only 11 years of age to a 50-year-old white man. The prognostic validity of this novel approach is still awaiting confirmation in prospective studies.

4.6.9 The Value of Coronary Artery Calcium in the Elderly Population

The assessment of coronary calcification may have particular value in the elderly population. The potential for prevention of coronary heart disease (CHD) in older adults is large, since even a small reduction in risk factor levels results in a considerable reduction in event rates. However, to identify asymptomatic elderly in the population at the highest risk of CHD is challenging. Office-based risk score algorithms like the Framingham risk score (Wilson et al. 1998) and the European SCORE (Conroy et al. 2003) have an upper age threshold that limits their applicability to older adults. Furthermore, the predictive power of risk factors diminishes with increasing age (Anderson et al. 1987; Glynn et al. 1995; Kannel et al. 1997). Finally, age becomes the predominant factor in the algorithm in older adults, despite the fact that a fixed weight attributed to age does not take into account the individual variation in coronary plaque burden. On the basis of risk factors and age, the true CHD risk may be miscalculated, and this may lead to inaccurate selection of elderly for aggressive risk factor modification.

CAC reflects the lifetime impact of all atherosclerosis risk factors, both known and unknown, on the arterial wall (Thompson and Partridge 2004). Thus, this non-invasive measurement can provide a more accurate estimate of the accumulated plaque burden and CHD risk. So far, one population-based study has focused on the predictive value of CAC in the elderly: the Rotterdam Coronary Calcification Study (mean age, 71 years) (Vliegenthart et al. 2005). During a mean follow-up period of 3.3 years, 50 of the 1795 initially asymptomatic subjects had a coronary event. Increasing CAC score categories showed relative risks for CHD up to 8.2 (95% confidence interval, 3.3–20.5) for a CAC score above 1000, compared to absent or low CAC score (0–100). Similar relative risks were found after adjustment for risk factors and in asymptomatic individuals over 70 years of age. Of interest, there was a very low probability of events in subjects with a low CAC score (0–100). Furthermore, irrespective of the Framingham risk category (low-to-intermediate or high risk), increasing CAC score categories were strongly associated with the risk of events. Thus, a low CAC score in elderly may be as valuable a finding as in younger subjects. These results indicate that the CAC score is a very promising measurement to improve cardiovascular risk stratification in the elderly. In a recent publication, Abbott et al. (2007) reported on 224 very old (age 84–96) Japanese men living in Hawaii followed for an average of 2.5 years after CAC imaging. A total of 17 deaths occurred during 2.5 years of follow-up and no death occurred in patients with a CAC score <10. As shown in the study by Vliegenthart et al. (2005), the death rate increased significantly as the CAC score increased ($p<0.001$). Finally, Newman et al. (2008) measured CAC and carotid intima-media thickness in 559 patients (336 women) age 70–99 years. The top quartile of each measurement was associated with ~two-fold increased risk of a combined cardiovascular disease end-point.

Other population prospective studies have been conducted in a wide age range (Greenland et al. 2004; Kondos et al. 2003; LaMonte et al. 2005; Raggi et al. 2000a; Arad et al. 2005; Budoff et al. 2007). Most of these studies did not specifically address the predictive value of CAC in older age. In a study by LaMonte et al. (2005), CHD event rates adjusted for gender were presented in different age groups. In subjects over 65 years of age, a graded increase in event rates was seen for CAC scores ≥100 and ≥400 (7.1 and 8.2 per 1000 person-years, respectively). Conversely, absence of CAC was associated with a very low event rate (0.9 per 1000 person-years).

4.6.10 Summary

These data support the notion that CAC screening may be used in all age groups to adjust the relative risk level. They must, however, be considered preliminary; more research will be needed to demonstrate that expensive medical therapies can be withheld in the elderly with risk factors in the absence of CAC and to establish the best approach to managing older, asymptomatic patients with extensive CAC.

4.6.11 Diabetes Mellitus and Coronary Artery Calcium

Patients suffering from diabetes type-2 have been shown to harbor larger amounts of CAC than non-diabetic patients with the metabolic syndrome (Wong et al. 2003) and subjects of similar age and otherwise similar risk factor profile (Wong et al. 2003; Schurgin et al. 2001). The extent of CAC in patients with type-2 diabetes is similar to that of patients with established CAD but without diabetes, diabetic women harbor as much CAC as diabetic men (Khaleeli et al. 2001; Mielke et al. 2001), and younger diabetic individuals have a plaque burden comparable to that of older non-diabetic individuals (Hoff et al. 2003). All of this confirms the clinical evidence that diabetes mellitus is associated with a very high prevalence of CAD; it negates the advantage of women over men and of youth over older age in prevalence and extent of atherosclerosis. Hoff et al. (2003) utilized a large database to calculate the age and gender normative (percentile) distribution of calcium scores in asymptomatic (self-reported) diabetic individuals.

Olson et al. (2000) investigated the presence of CAC and prior CAD in 302 patients with diabetes mellitus type-1 and a history of myocardial infarction, angina, or evidence of ischemia on stress testing or surface electrocardiograms. Among the subjects free of clinical CAD, 5% had a CAC score ≥400 (large atherosclerosis burden), as opposed to 25% of the subjects with prior angina or objective evidence of myocardial ischemia and 80% of the patients with myocardial infarction or luminal stenoses on invasive angiography. CAC showed a sensitivity of 84% and 71% for clinical CAD in men and women, respectively, and 100% sensitivity for myocardial infarction (MI) and obstructive CAD.

Limited data exist on outcome related to CAC in diabetic patients. Wong et al. (2005) performed CAC screening and stress myocardial perfusion imaging (MPI) in 1043 patients, 313 of whom were affected by either diabetes mellitus ($n = 140$) or the metabolic syndrome ($n = 173$). In patients with a CAC score < 100, the prevalence of stress induced MPI abnormalities was very low (~2%). However, in the presence of a metabolic disorder (diabetes mellitus or the metabolic syndrome) a CAC score between 100–399 or greater than 400 was associated with a greater incidence of ischemia than in patients without a metabolic disorder (13% vs. 3.6%, $p < 0.02$, and 23.4% vs. 13.6%, $p = 0.03$, respectively). Similarly, Anand et al. (2006) performed sequential CAC screening and MPI in 180 type-2 diabetic patients. The incidence of myocardial ischemia was directly proportional to the CAC score. For type-2 diabetic patients with a CAC score of 0, 11–100, 101–400, 401–1000, and >1000, the incidence of myocardial ischemia on stress MPI was 0%, 18%, 23%, 48%, and 71%, respectively. In summary, based on the data from Wong et al. (2005) and Anand et al. (2006), type-2 diabetic patients with a CAC score > 100 are expected to have an increased frequency of ischemia on MPI.

Two outcome studies addressed the question of whether CAC constitutes a risk for events in asymptomatic patients but came to opposite conclusions. The South Bay Heart Watch (SBHW) was a prospective cohort study designed to determine the relation between radiographically detectable CAC and cardiovascular outcome in high-risk asymptomatic adults (Qu et al. 2003). A total of 1312 asymptomatic subjects ≥45 years old with cardiac risk factors were recruited via mass-mailing advertisement in the Los Angeles area; of these 19% were diabetic patients. In a sub-analysis of the main database after a mean follow-up of 6 years, Qu et al. (2003) found an increased risk of cardiovascular events (death, myocardial infarction, stroke and revascularizations) in diabetic patients compared to non-diabetic subjects in the presence of CAC. However, the risk did not increase significantly as the CAC score increased. Raggi et al. (2004a) utilized a database of 10,377 asymptomatic individuals (903 diabetic patients), followed for an average of 5 years after CAC screening. The primary end-point of the study was all-cause mortality. The authors showed that the risk of all-cause mortality was higher in diabetic patients than non-diabetic subjects for any degree of CAC and the risk increased as the score increased. Additionally, the absence of CAC predicted a low short-term risk of death (~1% at 5 years) for both diabetic patients and non-diabetic subjects [67]. Hence, both the presence and absence of CAC were important modifiers of risk even in the presence of established risk factors for atherosclerosis such as diabetes mellitus. This suggests that there is a great heterogeneity among diabetes mellitus patients and that risk stratification may be of benefit even in patients considered to be at high-risk of atherosclerosis complications.

4.6.12 Summary

The preceding discussion suggests that CAC imaging techniques may be very helpful to the practicing physician faced with the dilemma of accurate risk assessment even in diabetic patients at high risk. However, as is the case with other subsets of patients, further research will be needed to confirm the prognostic role of CAC in diabetes mellitus.

4.6.13 Renal Failure and Coronary Artery Calcium

Both EBT and MSCT have been utilized in the recent past to investigate the natural history and pathogenesis of CAC, as well as the impact of different therapeutic strategies in chronic kidney disease (CKD). Evidence indicates that as the estimated glomerular filtration rate (eGFR) declines the prevalence of CAC increases. In fact, the prevalence of CAC was reported to be 40% in 85 pre-dialysis patients as opposed to 13% in controls with normal renal function (Russo et al. 2004). In a prospective study of 313 high-risk hypertensive patients a reduced eGFR was shown to be the major determinant of the rate of progression of CAC (odds ratios for calcium progression in the group with eGFR ≤60 ml/min: 2.1; 95% CI 1.2–3.7) (Bursztyn et al. 2003). Consistent with these findings, Sigrist et al. (2006) reported a prevalence of CAC of 46% in 46 pre-dialysis patients compared to 70% and 73%, respectively, in 60 hemodialysis and 28 peritoneal dialysis patients ($p = 0.02$). Hence, it appears that the prevalence of CAC increases with declining renal function and after initiation of dialysis. Of note, CAC was reported in ~60% of patients new to hemodialysis (Block et al. 2007) and in as many as 80%–85% of adult prevalent hemodialysis patients (Raggi et al. 2002) in two prospective, randomized studies. In a small longitudinal study, the baseline CAC score measured by EBT in 49 prevalent hemodialysis patients was on average two- to five-fold higher than in age and sex matched individuals with established CAD. A repeat CT after an interval of 12 months showed significant progression of CAC ($p < 0.05$) (Braun et al. 1996).

A number of factors have been associated with progression of CAC in dialysis patients. Associations with age and duration of dialysis (Raggi et al. 2002; Goodman et al. 2000), diabetes mellitus (Raggi et al. 2002) abnormalities of mineral metabolism (Oh et al. 2002; Wang et al. 2003; Chertow et al. 2004) as well as use and dose of calcium based phosphate binders (Chertow et al. 2002; Guerin et al. 2000) have all been reported. To investigate the impact of therapy for hyperphosphatemia on the progression of CAC a randomized clinical trial compared the effect of Sevelamer (Genzyme, Cambridge, MA USA – a non absorbable polymer with gut phosphate binding ability) and calcium-based phosphate binders in 200 hemodialysis patients for 1 year (Chertow et al. 2002). Throughout the study both drugs provided a comparable phosphate control (mean phosphate = 5.1 mg/dl), although a significantly higher serum calcium concentration ($p = 0.002$) was noted in the calcium-salts treated arm. At study completion Sevelamer treated subjects were less likely to experience CAC progression (median absolute progression of CAC score 0 vs. 36.6, $p = 0.03$ and aorta 0 vs. 75.1, $p = 0.01$, respectively) (Chertow et al. 2002).

In a smaller series of 129 patients new to hemodialysis (Block et al. 2005), subjects treated with calcium containing phosphate binders showed a more rapid and more severe increase in CAC score compared with those receiving Sevelamer ($p = 0.056$ at 12 months, $p = 0.01$ at 18 months) (Block et al. 2005). In the same series, all cause mortality was strongly associated with the baseline CAC score, and was significantly lower in the Sevelamer arm after 4.5 years of follow up ($p = 0.02$) (Block et al. 2007). Even more surprisingly mortality was extremely low (3.9%/year) in patients with 0 calcium score. This stands in contrast with a reported mortality of ~20–25%/year in patients undergoing hemodialysis. CAC scores were also shown to be predictive of an unfavorable outcome in dialysis patients by Matsuoka et al. (2004). The authors followed 104 chronic hemodialysis patients for an average of 43 months after a screening EBT. Patients were divided into two groups according to a baseline CAC score falling below or above the median for the group (score = 200). The 5-year cumulative survival was significantly lower for patients with a CAC score >200 than for those with a score <200 (67.9% vs. 84.2%, $pV \geq = 0.0003$).

4.6.14 Summary

CAC appears to be predictive of an adverse outcome in CKD patients and its absence has been linked with a very low event rate.

4.6.15 The Value of the ZERO Calcium Score – Asymptomatic Patients

The presence of coronary calcification is, especially with advancing age, a sensitive but unspecific finding. As discussed above, many studies have emphasized the graded increase in CHD risk with increasing calcium scores. However, an even more clinically relevant finding may be the absence of CAC. In a large population of over 10,000 individuals screened for CAC, all-cause mortality was assessed during a 5-year follow-up period. With a zero or very low (<10) calcium score, the investigators reported a very low probability of mortality, ~1.0% at the end of follow-up (Shaw et al. 2003). This finding was confirmed in a study by Budoff et al. (2007) in 25,253 individuals, in which only 0.4% of the individuals with a negative calcium score died during almost 7 years of follow-up, compared to 3.3% of individuals with a positive CAC score. In prospective studies in which coronary heart disease was used as outcome measure, a zero or very low calcium score was associated with a very low probability of events during follow-up (Kondos et al. 2003; Taylor et al. 2005a; Raggi et al. 2000a; Arad et al. 2005; Church et al. 2007). Church et al. (2007) reported a relative risk of coronary events in subjects without CAC compared to those with a positive calcium score of 0.13 (95% confidence interval, 0.06–0.30). Cumulative incidences in studies with a follow-up period of 3–5 years ranged between 0.1% and 0.7% (Table 4.6.2). One study showed a somewhat higher cumulative incidence of 4.4% during more than 6 years (Greenland et al. 2004). This may be partly explained by the different CT protocol (6-mm slicing) which may have resulted in missing calcified lesions.

Four studies have specifically compared the prognosis for men and women in the absence of CAC. Raggi et al. (2004a) found no difference in all-cause mortality after 5 years of follow-up in over 4000 women and over 6000 men with a very low CAC score (<10): 1.6% vs. 1.5%. Recently, the results from three studies in which coronary heart disease was the outcome (Kondos et al. 2003; LaMonte et al. 2005; Taylor et al. 2005a), were used in a meta-analysis (Bellasi et al. 2007). In total, the analysis included 3862 women and 5548 men with absent or minimal CAC. The annual CHD event rate was very similar in women and men: 0.2% vs. 0.3%. When only women and men with no CAC were studied, rates were somewhat lower (0.16% vs. 0.27%) but again not significantly different. Thus, absent or very low CAC score carries the same prognostic value in both genders.

Interestingly, even in the presence of cardiovascular risk factors, the negative predictive value of absent or minimal CAC appears to be very high. In the aforementioned study in which all cause mortality was the outcome (Shaw et al. 2003), further investigations were performed according to smoking status and diabetes status of the participants (Shaw et al. 2006; Raggi et al. 2004b). Absence of CAC was

Table 4.6.2. Absent or very low calcium score and events in asymptomatic populations

Author (year)	Total (n)	Subgroups (n)	Mean age ± SD (years)	Lowest calcium score category	Percentage in lowest category	Mean follow-up ± SD (years)	Outcome	Cumulative incidence (%)
Raggi et al. (2000a)	632		52±9	0	46%	2.7±0.6	MI/cardiac death	0.3
Shaw et al. (2003)[a]	10377		53±10	0–10	57%	5.0±3.5	All-cause mortality	1.0
Raggi et al. (2004a)[a]	10377	4191 Women 6186 Men	55±11 52±11	0–10	68% 50%	5.0±3.5	All-cause mortality	1.6 1.5
Raggi et al. (2004b)[a]	10377	903 Diabetics 9474 Non-diabetics	57±10 53±10	0	30% 51%	5.0±3.5	All-cause mortality	1.2 0.6
Shaw et al. (2006)[a]	10377	4113 Smokers 6264 Non-smokers	53±10 54±11	0–10	about 49% about 63%	5.0±3.5	All-cause mortality	0.5 0.3
Kondos et al. (2003)	5635	1484 Women 4151 Men	54±9 50±9	0	49% 26%	3.0±1.0	MI/CHD death	0.3 0.3
Greenland et al. (2004)	1029		66±8	0	31%	6.3±1.5	MI/CHD death	4.4
Arad et al. (2005)	4613		59±6	0	33%	4.3	MI/CHD death/ revascularizations	0.5
Vliegenthart et al. (2005)	1795		71±6	0–100	50%	3.3±0.8	MI/CHD death	0.7
Taylor et al. (2005a)	1983	356 Women 1627 Men	43±3	0	92% 78%	3.0±1.4	MI/CHD death/ unstable angina	0.0 0.2
Church et al. (2007)[b]	10746		54±10	0	53%	3.5±1.4	MI/CHD death	0.1
LaMonte et al. (2005)[b]	10746	3911 Women 6835 Men	54±10 53±10	0	71% 39%	3.5±1.4	MI/CHD death	0.1 0.1
Budoff et al. (2007)	25253		56±11	0	44%	6.8±3.0	All-cause mortality	0.4

[a] Same study, analysis in different subgroups.
[b] Same study, analysis in different subgroups. CHD, coronary heart disease; MI, myocardial infarction; SD, standard deviation. Cumulative incidence derived from published data or calculated

noted in about 30% of individuals with diabetes, and in 50% of smokers. Little or no CAC was associated with a near 100% survival in non-smokers as well as smokers, and non-diabetic as well as diabetic subjects.

As discussed in the previous section, Block et al. (2007) reported a very low mortality rate for hemodialysis patients without evidence of CAC (3.9%/year); this is in contrast with the extremely high mortality rate (~25%–30%/yearly), typically quoted for this category of patients. Thus, the absence of CAC may be an important modifier of the risk of events even in the presence of cardiovascular risk factors. The high negative predictive value of a zero CAC score is extremely valuable, considering that a large number of asymptomatic individuals have no CAC. In various studies, absence of CAC was noted in 26%–92% of individuals, depending on the age of the individuals. Hence, a zero CAC score may have important implications in daily clinical practice and on a population level. The most important question from a population and societal point of view is whether individuals without CAC should be considered at low risk, even in the presence of cardiovascular risk factors, and therefore be spared therapies such as aspirin and cholesterol-lowering medications. Although the current evidence is substantial, such a notion cannot be endorsed at this time in the absence of prospective, randomized trials.

4.6.16 The Value of ZERO Calcium Score – Symptomatic Patients

4.6.16.1 Calcium Score and Prediction of Obstructive Coronary Artery Disease on Angiography

As outlined above, a negative CAC score has a high negative predictive value in asymptomatic patients of both genders and even in patients with risk factors such as smoking, diabetes or renal failure. In symptomatic patients where CAD is suspected, can a zero or a minimal CAC score (e.g., < 10) be used as a filter to rule out obstructive CAD? Several investigators have addressed this point. Becker et al. studied 1347 symptomatic subjects with suspected CAD (Becker et al. 2007a). Sensitivity, specificity and predictive accuracy were calculated for different calcium thresholds for prediction of CAD. In 720 (53%) subjects, invasive angiography revealed a lumen diameter stenosis greater than 50%. Patients with obstructive CAD had significantly higher total calcium scores than patients without CAD ($p = 0.001$). The overall sensitivity of any CAC score to predict stenosis was 99%, with a specificity of 32%. An absolute score cutoff ≥ 100 and an age and sex specific score $> 75^{th}$ percentile were identified as the cutoff levels with the highest sensitivities (86%–89%) and lowest false positive rates (20%–22%). Absence of CAC was highly accurate for exclusion of CAD in subjects older than 50 years (negative predictive value = 98%). The authors concluded that the presence of CAC on MDCT in symptomatic patients is accurate for prediction of obstructive CAD and that its absence is associated with a high negative predictive value for exclusion of CAD.

Several other studies investigated the presence of non-calcified plaques and obstructive lesions in patients with a low or zero CAC score. Cheng et al. (2007) assessed the presence and severity of non-calcified coronary plaques on 64-MDCT coronary angiography in 554 symptomatic patients with low to intermediate pre-test likelihood for CAD and zero or low CAC score (low score: men, score < 50; women, score < 10). The authors intended to elucidate how well absence of CAC predicts the absence of obstructive non-calcified coronary artery plaque (NCAP). Compared with patients with absent CAC, those with a low CAC score had markedly increased rates of critical luminal stenoses (8.7% vs. 0.5%, $p < 0.001$). The authors concluded that in symptomatic patients with low to intermediate pre-test probability of CAD, absence of CAC predicts very low prevalence of occlusive NCAP. Nonetheless, low but detectable CAC scores were significantly less reliable in excluding the presence of plaque that at times could be obstructive.

Leschka et al. (2007) recently studied the potential of using the CAC score to improve the diagnostic accuracy of MDCT angiography. They evaluated 74 consecutive patients who underwent CAC scoring, MDCT angiography and invasive angiography. Segments that were not evaluable on MDCT angiography were considered to be false-positive. When using CAC scores of 0 to exclude stenoses and ≥ 400 to predict stenosis for segments with non-evaluative segments, the per-patient sensitivity and specificity improved from 98% and 87% to 98% and 100%, respectively. Only the 0 CAC score was found to be helpful to exclude stenoses as a high CAC score often corresponds to more than one stenosis in the coronary artery tree.

In a study by Rubinshtein et al. (2007), the severity of CAD was examined using 64-MDCT angiography in patients who underwent testing due to chest pain syndromes and had a zero or low CAC score. Of 668 consecutive patients, 231 had a low score (< 100) or absent CAC. Obstructive CAD was present in nine of 125 patients (7%) with a 0 CAC score, and in 18 of 106 (17%) with a low score (CAC: 1 to 100).

4.6.17 Summary

In conclusion, absent CAC seems to be an excellent filter for exclusion of obstructive CAD in symptomatic patients with intermediate to high pre-test likelihood of obstructive CAD. A low CAC score, however, is more controversial as a number of studies showed that the presence of non-calcified and potentially obstructive lesions is higher in patients with low CAC scores and symptoms compared to patients with a score of zero.

4.6.17.1 The Value of Zero Calcium Score to Rule Out CAD in Symptomatic Patients: Comparison to Treadmill Stress Testing and Nuclear Stress Tests

In discussing the potential value of a zero CAC score in symptomatic patients for a reliable exclusion of CAD, other non-invasive tests like ECG stress testing or nuclear stress testing have to be considered. Exercise stress testing is often used as the initial non-invasive diagnostic test in symptomatic patients with suspected obstructive CAD. Positive standard ECG criteria are quite specific for obstructive CAD, but there may be a substantial number of false negative tests, including patients with severe disease. Also, exercise stress tests frequently yield equivocal results. Lamont et al. (2002) assessed the value of combining CAC screening with a stress test to reduce the high false-positive rate seen with treadmill stress test (TMST) alone. A CAC score was obtained by EBT in 153 symptomatic patients who underwent coronary angiography because of a positive TMST. The TMST false-positive rate was 27% (41 of 153). In these patients, a CAC score of zero resulted in a negative predictive value of 93%. The authors concluded that the absence of CAC reliably identified patients with a false-positive TMST result. Raggi et al. (2000b) showed that in symptomatic patients with low to intermediate pretest probability of disease (5%–50%), a CAC score of zero can be reliably used to exclude obstructive CAD and that calcium scoring as the initial test to investigate presence of CAD provides a substantial cost benefit over a pathway based on exercise stress testing. Berman et al. (2004) described the relationship between stress-induced myocardial ischemia on single-photon emission computed tomography (SPECT) perfusion studies and CAC. Including a total of 1195 patients without known CAD, 51% asymptomatic, the frequency of ischemia by SPECT was compared to the magnitude of CAC. The frequency of ischemic SPECT was <2% with CAC scores <100 and increased progressively with CAC >100 (p for trend <0.0001). Patients with symptoms and CAC scores >400 had higher likelihood of myocardial ischemia versus those without symptoms ($p<0.025$). The authors concluded that ischemic SPECT is associated with a high likelihood of subclinical atherosclerosis by CAC, but it is rarely seen for CAC scores <100. In most patients, low CAC scores appear to obviate the need for subsequent noninvasive testing. Patients with normal perfusion studies, however, frequently had extensive non-obstructive atherosclerosis by CAC criteria.

Geluk et al. (2007) determined the efficiency of a screening protocol based on CAC scores compared with exercise testing in patients with suspected CAD, a normal ECG and troponin levels. A total of 304 patients were enrolled in a screening protocol that included CAC scoring by EBT, and exercise testing. Decision-making was based on CAC scores. When the CAC score was ≥400, coronary angiography was recommended. When the CAC was <10, patients were discharged. Exercise tests were graded as positive, negative or nondiagnostic. The combined endpoint was defined as coronary event or obstructive CAD at coronary angiography. During 12±4 months, CAC ≥400, 10–399 and <10 were found in 42, 103 and 159 patients and the combined endpoint occurred in 24 (57%), 14 (14%) and 0 patients (0%), respectively. In 22 patients (7%), myocardial perfusion scintigraphy was performed instead of exercise testing due to the inability to perform an exercise test. A positive, nondiagnostic and negative exercise test result was found in 37, 76 and 191 patients, and the combined endpoint occurred in 11 (30%), 15 (20%) and 12 patients (6%), respectively. Receiver-operator characteristics curves showed that the area under the curve of 0.89 (95% CI: 0.85–0.93) for CAC was superior to 0.69 (95% CI: 0.61–0.78) for exercise testing ($p<0.0001$). The authors concluded that measurement of CAC is an appropriate initial screening test in a well-defined low-risk population with suspected CAD.

4.6.17.2 The Value of Zero Calcium Score in Patients Presenting with Acute Chest Pain to the Emergency Department

The use of CAC assessment was briefly discussed in a recent consensus paper on the use of MDCT for acute chest pain (STILLMAN et al. 2007a,b). The use of CAC screening has been described in patients with angina-like symptoms and negative cardiac enzymes presenting to the emergency department (ED). LAUDON et al. (1999) performed CAC scoring in the emergency department in 104 patients, and noted a negative predictive value for CAD of 100% for a CAC score of zero. MCLAUGHLIN et al. (1999) reported a negative predictive value of 98% in 134 patients in a similar ED setting. GEORGIOU et al. (2001) followed 198 patients presenting to the ED with chest pain and normal ECG and cardiac enzymes and found that the presence of any CAC is a strong predictor for future cardiac events. Conversely, patients without CAC may safely be discharged from the ED given the extremely low rate of future events (~0.1%/year). Nonetheless, after reviewing the available evidence, ANDREWS (2000) concluded that currently existing data do not sufficiently support the widespread use of CAC CT in patients with acute chest pain syndromes. Even so, in patients at low pre-test likelihood of CAD presenting with angina-like symptoms to the ED, a negative CAC score can possibly be used to rule out an acute coronary syndrome. In conclusion, the available single center studies based on a limited number of patients indicate that the negative predictive value of a zero CAC is high (>90%). However, the positive predictive value is somewhat lower, rendering CAC screening a highly sensitive, but poorly specific modality for the diagnosis of acute coronary syndromes.

4.6.18 Calcium Score Progression: Interpretation

Serial changes in CAC score may have important implications for monitoring the response of atherosclerotic disease to the initiation of or changes in plaque-altering medical therapy as well as for identifying patients with more aggressive disease who are at high risk for incident CAD (GREENLAND et al. 2007). In this section, we will discuss the methodological approaches to calculating CAC progression as well as provide a synopsis of the available literature on the utility of sequential CT imaging to evaluate atherosclerotic disease progression.

4.6.19 Serial Testing Paradigm

Serial testing is based on the concept that changes in CAC are valid markers of varying atherosclerotic disease states (VILLINES and TAYLOR 2005). Furthermore, a change in CAC may serve as a surrogate for clinical outcomes or disease activity and, as such, provides clinically useful information to guide further patient management (RAGGI et al. 2003, 2004c, 2005a–c; TAYLOR et al. 2005b). The paradigm of using imaging as a surrogate outcome has been advanced in the oncologic PET literature (THERASSE et al. 2000). The Response Evaluation Criteria In Solid Tumors (RECIST) provide definable criteria for partial or complete response to therapies of target and non-target lesions.

Using this type of sequential monitoring, a positive change in CAC score above a given threshold signifies progressive disease, minimal or no changes in CAC score identify patients with stable disease, while a reduction in CAC score beyond a given limit defines patients exhibiting regression in their underlying disease. With regards to the latter, it is still very controversial whether CAC truly regresses. As such, this document will focus on defining rapidly and slowly progressive disease states.

4.6.20 Reproducibility of CAC CT and Its Determinants

A major consideration for interpretation of changes in CAC between serial CT examinations is the variability of repeat imaging. Inter-examination variability is affected by image artifacts including motion, noise, and partial volume averaging that are highly dependent on the specific imaging protocol as well as the extent of CAC burden. Optimal timing of ECG triggering can reduce variability of Agatston scores >30% to <15% with EBT (BUDOFF and RAGGI 2001; LU et al. 2002; MAO et al. 2001). The correlation coefficients across CAC measurements, including Agatston score (AU), calcium volume score (CVS), or MS, are excellent ($r \geq 0.96$, $n = 161$) (HORIGUCHI et al. 2004; HOFFMANN et al. 2006). CVS's improve reproducibility only marginally compared to Agatston scores. The square root of the CVS has, however, been suggested to reduce inter-examination variability (Hokanson et al. 2004).

Differences between types of CT systems are very small after adjustment for body mass index and CAC burden (Detrano et al. 2005). In the MESA study, mean relative differences between CT examinations at different times were 20.1% for the Agatston score, and 18.3% for the interpolated CVS ($p<0.01$) (Detrano et al. 2005), which are in line with previous reports. Of note these data were obtained from CT performed at 80% of the RR-interval, which is associated with a lower reproducibility as compared to earlier triggering.

Data acquired with four-slice CT systems were reported to have higher rates of mis-registration compared with EBT (Detrano et al. 2005). Motion artifacts were also higher in these CT systems compared to EBT machines, while image noise was lower (Detrano et al. 2005). The reproducibility of the calcium score has improved with the introduction of 16-slice and more recently 64-slice MDCT systems. The variability is best with thinner slices, higher calcium scores and with retrospective acquisition mode, although this is associated with a higher radiation dose for the patient. Currently, the reported variability of the Agatston, volume and mass score on 16- to 64-slice MDCT ranges between 8%–18% (lower end of the range with 64-slice MDCT) on sequential examinations performed within minutes of each other (Groen et al. 2007; Horiguchi et al. 2006, 2008). Given the radiation exposure, especially with MDCT systems, the benefit-risk ratio and time intervals of repeat CT must be considered individually, especially when women and young men are examined.

4.6.20.1 Clinical Thresholds of Coronary Artery Calcium Progression

Progression of CAC is generally calculated as a percent or absolute change from the baseline score using either the Agatston score, CVS, or MS (Raggi et al. 2005a; Budoff and Raggi 2001; Becker et al. 2007b; Budoff et al. 2005a; Gopal et al. 2007; Hsia et al. 2004; Rasouli et al. 2005; Shemesh et al. 2001; Sutton-Tyrrell et al. 2001; Yoon et al. 2002). Raggi et al. (2005a) defined a change >15% as true progression, while Hokanson et al. (2004) suggested a CAC progression $\geq 2.5\ mm^3$ of the square root of the initial volume score as a useful threshold of progression.

The absolute change in CAC is expected to be greater in patients with a higher baseline score (Figs. 4.6.3 and 4.6.4) (Raggi et al. 2005a; Hsia et al. 2004; Rasouli et al. 2005), although the absolute differences reflect minor changes compared to baseline. Larger percent score changes are expected in patients with a low index CAC score (e.g., index CAC score of 10 to repeat score of 20 = progression of 100%) and do not necessarily reflect a clinically relevant change.

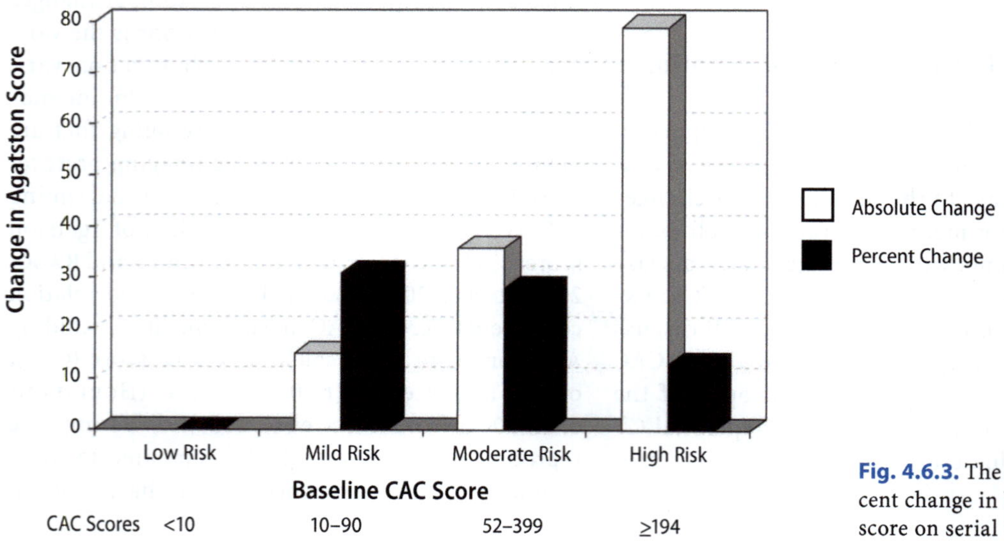

Fig. 4.6.3. The absolute and percent change in baseline Agatston score on serial CT imaging

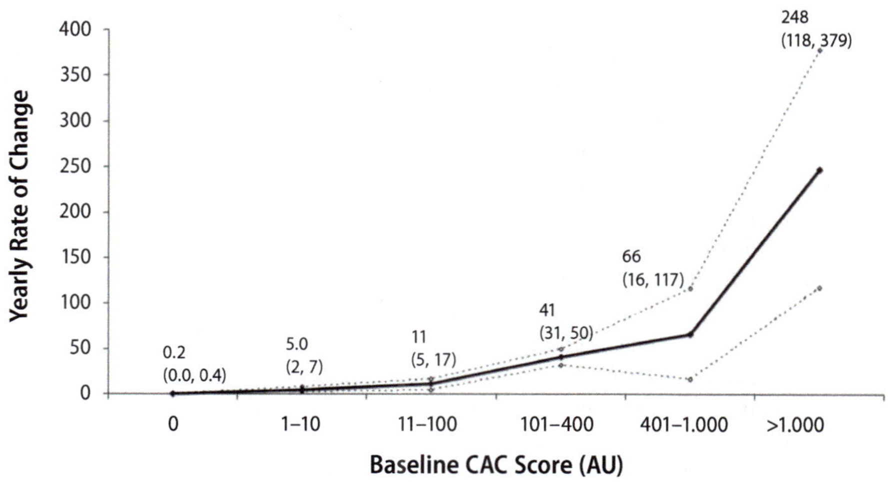

Fig. 4.6.4. Expected yearly rate of change (95% confidence intervals) from baseline for coronary artery calcium scores ranging from 0 to ≥ 1000 Agatston units (AU)

4.6.21 Clinical Interpretation of Changes in Coronary Artery Calcium

For most patients within the various risk groups in Figure 4.6.5, the error in score reproducibility would not affect their clinical management, unless scores are close to adjacent risk groups. Variability increases with CAC score and may be as much as 200–380 units for scores of 400 or higher (Fig. 4.6.5) (Sevrukov et al. 2005). As scores of 100 or 400 may trigger more aggressive post-screening management or follow-up ischemia testing, clinicians should rely less on the absolute thresholds and more on a combination of CAC score with the patient's clinical presentation and cardiac risk factor profile. Aggressive management is indicated for scores of 1000 or higher (very high risk CAC) and it is unlikely that the expected variability about this point estimate will change clinical care (Raggi et al. 2003; Budoff and Raggi 2001; Becker et al. 2007b; Budoff et al. 2005a; Gopal et al. 2007; Hsia et al. 2004; Rasouli et al. 2005; Shemesh et al. 2001; Sutton-Tyrrell et al. 2001; Yoon et al. 2002).

4.6.21.1 Rates of Coronary Artery Calcium Progression and Its Determinants

In subjects at average Framingham risk the annual CAC progression rates typically range from 20% to 24% per year using either the Agatston or the CVS (Raggi et al. 2003; Budoff and Raggi 2001; Becker et al. 2007b; Budoff et al. 2005a; Gopal et al. 2007; Hsia et al. 2004; Rasouli et al. 2005;

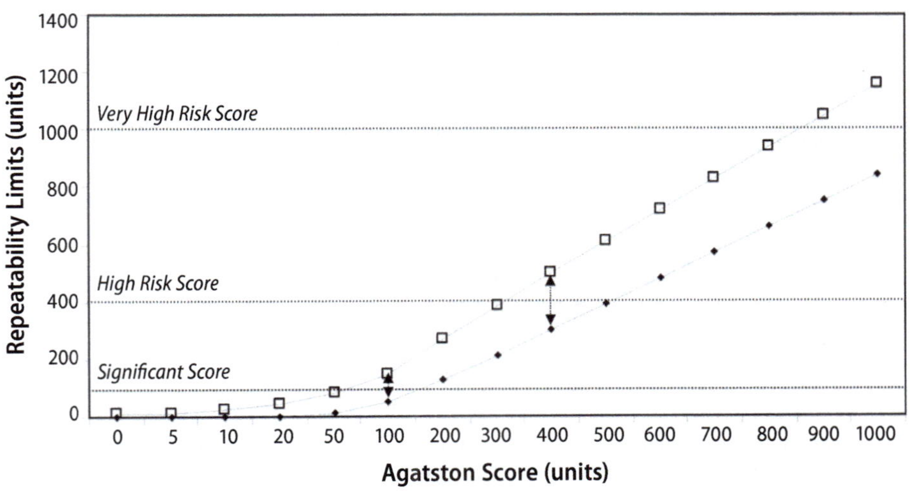

Fig. 4.6.5. 95% Confidence intervals for repeatability of coronary artery calcium scores from 0 to ≥1000

Shemesh et al. 2001; Sutton-Tyrrell et al. 2001; Yoon et al. 2002). Factors that may significantly modify rate of change include the patient's baseline CAC score, gender, age, family history of premature CAD, ethnicity, diabetes and glycemic control, body mass index, hypertension, and renal insufficiency (Raggi et al. 2005a; Cassidy et al. 2005; Kawakubo et al. 2005; Kronmal et al. 2007; Mehrotra et al. 2004; Snell-Bergeon et al. 2003). Furthermore, the longer the interval from baseline to repeat CAC CT, the greater the expected change (Shemesh et al. 2001). However, the absolute change will be greater but the relative change may be smaller. The score does not continue to grow exponentially and the rate of growth eventually tapers off. Most patients exhibit a positive change in CAC scores over time (Raggi et al. 2003; Becker et al. 2007b; Budoff et al. 2005a; Gopal et al. 2007; Rasouli et al. 2005; Sutton-Tyrrell et al. 2001), although some patients (29%–34%) exhibit no change if they are at low Framingham risk, including women, or have a baseline score of 0 (38%) (Gopal et al. 2007). In patients with an initial 0 score, a repeat CT < 5 years after the initial examination may not be useful for clinical purposes (Gopal et al. 2007).

4.6.21.2 Results of Randomized Clinical Trials on Effect of Statin Therapy on Coronary Artery Calcium Progression

A number of observational studies (Table 4.6.3) and randomized clinical trials (Fig. 4.6.6) have evaluated change in CAC following treatment with statin therapy. In four observational reports untreated patients had an average CAC score progression of 36% (Raggi et al. 2005a; Budoff et al. 2000, 2005b; Callister et al. 1998). By comparison, statin therapy attenuated changes in CAC scores averaging 13% (Table 4.6.3) (Raggi et al. 2005a; Budoff et al. 2000, 2005; Callister et al. 1998).

Table 4.6.3. Percent yearly progression from observational cohorts of consecutive patient series, with average Framingham risk, and evidence of coronary artery calcium (CAC) on Baseline CT

Author/year	No. of patients	Entry criteria	Score	Testing period (in years)	Percent change CAC Score/year[a]
Budoff et al. (2000)	299	Consecutive patients	AU	≥1	33%
Shemesh et al. (2001)	116	Asymptomatic Hypertensive patients	AU	1, 2, 3	Year. 1: 18% Year 2: 31% Year 3: 41%
Sutton-Tyrrell et al. (2001)	80	Middle-aged women	AU	1.5	11%
Yoon et al. (2002)	217	Consecutive subjects	AU CVS	2.1	34% 29%
Raggi et al. (2003)	772	Consecutive patients	CVS	2.2	26%
Hsia et al. (2004)	94	Healthy post-menopausal women CAC ≥10	AU	3.3	27%
Budoff et al. (2005)	177	Post-menopausal patients	AU	≥1	15%–22%
Rasouli et al. (2005)	133	Asymptomatic patients	AU	1.7	17%–22%
Gopal et al. (2007)	710	Consecutive patients. w/ CAC = 0	AU	≥1	Mean±SD: 1±3 Median (IQR): 0 (0–0.8)
Becker et al. (2007b)	277	Post-menopausal women	CVS	3.3	18%
Summary Data	2875		AU CVS		20% 24%

[a] Or mean±standard deviation (SD), median, interquartile range (IQR) in the Gopal series.
CAC, coronary artery calcium; yr, year; AU, Agatston units; CVS, calcium volume score; SD, standard deviation.

RCTs of Statin Therapy vs. Placebo

			Baseline CAC	Change/yr
Studies	N	CAC	Control: Active	Control: Active
ACHENBACH et al. 2002	66	CVS	155*	25:11 relative
ARAD et al. 2000	1,005	AU	563:527	240:192 abs

Rate Difference (95% CI)

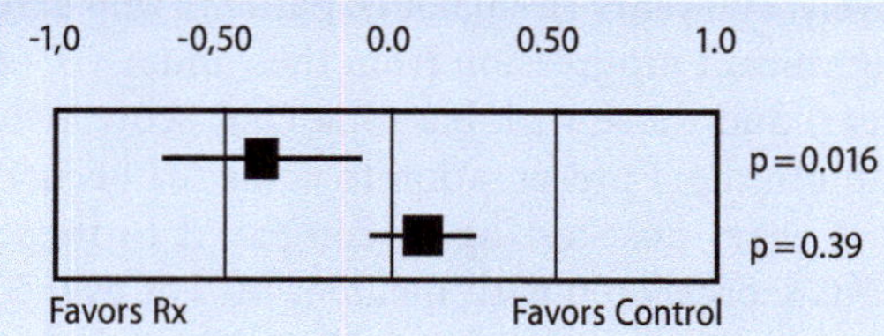

* Achenbach – Patients had a Treated and Untreated Time Period. Thus, there is no RCT of Statin vs. Placebo and no summary effect was clculated

RCTs of Moderate vs. Intensive Statin Therapy

			Baseline CAC	Change/yr
Studies	N	CAC	Moderate: Intensive	Moderate: Intensive
RAGGI et al. 2005a	614	CVS	371:434	23:38 relative
SCHMERMUND et al. 2006	366	CVS	267:205	31:28 relative
Summery Effect				

Rate Difference (95% CI)

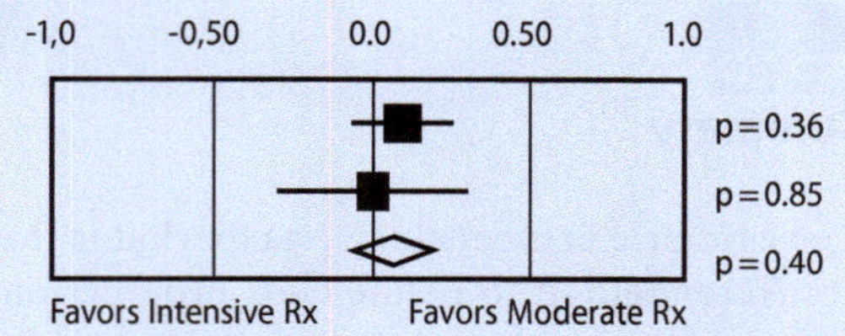

Abbreciations: CAC=Coronary Artery Clcium, CVS=Calcium Volume Score, AU=Agatston Units, RCT=Randomized Clinical Trial, Yr=Year

Fig. 4.6.6. Summary meta-analysis of randomized control trials (*RCT*) on the effect of statin therapy (*Rx*) on CAC progression

However, these promising observational data were contradicted by large randomized clinical trials showing similar changes in CAC scores following placebo and/or moderate-intensive statin therapy (Fig. 4.6.6). Except for a preliminary pilot trial (ACHENBACH et al. 2002), all other randomized trials have failed to confirm the preliminary observational findings (Fig. 4.6.6). Comparison of intensive vs. moderate statin therapy showed no difference in CAC progression (Fig. 4.6.6) (RAGGI et al. 2005b; SCHMERMUND et al. 2006). The lack of an effect in these clinical trials suggests that a longer observational time period may be warranted and that statins may reduce cardiac events independent of an effect on calcified plaque (GREENLAND et al. 2007). Further, these trials often did not consider or plan the management of other CV risk factors that may confound the lack of therapeutic benefit (GREENLAND et al. 2007). There are ongoing trials using CAC as a surrogate where additional evidence may be put forth on the benefit in serial imaging (HARMAN et al. 2005; KULLER et al. 2007). Finally, other treatments have been tested as far as an effect on CAC progression. In the Women's Health Initiative (WHI), menopausal women between the ages of 50–59 years were randomized to treatment with conjugated estrogens or placebo (MANSON et al. 2007). In a sub-study of the WHI, 1064 women were submitted to CAC screening after 8.7 years from trial initiation. Women receiving estrogens showed a lower CAC score compared those receiving placebo (83.1 vs. 123.1, $p = 0.02$).

4.6.22 Cardiovascular Prognosis Related to Coronary Artery Calcium Progression

Despite the lack of an effect of statins on CAC progression, several reports have noted that a rapid change in CAC score is associated with worse clinical outcomes including incident MI (RAGGI et al. 2003, 2004c). In one report of 495 patients, subjects who experienced an acute MI experienced greater degrees of CAC progression compared to event-free survivors (42% ± 23% vs. 17% ± 25%, $p < 0.0001$) [97].

Patients with and without >15%/year change in CAC score had 66% and 97% MI-free survival, respectively, at 6 years ($p<0.0001$). Patients who exhibited significant progression from their index CT (≥15%/year) and those with baseline CAC score ≥400 had a more rapid presentation to acute MI occurring at 2–4 years post-testing as compared to those with CAC scores ≤100 with incident MI's at over 5 years from baseline testing ($p<0.0001$). Thus, the baseline CAC score provides an insight into not only the expected rate of progression but also the timeline of conversion to symptomatic CAD.

4.6.23 Summary

The evidence is inconclusive as to what is the most accurate method to define CAC progression (percent vs. absolute vs. square root change). Further research is indicated as to documenting meaningful changes in the various scores. For the patient with an average Framingham risk score, the yearly increase in CAC score is approximately 15%–20%. Absolute changes are greater in patients whose baseline score exceeds 100. To date, published randomized trials have failed to demonstrate a benefit of statin therapy to attenuate CAC progression. Despite this, rapidly increasing CAC scores may be used to define higher risk patients. Further insight into the prognostic implications of serial CT examinations is warranted to further guide optimal patient management. This writing committee does not recommend the systematic performance of serial CAC scoring in every patient that has undergone a baseline CT and is receiving treatment for factors related to atherosclerosis. An individualized approach to assess rate of progression in specific situations may be taken into consideration.

4.6.24 Standardization of the Calcium Score Measured Using Different CT Systems

The utilization of CAC scores for outcomes data, risk stratification, and particularly, the serial assessment of patients over time demands accurate measurements. Accurate measurement of MDCT derived CAC scores requires implementation of standardized imaging and quantification methods on many different types of commercially available MDCT systems. This formidable goal can be achieved by selecting CT parameters that fulfill minimum requirements for temporal resolution, spatial resolution, and noise and by applying a physically-meaningful, calibration-based calcium quantification algorithm.

A standard for CAC quantification was recently proposed by the Physics Task Group of the International Consortium on Standardization in Cardiac CT and is reviewed here (McCollough et al. 2007). Standardized CT protocols were developed for six CT models from five manufacturers (Aquilion, Toshiba Medical Systems, Nasu, Japan; Imatron, Imatron San Francisco, CA; LightSpeed Plus, General Electric Healthcare, Milwaukee, Wisconsin; MX8000, Philips Medical Systems, Best, The Netherlands; Volume Zoom, Siemens Medical Solutions, Erlangen, Germany; Sensation 64, Siemens) using an anthropomorphic cardiac phantom containing water and calcium inserts and capable of simulating three patient sizes. Manufacturer recommended protocols met the minimum requirements for imaging coronary calcium with MDCT: (1) acquisition of at least four slices per rotation, (2) rotation time less than or equal to 0.5 s, (3) ability to reference data acquisition or reconstruction to the ECG signal. Most protocols were, however, modified to achieve a target noise level (20–23 HU) in the water insert for each phantom size. This primarily required determination of CT model- and size-specific values for the tube current (mA) or tube-current time product (mAs). Small, medium, and large anthropomorphic phantoms were then examined on a total of ten different CT machines using these standardized CT protocols.

All image sets were scored using a single software package because, although not explicitly evaluated by the Consortium, differences among scoring packages are assumed to be non-negligible (but low compared to other sources of error; see next section). To address this issue, software manufacturers were asked to modify existing algorithms according to recommendations of the Consortium. Software packages will then be validated as they become available (at least three manufacturers have incorporated the Consortium recommendations into their software at this writing).

To quantify CAC, voxels containing calcium were first isolated from other tissue and image noise primarily by applying a standard 130-HU attenuation threshold to the reconstructed images. Agatston, volume, and mass scores were then calculated using standard quantification algorithms (McCollough et al. 2007). To obtain absolute values for calcium mass, a calibration measurement of a calcification with known hydroxyapatite (HA) density was carried out and a calibration factor determined. Because the CT number of all materials except water depends on the X-ray spectrum, a specific calibration factor exists for each machine and each CT protocol. Work by the Physics Group of the Consortium also showed that patient size changes the X-ray spectrum and impacts the value of the calibration factor significantly. Therefore, a unique calibration factor was determined for each of three broad categories of patient sizes for each CT model and each CT protocol using the cardiac phantom's water and calcium inserts.

The mass score (m_{ij}) was then computed as the product of the appropriate calibration factor (C_{HA}), the number of voxels containing calcium (N_{voxel}), the volume of one voxel (V_{voxel}), and the mean CT number for each lesion (CT_{ij}):

$$m_{ij} = C_{HA} \cdot N_{voxel} \cdot V_{voxel} \cdot CT_{ij}$$

The total mass score is the sum of the mass of all individual lesions.

Analysis of the mean and standard deviation of the calcium scores measured under ideal conditions from EBCT and MDCT systems demonstrated a coefficient of variation of 4.0% for Agatston scores, 7.9% for volume scores, and 4.9% for mass scores. The accuracy, or exact correspondence between measured and true values, could not be assessed for Agatston scores because this score represents only a mathematical construct and as such cannot be compared to a physical reference standard. However, calcium volume and mass scores could be compared to known values from the cardiac phantom. For the five MDCT systems, the total calcium mass score was within ±5 mg of the total known mass of calcium HA within the phantom (168.2 mg). The accuracy of EBT measurement was considerably worse (mean mass score equaled 182.7 mg). Therefore, the increased precision of the mass score as compared with the volume score and the ability to compare the measured mass score with a known physical standard motivated the Consortium to endorse the mass score approach as the preferred method of quantifying CAC.

Additional data have been collected by the Physics Group towards optimization of the mass score. Specifically, the requirements for calculation of a calibration factor were examined. Variation in the measured calibration factor from three sizes of the anthropomorphic cardiac phantom was assessed across CT machines, time, and patient sizes. Assessment across CT machines, revealed the coefficient of variation in the calibration factor was small for a specific CT manufacturer and CT model (0.13%–1.6%). Subsequent data analysis from the same CT systems over time has shown slightly higher variation for measurements made quarterly over a 4-year period from a single 16-slice CT machine (2.8%–3.2%) and over a 2-year period from a single 64-slice CT machine (2.5%–3.1%). The change in phantom (i.e., patient size), however, caused a much larger change in calibration factor both across CT systems (3.8%–5.1%) and over time (3.4%–5.0%). Therefore, determination of a calibration factor for a given CT machine and patient size from quarterly CT of an anthropomorphic phantom should be sufficiently stable over time to permit 3% or less variation in the measurement. It has been suggested that inclusion of a calibration insert with each patient is necessary for precise measurement of a calibration factor. However, this seems unnecessary based on the low variability in calibration estimation with quarterly anthropomorphic CT.

Because of the variation in calibration measurements, particularly across patient sizes, the consortium recommended identifying voxels containing calcium by applying a threshold based on a fixed density or concentration of calcium HA (100 mg/cc of calcium HA) rather than the traditional fixed attenuation (130 HU) that may not provide a consistent cutoff value for calcium across examinations.

In summary, the Physics Group demonstrated that standardized protocols and algorithms can provide accurate and precise calcium mass scores in phantoms independent of MDCT model and phantom (patient) size through the use of appropriate calibration factors. Implementation of these protocols should move the field of CAC scoring closer to the realization of meaningful quantitative comparisons of CAC scores measured over time within a patient and across patients even when imaging is performed using different MDCT models. An obvious output of the implementation of such standards should be reduced variability in CAC measurements although this remains a point of investigation.

The recommendations of the Consortium have largely been implemented by the CT manufacturers making adherence to these standardization procedures in clinical CT straightforward. Additional relatively tasks beyond current practice will, however, be required including measurement of lateral skin-to-skin width at mid-liver from an anteroposterior CT radiograph ("scout" image) to assess patient size, selection of appropriate patient-size specific mA/mAs to achieve the noise target, and selection of appropriate patient-size specific calibration factor to determine a density-based attenuation threshold and calculate absolute calcium mass.

The biggest obstacle to widespread use of the mass score is the paucity of data available for clinical decision-making. The CAC score is most clinically meaningful in the context of risk-stratification which requires referencing a patient's total CAC score to age- and sex-matched data. A patient is assigned to a percentile range of risk on the basis of his or her total CAC score; the percentile range is defined by flexible thresholds that take into account the independent effects of age and sex on the amount of total CAC. Most currently available databases, particularly those with a significant number of patients, contain only Agatston scores. An MDCT database founded upon standard protocols using the mass score is therefore necessary.

Implementation of a standardization procedure for the acquisition and analysis of CAC images permits the accumulation of scores from various MDCT systems in a single database. A web-based database has been developed through the efforts of the Consortium to allow collection of standardized MDCT patient risk factor and CAC data (https://clinapps.bio.ri.ccf.org/cascore/). A sufficient number of patients must be entered before assignment of a precise percentile ranking can be provided to an individual patient. Based on early data, it was determined that a total registry size of 4000 would be sufficient to estimate the percentile ranking of future patients in the age range of 45–70 years. To date, data from over 1000 patients have been collected. The Writing Group supports this standardization procedure and recommends that this registry be supported.

4.6.25 Influence of Scoring Parameter Settings of Underlying Software Algorithms on Calcium Scoring

All scoring methods used for the determination of CAC have a common denominator. This is the algorithm used to determine which areas above the threshold HU value are calcified lesions and which can be discarded as noise. To determine this very important distinction, common algorithms are used that are influenced by a number of different parameter settings which, as shown by van Ooijen et al. (2005) in 50 patients imaged with EBT, influence the resulting CAC score. The most common parameters are the HU threshold value, the connectivity, the lesion size threshold and the use of interpolation. Some commercially available software packages provide the user with the parameter settings and even allow changing these parameters. Others hide the default settings and determining the settings used can be very difficult. Mean variability can be up to 15–16 points for the Agatston score with the largest influence coming from changing the lesion size threshold between two and four pixels. For the CVS, mean variability can be up to 20–30 points largely due to the effect of changing the lesion size threshold between two and four pixels and from turning interpolation on and off. It could well be that the effect of interpolation will be less prominent when using MDCT instead of EBT because of the use of slice overlap. There are no published data for the mass scoring method, but since this method also relies on algorithms to determine what regions are lesions and what regions are not, it is likely that similar results will be found.

In conclusion, when performing CAC scoring based on the volume or Agatston score, software parameter settings affect the outcome. Furthermore, the use of new software versions or other software packages and the use of data acquired in other institutes in the follow-up of patients could also affect the measured progression or regression of CAC because of different parameter settings. These data show, therefore, that not only standardization of CT protocols is obligatory, but CAC scoring parameters also need to be standardized. Further research is required to determine whether using phantom data or test patient datasets can help standardizing settings across software and help selecting the appropriate settings of a certain software package when they are unclear.

4.6.26 Radiation Exposure

A broad implementation of CAC screening may be limited by factors such as cost, patient access and demonstration of altered medical outcomes. In addition, risks associated with the use of ionizing radiation must be taken into account, especially for younger or female patients or when considering additional radiological tests such as CT and MPI. CAC screening delivers a relatively low radiation dose (effective dose of 0.7 mSv with EBT and 1.0–4.1 mSv with MDCT) (Morin et al. 2003), while coronary CT angiography (outside of the scope of this writing) delivers somewhat increased levels of radiation dose (effective dose of 9.4–14.8 mSv) (Hausleiter et al. 2006). The dose to any one individual depends both on the imaging protocol used and the patient's body habitus. The radiation exposure provided by CAC screening is substantially lower than that of MPI studies (effective dose range of 13-16 mSv), especially those conducted using Thallium-201 or dual isotope techniques (effective dose of 27.3 mSv) (Thompson and Cullom 2006) or invasive diagnostic coronary catheterization (effective dose of 3–10 mSv) (Einstein et al. 2007a).

Much of our knowledge on the carcinogenic effects of low doses of radiation (whole body exposures of 5–150 mSv) derives from follow-up data on the survivors of the atomic bombings in Japan. Although quite small, there appears to be an increase in incidence of cancer in subjects exposed to low doses of radiation, especially in children – because of the higher radiation sensitivity and the longer available time for cancer development after exposure. Using the linear non-threshold model of radiation induced risk and the organ specific risk from Biological Effects of Ionizing Radiation (BEIR VII) (National Research Council, US, 2006), the data presented by Einstein et al. (2007b) can be linearly scaled to predict the lifetime risk of cancer. Assuming a factor of 10 reduction of dose from a coronary CTA exam, the lifetime risk of cancer for a CAC CT in a 50-year-old individual is 0.04% for a man and 0.12% for a woman. To properly interpret these data, the individual's complete risk profile must be considered, including the background risk of cancer incidence in the general population and any individual-specific risks such as diabetes, high blood pressure or a family history of cancer or heart disease. According to statistics from the American Cancer Society, the lifetime risk of cancer at any site is 45% for men and 38% for women; the respective death rates are 23% and 20% (Jemal et al. 2007). Thus, taking into account the patient's specific medical risks, particularly of coronary artery disease, and the background population risks, the additive cancer risk from a CAC exam is negligible, provided that some benefit may be gained from the examination. Thus, this committee of experts does not support the application of CAC screening to individuals at low risk of coronary artery disease, where medical benefit is not expected. For individuals at intermediate risk of coronary artery disease, the small statistical risk of cancer induction and death is very low relative to the patient's complete risk profile. In these patients, the potential benefit to the patient from knowledge obtained in the CAC exam greatly exceeds the small potential risk of cancer and the use of CAC screening is recommended in several clinical scenarios.

Further, in contrast to alarming media reports regarding the risks associated with ionizing radiation, the radiation biology and epidemiology community is divided as to the actual degree of risk at the low doses associated with medical imaging examinations. Considering the error bars associated with the data from the Japanese bomb survivors, the difficultly in transferring risk estimates between population cohorts and irradiation dose rates and types (high vs. low dose rates, whole body vs. partial body exposures, etc.), and the conflicting reports from medically exposed populations that show no increase in risk at medical imaging dose levels, it is the official position of the Health Physics Society that meaningful risk estimates are not possible below effective doses of 100 mSv (Health Physics Society 2004). Thus, CAC exams, with effective doses of 1–4 mSv, may in fact be associated with no additional risk and hence should not be avoided when information important to the patient's medical management may be obtained.

4.6.27 Conclusions

The writing committee would like to summarize in a series of conceptual points the evidence discussed herein as follows.

We know and support the conclusion that:

- CAC is a good predictor of events in Caucasians and adds incremental prognostic value to risk factors in intermediate risk populations
- There is significant variability between ethnicities in the prevalence and extent of coronary calcium.
- Absence of CAC is associated with very low event rates in most risk categories
- Rapid CAC progression is associated with higher risk of events
- CAC is a strong predictor of events in end stage renal disease
- A zero calcium score is associated with a very low prevalence of ischemia on functional stress testing and obstructive disease on angiography

We are beginning to understand that:

- CAC may have good predictive value in the elderly, in diabetic patients and in patients of different ethnic background
- CAC scores can be used to predict presence of obstructive CAD but despite a high sensitivity this tool demonstrates a low specificity; hence the main utilization of CAC should be assessment of risk of cardiovascular events rather than the detection of severe CAD

We still need to prove that:

- We can alter CAC progression with medical interventions
- Altering CAC progression with medical interventions impacts patients' outcome
- We may not need to treat patients with risk factors in the absence of CAC

Finally, standardized procedures for both image acquisition and CAC scoring should be followed so that we might best advance our knowledge using MDCT.

Disclosure of Support

Author	Disclosure of Support
SSH	None
WAK	Siemens Medical Solutions
CHM	Bayer Healthcare, Siemens Medical Solutions, RTI Electronics, Inc
SM	None
MO	None
PMAO	None
PR	None
AES	Astellas, Siemens Medical Solutions
LJS	None
WS	None
AJT	None
RV	None
LW	None

References

Abbott RD, Ueshima H, Masaki KH et al. (2007) Coronary artery calcification and total mortality in elderly men. J Am Geriatr Soc 55:1948–1954

Achenbach S, Ropers D, Pohle K et al. (2002) Influence of lipid-lowering therapy on the progression of coronary artery calcification: a prospective evaluation. Circulation 106:1077–1082

Anand DV, Lim E, Hopkins D et al. (2006) Risk stratification in uncomplicated type 2 diabetes: prospective evaluation of the combined use of coronary artery calcium imaging and selective myocardial perfusion scintigraphy. Eur Heart J 27:713–721

Anderson KM, Castelli WP, Levy D (1987) Cholesterol and mortality. 30 years of follow-up from the Framingham study. JAMA 257:2176–2180

Andrews TC (2000) Electron-beam computed tomography in the evaluation of patients with chest pain. Am J Cardiol 85:386–387

Arad Y, Spadaro LA, Goodman K, Newstein D, Guerci AD (2000) Prediction of coronary events with electron beam computed tomography. J Am Coll Cardiol 36:1253–1260

Arad Y, Goodman KJ, Roth M, Newstein D, Guerci AD (2005) Coronary calcification, coronary disease risk factors, C-reactive protein, and atherosclerotic cardiovascular disease events: the St. Francis Heart Study. J Am Coll Cardiol 46:158–165

Assmann G, Cullen P, Schulte H (2002) Simple scoring scheme for calculating the risk of acute coronary events based on

the 10-year follow-up of the prospective cardiovascular Munster (PROCAM) study. Circulation 105:310–315
Becker CR, Kleffel T, Crispin A et al. (2001) Coronary artery calcium measurement: agreement of multirow detector and electron beam CT. AJR Am J Roentgenol 176:1295–1298
Becker A, Leber A, White CW, Becker C, Reiser MF, Knez A (2007a) Multislice computed tomography for determination of coronary artery disease in a symptomatic patient population. Int J Cardiovasc Imaging 23:361–367
Becker A, Leber A, von Ziegler F, Becker C, Knez A (2007b) Comparison of progression of coronary calcium in postmenopausal women on versus not on estrogen/progestin therapy. Am J Cardiol 99:374–378
Bellasi A, Lacey C, Taylor AJ et al. (2007) Comparison of prognostic usefulness of coronary artery calcium in men versus women (results from a meta- and pooled analysis estimating all-cause mortality and coronary heart disease death or myocardial infarction). Am J Cardiol 100:409–414
Berman DS, Wong ND, Gransar H et al. (2004) Relationship between stress-induced myocardial ischemia and atherosclerosis measured by coronary calcium tomography. J Am Coll Cardiol 44:923–930
Bild DE, Detrano R, Peterson D et al. (2005) Ethnic differences in coronary calcification: the Multi-Ethnic Study of Atherosclerosis (MESA). Circulation 111:1313–1320
Block GA, Spiegel DM, Ehrlich J et al. (2005) Effects of sevelamer and calcium on coronary artery calcification in patients new to hemodialysis. Kidney Int 68:1815–1824
Block GA, Raggi P, Bellasi A, Kooienga L, Spiegel DM (2007) Mortality effect of coronary calcification and phosphate binder choice in incident hemodialysis patients. Kidney Int 71:438–441
Braun J, Oldendorf M, Moshage W, Heidler R, Zeitler E, Luft FC (1996) Electron beam computed tomography in the evaluation of cardiac calcification in chronic dialysis patients. Am J Kidney Dis 27:394–401
Budoff MJ, Lane KL, Bakhsheshi H et al. (2000) Rates of progression of coronary calcium by electron beam tomography. Am J Cardiol 86:8–11
Budoff MJ, Raggi P (2001) Coronary artery disease progression assessed by electron-beam computed tomography. Am J Cardiol 88:46E–50E
Budoff MJ, Diamond GA, Raggi P et al. (2002) Continuous probabilistic prediction of angiographically significant coronary artery disease using electron beam tomography. Circulation 105:1791–1796
Budoff MJ, Chen GP, Hunter CJ et al. (2005a) Effects of hormone replacement on progression of coronary calcium as measured by electron beam tomography. J Womens Health (Larchmt) 14:410–417
Budoff MJ, Yu D, Nasir K et al. (2005b) Diabetes and progression of coronary calcium under the influence of statin therapy. Am Heart J 149:695–700
Budoff MJ, Achenbach S, Blumenthal RS et al. (2006) Assessment of coronary artery disease by cardiac computed tomography: a scientific statement from the American Heart Association Committee on Cardiovascular Imaging and Intervention, Council on Cardiovascular Radiology and Intervention, and Committee on Cardiac Imaging, Council on Clinical Cardiology. Circulation 114:1761–1791
Budoff MJ, Shaw LJ, Liu ST et al. (2007) Long-term prognosis associated with coronary calcification: observations from a registry of 25,253 patients. J Am Coll Cardiol 49:1860–1870
Bursztyn M, Motro M, Grossman E, Shemesh J (2003) Accelerated coronary artery calcification in mildly reduced renal function of high-risk hypertensives: a 3-year prospective observation. J Hypertens 21:1953–1959
Callister TQ, Raggi P, Cooil B, Lippolis NJ, Russo DJ (1998) Effect of HMG-CoA reductase inhibitors on coronary artery disease as assessed by electron-beam computed tomography. N Engl J Med 339:1972–1978
Carr JJ, Crouse JR 3rd, Goff DC Jr, D'Agostino RB Jr, Peterson NP, Burke GL (2000) Evaluation of subsecond gated helical CT for quantification of coronary artery calcium and comparison with electron beam CT. AJR Am J Roentgenol 174:915–921
Cassidy AE, Bielak LF, Zhou Y et al. (2005) Progression of subclinical coronary atherosclerosis: does obesity make a difference? Circulation 111:1877–1882
Cheng VY, Lepor NE, Madyoon H, Eshaghian S, Naraghi AL, Shah PK (2007) Presence and severity of noncalcified coronary plaque on 64-slice computed tomographic coronary angiography in patients with zero and low coronary artery calcium. Am J Cardiol 99:1183–1186
Chertow GM, Burke SK, Raggi P (2002) Sevelamer attenuates the progression of coronary and aortic calcification in hemodialysis patients. Kidney Int 62:245–252
Chertow GM, Raggi P, Chasan-Taber S, Bommer J, Holzer H, Burke SK (2004) Determinants of progressive vascular calcification in haemodialysis patients. Nephrol Dial Transplant 19:1489–1496
Church TS, Levine BD, McGuire DK et al. (2007) Coronary artery calcium score, risk factors, and incident coronary heart disease events. Atherosclerosis 190:224–231
Conroy RM, Pyorala K, Fitzgerald AP et al. (2003) Estimation of ten-year risk of fatal cardiovascular disease in Europe: the SCORE project. Eur Heart J 24:987–1003
Daniell AL, Wong ND, Friedman JD et al. (2005) Concordance of coronary artery calcium estimates between MDCT and electron beam tomography. AJR Am J Roentgenol 185:1542–1545
Detrano RC, Anderson M, Nelson J et al. (2005) Coronary calcium measurements: effect of CT scanner type and calcium measure on rescan reproducibility – MESA study. Radiology 236:477–484
Detrano R, Guerci AD, Carr JJ et al. (2008) Coronary calcium as a predictor of coronary events in four racial or ethnic groups. N Engl J Med 358:1336–1345
Doherty TM, Tang W, Detrano RC (1999) Racial differences in the significance of coronary calcium in asymptomatic black and white subjects with coronary risk factors. J Am Coll Cardiol 34:787–794
Einstein AJ, Moser KW, Thompson RC, Cerqueira MD, Henzlova MJ (2007a) Radiation dose to patients from cardiac diagnostic imaging. Circulation 116:1290–1305
Einstein AJ, Henzlova MJ, Rajagopalan S (2007b) Estimating risk of cancer associated with radiation exposure from 64-slice computed tomography coronary angiography. JAMA 298:317–323
Erbel R, Mohlenkamp S, Lehmann N et al. (2007) Sex related cardiovascular risk stratification based on quantification of atherosclerosis and inflammation. Atherosclerosis 197:662–672

Fleischmann KE, Hunink MG, Kuntz KM, Douglas PS (2002) Exercise echocardiography or exercise SPECT imaging? A meta-analysis of diagnostic test performance. J Nucl Cardiol 9:133–134

Geluk CA, Dikkers R, Perik PJ et al. (2007) Measurement of coronary calcium scores by electron beam computed tomography or exercise testing as initial diagnostic tool in low-risk patients with suspected coronary artery disease. Eur Radiol 18:244–252

Georgiou D, Budoff MJ, Kaufer E, Kennedy JM, Lu B, Brundage BH (2001) Screening patients with chest pain in the emergency department using electron beam tomography: a follow-up study. J Am Coll Cardiol 38:105–110

Gibbons RJ, Balady GJ, Bricker JT et al. (2002) ACC/AHA 2002 guideline update for exercise testing: summary article: a report of the American College of Cardiology/American Heart Association Task Force on Practice Guidelines (Committee to Update the 1997 Exercise Testing Guidelines). Circulation 106:1883–1892

Glynn RJ, Field TS, Rosner B, Hebert PR, Taylor JO, Hennekens CH (1995) Evidence for a positive linear relation between blood pressure and mortality in elderly people. Lancet 345:825–829

Goodman WG, Goldin J, Kuizon BD et al. (2000) Coronary-artery calcification in young adults with end-stage renal disease who are undergoing dialysis. N Engl J Med 342:1478–1483

Gopal A, Nasir K, Liu ST, Flores FR, Chen L, Budoff MJ (2007) Coronary calcium progression rates with a zero initial score by electron beam tomography. Int J Cardiol 117:227–231

Graham I, Atar D, Borch-Johnsen K et al. (2007) European guidelines on cardiovascular disease prevention in clinical practice: executive summary. Fourth Joint Task Force of the European Society of Cardiology and other societies on cardiovascular disease prevention in clinical practice (constituted by representatives of nine societies and by invited experts). Eur J Cardiovasc Prev Rehabil 14 Suppl 2:E1–40

Greenland P, LaBree L, Azen SP, Doherty TM, Detrano RC (2004) Coronary artery calcium score combined with Framingham score for risk prediction in asymptomatic individuals. JAMA 291:210–215

Greenland P, Bonow RO, Brundage BH et al. (2007) ACCF/AHA 2007 clinical expert consensus document on coronary artery calcium scoring by computed tomography in global cardiovascular risk assessment and in evaluation of patients with chest pain: a report of the American College of Cardiology Foundation Clinical Expert Consensus Task Force (ACCF/AHA Writing Committee to Update the 2000 Expert Consensus Document on Electron Beam Computed Tomography). Circulation 115:402–426

Greuter MJ, Dijkstra H, Groen JM et al. (2007) 64 slice MDCT generally underestimates coronary calcium scores as compared to EBT: a phantom study. Med Phys 34:3510–3519

Groen JM, Greuter MJ, Schmidt B, Suess C, Vliegenthart R, Oudkerk M (2007) The influence of heart rate, slice thickness, and calcification density on calcium scores using 64-slice multidetector computed tomography: a systematic phantom study. Invest Radiol 42:848–855

Grundy SM, Cleeman JI, Merz CN et al. (2004) Implications of recent clinical trials for the National Cholesterol Education Program Adult Treatment Panel III Guidelines. J Am Coll Cardiol 44:720–732

Guerin AP, London GM, Marchais SJ, Metivier F (2000) Arterial stiffening and vascular calcifications in end-stage renal disease. Nephrol Dial Transplant 15:1014–1021

Haberl R, Becker A, Leber A et al. (2001) Correlation of coronary calcification and angiographically documented stenoses in patients with suspected coronary artery disease: results of 1,764 patients. J Am Coll Cardiol 37:451–457

Harman SM, Brinton EA, Cedars M et al. (2005) KEEPS: The Kronos Early Estrogen Prevention Study. Climacteric 8:3–12

Hausleiter J, Meyer T, Hadamitzky M et al. (2006) Radiation dose estimates from cardiac multislice computed tomography in daily practice: impact of different scanning protocols on effective dose estimates. Circulation 113:1305–1310

Health Physics Society (2004) Radiation Risk in Perspective. Available at: http://hps.org/documents/risk_ps010-1.pdf. Accessed March 18

Hendel RC, Patel MR, Kramer CM et al. (2006) ACCF/ACR/SCCT/SCMR/ASNC/NASCI/SCAI/SIR 2006 appropriateness criteria for cardiac computed tomography and cardiac magnetic resonance imaging: a report of the American College of Cardiology Foundation Quality Strategic Directions Committee Appropriateness Criteria Working Group, American College of Radiology, Society of Cardiovascular Computed Tomography, Society for Cardiovascular Magnetic Resonance, American Society of Nuclear Cardiology, North American Society for Cardiac Imaging, Society for Cardiovascular Angiography and Interventions, and Society of Interventional Radiology. J Am Coll Cardiol 48:1475–1497

Hoff JA, Quinn L, Sevrukov A et al. (2003) The prevalence of coronary artery calcium among diabetic individuals without known coronary artery disease. J Am Coll Cardiol 41:1008–1012

Hoffmann U, Siebert U, Bull-Stewart A et al. (2006) Evidence for lower variability of coronary artery calcium mineral mass measurements by multi-detector computed tomography in a community-based cohort – consequences for progression studies. Eur J Radiol 57:396–402

Hokanson JE, MacKenzie T, Kinney G et al. (2004) Evaluating changes in coronary artery calcium: an analytic method that accounts for interscan variability. AJR Am J Roentgenol 182:1327–1332

Horiguchi J, Yamamoto H, Akiyama Y, Marukawa K, Hirai N, Ito K (2004) Coronary artery calcium scoring using 16-MDCT and a retrospective ECG-gating reconstruction algorithm. AJR Am J Roentgenol 183:103–108

Horiguchi J, Yamamoto H, Hirai N et al. (2006) Variability of repeated coronary artery calcium measurements on low-dose ECG-gated 16-MDCT. AJR Am J Roentgenol 187:W1–6

Horiguchi J, Matsuura N, Yamamoto H et al. (2008) Variability of repeated coronary artery calcium measurements by 1.25 mm and 2.5 mm thickness images on prospective electrocardiograph-triggered 64-slice CT. Eur Radiol 18:209–216

Hsia J, Klouj A, Prasad A, Burt J, Adams-Campbell LL, Howard BV (2004) Progression of coronary calcification in healthy postmenopausal women. BMC Cardiovasc Disord 4:21

Jain T, Peshock R, McGuire DK et al. (2004) African Americans and Caucasians have a similar prevalence of coronary calcium in the Dallas Heart Study. J Am Coll Cardiol 44:1011–1017

Jemal A, Siegel R, Ward E, Murray T, Xu J, Thun MJ (2007) Cancer statistics, 2007. CA Cancer J Clin 57:43–66

Kalia NK, Miller LG, Nasir K, Blumenthal RS, Agrawal N, Budoff MJ (2006) Visualizing coronary calcium is associated with improvements in adherence to statin therapy. Atherosclerosis 185:394–399

Kannel WB, D'Agostino RB, Silbershatz H (1997) Blood pressure and cardiovascular morbidity and mortality rates in the elderly. Am Heart J 134:758–763

Kawakubo M, LaBree L, Xiang M et al. (2005) Race-ethnic differences in the extent, prevalence, and progression of coronary calcium. Ethn Dis 15:198–204

Khaleeli E, Peters SR, Bobrowsky K, Oudiz RJ, Ko JY, Budoff MJ (2001) Diabetes and the associated incidence of subclinical atherosclerosis and coronary artery disease: Implications for management. Am Heart J 141:637–644

Knez A, Becker C, Becker A et al. (2002) Determination of coronary calcium with multi-slice spiral computed tomography: a comparative study with electron-beam CT. Int J Cardiovasc Imaging 18:295–303

Knez A, Becker A, Leber A et al. (2004) Relation of coronary calcium scores by electron beam tomography to obstructive disease in 2,115 symptomatic patients. Am J Cardiol 93:1150–1152

Kondos GT, Hoff JA, Sevrukov A et al. (2003) Electron-beam tomography coronary artery calcium and cardiac events: a 37-month follow-up of 5635 initially asymptomatic low-to intermediate-risk adults. Circulation 107:2571–2576

Kronmal RA, McClelland RL, Detrano R et al. (2007) Risk factors for the progression of coronary artery calcification in asymptomatic subjects: results from the Multi-Ethnic Study of Atherosclerosis (MESA). Circulation 115:2722–2730

Kuller LH, Kriska AM, Kinzel LS et al. (2007) The clinical trial of Women On the Move through Activity and Nutrition (WOMAN) study. Contemp Clin Trials 28:370–381

Lamont DH, Budoff MJ, Shavelle DM, Shavelle R, Brundage BH, Hagar JM (2002) Coronary calcium scanning adds incremental value to patients with positive stress tests. Am Heart J 143:861–867

LaMonte MJ, FitzGerald SJ, Church TS et al. (2005) Coronary artery calcium score and coronary heart disease events in a large cohort of asymptomatic men and women. Am J Epidemiol 162:421–429

Laudon DA, Vukov LF, Breen JF, Rumberger JA, Wollan PC, Sheedy PF 2nd. (1999) Use of electron-beam computed tomography in the evaluation of chest pain patients in the emergency department. Ann Emerg Med 33:15–21

Leschka S, Scheffel H, Desbiolles L et al. (2007) Combining Dual-Source Computed Tomography Coronary Angiography and Calcium Scoring: Added Value for the Assessment of Coronary Artery Disease. Heart

Lu B, Zhuang N, Mao SS et al. (2002) EKG-triggered CT data acquisition to reduce variability in coronary arterial calcium score. Radiology 2002; 224:838–844

Manson JE, Allison MA, Rossouw JE et al. (2007) Estrogen therapy and coronary-artery calcification. N Engl J Med 356:2591–2602

Mao S, Bakhsheshi H, Lu B, Liu SC, Oudiz RJ, Budoff MJ (2001) Effect of electrocardiogram triggering on reproducibility of coronary artery calcium scoring. Radiology 220:707–711

Matsuoka M, Iseki K, Tamashiro M et al. (2004) Impact of high coronary artery calcification score (CACS) on survival in patients on chronic hemodialysis. Clin Exp Nephrol 8:54–58

McCollough CH, Ulzheimer S, Halliburton SS, Shanneik K, White RD, Kalender WA (2007) Coronary artery calcium: a multi-institutional, multimanufacturer international standard for quantification at cardiac CT. Radiology 243:527–538

McLaughlin VV, Balogh T, Rich S (1999) Utility of electron beam computed tomography to stratify patients presenting to the emergency room with chest pain. Am J Cardiol 84:327–328, A328

Mehrotra R, Budoff M, Christenson P et al. (2004) Determinants of coronary artery calcification in diabetics with and without nephropathy. Kidney Int 66:2022–2031

Mielke CH, Shields JP, Broemeling LD (2001) Coronary artery calcium, coronary artery disease, and diabetes. Diabetes Res Clin Pract 53:55–61

Morin RL, Gerber TC, McCollough CH (2003) Radiation dose in computed tomography of the heart. Circulation 107:917–922

Nasir K, Shaw LJ, Liu ST et al. (2007) Ethnic differences in the prognostic value of coronary artery calcification for all-cause mortality. J Am Coll Cardiol 50:953–960

National Research Council (US) (2006) Committee to Assess Health Risks from Exposure to Low Level of Ionizing Radiation. Health risks from exposure to low levels of ionizing radiation: BEIR VII Phase 2. Washington DC: National Academies Press

Newman AB, Naydeck BL, Ives DG et al. (2008) Coronary artery calcium, carotid artery wall thickness, and cardiovascular disease outcomes in adults 70 to 99 years old. Am J Cardiol 101:186–192

Oei HH, Vliegenthart R, Hofman A, Oudkerk M, Witteman JC (2004) Risk factors for coronary calcification in older subjects. The Rotterdam Coronary Calcification Study. Eur Heart J 25:48–55

Oh J, Wunsch R, Turzer M et al. (2002) Advanced coronary and carotid arteriopathy in young adults with childhood-onset chronic renal failure. Circulation 106:100–105

Olson JC, Edmundowicz D, Becker DJ, Kuller LH, Orchard TJ (2000) Coronary calcium in adults with type 1 diabetes: a stronger correlate of clinical coronary artery disease in men than in women. Diabetes 49:1571–1578

O'Rourke RA, Brundage BH, Froelicher VF et al. (2000) American College of Cardiology/American Heart Association Expert Consensus document on electron-beam computed tomography for the diagnosis and prognosis of coronary artery disease. Circulation 102:126–140

Patel MR, Spertus JA, Brindis RG et al. (2005) ACCF proposed method for evaluating the appropriateness of cardiovascular imaging. J Am Coll Cardiol 46:1606–1613

Pletcher MJ, Tice JA, Pignone M, Browner WS (2004) Using the coronary artery calcium score to predict coronary heart disease events: a systematic review and meta-analysis. Arch Intern Med 164:1285–1292

Qu W, Le TT, Azen SP et al. (2003) Value of coronary artery calcium scanning by computed tomography for predicting coronary heart disease in diabetic subjects. Diabetes Care 26:905–910

Raggi P, Callister TQ, Cooil B et al. (2000a) Identification of patients at increased risk of first unheralded acute myocardial infarction by electron-beam computed tomography. Circulation 101:850–855

Raggi P, Callister TQ, Cooil B, Russo DJ, Lippolis NJ, Patterson RE (2000b) Evaluation of chest pain in patients with low to intermediate pretest probability of coronary artery disease by electron beam computed tomography. Am J Cardiol 85:283–288

Raggi P, Boulay A, Chasan-Taber S et al. (2002) Cardiac calcification in adult hemodialysis patients. A link between end-stage renal disease and cardiovascular disease? J Am Coll Cardiol 39:695–701

Raggi P, Cooil B, Shaw LJ et al. (2003) Progression of coronary calcium on serial electron beam tomographic scanning is greater in patients with future myocardial infarction. Am J Cardiol 92:827–829

Raggi P, Shaw LJ, Berman DS, Callister TQ (2004a) Gender-based differences in the prognostic value of coronary calcification. J Womens Health (Larchmt) 13:273–283

Raggi P, Shaw LJ, Berman DS, Callister TQ (2004b) Prognostic value of coronary artery calcium screening in subjects with and without diabetes. J Am Coll Cardiol 43:1663–1669

Raggi P, Callister TQ, Shaw LJ (2004c) Progression of coronary artery calcium and risk of first myocardial infarction in patients receiving cholesterol-lowering therapy. Arterioscler Thromb Vasc Biol 24:1272–1277

Raggi P, Cooil B, Ratti C, Callister TQ, Budoff M (2005a) Progression of coronary artery calcium and occurrence of myocardial infarction in patients with and without diabetes mellitus. Hypertension 46:238–243

Raggi P, Davidson M, Callister TQ et al. (2005b) Aggressive versus moderate lipid-lowering therapy in hypercholesterolemic postmenopausal women: Beyond Endorsed Lipid Lowering with EBT Scanning (BELLES). Circulation 112:563–571

Raggi P, Taylor A, Fayad Z et al. (2005c) Atherosclerotic plaque imaging: contemporary role in preventive cardiology. Arch Intern Med 165:2345–2353

Rasouli ML, Nasir K, Blumenthal RS, Park R, Aziz DC, Budoff MJ (2005) Plasma homocysteine predicts progression of atherosclerosis. Atherosclerosis 181:159–165

Rubinshtein R, Gaspar T, Halon DA, Goldstein J, Peled N, Lewis BS (2007) Prevalence and extent of obstructive coronary artery disease in patients with zero or low calcium score undergoing 64-slice cardiac multidetector computed tomography for evaluation of a chest pain syndrome. Am J Cardiol 99:472–475

Russo D, Palmiero G, De Blasio AP, Balletta MM, Andreucci VE (2004) Coronary artery calcification in patients with CRF not undergoing dialysis. Am J Kidney Dis 44:1024–1030

Santos RD, Nasir K, Rumberger JA et al. (2006) Difference in atherosclerosis burden in different nations and continents assessed by coronary artery calcium. Atherosclerosis 187:378–384

Schmermund A, Achenbach S, Budde T et al. (2006) Effect of intensive versus standard lipid-lowering treatment with atorvastatin on the progression of calcified coronary atherosclerosis over 12 months: a multicenter, randomized, double-blind trial. Circulation 113:427–437

Schurgin S, Rich S, Mazzone T (2001) Increased prevalence of significant coronary artery calcification in patients with diabetes. Diabetes Care 24:335–338

Sevrukov AB, Bland JM, Kondos GT (2005) Serial electron beam CT measurements of coronary artery calcium: Has your patient‘s calcium score actually changed? AJR Am J Roentgenol 185:1546–1553

Shaw LJ, Raggi P, Schisterman E, Berman DS, Callister TQ (2003) Prognostic value of cardiac risk factors and coronary artery calcium screening for all-cause mortality. Radiology 228:826–833

Shaw LJ, Raggi P, Callister TQ, Berman DS (2006) Prognostic value of coronary artery calcium screening in asymptomatic smokers and non-smokers. Eur Heart J 27:968–975

Shemesh J, Apter S, Stolero D, Itzchak Y, Motro M (2001) Annual progression of coronary artery calcium by spiral computed tomography in hypertensive patients without myocardial ischemia but with prominent atherosclerotic risk factors, in patients with previous angina pectoris or healed acute myocardial infarction, and in patients with coronary events during follow-up. Am J Cardiol 87:1395–1397

Sigrist M, Bungay P, Taal MW, McIntyre CW (2006) Vascular calcification and cardiovascular function in chronic kidney disease. Nephrol Dial Transplant 21:707–714

Sirineni GK, Raggi P, Shaw LJ, Stillman AE (2008) Calculation of coronary age using calcium scores in multiple ethnicities. Int J Cardiovasc Imaging 24:107–111

Smith SC Jr, Amsterdam E, Balady GJ et al. (2000) Prevention Conference V: Beyond secondary prevention: identifying the high-risk patient for primary prevention: tests for silent and inducible ischemia: Writing Group II. Circulation 101:E12–16

Snell-Bergeon JK, Hokanson JE, Jensen L et al. (2003) Progression of coronary artery calcification in type 1 diabetes: the importance of glycemic control. Diabetes Care 26:2923–2928

Stillman AE, Oudkerk M, Ackerman M et al. (2007a) Use of multidetector computed tomography for the assessment of acute chest pain: a consensus statement of the North American Society of Cardiac Imaging and the European Society of Cardiac Radiology. Eur Radiol 17:2196–2207

Stillman AE, Oudkerk M, Ackerman M et al. (2007b) Use of multidetector computed tomography for the assessment of acute chest pain: a consensus statement of the North American Society of Cardiac Imaging and the European Society of Cardiac Radiology. Int J Cardiovasc Imaging 23:415–427

Sutton-Tyrrell K, Kuller LH, Edmundowicz D et al. (2001) Usefulness of electron beam tomography to detect progression of coronary and aortic calcium in middle-aged women. Am J Cardiol 87:560–564

Taylor AJ, Bindeman J, Feuerstein I, Cao F, Brazaitis M, O‘Malley PG (2005a) Coronary calcium independently predicts incident premature coronary heart disease over measured cardiovascular risk factors: mean three-year outcomes in the Prospective Army Coronary Calcium (PACC) project. J Am Coll Cardiol 46:807–814

Taylor A, Shaw LJ, Fayad Z et al. (2005b) Tracking atherosclerosis regression: a clinical tool in preventive cardiology. Atherosclerosis 180:1–10

Therasse P, Arbuck SG, Eisenhauer EA et al. (2000) New guidelines to evaluate the response to treatment in solid tumors. European Organization for Research and Treatment of Cancer, National Cancer Institute of the United States, National Cancer Institute of Canada. J Natl Cancer Inst 92:205–216

Thompson GR, Partridge J (2004) Coronary calcification score: the coronary-risk impact factor. Lancet 363:557–559

Thompson RC, Cullom SJ (2006) Issues regarding radiation dosage of cardiac nuclear and radiography procedures. J Nucl Cardiol 13:19–23

Ulzheimer S, Kalender WA (2003) Assessment of calcium scoring performance in cardiac computed tomography. Eur Radiol 13:484–497

van Ooijen PM, Vliegenthart R, Witteman JC, Oudkerk M (2005) Influence of scoring parameter settings on Agatston and volume scores for coronary calcification. Eur Radiol 15:102–110

Villines TC, Taylor AJ (2005) Non-invasive atherosclerosis imaging: use to assess response to novel or combination lipid therapies. Curr Drug Targets Cardiovasc Haematol Disord 5:557–564

Vliegenthart R, Oudkerk M, Hofman A et al. (2005) Coronary calcification improves cardiovascular risk prediction in the elderly. Circulation 112:572–577

Wang AY, Wang M, Woo J et al. (2003) Cardiac valve calcification as an important predictor for all-cause mortality and cardiovascular mortality in long-term peritoneal dialysis patients: a prospective study. J Am Soc Nephrol 14:159–168

Wexler L, Brundage B, Crouse J et al. (1996) Coronary artery calcification: pathophysiology, epidemiology, imaging methods, and clinical implications. A statement for health professionals from the American Heart Association. Writing Group. Circulation 94:1175–1192

Wilson PW, D'Agostino RB, Levy D, Belanger AM, Silbershatz H, Kannel WB (1998) Prediction of coronary heart disease using risk factor categories. Circulation 97:1837–1847

Wong ND, Sciammarella MG, Polk D et al. (2003) The metabolic syndrome, diabetes, and subclinical atherosclerosis assessed by coronary calcium. J Am Coll Cardiol 41:1547–1553

Wong ND, Rozanski A, Gransar H et al. (2005) Metabolic syndrome and diabetes are associated with an increased likelihood of inducible myocardial ischemia among patients with subclinical atherosclerosis. Diabetes Care 28:1445–1450

Yoon HC, Emerick AM, Hill JA, Gjertson DW, Goldin JG (2002) Calcium begets calcium: progression of coronary artery calcification in asymptomatic subjects. Radiology 224:236–241

Multi-Dimensional Computed Cardiac Visualization

5

PETER M. A. VAN OOIJEN, WISNU KRISTANTO, GONDA J. DE JONGE, CAROLINE KUEHNEL, ANJA HENNEMUTH, TOBIAS BOSKAMP, JAAP M. GROEN, and ANDRÉ BROEKEMA

CONTENTS

P. M. A. VAN OOIJEN, PhD; W. KRISTANTO, MSc; G. J. DE JONGE, MD; J. M. GROEN, MSc, PhD; A. BROEKEMA, BSc
Department of Radiology, University Medical Center Groningen, University of Groningen, Hanzeplein 1, P. O. Box 30.001, 9700 RB Groningen, The Netherlands
C. KUEHNEL, MSc; A. HENNEMUTH, MSc; T. BOSKAMP, PhD
MeVis Research, Universitätsallee 29, 28359 Bremen, Germany

5.1 Introduction

PETER M.A. VAN OOIJEN, WISNU KRISTANTO, GONDA J. DE JONGE, CAROLINE KUEHNEL, ANJA HENNEMUTH, TOBIAS BOSKAMP, and JAAP M. GROEN

Contemporary medical imaging modalities such as magnetic resonance imaging (MRI), electron-beam computed tomography (EBCT), and multi-detector computed tomography (MDCT) provide the clinician with a wealth of information. To be able to evaluate and diagnose the (projection and volumetric) data from modern non-invasive and invasive imaging modalities, new visualization techniques are increasingly used. These techniques have been described frequently both for coronary artery imaging (NAKANISHI et al. 1997; CHEN and CARROLL 1998; VAN OOIJEN et al. 1997, 2003a,b; LAWLER et al 2005), as well as for other applications in medicine (RANKIN 1999; KIRCHGEORG and PROKOP 1998; CALHOUN et al. 1999; DALRYMPLE et al. 2005; FISHMAN et al. 2006).

Visualization involves the process of transforming the acquired data to a format that enables data to be displayed on a computer screen or to be printed on film or paper in a representation that is clinically relevant. This process basically consists of two steps: image processing and rendering. Image processing involves the selection of the regions of interest in the database of voxels [or pixels in the case of a two-dimensional (2D) visualization], and rendering includes the conversion of this database representation into a (shaded) 2D image that can be displayed on a view surface (WATT 1993). After performing image processing and visualization, the following two steps are manipulation and analysis of the data (UDUPA 1999).

The data obtained from MRI, EBCT and MDCT basically consist of a three-dimensional (3D) matrix. To perform 3D image rendering and processing on such a dataset, the structure of interest needs to have gray values that are distinctly different compared to surrounding tissues. For vessels this is typically achieved by injecting an intravenous contrast medium to increase the radio-opacity of blood in MDCT and EBCT, or by, for example, using blood enhancement and fat suppression sequences in MRI. After image acquisition, the volumetric (3D) dataset can be evaluated by a variety of visualization techniques (Höhne et al. 1990; Ney et al. 1990a,b; Udupa and Hung 1990; Fishman et al. 1991; Rubin et al. 1995; Elvins 1992).

Recent advances in imaging techniques enable the acquisition of multiple 3D datasets (in a time sequence) to obtain a four-dimensional (4D) representation. This allows functional analysis of the heart by observing its motion, as well as perfusion analysis by observing the uptake and wash-out of contrast agent in the heart muscle tissue.

The quality of the acquired and reconstructed dataset is a very important issue for the 3D rendering of MRI, EBCT, or MDCT data, especially for coronary artery imaging. The quality of the dataset can be diminished by different factors:

- Incorrect timing of the intravenous contrast medium administration
- Incorrect scan start position (below the ostium of the left main coronary artery)
- Motion artifacts (due to inconsistent breath-holding, arrhythmia, patient movement)
- Overlapping veins that obscure the view on the coronary arteries
- Insufficient contrast to distinguish between the coronary arteries and the surrounding tissue (heart muscle, pericardial fat, veins, etc.)
- Blooming artifacts caused by strong calcifications, stents, or other metal implants such as surgical clips, ICDs or defibrillators

In the case of MRI, the data quality also heavily depends on the imaging protocol. When using MDCT or EBCT, raw data processing factors, such as the reconstruction phase and the reconstruction kernel, have a significant influence. When 4D data are acquired, the above-mentioned difficulties, as well as the requirements for a comprehensive visualization will increase.

5.2 Visualization Techniques

Peter M.A. van Ooijen, Wisnu Kristanto, Gonda J. de Jonge, Caroline Kuehnel, Anja Hennemuth, Tobias Boskamp, and Jaap M. Groen

In general, the visualization process converts the volumetric dataset into a 2D image that is suitable for display on a computer screen. Various visualization techniques are available with varying degrees of suitability for imaging of the coronary artery tree (Fishman and Ney 1993, Murakami et al. 1993; Rubin et al. 1994; Heath et al. 1995; Meyers et al. 1995; Soyer et al. 1996; Hany et al. 1998; Rankin 1999; Rensing et al. 1999a; Udupa 1999; Lawler et al. 2005).

5.2.1 Two-Dimensional Slice Viewing

Although we categorize multi-planar reformation (MPR) as a 3D technique, the resulting images are 2D slices. For viewing purposes MPR techniques transform the data located on an arbitrary surface within the volumetric dataset onto a 2D plane. A variety of surfaces are used in medical imaging. Besides the "normal", native MPR, oblique, double oblique, curved MPR and stretched MPR can be constructed.

5.2.1.1 Native Multi-planar Reformation

With the standard MPR visualization, planes orthogonal to the original data slices are defined in the volumetric dataset and displayed adjacently. In the common case of original data slices acquired in axial orientation, the additional views are chosen in sagittal and coronal orientation (Fig. 5.1). A small effective slice thickness (close to isotropic) is a prerequisite to obtain high quality orthogonal reformatted images. The use of MPR for evaluation of coronary artery disease in MDCT data with good sensitivity and specificity has been reported (Nakanishi et al. 1997; Ropers et al. 2003). Nakanishi et al. (1997) used cine loop viewing in order to avoid the delusive visualization of non-existing stenoses because of incorrect placement of the planes.

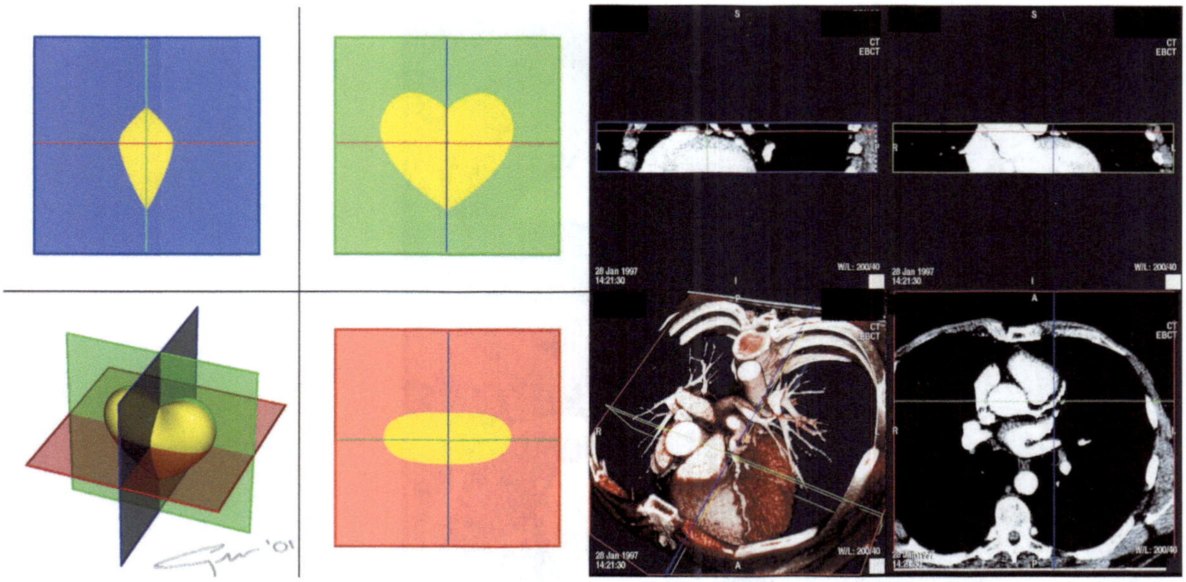

Fig. 5.1. The *bottom left* image shows a three-dimensional image with the definition of the planes that are reconstructed to obtain the other three images. All images are orthogonal to each other and in each image, the location of the other two is given by a *colored line*

5.2.1.2 Oblique Multi-planar Reformation

In oblique or double oblique MPR, one or two of the image planes are angulated in order to address a larger section of an artery in a single image (Fig. 5.2). The placement of the planes is critical for an adequate display of the data.

5.2.1.3 Curved Multi-planar Reformation

In the case of a curved MPR, a path is drawn along the trajectory of the artery, along which a curved surface is reconstructed. This enables visualization of an entire artery in one single image (Fig. 5.3). This method even allows us to display the full right coronary artery (RCA) and left anterior descending artery (LAD) in one single image (Fig. 5.4). Curved MPR has been evaluated by Achenbach et al. (1998) for use in EBCT imaging of the coronary arteries yielding a sensitivity of 89% and a specificity of 92% for the detection of significant stenoses and occlusions. An analysis by Ferencik et al. (2007) showed that 93% of the arteries could be evaluated and an accuracy of 81% for detecting stenosis using 16-slice MDCT. Scheffel et al. (2006) even showed a sensitivity of 96.4 and a specificity of 97.5 for evaluation of coronary artery disease using dual source computed tomography.

5.2.1.4 Stretched Multi-planar Reformation

Stretched MPR is very similar to curved MPR, but differs in the way it represents the artery as if it has been pulled straight. This view promotes simpler perception of a straight vessel, whereas a graph depicting one of the vessel's characteristics, such as lumen area, can be placed parallel to it.

MPR has several advantages. First, it is an algorithm with relatively low complexity and thus can be rendered quickly and accurately on most workstations. Second, distance measurements in MPR are accurate (with some restrictions in the case of curved and stretched MPR) and not subject to foreshortening due to projection. Third, different structures in MPR images do not overlap and 100% of the available data are incorporated in the images (no loss of voxel value information due to thresholding). Finally, longer trajectories of a vessel can be displayed in a single image by angulating the planes along the course of the vessel.

In contrast, MPR does have its drawbacks, as the image quality of an MPR is highly dependent on the resolution and the dataset anisotropy. False-

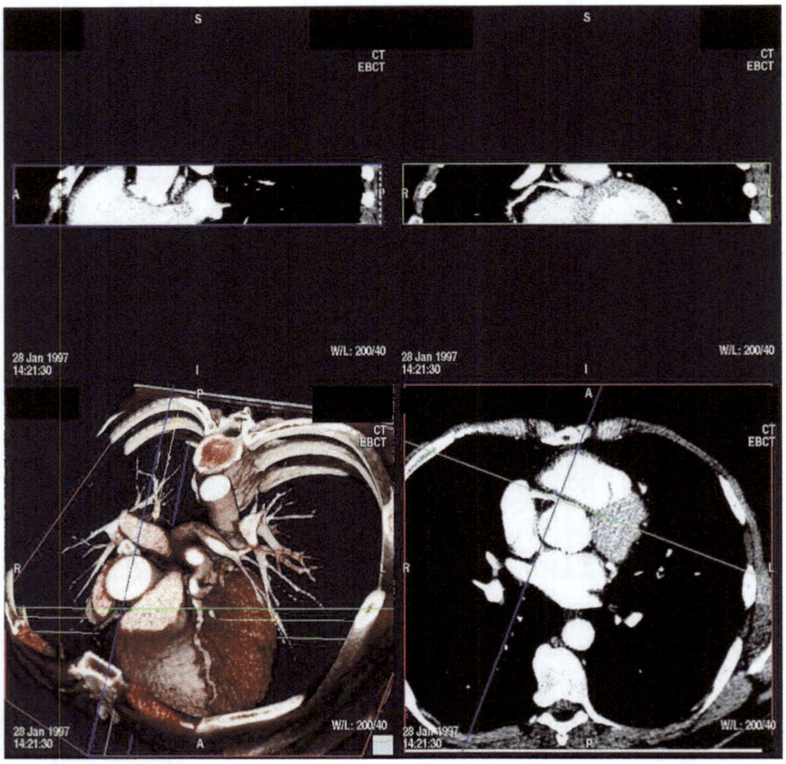

Fig. 5.2. Here a single oblique multiplanar reformation is shown with a rotation of the planes around the z-axis, resulting in a better depiction of the right coronary artery in the *upper right frame*

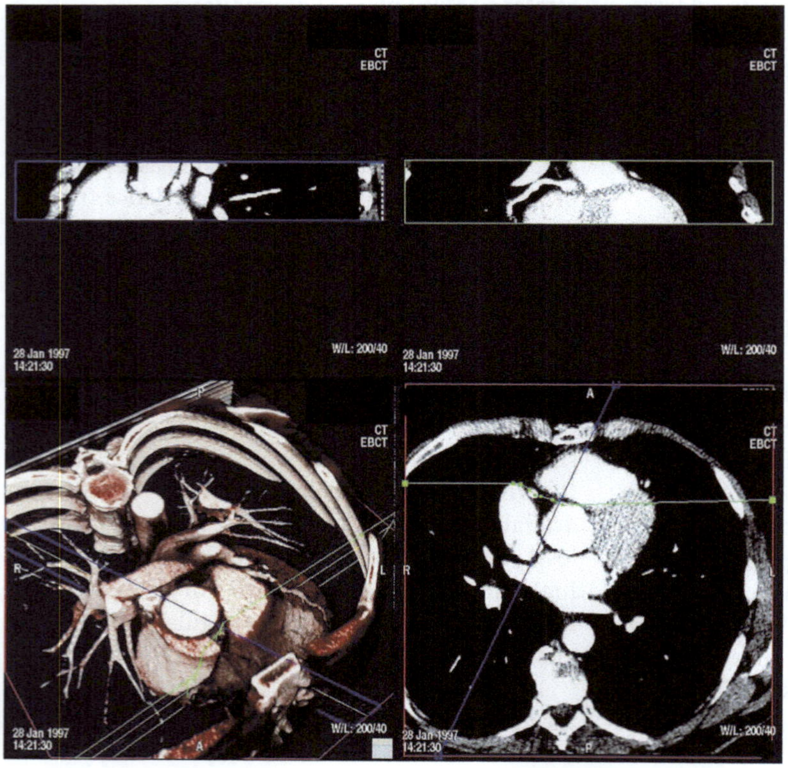

Fig. 5.3. A Curved multi-planar reformation (MPR) can be performed to obtain an even better depiction of the right coronary artery. If we compare the result in the *upper right frame* with the ones in the previous figures (Figs. 5.1 and 5.2) of the oblique MPR, a possible stenosis can be seen in the oblique MPR that proves to be false-positive in the thin slab oblique MPR and the curved MPR

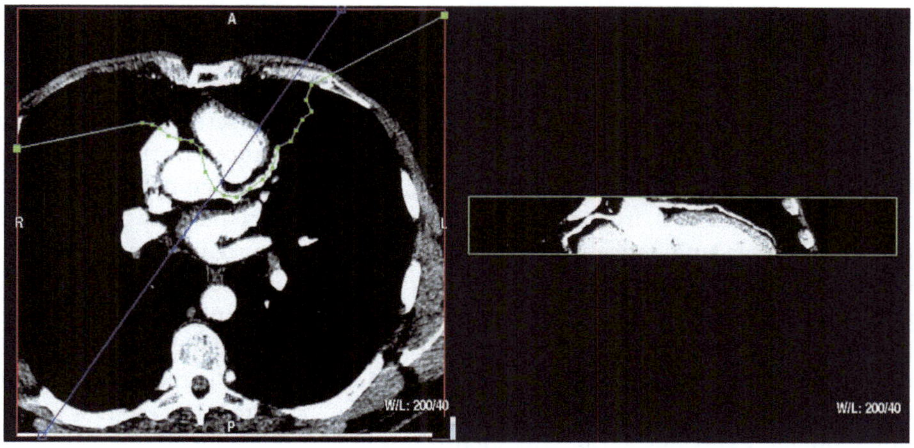

Fig. 5.4. Using a curved multi-planar reformation the depiction of right coronary artery, left main, and left anterior descending artery is possible

positive artery stenoses, introduced by inadequate breath-hold and other motion artifacts are more difficult to recognize in MPR compared to more 3D oriented visualization methods. However, the first two drawbacks are less prominent when using modern scanners with high spatial resolution (e.g. 16- or 64-detector CT). These scanners allow thin slice acquisition with accurate ECG gating providing excellent MPR images with reduced stair-step artifacts. A major additional drawback of MPR is, however, that the vessels have to be visualized selectively, one at a time, and side branches are not depicted unless a separate reconstruction is rendered for each side branch. Finally, an inaccurate definition of the reformation path for curved or stretched MPR can introduce false-positive stenoses if the curve deviates from the vessel centerline (Fig. 5.5). Such inaccuracies can arise if the reformation path is defined manually, or if non-optimal algorithms for the automatic centerline detection are used. State-of-the-art skeletonization algorithms, on the other hand, are able to compute the centerline with accuracy in the order of the voxel precision, as could be verified in phantom studies (Boskamp et al. 2005).

Recently developed and commercially available routines allow the automatic selection of a vessel or even of a branching vascular tree and visualization of this tree in a single reconstruction image (Selle et al. 2002). Applying these algorithms the user either selects only a small amount of points indicating

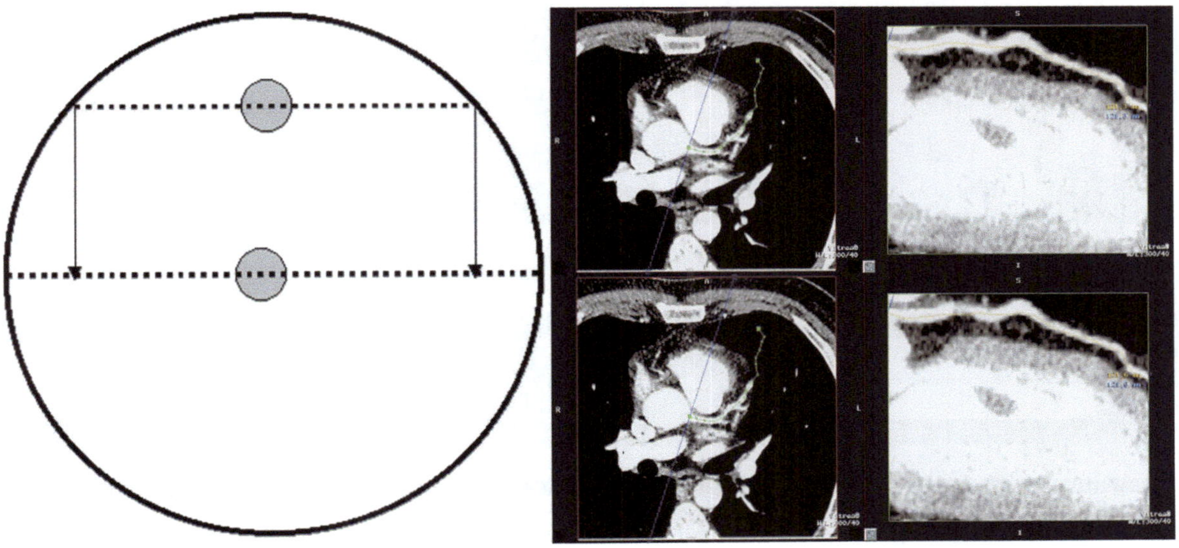

Fig. 5.5. Possible introduction of false positive stenoses using multi-planar reformation because of misplacement of control points

the vessel and the branches to be segmented or the algorithm detects the aorta and segments the aortic root and coronary arteries fully automatically. One implementation is the medial axis reformation (MAR) proposed by HE et al. (2001). This technique is based on a first coarse manual segmentation of the region of interest (ROI), from which the medial axis of a vessel tree is automatically extracted, generates curved sections along this axis and finally maps them on a 2D image plane. Other software methods are also available resulting in an automatic detection and reformation of a coronary artery tree (Fig. 5.6) (HENNEMUTH et al. 2005). Some of the drawbacks of the previous versions of the MPR algorithms are eliminated by these novel techniques.

In conclusion, MPR techniques provide fast, easy and user interactive means of visualization of the coronary artery tree.

5.2.2 Maximum Intensity Projection

As described earlier, vascular structures can be enhanced during data acquisition to attain higher contrast compared to surrounding voxels. The maximum intensity projection (MIP) technique uses this enhancement to select and display the vasculature from the volumetric data. MIP is a projection technique in which imaginary rays are cast through the 3D data volume from the viewpoint of the user (Fig. 5.7), and only the highest intensity voxels encountered by each ray are used to reconstruct the 2D projection image, comparable to a standard X-ray image (Fig. 5.8).

Advantages of MIP vascular imaging are the relatively short reconstruction time of the images and the generally excellent differentiation between vas-

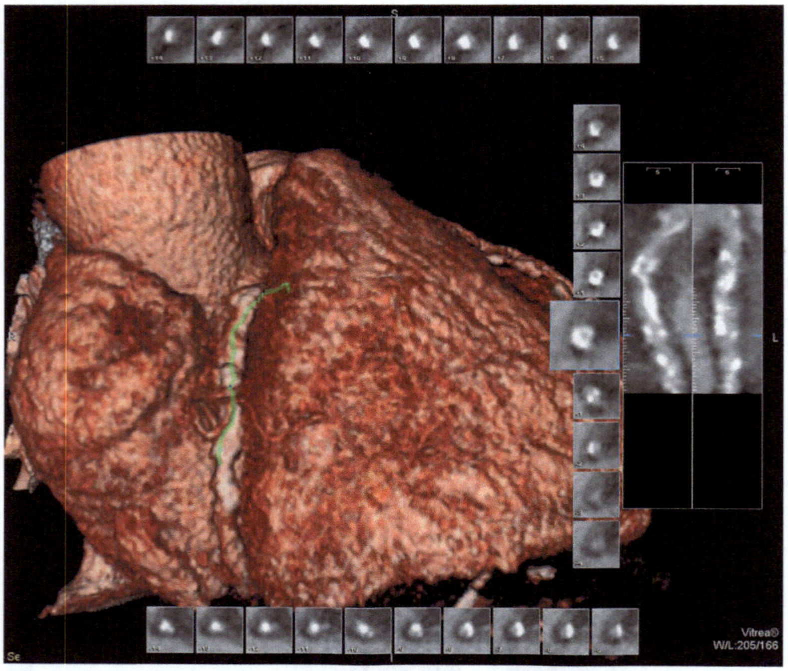

Fig. 5.6. New methods allow automatic reconstruction of a curved multi-planar reformation based on a starting point defined by the user. The reconstructed right coronary artery is shown in 3D view and at several points on the centerline 2D reconstructions are shown perpendicular to the centerline. In addition a view parallel to the centerline is also shown in two views that are 90° apart from each other.

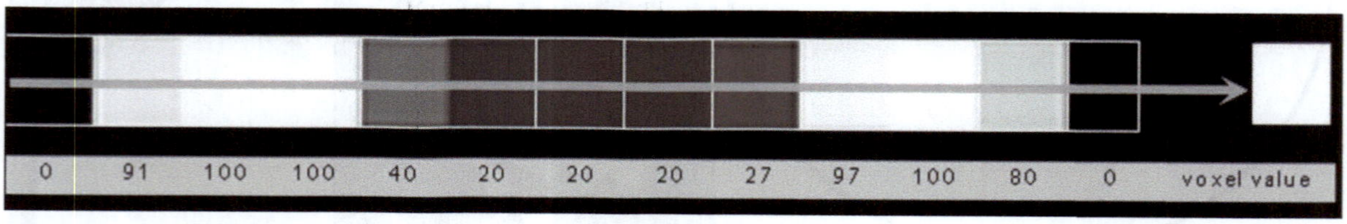

Fig. 5.7. Rays are cast through the volume to obtain the values for the image plane. Here, *row six* is selected from the example of Fig. 5.8 to demonstrate this. All voxels are traversed and the resulting pixel at the *right* of the image only shows the highest value encountered *(100)*

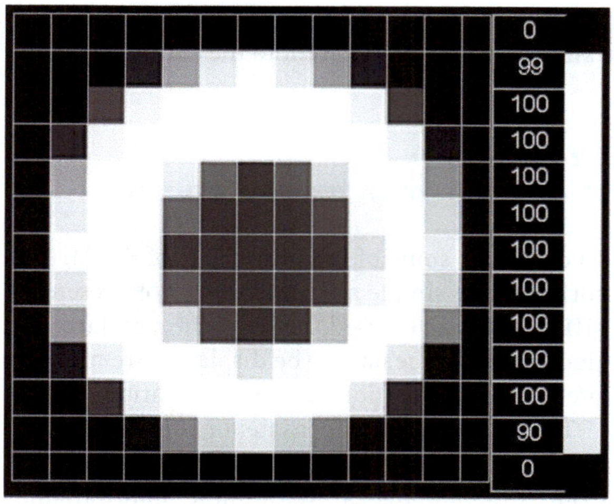

Fig. 5.8. The maximum intensity projection image that would represent this structure is shown in the *bar* at the *right side*, the highest voxel values encountered for each row are displayed to the *left* of this bar

cular and non-vascular structures. For EBCT it was shown by Lu et al. (2001) that this differentiation can be optimized when using an optimal window/level setting (level = 0.47 × coronary lumen attenuation - 47.70).

MIP used for vascular imaging introduces several artifacts and has certain shortcomings, which are inherent to the algorithm (Anderson et al. 1990; Marks et al. 1993; Heath et al. 1995; Verdonck 1996):

Low intensity of voxels at the edges of vessels compared to the center will cause the edges to disappear. The difference in voxel intensity of these edges compared to the background intensity is too small, which results in a (false) reduction of the apparent vessel diameter (Anderson et al. 1990). These low voxel intensities at the edges of vessels which decrease the total intensity of those vessels can be caused by so-called partial volume effects. Additionally, in flow dependent MRI scanning techniques, such as phase contrast angiography, the intensities of the voxels near the vessel wall can decrease due to low flow velocities.

Furthermore, in MIP images, the contrast is heavily dependent on the background noise. Anderson et al. (1990) states that the contrast will be excellent when the vessel intensity is two times larger than the standard deviation of the mean background noise. If more slices are selected for projection with vessel intensity 0.5 times the standard deviation above the background, eventually the resulting image will have a background intensity that will be higher than the intensity of the vessel.

MIP can also lead to striping or disappearance of vessel segments. Discontinuity is introduced, because the voxel intensities are adequately high for detection in one slice, but not in the next due to partial volume effects. This striping effect is most evident in smaller vessels. If the vessel is small enough, the voxel values will drop below the background intensity level and the vessel will disappear from the image (Fig. 5.9).

Because of the projection nature of the MIP algorithm, the resulting image will be three-dimensionally ambiguous when displayed without additional depth cues (Fig. 5.10).

MIP images are unable to display superimposed structures (e.g. vessel crossings) and lack vessel "depth" information (Fig. 5.11). Conventional angiograms, on the other hand, contain some depth information because of the additive nature of these images. A vessel crossing will be depicted as a region with higher intensity because of the additive contribution of both vessels to the resulting attenuation.

Despite its shortcomings MIP has played an important role in medical imaging (Anderson et al. 1990; Napel et al. 1992; Marks et al. 1993). Although this technique is widely used, it is not very useful for coronary imaging unless a large amount of segmentation is performed to obtain a dataset containing nothing but the coronary arteries (Achenbach et al. 2000). Further drawbacks of the method are the incapability of visualizing intra-luminal defects (Fig. 5.11) unless they coincide with the vessel wall, and the large influence of partial volume effects on

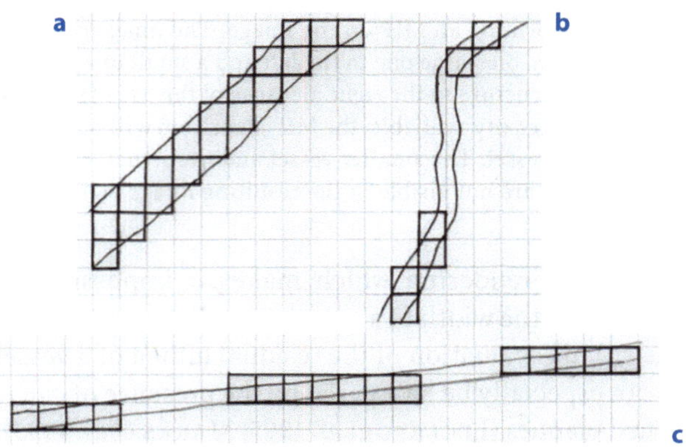

Fig. 5.9a–c. Due to partial volume effects several artefacts are introduced: **a,b** The vessel shows a staircase artefact; **a** vessels look smaller than they actually are; **b** vessels can have gaps or even disappear completely; **c** striping of vessels occurs

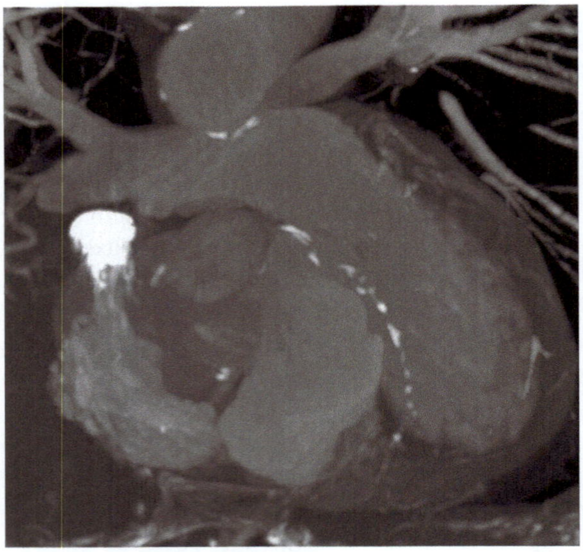

Fig. 5.10. Maximum intensity projection of the heart. Coronary calcifications, other calcified plaques, bony structures and highly concentrated contrast medium in the superior vena cava are visualized, but no depth can be perceived from the image

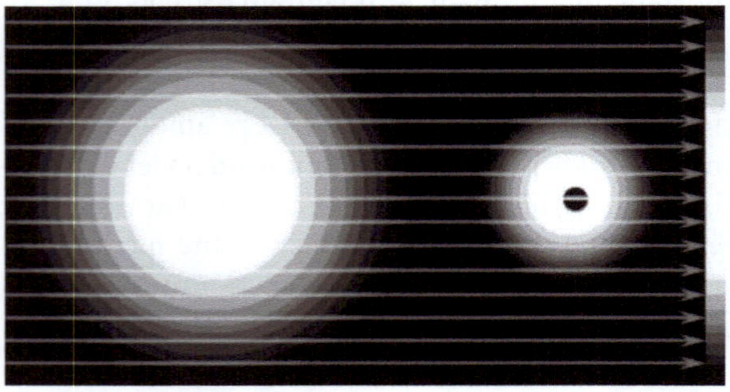

Fig. 5.11. Maximum intensity projection (MIP) rendering procedure. The *bar* at the *right* depicts the resulting image after performing an MIP on the image. The image contains two vessels, one large one to the *left* and a small one with an internal structure to the *right*. Because of the use of only the highest intensity available, the MIP algorithm will only show the large vessel. The smaller vessel and the structure inside this vessel are not visible in the resulting image at all

the MIP rendering which makes it impossible to measure the width of a vessel or to diagnose a stenosis. This evaluation of the residual lumen of a vessel can especially be hampered by the presence of calcified plaques (Leclerc et al. 1995; Marks et al. 1993), which often occurs in coronary artery imaging.

Summarized, the advantages of the MIP algorithm are its speed, the – in general – good differentiation between vascular and non-vascular structures, and the easy processing of the data. However, as described above, there are also some large disadvantages which are inherent to the algorithm.

5.2.3 Thin Slab Maximum Intensity Projection

To overcome some of the drawbacks of the MIP algorithm, two simple alternative ways of presenting MIP images can be used. Both use the standard MIP algorithm, but the data to be displayed are manipulated either by rotation or by segmentation.

The first way to compensate for some of the MIP specific drawbacks uses reconstruction MIP images from different angles. With these multi-angular MIP images, it is possible to target particular vessels without the need for additional acquisitions.

Superimposing structures in MIP can also be avoided by interactive sliding thin slab MIP (STS-MIP) rendering (Napel et al. 1993). Instead of the entire volume, only a slab consisting of a small number of slices of the volume is MIP rendered. This slab can be moved through the volume, typically with a step size less than the slab thickness (e.g. a 5-mm slab thickness with a 2.5-mm step size) (Fig. 5.12). The result of this procedure can either be viewed as separate images, or as a cine-loop movie. The STS-MIP procedure requires no pre-processing or user interaction. Because the thin slabs are more targeted, artifacts can be detected more easily than in full volume MIP. In particular, the artifacts introduced by using a large number of slices, which increase the background noise, are less prominent in the STS-MIP.

The STS-MIP is the preferred MIP algorithm for visualizing the coronary artery tree. Due to their dynamic nature, however, the multi-angular and STS-MIP do require more powerful graphic workstations, which are not always available to the clinician. Furthermore, it is claimed that MIP should only be analyzed together with the original axial slices due to the MIP related artifacts (Anderson et al. 1990; Prokop et al. 1997).

5.2.4 Surface Rendering

Surface rendering techniques are based upon geometrically approximated representations of, for example, anatomical objects derived directly from the source image or from segmentation results (Lorensen and Cline 1987; Gibson 1998; Ohtake

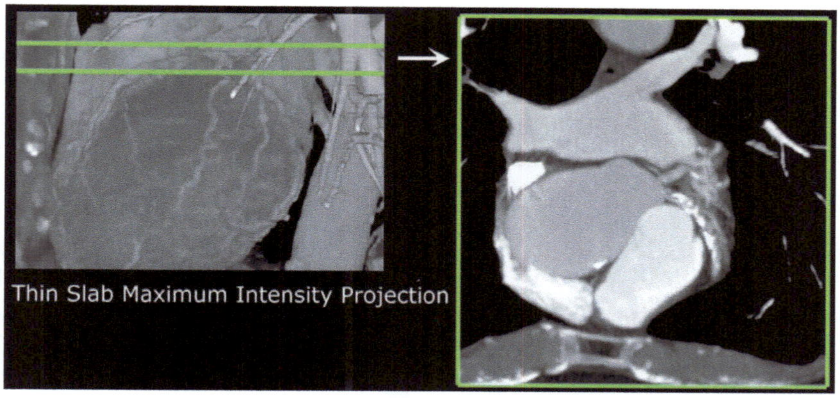

Fig. 5.12. Sliding thin slab maximum intensity projection (MIP). A small slab is selected from the complete volume data (*horizontal lines* in the image to the *left*) and used to perform the rendering. The *right* image shows MIP of the selected slab. High density calcifications are clearly visible in the MIP image. After rendering, the slab can be moved to another level within the volume and a new image can be reconstructed

et al. 2003; Schumann et al. 2007). These methods can be applied in cases where structure and parametric information are of main interest but not so much the exact voxel intensity information. The application to image data with relatively low resolution and high slice distance produces smooth approximations which give a good visual impression of 3D objects and their spatial relations. Furthermore, surface representations allow the visualization of parameters using color or opacity (Fig. 5.13).

In case of the visualization of vascular trees, model based methods are applied to generate artifact free, smooth representations of the interesting structures. These methods are based on a graph describing the tree's branching structure combined with the information on the segments' lengths and diameters. One realization of this approach assumes the segments to be cylinders (Gerig et al. 1993) or truncated cones (Hahn et al. 2001), while more complex approaches generate surface representations such as freeform surfaces (Ehricke et al. 1994), subdivision surfaces (Felkel et al. 2002), simplex meshes (Bornik et al. 2005) or convolution surfaces (Oeltze and Preim 2004).

The resulting surfaces can additionally be annotated with different features of the presented objects by using color, transparency, or shininess. As an example, color coding can be used to represent the vessel hierarchy, the main coronary branches (Fig. 5.14) or the local diameter of a branch, as well as local measurements of the myocardium including wall thickening or perfusion parameters (Beliveau et al. 2007) (Fig. 5.13).

5.2.5 Volume Rendering

Volume rendering (VR) has initially been applied to visualize pathology other than the coronary artery tree (Kuszyk et al. 1995; Johnson et al. 1997). Unlike other techniques, VR does not rely on surface information but all voxels in the volume are rendered. Based on its value [e.g. CT attenuation expressed in Hounsfield units (HU) in the case of CT data], a specific color and opacity is assigned to each voxel (Fig. 5.15). The intensity of each pixel in the image

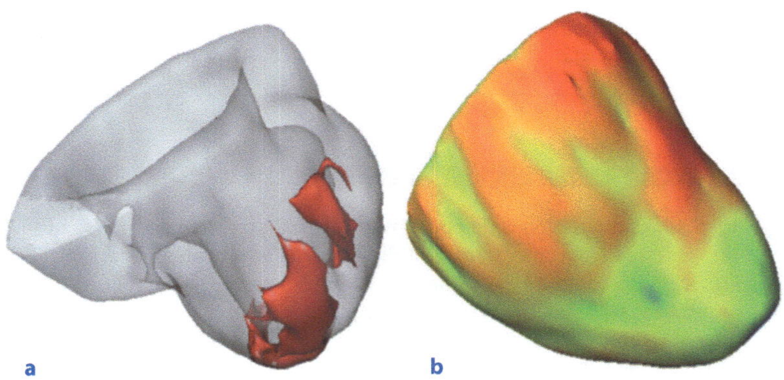

Fig. 5.13a,b. Surface representations. **a** The gray surface shows the segmented left ventricle. The transparency allows visualization of the location of a segmented infarction inside the ventricle. (Courtesy of Dr. M. Fenchel and Dr. A. Seeger, Department of Diagnostic Radiology, University of Tuebingen, Germany). **b** The color coding of the surface shows the parametric results of the wall thickness analysis. (Courtesy of Prof. Dr. S. Achenbach, Department of Medicine 2, University Hospital Erlangen, Germany)

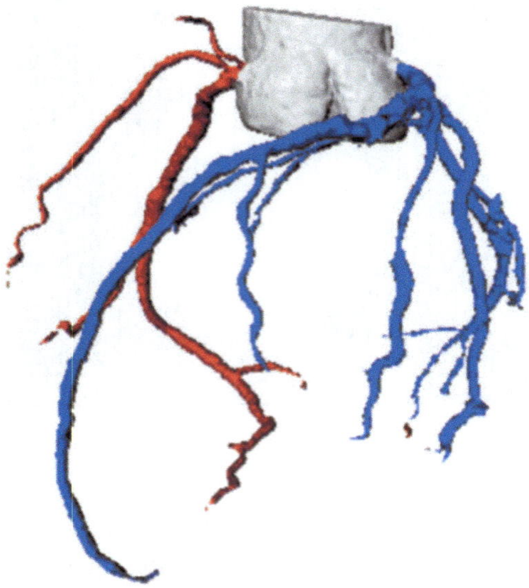

Fig. 5.14. Color coded surface visualization of the main coronary branches. (Courtesy of Prof. Dr. S. Achenbach, Department of Medicine 2, University Hospital Erlangen, Germany)

plane is then calculated based on the opacities and values of the voxels encountered along the viewing ray (Figs. 5.16 and 5.17). As with surface rendering, the use of an external light source may improve the perceptibility of small variations in the surface orientation.

Several types of algorithms are available to perform VR. Partial rendering can, other than binary rendering, have voxels with more than one assigned tissue type (with a certain percentage for each tissue type). Then, an object order (or compositing) projection method traverses all voxels from back to front and displays them on the screen while building the volume layer by layer. An image order (or ray-casting) technique, however, will cast rays through a volume from front to back and only display the complete image when finished. Image order techniques require more calculations than object order techniques. For a full description of this and other VR techniques, we refer to DREBIN et al. (1988) and ZUIDERVELD (1995).

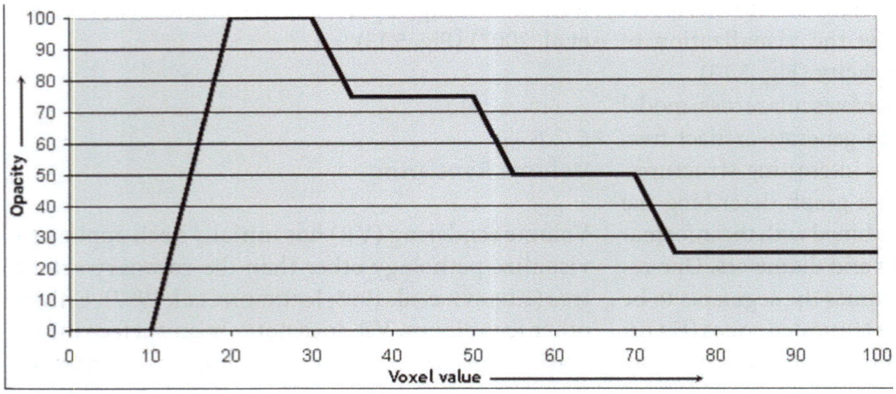

Fig. 5.15. Opacity assignment for each voxel value. The x-axis gives the voxel values, the y-axis the opacity value. The curve thus defines an opacity value for each voxel value. The example is again based on the example of Fig. 5.8. This curve assigns a high opacity to the internal (*dark*) structure

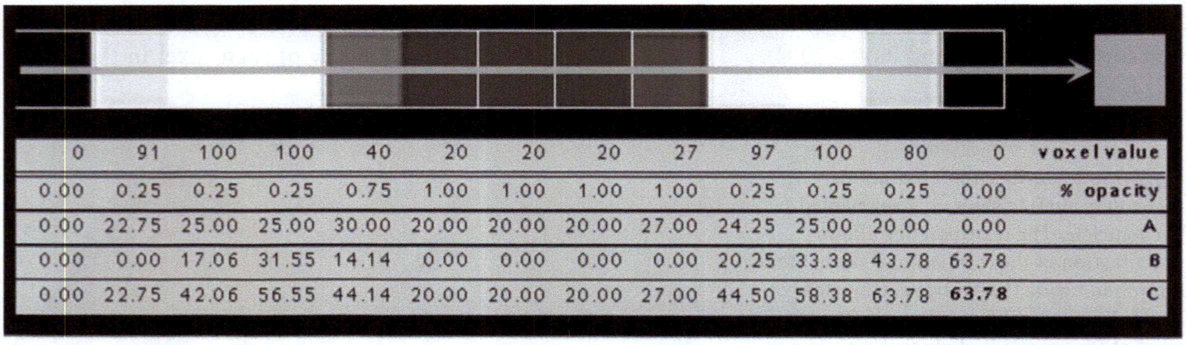

0	91	100	100	40	20	20	20	27	97	100	80	0	voxel value
0.00	0.25	0.25	0.25	0.75	1.00	1.00	1.00	1.00	0.25	0.25	0.25	0.00	% opacity
0.00	22.75	25.00	25.00	30.00	20.00	20.00	20.00	27.00	24.25	25.00	20.00	0.00	A
0.00	0.00	17.06	31.55	14.14	0.00	0.00	0.00	0.00	20.25	33.38	43.78	63.78	B
0.00	22.75	42.06	56.55	44.14	20.00	20.00	20.00	27.00	44.50	58.38	63.78	**63.78**	C

Fig. 5.16. Computation of the pixel values based on the voxel value and the opacity assignment. To demonstrate this, *row six* is selected from the example of Fig. 5.8. The voxel value of each pixel is determined as well as the opacity percentage (Fig. 5.15). To compute the value of the voxel (C (sum_n)), the following formula is used: C = A + B, where A = opacity × value and B = (1-opacity) × sum_{n-1}. The pixel value is calculated while passing through the row from *left* to *right*, the final value of C (approximately 78) is the value of the pixel in the resulting image. The corresponding gray level is shown in the square at the end of the *arrow*

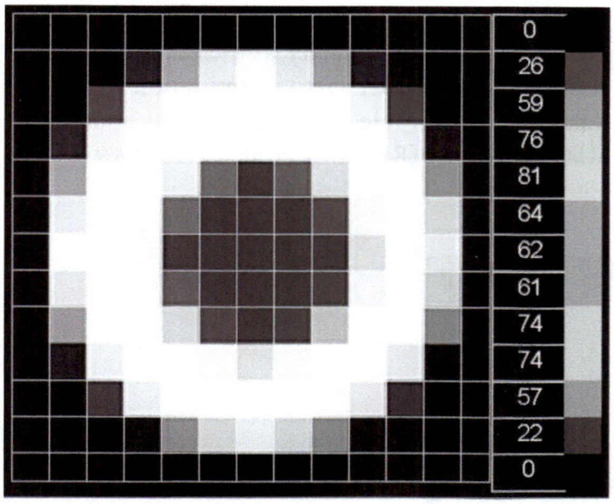

Fig. 5.17. The complete volume rendered example. It can be appreciated from the result (bar to the *right*) that, because of higher opacity of the lower intensity voxels in the center of the circle, they are still visible in the resulting image together with the outline of the complete circle´´

The greatest advantage of VR is the fact that it retains all voxels from the original 3D data set, thereby preserving all detail. Furthermore, VR allows partial transparency of superimposing structures to reveal other more opaque structures behind it (Figs. 5.18 and 5.19). Moreover, it produces three-dimensionally unambiguous images and it facilitates partial rendering and transparency, which in some cases makes segmentation obsolete.

Until recently, the main drawback of VR was the long computation time. However, with current (graphics) hardware and software, interactive 3D VR can be performed at acceptable speed. Adaptive refinement, which involves displaying the volume at a lower resolution during interaction and only showing it at full resolution in steady state, can produce VR with acceptable frame rates applicable to clinical practice. The frame rate is the number of images that can be displayed per second. For good interaction a minimal frame rate of 30 frames per second is required. Other drawbacks, which are harder to overcome, are the difficulty of obtaining the optimal settings because of the large amount of user definable

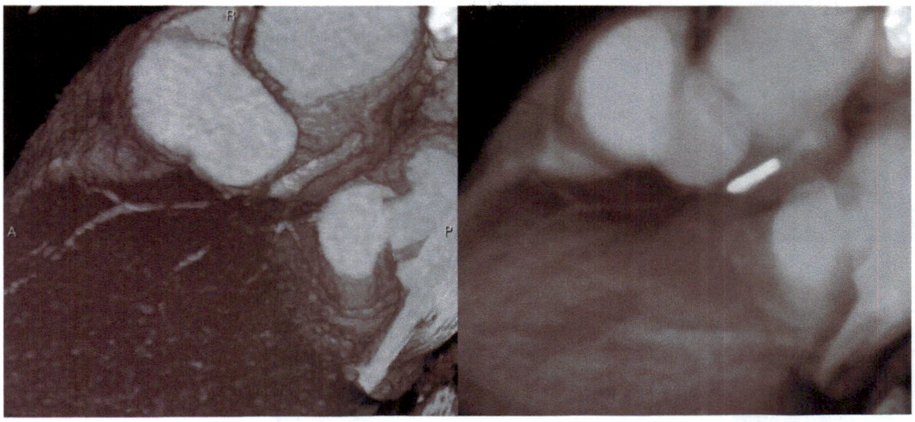

Fig. 5.18. Volume rendering of the left anterior descending artery. The *left image* shows a stenotic artery, the *right image* shows the cause of the stenosis, a large calcified region

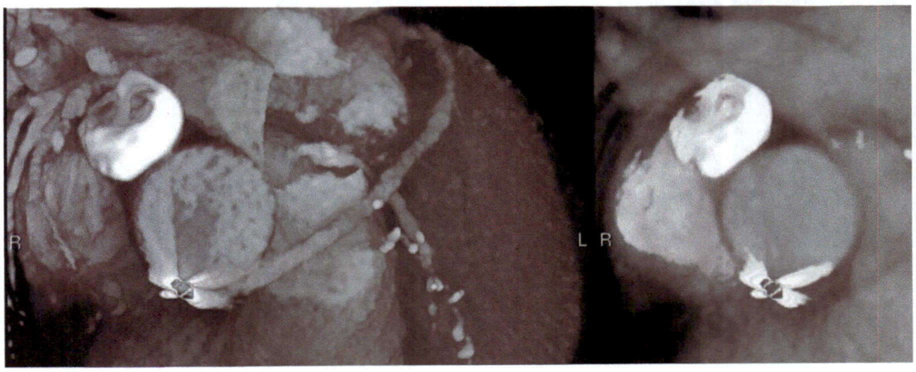

Fig. 5.19. Again, volume rendering of the coronary arteries. Using the opacity settings, calcified regions and surgical clips used for coronary artery bypass graft placement can be easily visualized

settings. This dependency on the defined parameter settings can also negatively influence the accuracy of VR for the evaluation of arterial stenoses, as the selection of window width, window level, brightness and opacity differs with each observer (EBERT et al. 1998) (Fig. 5.20).

VR is a very flexible rendering method and by assigning the right opacity and colors to different tissues we can ensure virtual simulation of the real anatomy comparable to pictures in an anatomical atlas (Fig. 5.21) (RENSING et al. 1999b; VAN GEUNS 1999).

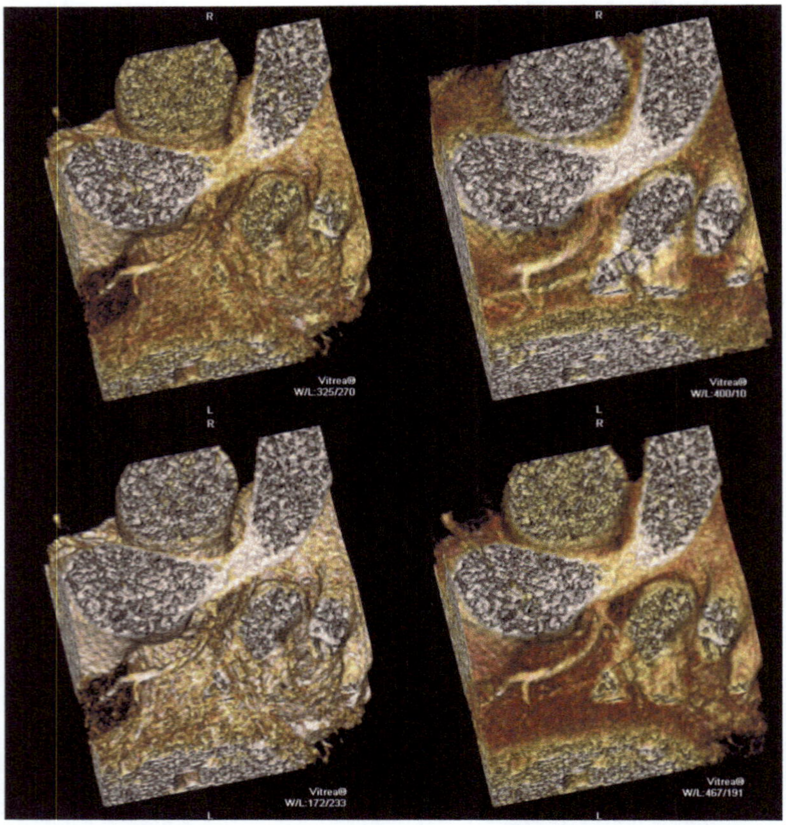

Fig. 5.20. Four different window level settings resulting in four different images. Window/level settings was set to 325/270 (*top left*), 400/10 (*top* right), 172/233 (*bottom left*) and 467/191 (*bottom right*) to demonstrate the possible effect on diagnosis of a left anterior descending artery of different settings

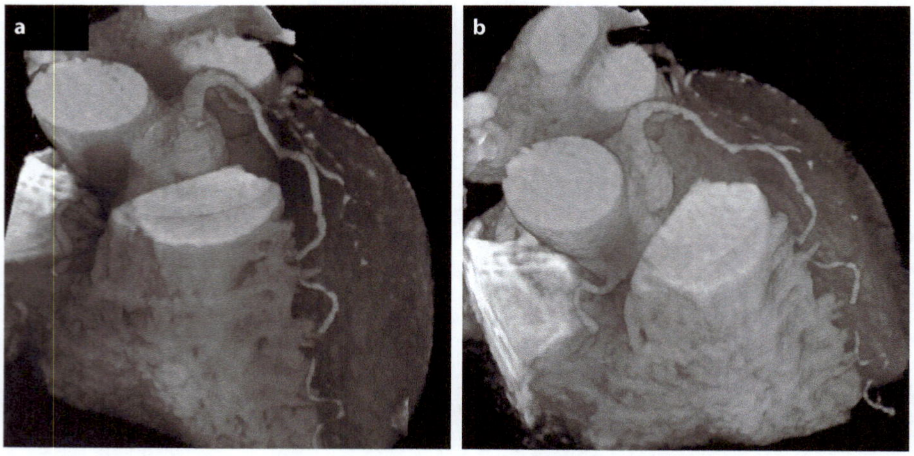

Fig. 5.21a,b. Volume rendered image of the heart

5.3 Intra-coronary Visualization

Peter M. A. van Ooijen, Wisnu Kristanto, Gonda J. de Jonge, Caroline Kuehnel, Anja Hennemuth, Tobias Boskamp, and Jaap M. Groen

Intra-coronary ultrasound and angioscopy enable invasive intravascular visualization of the coronary arteries. Advances both in data acquisition devices and visualization hard- and software allow us to visualize the interior of the coronary arteries non-invasively. This is achieved by means of virtual fly-through based non-invasive EBCT imaging (Nakanishi et al. 20000; van Ooijen et al. 2000a) or MDCT (Schroeder et al. 2002; van Ooijen et al. 2002; Traversie and Tramarin 2003) applying the same techniques as used in other fly-throughs of the human body (Terwisscha van Scheltinga 2001; Wiese and Rogalla 2001).

Coronary artery fly-through is another way to provide a comprehensive delineation of the lumen and the impact of vessel wall disease on the lumen. To perform coronary artery fly-through it is essential to have an EBCT or CT angiogram of the coronary arteries of adequate quality.

A fly-through (or intra-luminal visualization) can be looked upon as a virtual catheter mounted camera that is inserted into a vessel. Displaying images at consecutive positions along a certain path through the coronary creates the illusion of moving through this coronary. To perform a fly-through presentation, the vessels first have to be "hollowed out" by assigning voxels representing contrast media rich blood (usually voxel values of 100–250 HU) with zero opacity (= full transparency) (Fig. 5.22).

Consequently, surrounding tissues such as the vessel wall (voxel values of 80–100 HU) and calcifications in the arteries (voxel values of >250 HU) will have high opacity.

Second, the viewpoint is moved inside the aorta or a coronary artery. Next, a number of viewpoints can be selected, using either manual of automated centerline detection methods, positioned along the flight path. This flight path is then utilized to reconstruct a fly-through movie.

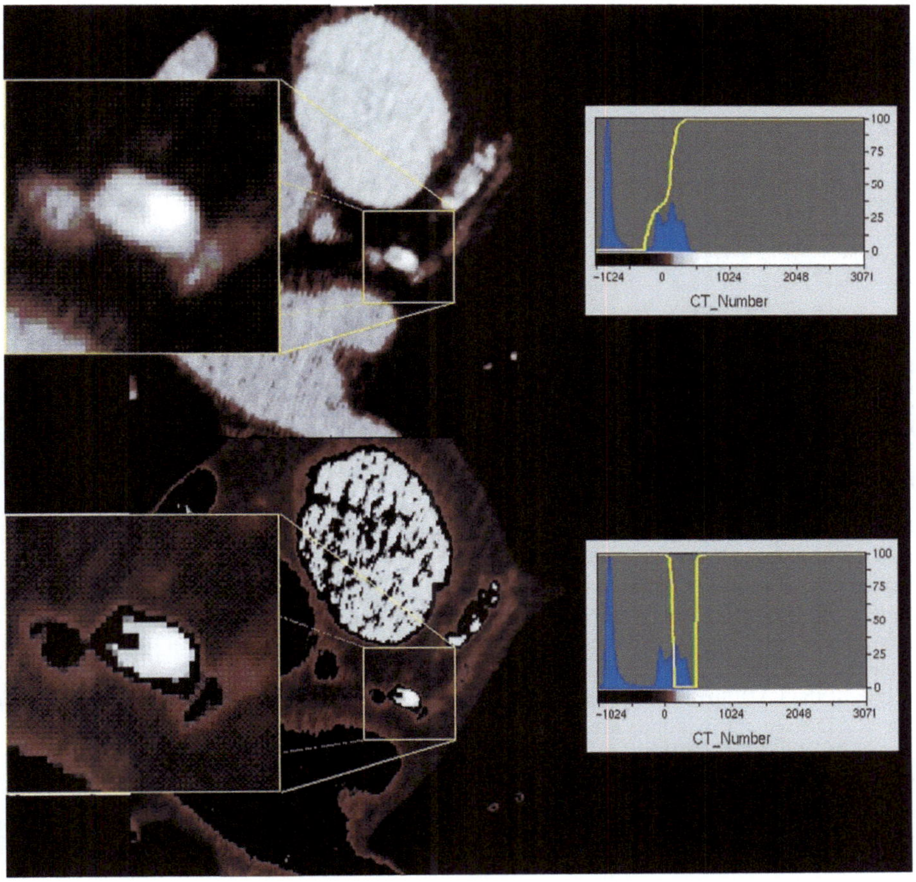

Fig. 5.22. At the *top right* a normal opacity curve is shown for the depiction of the coronary arteries using volume rendering, the resulting image is shown on the *top left*. The bottom histogram shows an opacity curve that assigns 100% opacity to both low CT numbers and high CT numbers, but a zero opacity to a range in the middle. This range represents the contrast enhanced blood in the heart. This setting results in a hollow vessel with the calcified plaques still opaque as shown in the *bottom left* image

For the reconstruction of fly-through movies, the image quality of the 3D datasets has to be very high. Special attention has to be paid to the inter-slice correlation quality, the lack of artifacts and the slice image quality. Even small irregularities may hamper a successful construction of a coronary artery fly-through. There are several issues that may lead to these irregularities. First, problems with breath-holding may reduce continuation of a coronary artery from one slice to another. Second, arrhythmia, or even a single premature complex may lead to images that are triggered at a slightly different time during the heart cycle, resulting in a displacement of 1–2 mm of a single slice with respect to the other slices. This phenomenon creates a discontinuation of the coronary arteries in 3D reconstructions. Third, vessels with a diameter smaller than 1.75 mm (cross-section of approximately 5×5 pixels) will not provide a smooth coronary fly-trough. Fourth, motion artifacts of the coronary arteries may hamper the construction of a fly-through movie.

Many of the difficulties stated here have been overcome in recent improvements in spatial and temporal resolution of the acquisition device and by improvements in visualization software. The recent introduction of dual source computed tomography (DSCT) (van Ooijen et al. 2007) enabled a 100% visualization of all major arteries, even at high heart rate, which is a major improvement compared to the results found in previous studies with only 76% assessable for EBCT and 84% assessable for four-MDCT (van Ooijen et al. 2002).

Furthermore, the time required for post-processing the data decreased from 6--13 min in 2002 to just 2.5 min in 2007. Considering that the time recorded in 2002 was only preparation time and did not conclude the actual computation time only increases this difference since the 2.5 min in 2007 is real-time including visualization.

Fly-through movies of venous bypass grafts are relatively easy to create because the vessel diameter is relatively large and cardiac motion of these vessels is limited. However, surgical clips or sternal wires may sometimes degrade the images because of the blooming artifacts they cause.

Calcifications of the vessel wall, having a very high voxel value, are retained in the fly-throughs and are visible as white blobs floating around in the artery (Fig. 5.23).

The preliminary findings published so far demonstrate the feasibility and potential of this method in coronary artery or bypass graft fly-through movies (Nakanishi et al. 2000; van Ooijen et al. 2000a,

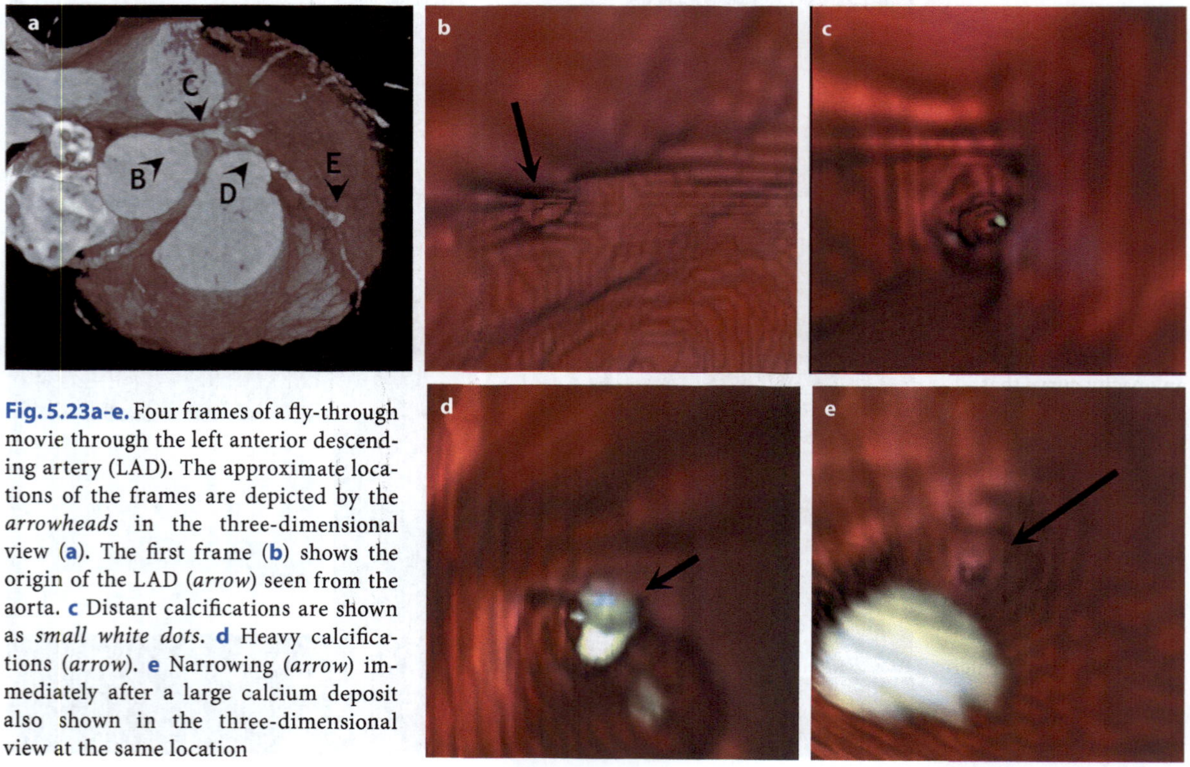

Fig. 5.23a-e. Four frames of a fly-through movie through the left anterior descending artery (LAD). The approximate locations of the frames are depicted by the *arrowheads* in the three-dimensional view (**a**). The first frame (**b**) shows the origin of the LAD (*arrow*) seen from the aorta. **c** Distant calcifications are shown as *small white dots*. **d** Heavy calcifications (*arrow*). **e** Narrowing (*arrow*) immediately after a large calcium deposit also shown in the three-dimensional view at the same location

2002, 2007; Schroeder et al. 2002; Traversie and Tramarin 2003). However, the technique of coronary artery fly-through cannot be considered as an alternative to traditional coronary angioscopy, since it does not provide us with any information about the color of the lumen wall or its contents such as plaque and thrombus.

Schroeder et al. (2002) reported direct comparison of virtual coronary angioscopy (VCA) in 16 MDCT scans with intravascular ultrasound, showing that all severe lesions were detected with virtual coronary angioscopy. However, non-calcified intermediate lesions could not be accurately distinguished from the vessel wall by VCA, but were recognized as vessel wall alterations without significant lumen narrowing.

Despite its shortcomings, coronary artery fly-through is an alternative evaluation method of non-invasive coronary angiography with several advantages. First, it provides delineation of the "true" three dimensions of the vessel lumen, unlike diagnostic angiography (lumenography) which is limited by foreshortening and overlapping structures. Second, fly-throughs may eliminate the time consuming segmentation of overlapping, obscuring anatomical structures (left atrium, coronary sinus) needed to visualize the coronary arteries from the outside. Third, fly-throughs may provide a more comprehensive delineation of bifurcation lesions, or anastomoses of grafts on native vessels, which are sometimes difficult to assess even with routine diagnostic angiography. Finally, fly-throughs may be helpful to assess the remaining coronary lumen in presence of a heavy calcified coronary plaque or in case of stented segments that may be invisible with traditional 3D rendering techniques.

Despite these advantages, conventional axial slices are still superior compared to VCA for the detection of coronary artery lesions, especially in non-significant lesions without calcifications. VCA is a method of compressing a huge amount of image data into a form of presentation that can be viewed in a short time.

5.4 Visualization of Four-Dimensional Data

Peter M. A. van Ooijen, Wisnu Kristanto, Gonda J. de Jonge, Caroline Kuehnel, Anja Hennemuth, Tobias Boskamp, and Jaap M. Groen

To visualize dynamic 4D data, all methods described above can be used to generate a time sequence of 2D or 3D visualizations. This allows an observation of dynamic processes in the so-called cine mode.

For a comprehensive visualization in 2D, information has to be derived from the 4D sequences. Thus, curves describing the dynamic changes of, for example, intensity values, wall thickness or flow velocity are computed (Fig. 5.24). These curves form

a

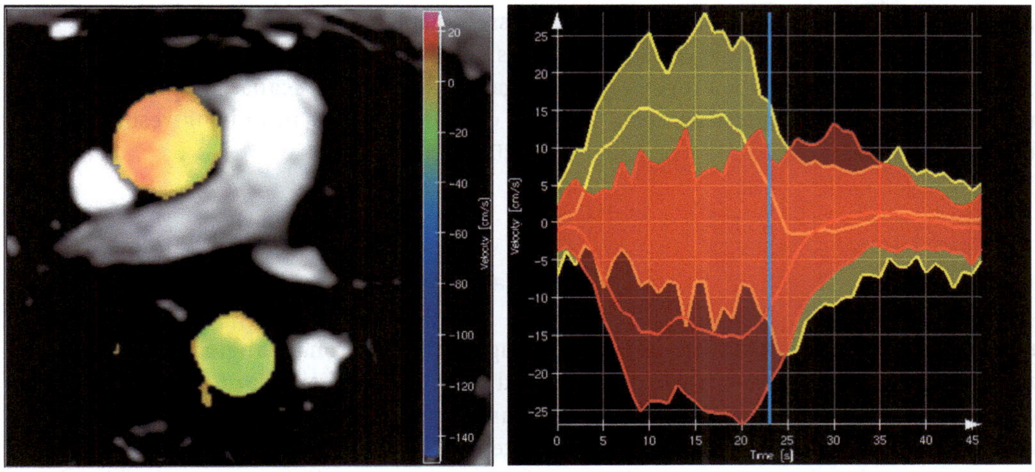

b

Fig. 5.24a,b. Flow visualization. The color coded overlay in (**a**) indicates the mean flow velocities per voxel. The diagram in (**b**) shows the maximum, minimum and averaged velocities for ascending (*yellow*) and descending (*red*) aorta covering the whole time sequence. The *blue line* in the diagram indicates the time point corresponding to the image in (**a**). (Courtesy of PD Dr. J. Lotz, Department of Diagnostic Radiology, Hannover Medical School, Germany) the basis for the computation of diagnostically relevant parameters, which are often visualized in the spatial context, as in parameter maps of perfusion or color coded surfaces in case of wall thickness analysis (Fig. 5.24).

5.5 Clinical Applications

Peter M.A. van Ooijen, Wisnu Kristanto, Gonda J. de Jonge, Caroline Kuehnel, Anja Hennemuth, Tobias Boskamp, and Jaap M. Groen

A 3D dataset acquired using CT or MRI to visualize the heart and coronary arteries will not only include those regions of interest, but the full thorax of the patient. Therefore, elaborate manual, semi-automatic, or automatic segmentation or selection is required to obtain a suitable visualization. However, the segmentation or selection effort is somewhat dependent on the visualization technique used (van Ooijen et al. 2003a).

Therefore, each clinical application, both for coronary evaluation and for left ventricle analysis, requires a different approach. When a user wants to address a certain clinical question, a careful decision has to be made about which software to use, which visualization technique to apply, and which protocol to follow. This requires insight in all those different subjects and understanding of the possibilities of the different techniques. In this section, several clinical applications are described together with the visualization and post-processing techniques available.

5.5.1 Coronary Calcification

Growing interest in coronary calcification screening has led to the introduction of software packages for the assessment of coronary calcification in non-contrast scans of the coronary arteries. In an axial view of the coronary arteries the software highlights pixels with a CT density above the calcium scoring threshold (usually 130 HU). Subsequently, the user selects regions in which calcifications are present. Using the marked calcifications a calcium score is calculated by the software. These software packages use fairly simple scoring techniques. The first uniform scoring method for coronary calcium was devised by Agatston et al. (1990) based on EBCT data and is called the Agatston score. It depends on the area of the calcification and the maximum Hounsfield value within that area per slice (Agatston et al. 1990). For each plaque, the size and maximum attenuation are determined in each slice. Based on the maximum attenuation, the size of the plaque is multiplied with a weight factor. The total score of a plaque is the summation over all slices. A second scoring method, known as the Volume Score, was proposed by Callister et al. (1998). The method showed better reproducibility than the traditional score and depends on the volume of the calcifications only. The total score represents the overall volume of the calcifications present in the coronary arteries. A third measure of coronary calcification is the determination of the equivalent mass. This method depends on the volume and the average Hounsfield value of the calcification per plaque and shows better reproducibility than the two other scores (Hoffmann et al. 2006). Here, the total score represents the summarized amount of coronary calcium mass in the coronary arteries. However, clinical data about risk of coronary artery disease in relation to coronary calcium is based prominently on the Agatston score, therefore this method is still most frequently used in practice.

Recent developments in computer aided diagnosis (CAD) have enabled the automatic segmentation of coronary calcifications enabling automatic risk assessment of coronary artery disease. First studies performed on the non-contrast enhanced, ECG-gated cardiac CT scans comprising a small group of patients show promising results (Isgum et al. 2007).

5.5.2 Coronary Anatomy

Although catheter coronary angiography is still considered to be the gold standard for the analysis of coronary artery anatomy, it has two major disadvantages.

First, there is a small, but not negligible, risk of major complications (mortality and morbidity). Second, only a 2D projection view of the coronary artery tree is provided. Thus evaluation of 3D course of the arteries is difficult even for experienced angiographers, especially with coronary anomalies (Klessen et al. 2000).

Normal coronary artery anatomy is clearly depicted using the new non-invasive techniques. For proper coronary evaluation, segmentation of the heart is required. With modern workstation software, in most cases this segmentation of overlapping structures can be done automatically or with little user interaction. Subsequently, semi-automatic or automatic segmentation of the coronary arteries is feasible.

The same procedure of segmentation is used to visualize coronary anomalies. Although coronary anomalies are rare, identification and definition of their exact anatomic course is crucial because they may cause myocardial ischemia and sudden cardiac death without stenotic coronary artery disease. When using invasive coronary angiography, misinterpretation of up to 50% of coronary anomalies is reported (Schmid et al. 2006). This misinterpretation is due to the difficult evaluation of the exact 3D course in the projection image and to the failure of positioning the catheter in the anomalous artery. Therefore, a good 3D visualization using volume rendered MRA (Klessen et al. 2000) or CTA data (Funabashi et al. 2001a,b) largely improves the interpretation of coronary anatomy and especially coronary anomalies (van Ooijen et al. 2004).

For the evaluation of the course of the anomalous artery, surface rendering (SR) or VR are very suitable because both really show the 3D course of the coronary artery tree. In some cases, such as the anomalous RCA shown in Figure 5.25, visualization of the shape of the ostium of the artery can be valuable (Funabashi et al. 2001a). To achieve this, intracoronary visualization can be used.

5.5.3 Coronary Stenosis and Atherosclerotic Plaque

Several image rendering techniques, such as MPR, SR, and VR, can be used for the visualization of coronary artery stenoses. High resolution data are required to allow correct grading of stenoses. If the length or width of a stenosis is below the resolution, the stenosis will become less visible because of partial volume effects, and thus will be underestimated. Furthermore, when the width of the stenosis is below the resolution it will appear to be a full occlusion. These partial volume effects negatively influence all rendering techniques mentioned before (Takahashi et al. 1997).

One of the main disadvantages in the use of SSD for the evaluation of coronary artery stenosis is the inability to differentiate between calcified plaque (200–700 HU) and contrast-enhanced lumen (90–250 HU) (Magnusson et al. 1991).

Because of the high attenuation of calcified plaques, VR is capable of differentiation between the two by assigning different properties (e.g. color) to voxel with a very high voxel value (e.g. >450 HU) (Fig. 5.26). However, because of the dependency of settings such as window width, window level, brightness and opacity (Figs. 5.27–5.30), measurement and grading of stenotic lesions are highly operator dependent (Ebert et al. 1998; Liu et al. 2000). MPR or axial slices provide the best evaluation of stenotic lesions at the site of calcifications because the extent of the calcifications is more easily perceived (Fig. 5.31). Newer methods, like automatic reconstruction of curved MPR or stretched MPR, even enhance the possibilities by reducing user dependence to a large extend.

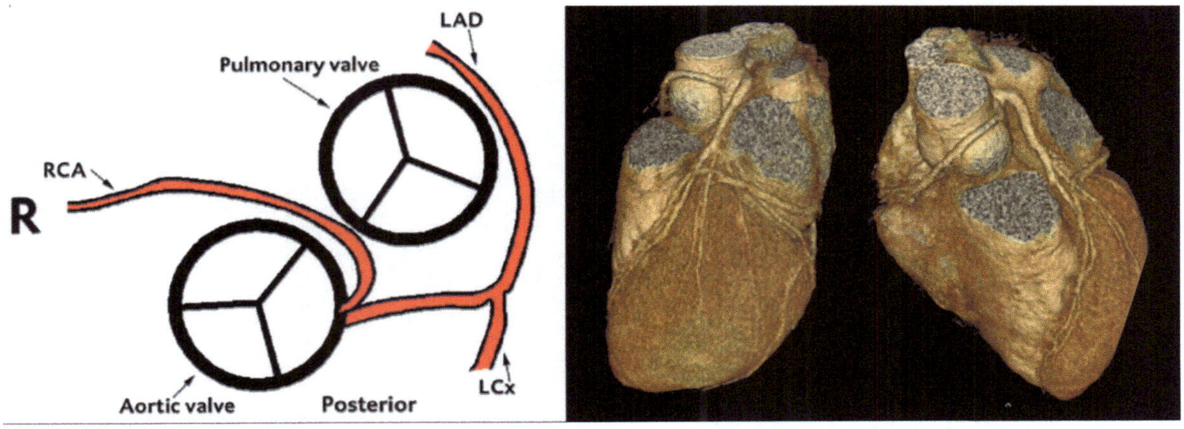

Fig. 5.25. Coronary anomaly in schematic representation (*left*) and three-dimensional volume rendering (*right*)

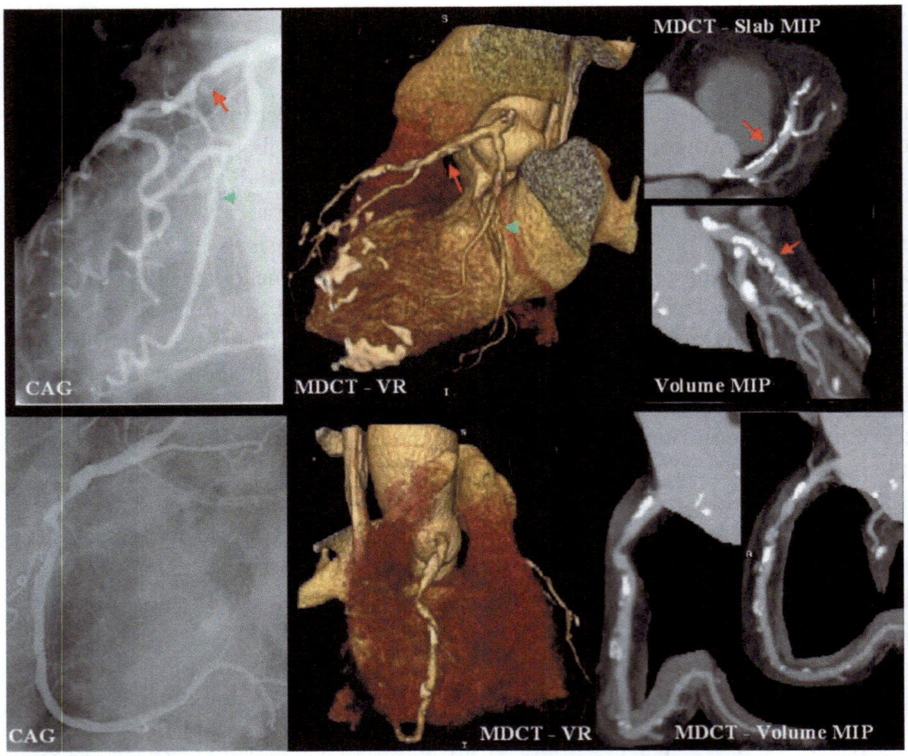

Fig. 5.26. Conventional angiogram (*left*), volume rendering (*middle*), and maximum intensity projection (*right*) of coronary artery stenoses in the right coronary artery

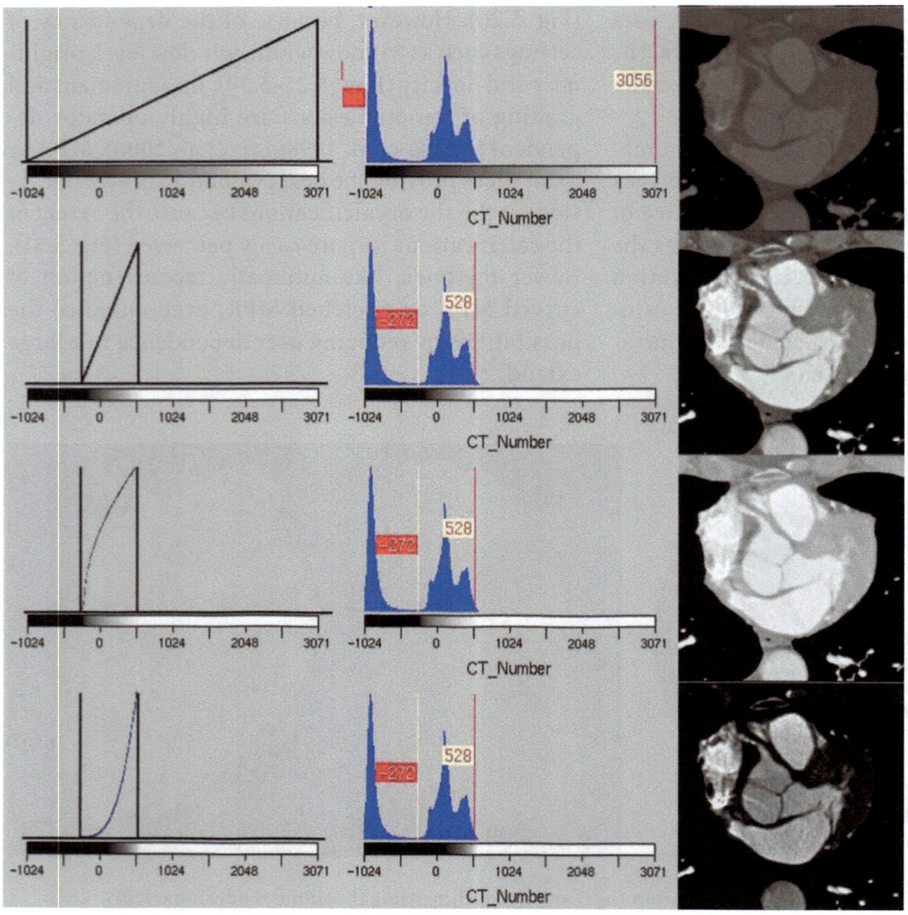

Fig. 5.27. The images in this figure show the shading curve. The extent and position of the shading curve is defined by the window and level settings (two *vertical lines* in the histograms). Between the boundaries of the window/level setting, the shading curve is applied (see images to the *left*). The shading will go from black (0) to white (256) using a certain curve. The first two settings apply a linear shading to the image, the other two a non-linear one

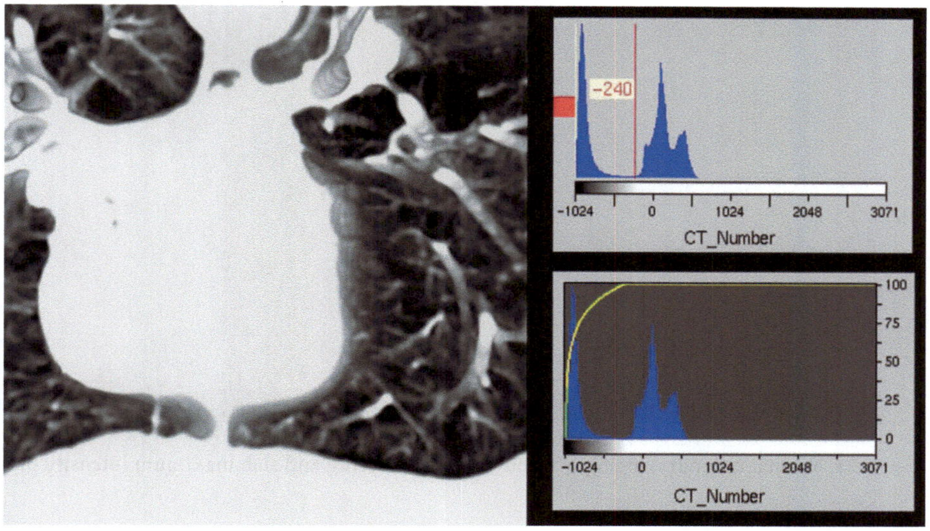

Fig. 5.28. Image with contrast stretch at levels –1024 and –240 HU, resulting in a window of 784 and a level of –632 with a linear shading curve. In the histogram, the peaks represent the number of voxels with the corresponding CT number (HU); the lines indicate the upper and lower levels for the stretch. With this setting, only air and lung tissue are highlighted

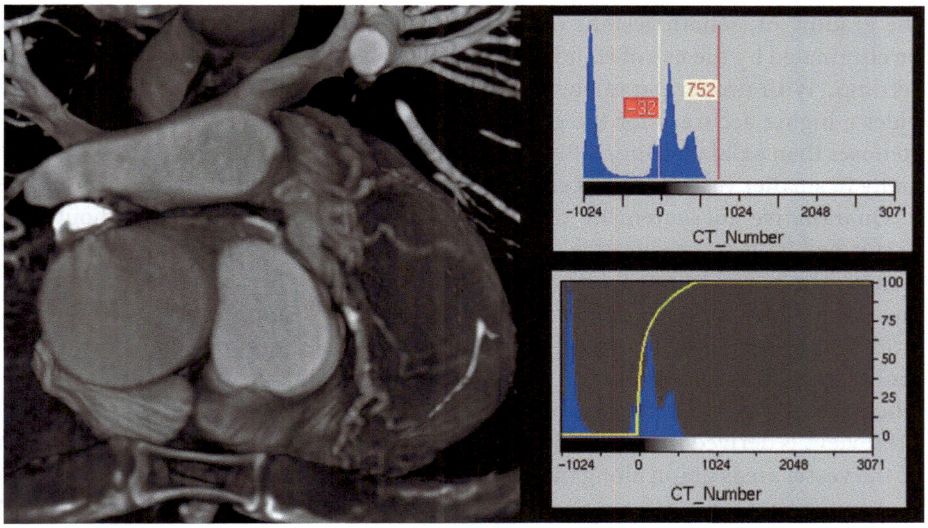

Fig. 5.29. The same data with contrast stretch at levels –32 and 752 HU, resulting in an image with window 784 and level 360 with a linear shading curve. The lines in the histogram are now positioned before and after the second peak, resulting in an image with enhanced fat and soft tissue. The line graph represents the percentage of opacity for the CT numbers (y-axis from 0% to 100%), in this case defining an image with opaque soft tissue and fat and transparent air

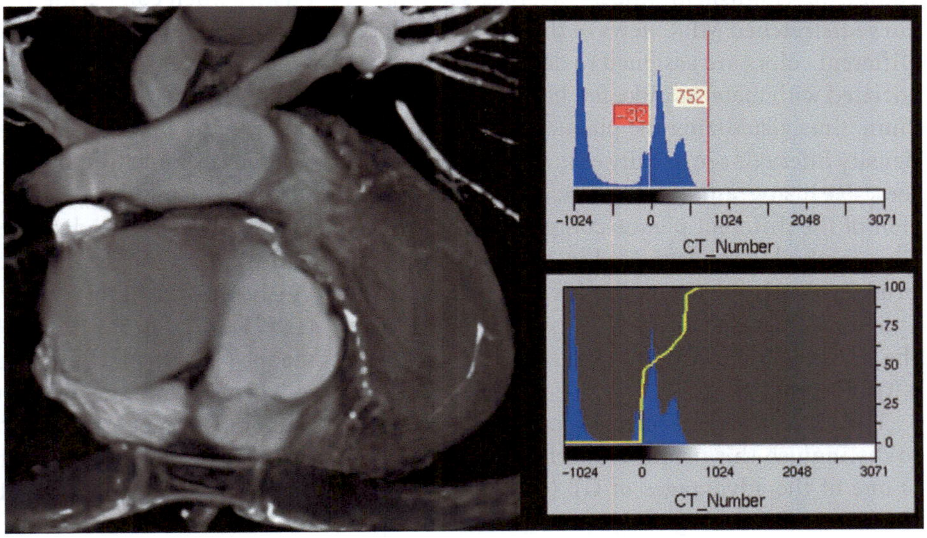

Fig. 5.30. Image with transparent soft tissue and fat, the intra-arterial calcifications in the left main and left anterior descending arteries can now be appreciated clearly. The line graph has been altered at the CT numbers of the second peak, giving these CT numbers a lower opacity resulting in partially transparent fat and soft tissue

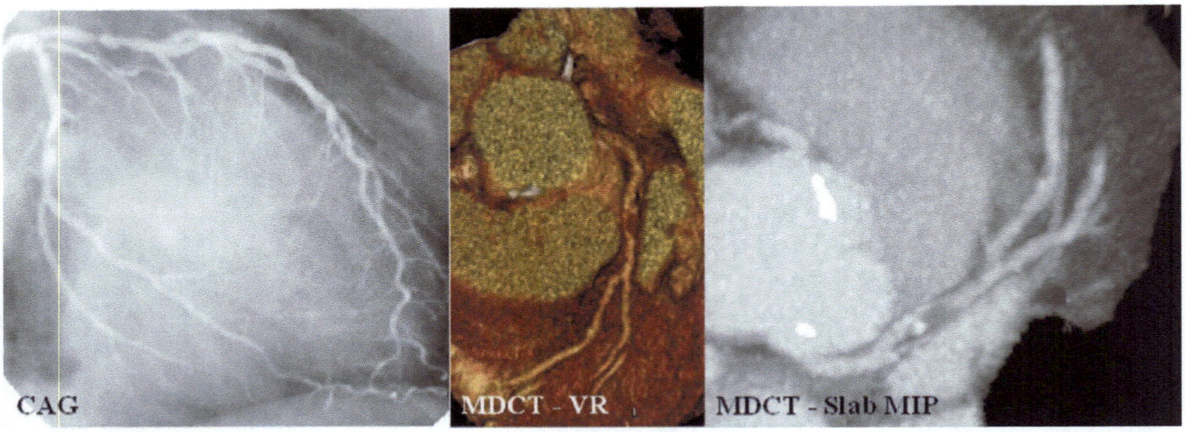

Fig. 5.31. Normal coronary angiogram and volume rendering and slab maximum intensity projection

However, when using CT data the dependency of the grading of stenotic lesions on the settings can be eliminated by the use of standardized parameter settings. With proper parameter settings, VR provides a higher accuracy for the grading of vascular stenoses than axial viewing, MPR, MIP or SSD especially in smaller vessels (ADDIS et al. 2001).

Quantitative measurement of stenoses can be performed with some software tools by first determining the normal lumen area or diameter reference. Some tools provide manual depiction of such a reference point along the vessel length while other tools can automatically generate a reference for the whole vessel length. The latter, available in stretched MPR view, is derived from the linear approximation of the vessel areas graph along the vessel length.

A common technique for supporting the diagnosis of atherosclerotic plaques in MDCT data is the color coding of Hounsfield values in cross-sections or curved/stretched MPR views of the affected branch. Different colors are assigned to density intervals associated with materials like fat, fibrous tissue or calcium, thus visualizing the plaque composition. The density intervals are usually editable utilizing an interactive histogram and, thus, enable the quantification of the different plaque components (Fig. 5.32). This method is implemented in clinically available products such as the Aquarius Workstation, the Syngo Circulation software (ABDALA et al. 2006) or the SUREPlaque application (HEIN et al. 2006) of the Vitrea Workstation.

The ability to detect coronary calcified plaque and to distinguish this plaque from the coronary lumen is one of the advantages of CT (KNEZ et al. 2002). However, when using contrast medium for depiction of the coronary arteries, partial volume effects will cause the edges of the plaque to have a similar attenuation as the contrast enhanced blood, which can lead to misinterpretation of the size of the coronary plaque and thus of the severity of a stenosis at that location (TAKAHASHI et al. 1997). Therefore, to evaluate the calcified plaque load in patients, scans are performed without contrast enhancement (see Sect. 5.5.1).

Besides the scoring of coronary calcification, a more precise classification of coronary plaques is gaining interest because of the enhanced imaging possibilities using contrast-enhanced CT scanning with high spatial and temporal resolution (SCHROEDER et al. 2001; LEBER et al. 2003; HOFFMANN and BUTLER 2005; REIMANN et al. 2007). A coronary plaque phantom study by REIMANN et al. (2007) showed a significant improvement of plaque image quality when comparing DSCT with 64-MDCT. The main reason for this improved plaque image quality was the increase in temporal resolution from 165 ms in 64-MDCT to 83 ms in DSCT. The proper way to analyze the plaque contents would be using MPR. A good visualization of plaque morphology can be obtained using the longitudinal and axial view of MPR. Moreover, the data are represented in its original value so the plaque components can be distinguished based on their HU value ranges: soft plaque (14±26 HU), fibrous tissue (91±21 HU) and calcified plaque (419±194 HU) (SCHROEDER et al. 2001).

There is an ongoing interest in the detection of vulnerable plaque, in particular lipid pool. Such a structure is hard to detect because of its small dimension and overlapping HU values with the surrounding soft tissue. LEBER et al. (2006) proposed

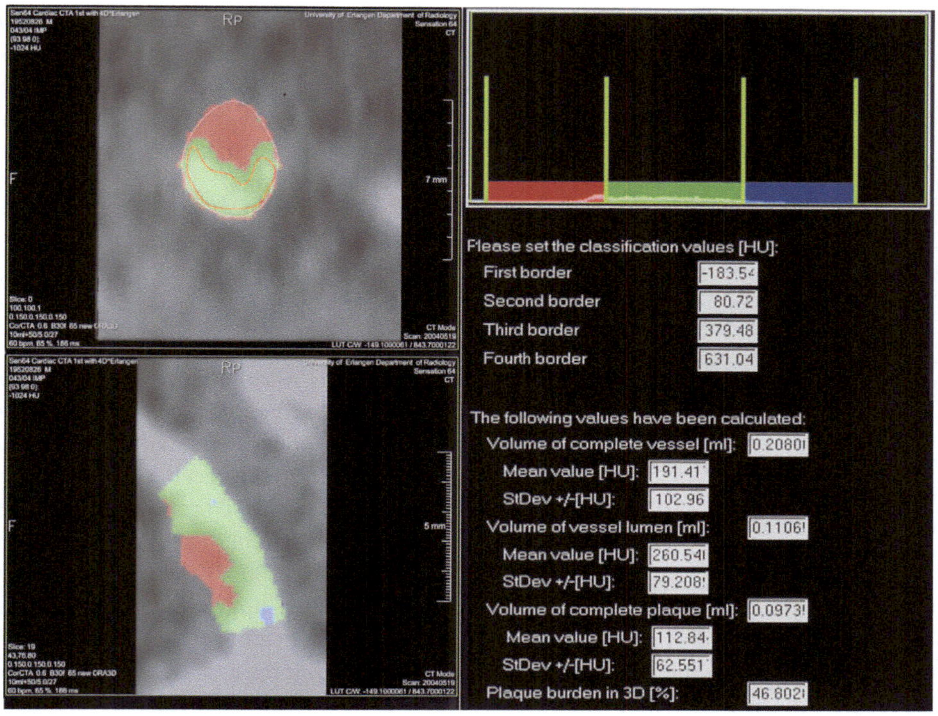

Fig. 5.32. Visualization and quantification of plaque composition. (Courtesy of Prof. Dr. S. Achenbach, Department of Medicine 2, University Hospital Erlangen, Germany)

a way to detect the lipid pool by searching on MPR images for the area inside non-calcified plaque for a structure with a minimal area of 2 mm^2 and a value of at least 20 HU below its surrounding. Using this manual method, seven of ten lipid pools (70%) could be detected.

5.5.4 Coronary Stent Evaluation

Since their introduction by Sigwart et al. in 1987 stents are commonly used to reduce restenosis rates in the coronary artery, to prevent myocardial infarction, and therefore to improve long-term prognosis. Nevertheless, it has been reported that in-stent restenosis occurs in about 10%–60% of the cases (Hoffmann and Mintz 2000). As invasive techniques such as coronary angiography are less suited for frequent follow-up, a noninvasive diagnostic modality would be highly desired.

Due to their metallic composition, stents cause blooming artefacts (scattering) that may obscure the Hounsfield units in the lumen, and therefore the detection of stenoses (Fig. 5.33).

To achieve a better understanding of how this scattering may affect the Hounsfield value, a Lekton stent was put in water and scanned on MDCT. An acquired slice is shown in Figure 5.34 where it can be clearly seen how artificial patterns are generated by the scattering effects of the stent. These patterns disturb the Hounsfield value of the surrounding tissue which (in this case) should be zero.

Studies on various coronary artery stents of different material and design have been done, and can be found in (Maintz 2003, 2006) and the references therein.

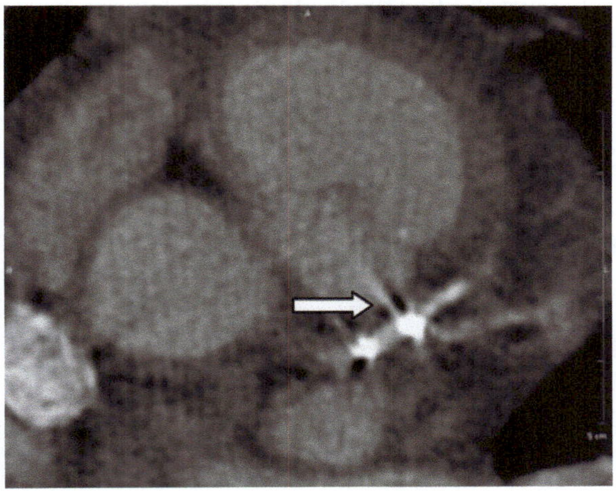

Fig. 5.33. Artifacts in an MDCT image caused by high signal density (scattering effect) of a stent (*arrow*)

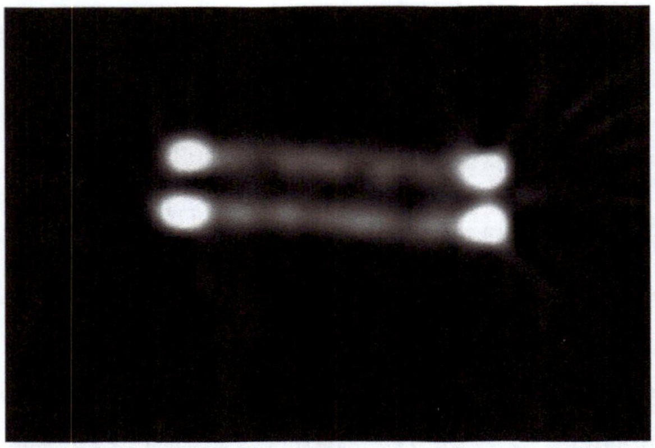

Fig. 5.34. A Lekton stent was put in water and scanned using MDCT. The four bright areas correspond to the four markers originated in the stent itself. Scatter effects are visible, and disturb the Hounsfield Units of water which should be zero

For the evaluation of coronary artery stents the preferred evaluation method is the use of a curved MPR through the stent. After this curved MPR is defined, planes perpendicular to the centerline of the curved MPR can be used to evaluate the lumen in more detail (Fig. 5.35). A curved MPR suffers least from scattering and the effects of the scattering can be easily recognized in the resulting images.

Although in-stent restenosis has developed into a significant clinical as well as technical problem, consistent and reliable predictors and detectors are still not available.

This is because coronary artery stents, and especially those plated with gold or markers, cause serious artifacts on MDCT scanning. These artifacts hinder any measurements based on the Hounsfield value surrounding the stents causing stenoses detection to be unreliable or even impossible. The use of a dedicated edge enhancing reconstruction kernel reduces the artifacts associated with stents significantly (Seifarth et al. 2005; Mahnken et al. 2004). Extensive studies are being carried out to compensate for these artifacts by using post-processing algorithms.

Besides the scattering effects the image quality of coronary stents is also hampered by motion artifacts due to cardiac motion. A low heart rate increases the visibility of the lumen of the stent (Groen 2006, 2007).

Although the literature shows that four-MDCT was not sufficient for adequate determination of in-stent restenosis (Chabbert et al. 2007; Ligabue et al. 2007), recent publications claim that with 16- and 64-MDCT scanners the assessment of stent patency is reliable (de Feyter and Krestin 2005; Kefer et al. 2007), clearly showing increasing capabilities with upgraded scanner generation. Furthermore, Sheth et al (2007) showed in 54 stents in 44 patients that the assessability of a stent is mainly determined by the stent size. According to their results, stents with nominal size of >3 mm are more consistently assessable than stents <3 mm. Current reports show up to 78% sensitivity and 100% specificity in 16-MDCT. However, the fact that the percentage of non-accessibility can be up to 40% in the same studies shows that the routine diagnostic evaluation of coronary stents using CT is still far away. For reliable diagnosis of coronary in-stent restenosis higher spatial and temporal resolution is required and dedicated filtering to reduce high-density blooming artifacts. Another solution is in the use of different stent types, such as biodegradable stents or stents of less radiopaque material, since previous studies show that stent configuration and material influence the visibility of the lumen.

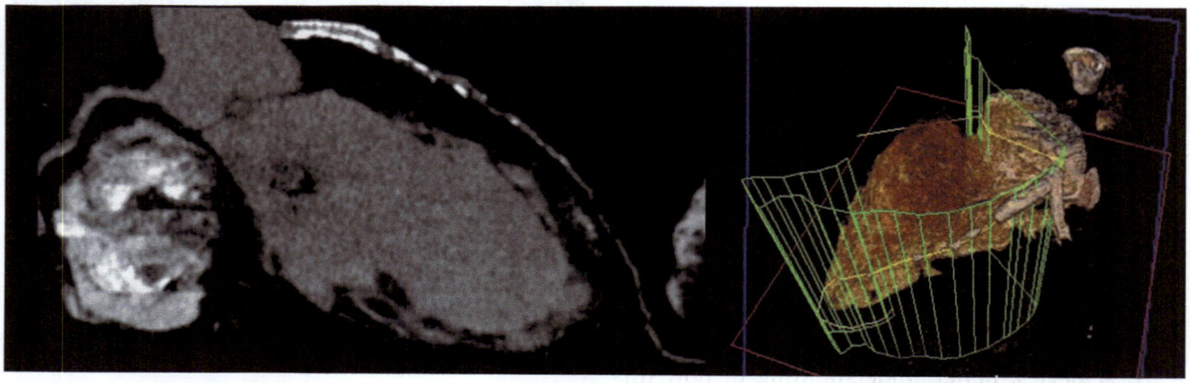

Fig. 5.35. Curved multi-planar reformation showing stent lumen (*left*) and the selected curve displayed within a three-dimensional visualization (*right*)

5.5.5 Cardiac Function

The acquisition of the entire heart during complete heart cycle enables functional analysis of the heart chambers and muscle. Parameters such as end-systolic volume, end-diastolic volume, ejection fraction, stroke volume, cardiac output, stroke index, cardiac index, myocardial volume and mass can be easily obtained from the acquired dataset. Both MDCT and MRI can be used for functional analysis.

In most software systems the only user interaction is the selection of end-systolic and end-diastolic phases, after which the segmentation is semiautomatic with minor user interaction (Fig. 5.36). Fine tuning of the segmentation can be performed manually by the user before the final computations. Figure 5.37 shows an example of functional MRI in which a mesh is built and tracked automatically in a fraction of a minute. Software is used for dividing the heart into segments in which a number of measurements such as regional strains, twist, mesh ejection fraction and wall thickening are computed. These quantitative results, evaluated according to the 17-segment model of the American Heart Association (AHA) (Cerqueria et al. 2002), are gener-

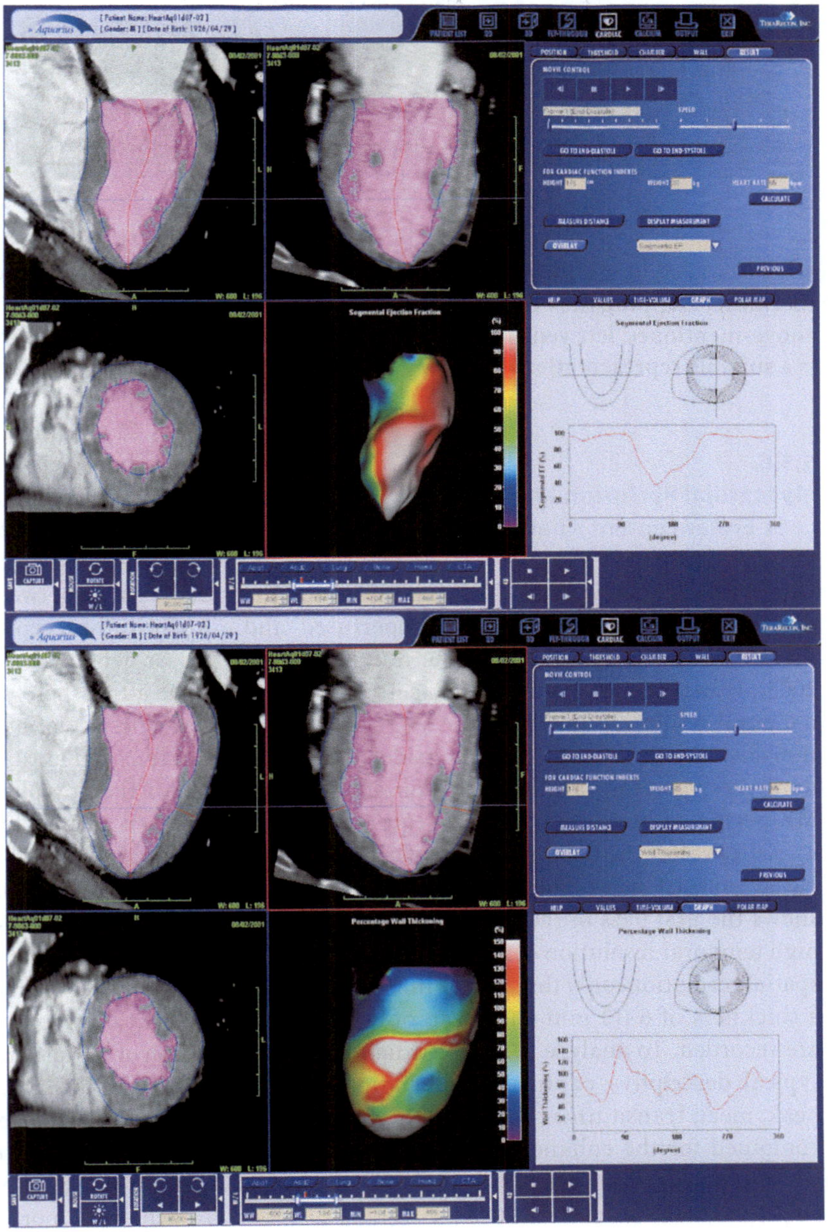

Fig. 5.36. Results of a functional analysis of a CT dataset showing screenshots of both ejection fraction (*top*) and wall thickening (*bottom*). (Image courtesy of TeraRecon, San Mateo, CA)

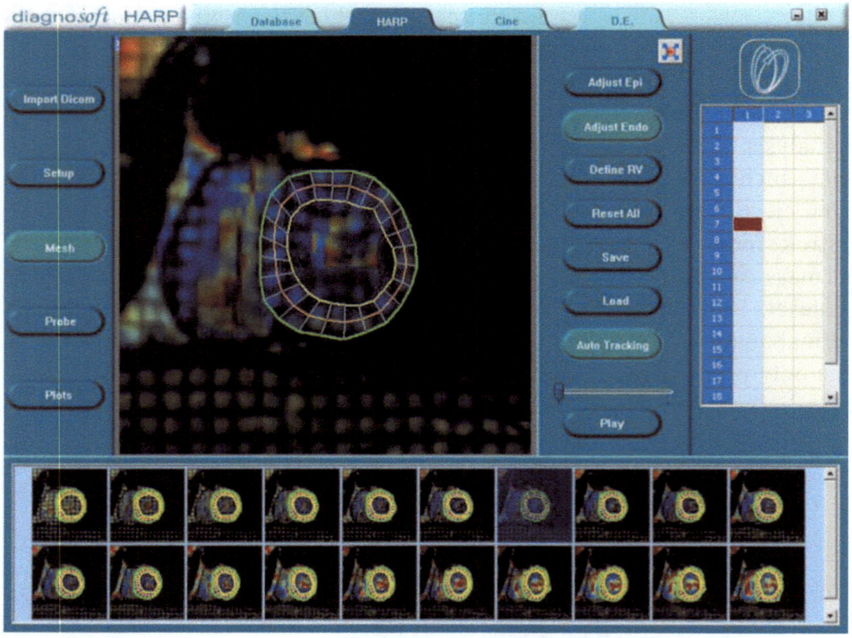

Fig. 5.37. A software where mesh can be easily built and tracked in a fraction of a minute. It is used for segmenting the heart scanned using MRI into segments. (Courtesy of Diagnosoft Inc., Palo Alto, CA)

ally visualized using bull's eye plots (Fig. 5.38). Furthermore, mapping the evaluated parameters on the above-mentioned left ventricular surface rendering is a suitable representation.

5.5.6 Myocardial Perfusion and Late-Enhancement Analysis

Recent studies show that CT can be used for the detection and the analysis of hypoperfused and scarred tissue (George et al. 2006; Buecker et al. 2005). However, a major drawback is its insufficient temporal resolution as well as the associated radiation dose. For this reason, MR is considered the standard modality for cardiac perfusion studies. The MR perfusion images are usually acquired in short axis slices after the bolus injection of a gadolinium-based contrast agent. The resulting image sequence shows the first pass of the contrast agent and has a high temporal resolution of about 1 s. Due to the low spatial resolution, only three to six image slices with a thickness of 6–10 mm and a gap of about 6 mm are recorded. To analyze the myocardial perfusion, typical descriptive parameters, including time to peak, mean transit time or maximum up-slope, are computed for the enhancement curves of myocardial segments (Breeuwer et al. 2003), as well as for single voxels (Nagel et al. 2003).

Acute or chronically infarcted tissue exhibits an increased distribution volume for the contrast agent Gd-DTPA, and hence shows high signal intensities several minutes after the bolus injection. Accordingly, so-called late enhancement image acquisition starts 10--30 min after bolus injection, again delivering short axis slices with about 8 mm thickness with or without spacing. For analysis purpose, the detection of the enhanced, scarred tissue requires the definition of a suitable threshold in order to distinguish between healthy and infarcted tissue. A clinically accepted method uses the histogram of a user defined, healthy myocardial region to determine a threshold at $\mu + 2\sigma$ (μ, mean grey value; σ, standard deviation) (Kim and Hillenbrand 2000; Kolipaka et al. 2005).

For therapy planning, especially the distinction between normal, hypoperfused, and infarcted myocardium is of high interest, which requires a combination of the results from the first pass perfusion and the late enhancement analysis. A common approach makes use of the AHA segment model and compares segment based perfusion parameters with the portion of infarction in the corresponding image region of the late enhancement image (Breeuwer et al. 2003) (Fig. 5.38).

As the image regions and slice orientations in perfusion and late enhancement images differ, this method can only provide very coarse information. To achieve a more accurate comparison and to vi-

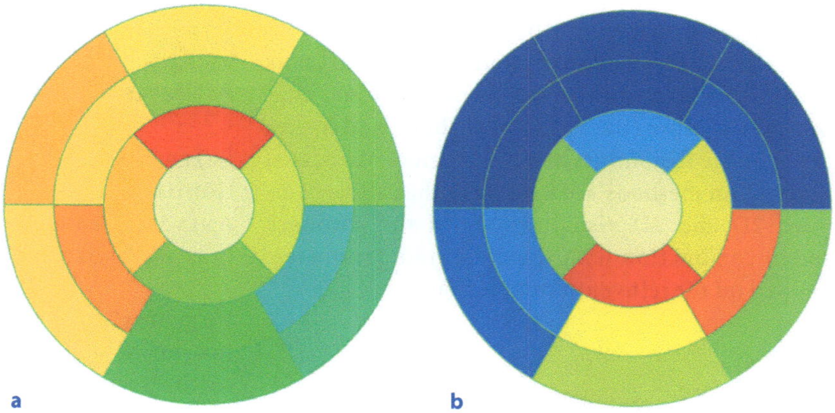

Fig. 5.38a,b. Bulls-eye-plot visualizations. **a** Peak enhancement parameter values of perfusion curves (*green* indicates low values) **b** Late enhancement portions per segment in percent (*red* indicates a high LE portion). (Courtesy of Dr. M. Fenchel and Dr. A. Seeger, Department of Diagnostic Radiology, University of Tübingen, Germany)

sualize topological relations, a registration has to be performed (Hennemuth et al. 2007a). The morphological information from the late enhancement analysis can then be combined with the perfusion parameter information (Fig. 5.39).

5.5.7 Combined Analysis of Coronary Arteries and Myocardium

Especially in the diagnosis and therapy planning for coronary artery disease the knowledge of both cause and effect of perfusion defects is very important. Only few software tools support a combined examination of the coronary arteries and the supplied myocardium for data acquired with a single machine like a PET-CT, CT or an MR scanner, where data are represented in a single reference coordinate system (Namdar et al. 2005; Hennemuth et al. 2007b; Kühnel et al. 2006).

Recent academic approaches combine results of different modalities, as, for example, MR and CT (Sturm et al. 2003). In particular, morphological information of the coronary tree is correlated with dynamic, functional information of the myocardium using the AHA segment model. Using this standardized scheme, a coarse estimation of the coronary main branches' supply territories is achieved, and thus myocardial segment based results from the analysis of cardiac function, perfusion or late enhancement can be inspected together with the

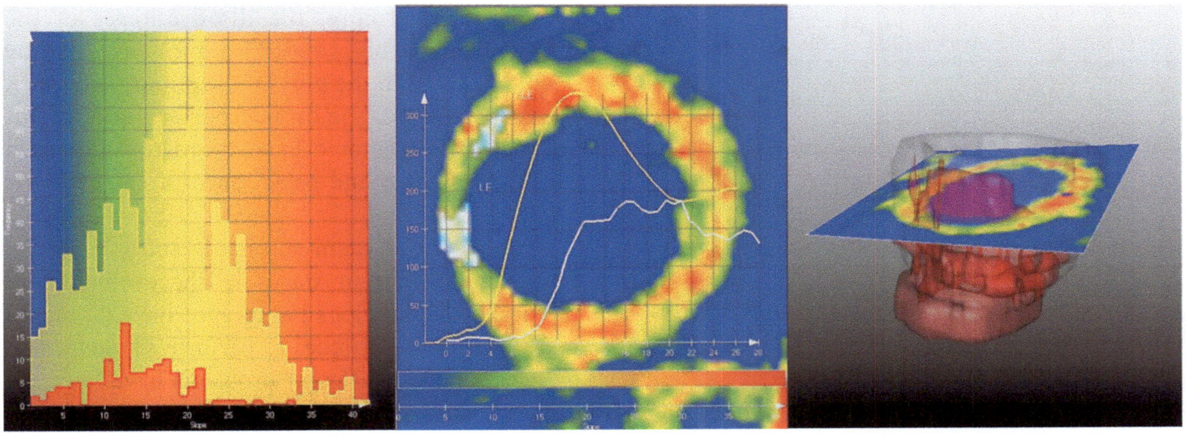

Fig. 5.39. Comparison of late enhancement segmentation with myocardial perfusion *Left* image: The slope parameter distribution of the whole myocardium (*yellow*) and the segmented late enhancement region (red). *Middle* image: Parameter image showing the up-slope of the enhancement curves, the white overlay shows the segmented late enhancement region. The lower curve shows the enhancement curve corresponding to the overlay region while the upper curve represents the enhancement curve of the segmented myocardium. *Right* image: 3D surface representation of the segmentation results from the late enhancement image combined with a texture representation of the transformed parameter image slice. (Courtesy of Dr. A. Seeger, Department of Diagnostic Radiology, University of Tübingen, Germany)

associated coronary branches (Oeltze et al. 2006) (Fig. 5.40). This standardization of supply areas is restricted in terms of the variety of individual anatomical structure (Beliveau et al. 2007) and makes direct image fusion inevitable. Therefore, dedicated registration methods are necessary that allow combined 2D and 3D visualizations of the coronary tree in conjunction with the measured parameters mapped on the left ventricular surface.

a
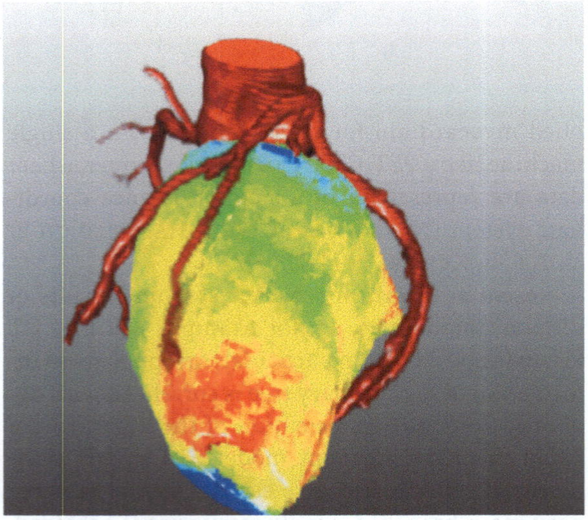

b
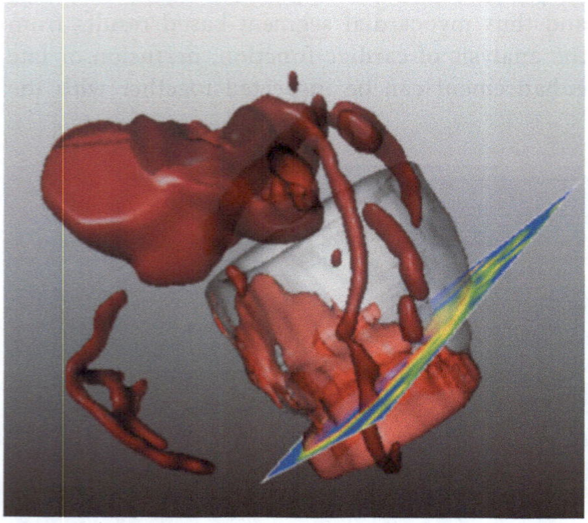

Fig. 5.40a,b. Combined visualizations of coronary arteries and myocardial examination results. **a** CT: Coronary tree segmentation combined with the results of the wall thickness analysis mapped on the ventricle surface. (Courtesy of Prof. Dr. S. Achenbach, Department of Medicine 2, University Hospital Erlangen, Germany). **b** MR: Coronary tree segmentation combined with late enhancement segmentation and perfusion parameter map. (Courtesy of Dr. A. Seeger, Department of Diagnostic Radiology, University of Tübingen, Germany)

5.6 Artifacts and Pitfalls

Peter M.A. van Ooijen, Wisnu Kristanto, Gonda J. de Jonge, Caroline Kuehnel, Anja Hennemuth, Tobias Boskamp, and Jaap M. Groen

In general, an artifact can be defined as a distortion or error in an image that is not related to the structure being imaged (de Feyter and Krestin 2005). The use of new and advanced visualization software tools for medical imaging also introduces a large number of artifacts and pitfalls (Nakanishi et al. 2005). These artifacts and pitfalls can either be related to the properties of the techniques used to perform the visualization or to the user interaction. Artifacts and pitfalls can be caused by the acquisition technique, the visualization technique, or the (semi)automatic post-processing technique (including computer aided diagnosis).

5.6.1 Technique-Related Problems

The technical aspects of the acquisition techniques such as misregistration, motion artifacts, beam hardening, noise, etc., are covered in a different chapter. Furthermore, the disadvantages of the different post-processing techniques have already been described in the previous sections; therefore, the focus will now be on bad performance of advanced (semi-) automatic software routines used for segmentation and selection of areas of interest.

Automatic and semi-automatic software is developed for different stages in the evaluation of the heart. The previous paragraphs have discussed many of these techniques to perform segmentation or selection, and different problems have been addressed. Current commercially available software systems provide the following semi-automatic and automatic procedures: segmentation of the heart, segmentation of the coronary artery tree, automatic determination of vessel lumen boundaries, and determination of the lumen and mass of the left ventricle. Although these techniques work in a considerably robust manner, automatic approaches in particular are still limited due to the varying character of the data.

With the automatic segmentation of the coronary arteries, for example, problems may occur due to the small size of the arteries and the presence of high density structures such as calcified plaques. One example is the incorrect classification as a calcified lesion being part of the vessel lumen leading to a missed coronary stenosis (Figs. 5.41 and 5.42).

Severe calcifications can also mislead automatic segmentation of the coronary artery lumen completely and hamper evaluation of the coronary arteries (Fig. 5.43).

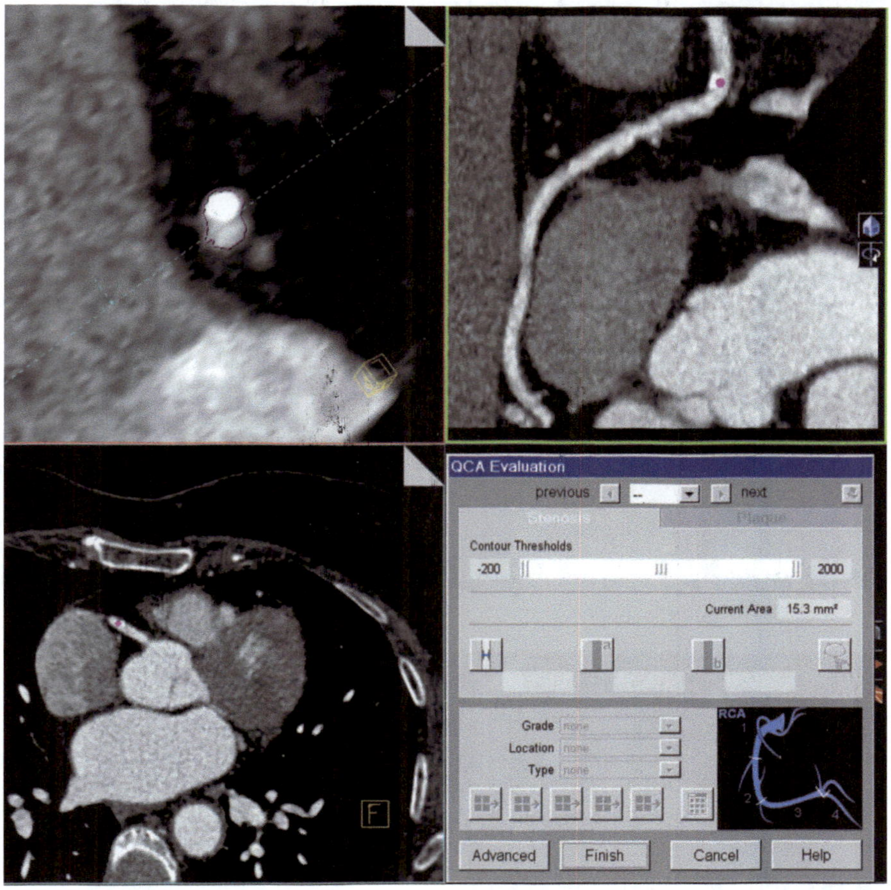

Fig. 5.41. Automatic segmentation of the right coronary artery showing the location of a severe calcification that was incorrectly added to the lumen of the artery (*purple* outline in the top *left panel*)

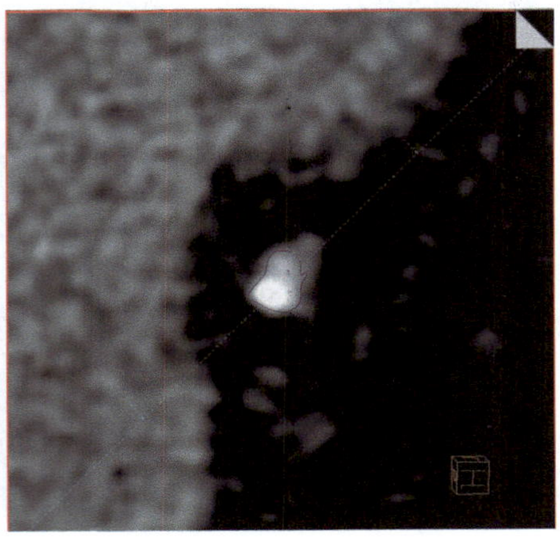

Fig. 5.42. Another example of a severe calcification that is included in the vessel lumen segmentation (*purple outline*) and thus results in a false negative evaluation. Severe calcifications can also mislead the automatic segmentation of the coronary artery lumen completely and hamper the evaluation of the coronary arteries (Fig. 5.43)

An example in left ventricular function analysis is the incorrect determination of the contour of myocardium for left ventricular analysis (Figs. 5.44 and 5.45). Even complete failure to select the left ventricle in a left ventricular function analysis can occur (Fig. 5.46).

The software failures demonstrated here clearly emphasize the requirement for interactive review of the images before making any diagnosis (Nakanishi et al. 2005) and that one should never rely on the computer generated results without checking.

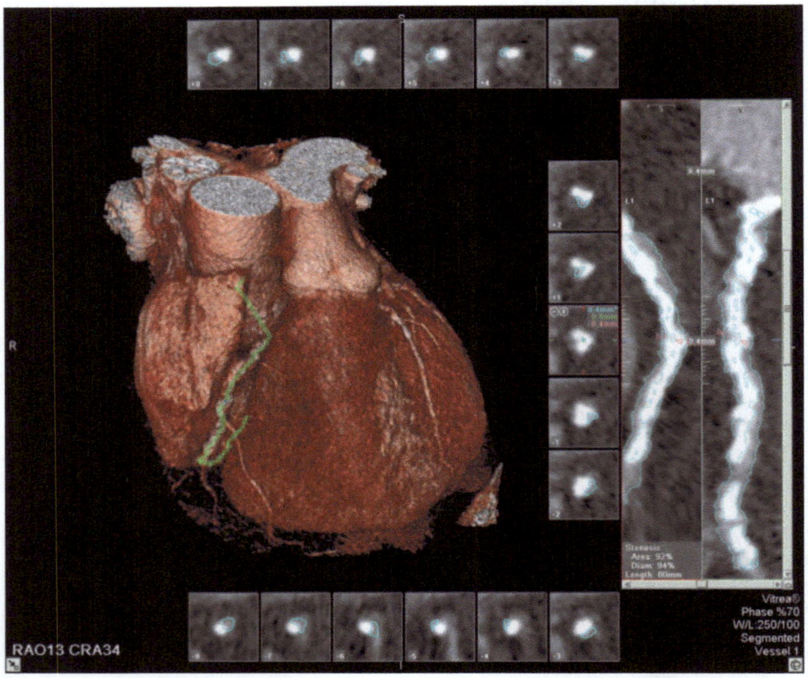

Fig. 5.43. Automatic vessel detection is unable to accurately determine the remaining lumen in a severely calcified coronary artery. The longitudinal views in particular provide very confusing images. An example in left ventricular function analysis is the incorrect determination of the contour of myocardium for left ventricular analysis (Figs. 5.44 and 5.45). Even a complete failure to select the left ventricle in a left ventricular function analysis can occur (Fig. 5.46).

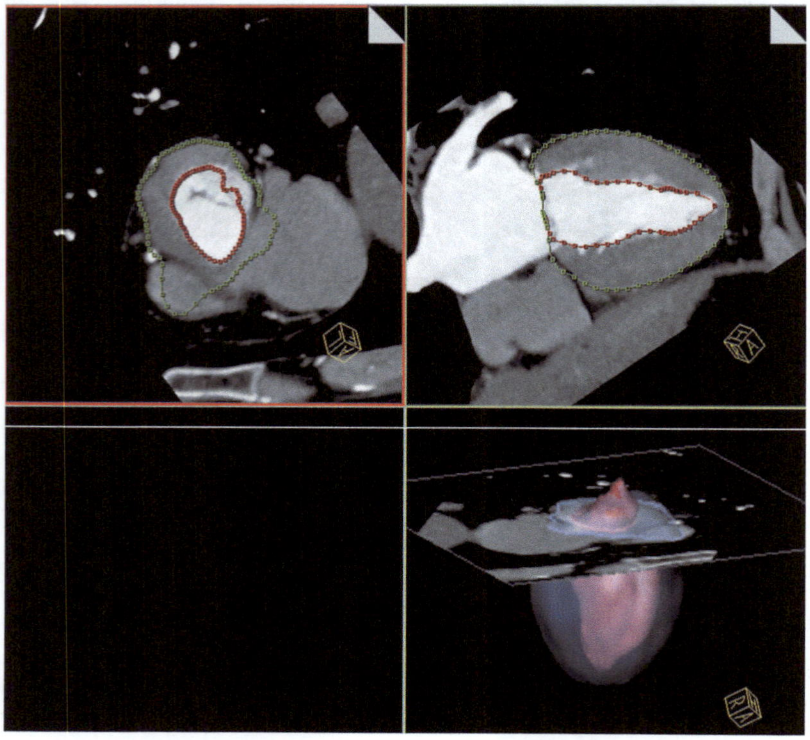

Fig. 5.44. Incorrect determination of the outlines of the left ventricular mass and lumen in the short axis view (*top left*) although the long axis view shows acceptable segmentation (*top right*)

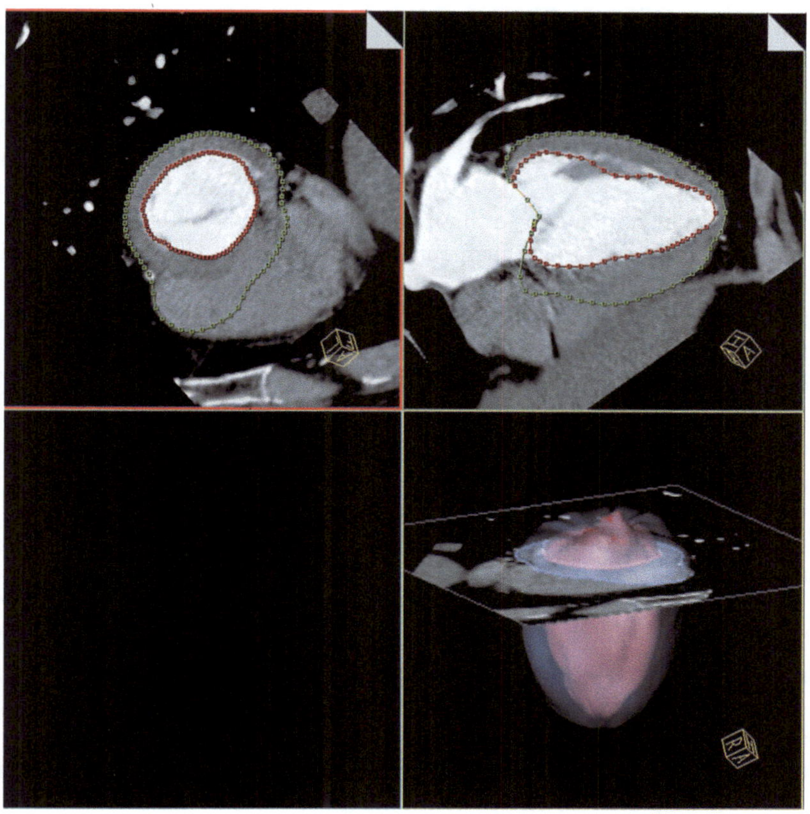

Fig. 5.45. Same patient as in Fig. 5.44, but with the short axis view at a different level. Again, incorrect determination of the outlines of the left ventricular mass and lumen in the short axis view (*top left*) although the long axis view shows acceptable segmentation (*top right*)

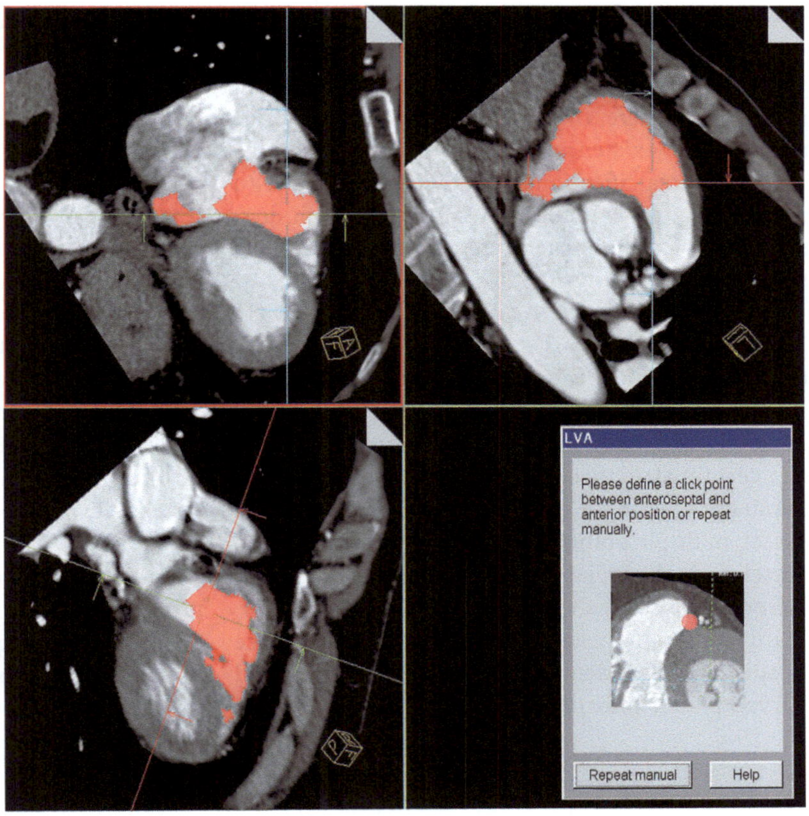

Fig. 5.46. Erroneous selection of the right instead of the left ventricle using automatic segmentation

5.6.2 User-Related Problems

5.6.2.1 Missegmentation

Segmentation can be done at many different levels. With user related, manual, segmentation techniques mistakes are easily made. When using MIP imaging the selection of the slab thickness is very important for the correct visualization of the area of interest. With more advanced segmentation mistakes are made even more often. Misplacement of manually drawn lines, incorrect placement of selection points are just two very obvious examples.

5.6.2.2 Improper Choice of Techniques

The availability of many different workstations and many different rendering and post-processing software tools introduces problems that are caused by the improper selection of those workstations and tools for a certain task.

One example is the choice of the thickness of a slab. In case of the coronary arteries, choosing slab thickness too small or too large will cause apparent stenoses or missing vessels.

Another example is the application of settings to volume rendering that obscure or erase certain structures, where the volume rendering settings obscure the existence of heavily stenotic lesions with severe calcifications. Another problem due to improper settings is the visualization of high density, intra-vascular structures, such as, for example, stents.

5.6.6.3 Misplacement of Selection Tools

In some cases user interaction is required to select certain structures of interest. For example, for manually creating a curved or stretched MPR of a vessel, multiple points have to be selected along the vessel path. Artificial stenotic lesions can be easily introduced by only a very small error of the operator. Many authors have commented on the occurrence of operator dependent artifacts in manually created curved planar reformations. The presence of these artifacts is unavoidable in normal clinical practice, not only because of human errors but also because of the limitations of manual pointing devices. In addition, only few points are used to define a manually created curved planar reformation. Linear or higher order interpolation is used to define the centerline between manually selected points, which may lead to artifacts if the interpolated line passes nearby or intersects the vessel wall (Rankin 1998; Rubin et al. 1995; Ochi et al. 1999; Achenbach et al. 1998; Rubin 1994).

5.7 Conclusion

Peter M.A. van Ooijen, Wisnu Kristanto, Gonda J. de Jonge, Caroline Kuehnel, Anja Hennemuth, Tobias Boskamp, and Jaap M. Groen

3D and 4D Imaging is slowly but increasingly being implemented in clinical medicine. In general, clinicians, including radiologists, are unfamiliar with volumetric representation of medical scans and often struggle with the interpretation of the 3D images. Another obstacle in the way of clinical acceptance of 3D rendering in medicine is the dependence on the numerous rendering properties that greatly affect the quality of the rendered images.

We believe that the application of three- and more dimensional imaging in medicine will increase, powered by the current developments in hard- and software. Therefore, clinicians need to be acquainted with these techniques, which is a pre-requisite for proper interpretation of the images acquired with volumetric scanners like CT and MRI (Nakanishi et al. 2005). Furthermore, automated segmentation and computer aided diagnosis are finding their way into the field of cardiac evaluation which facilitates an easy evaluation requiring less training of the user.

In order to avoid the pitfalls arising with modern visualization methods, an adequate standardization of analysis techniques and standardized procedures for their evaluation and validation have to be considered.

5.8 Digital Storage and Distribution

PETER M. A. VAN OOIJEN and A. BROEKEMA

To be able to perform 2D and 3D image processing, standardization and archiving of these data are essential. The standardization of the image data is realized by the world standard DICOM (digital image communication in medicine), which is adapted by the medical hardware and software industry and also specially tailored for use in catheterization laboratories. Digital archiving is performed on a so-called PACS (picture archiving and communication system). The PACS is responsible for the storage and retrieval of the image data and facilitates easy post-processing of the data. Driven by this digital standardization and archiving, the storage of acquired data in cardiologic examinations has moved from analog to digital. A major advantage of digital storage compared to analog storage is that there is no deterioration of the stored data, not even when making copies. Every digital copy is exactly identical to the original (THOMAS and NISSEN 1996).

5.9 History of Cardiac X-Ray Management

PETER M. A. VAN OOIJEN and A. BROEKEMA

Image management of cardiac X-ray images gradually evolved from analog storage on cine-film and VHS tape to the modern digital DICOM 3.0 storage on a PACS or portable media such as CD-R (BITTL and LEVIN 1997; GOEDHART and REIBER 1998; SCHMIDT 1999).

For a long time the medium of choice for recording and storage of coronary arteriograms was 35-mm cine-film (Fig. 5.47). The big advantage of cine-film was that it was a universal standard. Independent of from which hospital or vendor the cine-film came, every cardiologist could view it on his own system. Also, as long as quality control in cine-film development is adequate, spatial resolution (five line pairs/mm) and dynamic contrast range are very high. Furthermore, at that time, digital storage of the amount of data produced by digitalization of the cine-film (500--700 MB per study with a 512×512 matrix) was simply not possible or extremely expensive, and thus cine-film was the only option.

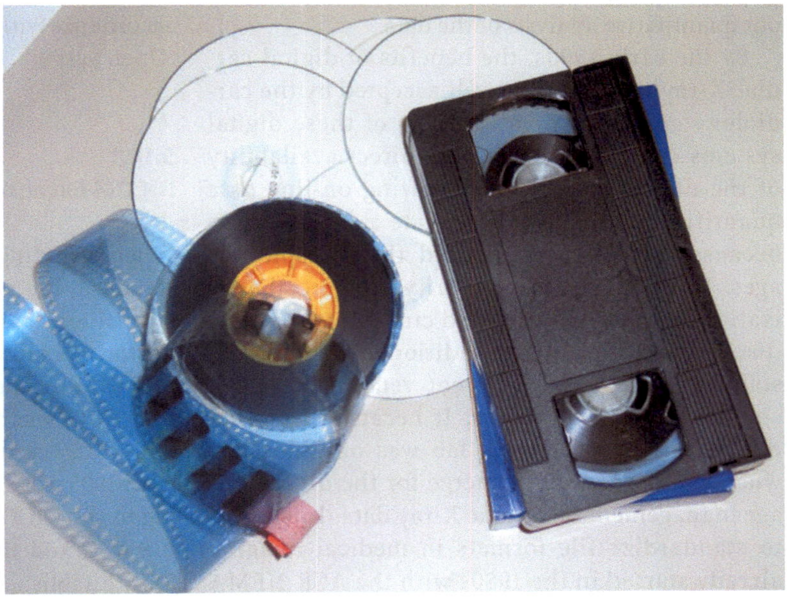

Fig. 5.47. Storage of conventional coronary angiograms has moved from 35-mm cine film to VHS video tape to CDs over the past decades

There were, however, some major disadvantages of cine-film. First, it was very expensive. Second, the sequential nature of the film required reeling to find the images of interest which could be quite time-consuming. Furthermore, cine-film quality was hampered by fogged, torn and improperly processed film. Because of the high cost, duplication was also expensive and inconvenient. This led to the situation where each cine-film was a unique copy which could easily become lost or even destroyed. Finally, a large storage space is required to retain all the cine-films.

In the 1980s alternatives to cine-film were marketed using super-VHS video tapes for the exchange of data. Although these video tapes were cheap compared to cine-film, their quality was also less optimal, and thus less suitable for clinical decision making, because of the poor signal to noise ratio and the limited bandwidth of a video tape.

Furthermore, no universal standard existed. Another alternative that gave rise at the same time was the use of (analog) optical discs reducing per patient media cost because multiple patients could be stored on one disc. Another advantage was the reduction in required storage space when using optical discs. Although all images were stored on optical discs, this storage was analog and all data was stored after edge-enhancement. To review the data on a viewing station, it had to be converted to digital again. Because of the edge-enhancement it was, however, impossible to go back to the raw data, thus ruling out quantitative analysis of the data.

By the early 1990s, the benefits of digital cardiac X-ray systems were well accepted by the cardiology community. Advantages of these digital systems could be found in the direct availability of the digital image data, allowing on-line data quantification and more accurate catheterization because of digitally enhanced fluoroscopic images. However, a large majority of the catheterization laboratories still used cine-film or optical disc to store their data. Additionally, the digital solutions offered by different vendors were not standardized at that time. It became clear that digitalization of the cath lab was only possible when standards would emerge for the digital image management of cardiac X-ray data. Initiatives to standardize file formats in medical imaging already started in the 1980s with the ACR-NEMA standard, but it was not until 1995 that the standardization for the cath lab was established using DICOM 3.0 and CD-R.

5.10 Standardized File Formats

Peter M. A. van Ooijen and A. Broekema

In 1983 the ACR (American College of Radiology) and the NEMA (National Electrical Manufacturers Association) defined a standard for the interconnection of medical imaging devices, known as ACR-NEMA Version 1.0. The standard included a list of required data elements and a specification of the physical hardware for connecting the devices. This first version was released at the RSNA in 1985, followed by Version 2.0 at the RSNA in 1988. Up to then only point-to-point networking was specified. However, in 1990 work was started to add a network standard. This resulted in a combination of these network standards and the ACR-NEMA Version 2.0 to lay the foundation of the current DICOM standard (Version 3.0) (Hindel 1994).

The three main goals of the DICOM standard are defined as (Pelanek 1997):

1. Establishing a standard for communication in a networked environment
2. Setting minimum requirements for claiming performance to the standard
3. Allowing interoperability, not just interconnection, between multiple vendors' equipment.

To meet these main goals, DICOM is defined in accordance with layer 7 (application level) of the OSI (Open System Interconnect) reference model.

5.10.1 DICOM Extensions for Cardiology Data

When including angiographic data into the DICOM standard, the main difference from other types of acquisition data within DICOM was the requirement of storing cine loops. In 1992, cooperation between ACR-NEMA and the American College of Cardiology (ACC) was started to develop the standards required for cardiac X-ray image management. Not until 1995 was an international agreement conforming to the DICOM 3 standard (with participation of the ACC and the European Society of Cardiology, ESC) established to include angiographic data into the DICOM 3 standard.

The use of CD-Recordable (CD-R) as a storage medium with a defined data structure was chosen to replace the cine-film. This also required the replacement of the traditional mechanical cine-projector by digital viewers. These digital viewers should minimally satisfy the same requirements as the conventional cine-film projectors, which involved displaying an enormous amount of data on the computer screen at high frame rates (12.5–30 frames per second). Also, display of the images at the maximum resolution without loss of information is required. Advantages of using digital displays are the ability to manipulate the images (contrast, brightness, region-of-interest zoom, thumbnail overview of runs, and quantitative measurements). CD-R met the functionality requirement and provided additional benefits and was accepted as a standard medium for digital viewing. With this introduction of CD-R, a long-term archiving capability (of raw data) was obtained that satisfied the legal requirements and allowed long-term storage without any data loss or deterioration with age. Other benefits were the decrease in storage space requirement, the elimination of chemical processing, the possibility of random access, and low cost per patient study.

However, storing the CD-R discs off-line still maintains some of the disadvantages of traditional cine-film. It is still possible that CD-R discs are misplaced in the archive, the storage takes up a lot of space, only one cardiologist can review a patient at the same time, and retrieving the data from the archive can take some time.

The DICOM standard defines four different ways of storing the images of an angiographic examination.

1. *Original.* Raw data without any image processing performed on it.
2. *Derived.* Image data derived from the original data by performing image processing techniques like zoom, pan, edge enhancement, window/level setting.
3. *Primary.* Identification of an image as the actual exam data, produced at the time of the actual angiographic procedure.
4. *Secondary.* Image produced after the actual angiographic procedure, e.g. overlays or annotations added to the image.

In 1998, additions to the standard were accepted in order to facilitate the exchange of angiographic and cardio-angiographic data on digital networks. Through these additional definitions within the DICOM protocol, manufacturers were able to meet the clinical demands about the management of large amounts of data in a satisfactory and cost-effective way. The demands on the network bandwidth are enormous. Typically, diagnostic examinations of about 2000 images have to be displayed at up to 30 frames per second. This involves a network transfer of approximately 250 MB of lossless compressed data at 4 MB/s. Current networks are capable of handling such data traffic at acceptable prices.

5.10.2 Image Compression

In the digitalization of cine-film the image quality is a crucial factor which is dictated by the storage capacity and the transfer capacity. One cine-film will show 2000 images per patient exam in the majority of examinations (Fig. 5.48) at a frame rate of 30 images

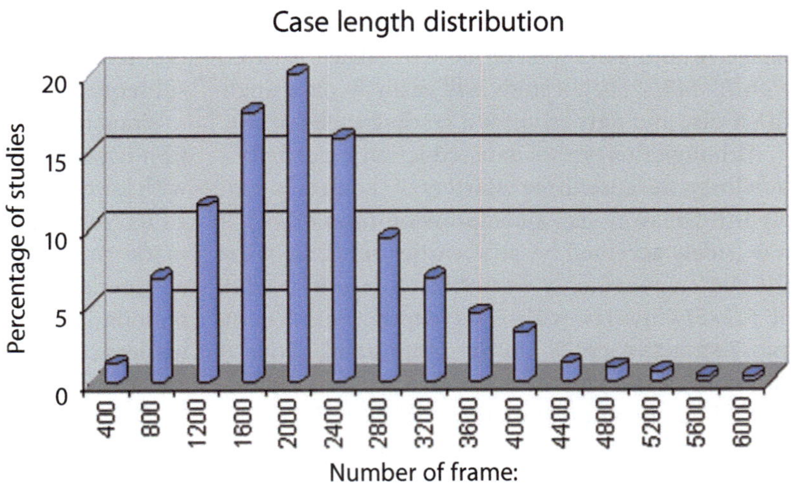

Fig. 5.48. Distribution of the number of frames per examination. The horizontal axis shows the number of frames, the vertical axis shows the percentage of studies with that particular number of frames

per second with a spatial resolution of four line pairs per millimeter (Brennecke and Kerensky 1997). To approach this with digital images we would need images with a resolution of 1024×1024 pixels (1 MB of data with 256 gray levels) displayed at 30 images per second (thus 30 MB/s). A complete patient exam would exist of 2000 MB of data. This would require three or four CD-R discs (depending on the use of 650 MB or 700 MB CD-R disks) per patient and a reading speed of 200× (max 52× commercially available, 1× equals a data transfer rate of 150 Kbyte per second) (Brennecke and Kerensky 1997).

The conclusion from this example is that for practical use of digital images, data size has to be reduced using data compression. Data compression can be either lossless or lossy. In most cases medical images used for evaluation and diagnosis of patients are compressed using a lossless compression that decreases the data size (at maximum a reduction by a factor of about 2 to 4 can be achieved) without decreasing the image information and quality. In the case of lossy compression, much higher reduction factors can be achieved, but some information of the data will be lost and data quality will possibly be reduced.

This kind of compression is frequently used, but careful evaluation of the trade-off between compressed data size and quality has to be made to obtain images that are suitable for clinical use.

5.10.3 Matrix Size Reduction

Digital cameras in a cath lab are typically capable of acquiring data in a 1024×1024 matrix. However, in practice these digital coronary angiograms are recorded using a 512×512 matrix. This already provides a different situation with only 0.25 MB of data per image, resulting in a total of 500 MB of data displayed with 7.5 MB/s. Such a study will easily fit on a single CD-R disc and only requires a reading speed of 50×.

Although this type of data reduction is per definition lossy, because three quarters of the data is simply thrown away (i.e. a compression ratio of 4:1), it was widely accepted because earlier versions of the DICOM standard only described storage of images of 512×512 matrix with 8-bit depth (Brennecke and Kerensky 1997). On the other hand, modern data compression methods are able to obtain significantly higher compression ratios while maintaining the original image size and introducing only a negligible reduction in image quality.

5.10.4 Data Size Reduction

Lossless compression can be performed on all data and is defined in the DICOM standard. For most images, this type of compression is able to reduce the data size by a factor of about 2 to nearly 4, by using a two-step lossless compression process consisting of predictive encoding followed by statistical encoding. With predictive encoding only the change in pixel value of one pixel compared to its neighbor, which is typically rather small, is stored. This results in a data reduction of close to a factor of 2 because for about 80% of the pixels only 4 bits are required (sign bit plus 3 data bits).

Statistical encoding involves the coding of data elements in which data elements that occur frequently are assigned a shorter code than data elements that are only used occasionally (e.g. one-bit code compared to a four-bit code). Statistical encoding is especially useful when predictive encoding was performed previously.

If higher data size reduction factors are required, this can only be achieved by lossy compression methods. By removing irrelevant information from an image, such as noise and small scale image details, reduction factors of 15:1 or more can easily be realized. In general, lossy compression methods allow adjusting the compression ratio or the amount of information reduction. To decide which lossy compression method and which compression factor is optimal, one has to consider the type of data to be compressed, the goal for which they will be used (diagnostic or communicative quality), and the lowest data quality clinically acceptable.

Within DICOM, lossy JPEG (Joint Photographic Experts Group) compression has been defined as the standard compression technique. This compression is based on two main steps: transform encoding and subsequent quantization.

Transform encoding will separate image information based on the variation in brightness. Regions with lower variation are separated from regions with a high variation. In the quantization step, the information on low variation regions is transferred virtually lossless while the information on high variation regions is reduced and transferred lossy. As with lossless compression, statistical encoding is used to encode the resulting quantized information.

The JPEG compression is primarily performed on blocks of 8×8 pixels. Higher compression factors (more blocks are transferred lossy), give rise to artifacts at the edges of those blocks, the so-called blocking artifacts.

5.11 PACS Development

PETER M. A. VAN OOIJEN AND A. BROEKEMA

Most cardiology departments and cath labs are using very small PACS systems (mini PACS) or even none at all for their permanent storage. This is not the case in radiology where large PACS installations have been installed over the past years. These large PACS installations are crucial for the acquisition, storage and processing of the enormous amounts of data produced by MRI and CT systems for evaluation of cardiovascular disease and function. Therefore PACS installations also become more and more important for cardiology, not only to store their own data, but also to be able to retrieve the data acquired and processed at the radiology department.

In order to be able to handle cardiac studies other than the X-ray studies performed in the cath lab, a PACS will have to be capable of storing a lot of different data. Not only the data from the digital modalities like MRI and CT have to be stored in the PACS, but also images from other modalities such as the coronary angiography (CAG) and IVUS. Preferably, the ECG and the triggering moments on this ECG should also be stored. As mentioned before, not only the wide variety of data is important in cardiac imaging, but also the amount of data that is produced during the acquisition. The amount of data stored ranges from a couple of Megabytes for a typical IVUS investigation to hundreds of Megabytes for a full angiographic investigation or a MDCT investigation (see Table 5.1).

In order to be able to store all this data and to retrieve it, large storage capacity is necessary. Moreover, fast retrieval of the stored data is obligatory. The only way to achieve data retrieval at a sufficiently high speed is by organizing the PACS in such a way that all data is always on-line. This is not only the case when using cardiac imaging data, but it also holds for the radiology department in general (VAN OOIJEN 2000b).

With the digitalization of a radiology department, four prerequisites can be defined that are partly based on the requirements mentioned before. First the system has to be extremely easy to use. Second, easy access to external resources should be possible at the user level. Third, the archived images must be on-screen extremely fast and in the case of cardiac data it should be also possible to display the images in cine loop with a frame-rate of up to 30 frames per second. Finally, this fast access should not only be implemented for recent studies, but also for old ones to be able to perform comparative diagnosis.

The first prerequisite about ease of use implies the demands on the user interface of the diagnostic viewing station. Easy interaction with the workstation providing only the required capabilities is essential.

A large number of viewing stations are available on the market nowadays, but judging the test results published in literature, the optimal workstation has yet to be developed (BAZAK et al. 2000; HONEA et al. 1998; POLLAK et al. 2000). Two of those publications together show rated comparisons of eight different workstations (BAZAK et al. 2000; POLLAK et al. 2000).

Table 5.1. Storage required for typical examinations of the coronary arteries using different acquisition techniques

Acquisition device	Matrix size	Bytes per pixel	MB per slice	No. of slices	Total storage needed
CAG	512	1	0.250	2000	500.0
IVUS	256	1	0.063	150	9.4
MRA	256	2	0.125	800	100.0
EBT	512	2	0.500	60	30.0
MDCT	512	2	0.500	500	25.0

CAG, coronary angiography; IVUS, intravenous ultrasound; MRA, magnetic resonance angiography; EBT, electron-beam tomography; MDCT, multi-detector computed tomography.

The basic features of a PACS workstation are patient selection and some basic viewing possibilities. Several search criteria can be selected to find the required patient, and after the patient study selection, the retrieved images are displayed using a standard viewing protocol. A simple user interface is obligatory for the acceptance of the PACS by the users. Another important aspect for the acceptance is the speed of the PACS, which allows every requested image to be available and on-screen within seconds. A viewing workstation fit for cardiovascular studies does not just need the standard radiological possibilities used for displaying axial data, but also additional features that are needed for cardiac evaluation. The first requirement is the possibility to display cardio DICOM coronary angiography data, which involves the ability to read the data, to display it in cine mode and to perform the common processing algorithms on the data (e.g. edge enhancement). Other requirements involve the possibility for comparison of catheter angiographic data with other data and to be able to compare old and new studies in a fast way.

To retrieve all additional information besides the images in the PACS (such as patient reports and medication), either multiple workstations have to be used, or the administration has to perform extra work to retrieve the information. However, a more desirable solution is to integrate all resources in one workstation. The HIS/RIS can be inquired within a window and other resources like an anatomical atlas and access to other information sources can also be made available (Fig. 5.49).

An implementation that meets all prerequisites mentioned before is the Everything On-Line (EOL) PACS developed in the late 1990s. The basic idea of the EOL principle is that all data should be always available within seconds after the request on any workstation. To be able to conform to this idea, the architecture of the whole PACS system is adapted.

A PACS based on the EOL principle consists of a very large on-line archive that contains all the information acquired over several years. The number of years on-line (preferably 5–10 years) has to be chosen such that only a small portion of the data not on-line is still requested for evaluation. This system makes all this data directly accessible to the radiologist and assures that it will be on-screen within seconds (Fig. 5.50). This on-line archive is based on a multi-terabyte storage system (storage area network, SAN). The capacity of the on-line archive can be easily expanded by expanding the storage capacity of the SAN. The ever decreasing costs of hard disk space with simultaneous increase in capacity per disk allows for large, multi-teraByte storage systems. This assures that the storage capacity of the PACS can grow based on the data production of the radiology department.

From the basics of the EOL archive the so-called MASS archive was developed by Rogan Medical Systems in 2001. This MASS concept takes the advantages of the EOL principle as described before and adds flexibility, scalability and redundancy. In addition, it increases data handling power and retrieval speed dramatically (Langenhuysen and Philipse

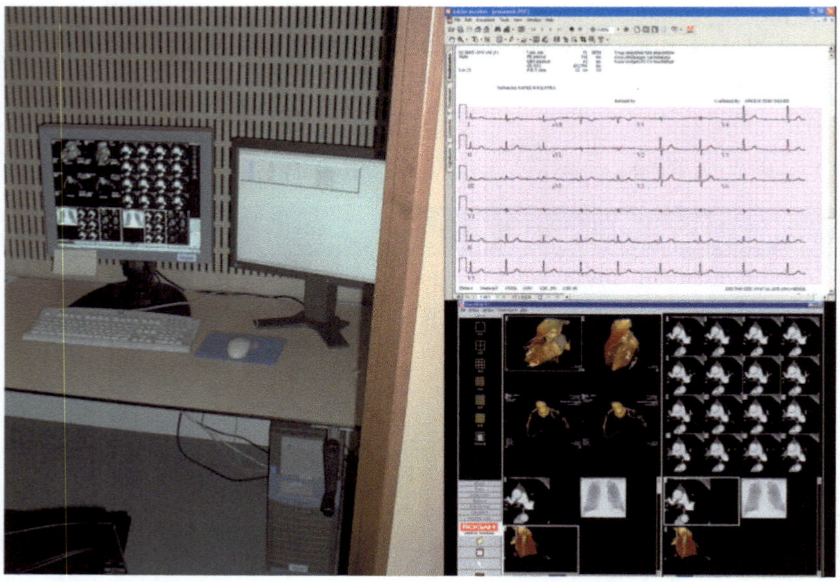

Fig. 5.49. Example of a diagnostic setup. To the *left* the two-screen setup of a diagnostic workstation. The left screen is used for the diagnostic images, the right screen is used to access other sources. To the *right* screen captures are shown. The *top image* shows an example of a cardiac ECG, while the *bottom image* shows the image data (CT, 3D reconstructions, and thorax X-ray)

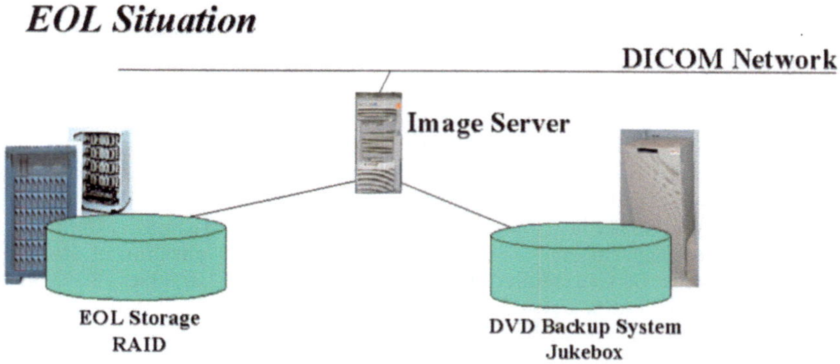

Fig. 5.50. In the EOL situation the schedule is slightly changed; basically, the size of the short-term storage now grows with the amount of data and thus the short-term storage now contains all available data. As a result, everything is available fast and the long-term storage (in our case on DVD-R) is now only used for on-line backup and is only accessed occasionally

2001). This MASS archive consists of a scalable DICOM server cluster using 'off the shelf' hardware and software. All servers in this cluster act as one virtual DICOM node. This recent development has enabled the realization of a large-scale PACS system that can easily be adapted to the growing needs using minor investments.

5.12 Conclusion

Peter M. A. van Ooijen and A. Broekema

Although most cardiology departments still use CD-R for long-term storage of their data, a gradual shift towards PACS storage will become visible in the next few years. The large amounts of data can be stored on-line and very short access times are feasible. Furthermore, full quality data is preserved indefinitely enabling quantification and evaluation at any time. One of the main questions will not be whether to archive X-ray coronary angiography or not, but whether to archive this in a separate PACS at the cardiology department or to include this data in the radiology PACS where MRI and CT studies are also stored.

A couple of years ago, developments tended towards dedicated cardio PACS with dedicated clinical viewing software (van der Putten et al. 1997; Bruski and Cutler 2003). The current trend, however, is leaning towards the integration of these cardio dedicated features into the general hospital-wide PACS to obtain a cost-effective solution that allows easy integration into the electronic patient record (Brandon et al. 2005) with full integration of all cardiology modalities into the radiology PACS and different workstations based on the application (Meinhardt 2006).

References

Abdala N, Achenbach S, Ropers D, Anders K, Ropers U, Bautz W et al. (2006) Syngo circulation the next generation. Somatom Sessions [18], 8–9. Siemens AG, Medical Solutions, Forchheim

Achenbach S, Moshage W, Ropers D, Bachmann K (1998) Curved multiplanar reconstructions for the evaluation of contrast-enhanced electron beam CT of the coronary arteries [see comments]. AJR Am J Roentgenol 170:895–899

Achenbach S, Ropers D, Regenfus M, Muschiol G, Daniel WG, Moshage W (2000) Contrast enhanced electron beam computed tomography to analyse the coronary arteries is patients after acute myocardial infarction. Heart 84:489–493

Addis KA, Hopper KD, Iyriboz TA, Liu Y, Wise SW, Kasales CJ, Blebea JS, Mauger DT (2001) CT angiography: in vitro comparison of five reconstruction methods. AJR Am J Roentgenol 177:1771–1776

Agatston AS, Janowitz WR, Hildner FJ, Zusmer NR, Viamonte M Jr, Detrano R (1990) Quantification of coronary artery calcium using ultrafast computed tomography. J Am Coll Cardiol 15:827–832

Anderson CM, Saloner D, Tsuruda JS, Shapeero LG, Lee RE (1990) Artifacts in maximum-intensity-projection display of MR angiograms. AJR Am J Roentgenol 154:623–629

Bazak N, Stamm G, Caldarone F, Lotz J, Leppert A, Galanski M (2000) PACS Workstations 2000: evaluation, usability and performance. Gell G, Holzinger A, and Wiltgen M 144, 133–142. Graz, Österreichische Computer Gesellschaft. Proceedings of the 18th International EuroPACS Conference

Beliveau P, Setser R, Cheriet F, O'Donnell T (2007) Patient-specific coronary territory maps. Proceedings of SPIE, SPIE, 6511

Bittl JA, Levin DC (1997) Coronary arteriography. In: Braunwald E (ed) Heart disease – a textbook of cardiovascular medicine, vol 1, chap 8. Saunders, Philadelphia, pp 240–272

Bornik A, Reitinger B, Beichel R (2005) Reconstruction and representation of tubular structures using simplex meshes. Proc of WSCG 2005, Short Papers 61–65

Boskamp T, Hahn H, Hindennach M, Oeltze S, Preim B, Zidowitz S, Peitgen HO (2005) Geometrical and structural analysis of vessel systems in 3D medical image datasets. In: Leondes CT (ed) Medical imaging systems. World Scientific, Singapore, October

Brandon D, Lovis C, Geissbühler A, Vallée J-P (2005) Enterprise-wide PACS: beyond radiology, and architecture to manage all medical images. Acad Radiol 12:1000–1009

Breeuwer M, Paetsch I, Nagel E, Muthupillai R, Flamm S, Plein S et al. (2003) The detection of normal, ischemic and infarcted myocardial tissue using MRI. International Congress Series 1256:1153–1158. CARS

Brennecke R, Kerensky R (1997) Image compression. In: A Primer; Kennedy TE, Nissen SE, Simon R, Thomas JD, Tilkemeier PL (eds) Digital cardiac imaging in the 21st Century. The Cardiac and Vascular Information Working Group, Bethesda, Maryland

Bruski GB, Cutler S (2003) Cardiac PACS: strategies for planning, integration and vendor selection. J Cardiovasc Manag 14:22–26

Buecker A, Katoh M, Krombach GA, Spuentrup E, Bruners P, Gunther RW et al. (2005) A feasibility study of contrast enhancement of acute myocardial infarction in multislice computed tomography: comparison with magnetic resonance imaging and gross morphology in pigs. Invest Radiol 40:700–704

Calhoun PS, Kuszyk BS, Heath DG, Carley JC, Fishman EK (1999) Three-dimensional volume rendering of spiral CT data: theory and method. Radiographics 19:745–764

Callister TQ, Cooil B, Raya SP et al. (1998) Coronary artery disease: improved reproducibility of calcium scoring with an electron-beam CT volumetric method. Radiology 208:807–14

Cerqueira MD, Weissman NJ, Dilsizian V, Jacobs AK, Kaul S, Laskey WK et al. (2002) Standardized myocardial segmentation and nomenclature for tomographic imaging of the heart: a statement for healthcare professionals from the Cardiac Imaging Committee of the Council on Clinical Cardiology of the American Heart Association. Circulation 105:539–542

Chabbert V, Carrie D, Bennaceur M, Maupas E, Lauwers V, Mhem M, Lhermusier T, Elbaz M, Joffre F, Rousseau H, Puel J (2007) Evaluation of in-stent restenosis in proximal coronary arteries with multidetector computed tomography (MDCT). European Radiology 17:1452–1463

Chen SJ, Carroll JD (1998) 3D Coronary angiography: improving visualization strategy for coronary interventions. In: Reiber JHC, Wall E (eds) What's new in cardiovascular imaging? Kluwer Academic Publishers, Dordrecht, pp 61–78

Dalrymple NC, Prasad SR, Freckleton MW, Chintapalli KN (2005) Introduction to the language of three-dimensional imaging with multidetector CT. Radiographics 25:1409–1428

de Feyter PJ, Krestin GP (2005) Computed tomography of the coronary arteries. Taylor & Francis, London, ISBN 1-84184-439-X

Drebin RA, Carpenter L, Hanrahan P (1988) Volume rendering. Proceedings Siggraph '88, Computer Graphics, 22:65–74

Ebert DS, Heath DG, Kuszyk BS, Edwards L, Shaw CD, Kukla J, Bedwell T, Fishman EK (1998) Evaluating the potential and problems of three-dimensional computed tomography measurements of arterial stenosis. J Digit Imaging 11:151–157

Ehricke HH, Donner K, Koller W, Strasser W (1994) Visualization of vasculature from volume data. Computers Graphics 18:395–406

Elvins TT (1992) A survey of algorithms for volume visualization. Computer Graphics 26:194–201

Felkel P, Fuhrmann A, Kanitsar A, Wegenkittl R (2002) Surface reconstruction of the branching vessels for augmented reality aided surgery. BIOSIGNAL 16:252–254

Ferencik M, Ropers D, Abbara S, Cury RC, Hoffmann U, Nieman K, Brady TJ, Moselewski F, Daniel WG, Achenbach S (2007) Diagnostic accuracy of image postprocessing methods for the detection of coronary artery stenoses by using multidetector CT. Radiology 243:696–702

Fishman EK, Magid D, Ney DR, Chaney EL, Pizer SM, Rosenman JG, Levin DN, Vannier MW, Kuhlman JE, Robertson DD (1991) Three-dimensional imaging. Radiology 181:321–337 [Published erratum appears in Radiology 182:899, 1992]

Fishman EK, Ney DR (1993) Advanced computer applications in radiology: clinical applications. Radiographics 13:463–475

Fishman EK, Ney DR, Heath DG, Corl FM, Horton KM, Johnson PT (2006) Volume rendering versus maximum intensity projection in CT angiography: what works best, when, and why? Radiographics 26:905–922

Funabashi N, Kobayashi Y, Rubin GD (2001a) Utility of three-dimensional volume rendering images using EBT to evaluate possible causes of ischemia from an anomalous origin of the RCA from the left sinus of valseva. Jpn Circ J 65:575–578

Funabashi N, Kobayashi Y, Rubin GD (2001b) Three-dimensional images of coronary arteries after heart transplantation using electron-beam computed tomography data with volume rendering. Circulation 103:e25–e26

George RT, Silva C, Cordeiro MA, DiPaula A, Thompson DR, McCarthy WF et al. (2006) Multidetector computed tomography myocardial perfusion imaging during adenosine stress. J Am Coll Cardiol 48:153–160

Gerig G, Koller T, Székely G, Brechbühler C, Kübler O (1993) Symbolic description of 3-D structures applied to cerebral vessel tree obtained from MR angiography volume data. Proceedings of the 13th International Conference on Information Processing in Medical Imaging, pp 94–111

Gibson S (1998) Constrained elastic surface nets: generating smooth surfaces from binary segmented data. Proc MICCAI 98:888–898

Goedhart B, Reiber JHC (1998) How will DICOM change the cardiac catherisation environment? Cardiologie 5:148–153

Groen JM, Greuter MJ, van Ooijen PM, Willems TP, Oudkerk M (2006) Initial results on visualization of coronary artery stents at multiple heart rates on a moving heart phantom using 64-MDCT. J Comput Assist Tomogr 30:812–817

Groen JM, Greuter MJ, van Ooijen PM, Oudkerk M (2007) A new approach to the assessment of lumen visibility of coronary artery stent at various heart rates using 64-slice MDCT. Eur Radiol 17:1879–1884. Epub Feb 16

Hahn HK, Preim B, Selle D, Peitgen HO (2001) Visualization and interaction techniques for the exploration of vascular structures. Visualization, VIS'01. Proceedings, pp 395–402

Hany TF, Schmidt M, Davis CP, Gohde SC, Debatin JF (1998) Diagnostic impact of four postprocessing techniques in evaluating contrast-enhanced three-dimensional MR angiography. AJR Am J Roentgenol 170:907–912

He S, Dai R, Lu B, Cao C, Bai H, Jing B (2001) Medial axis reformation: a new visualization method for CT angiography. Acad Radiol 8:726–733

Heath DG, Soyer PA, Kuszyk BS, Bliss DF, Calhoun PS, Bluemke DA, Choti MA, Fishman EK (1995) Three-dimensional spiral CT during arterial portography: comparison of three rendering techniques. Radiographics 15:1001–1011

Hein PA, Rogalla P, Mews J (2006) Analysis of a cardiac MSCT study employing the sure plaque software. Visions Magazine 10[13]:38–42. TOSHIBA Medical Systems

Hennemuth A, Bock S, Boskamp T, Fritz D, Kühnel C, Rinck D, Scheuering M, Peitgen HO (2005) One-click coronary tree segmentation in CT angiographic images. Computer Assisted Radiology and Surgery. Elsevier, pp 317–321

Hennemuth A, Behrens S, Kühnel C, Oeltze S, Konrad O, Peitgen H-O (2007a) Novel methods for parameter based analysis of myocardial tissue in MR-Images. SPIE Press, Bellingham, WA, pp 65111N-1--65111N-9

Hennemuth A, Seeger A, Kuehnel C, Boskamp T, Miller S, Konrad O et al. (2007b) A software tool for the combined analysis of angiographic and perfusion MRI datasets for an optimized diagnosis of coronary artery disease. Proc Intl Soc Mag Reson Med 15. MIRA Digital Publishing, p 3616

Hindel R (1994) Implementation of the DICOM 3.0 standard – a pragmatic handbook. Radiological Society of North America, Oak Brook, IL

Hoffmann R, Mintz GS (2000) Coronary in-stent restenosis – predictors, treatment and prevention. Eur Heart J 21:1739–1749

Hoffmann U, Butler J (2005) Noninvasive detection of coronary atherosclerotic plaque by multidetector row computed tomography. Int J Obes 29[Suppl 2]:s46–53

Hoffmann U, Siebert U, Bull-Stewart A et al. (2006) Evidence for lower variability of coronary artery calcium mineral mass measurements by multi-detector computed tomography in a community-based cohort – consequences for progression studies. Eur J Radiol Mar 57:396–402

Höhne KH, Bomans M, Pommert A, Tiede U (1990) Voxel based volume visualization techniques. Levoy M ACM Siggraph Course Notes 11 [Volume Visualization Algorithms and Architecture], pp 66–83

Honea R, McCluggage CW, Parker B, O'Neall D, Shook K (1998) An evaluation of commercial PC-based DICOM image viewers. J Digit Imaging 11:151–155

Isgum I, Rutten A, Prokop M, van Ginneken B (2007) Detection of coronary calcifications from computed tomography scans for automated risk assessment of coronary artery disease. Medical Physics 34:1450–1461

Johnson PT, Heath DG, Kuszyk BS, Fishman EK (1997) CT angiography: thoracic vascular imaging with interactive volume rendering technique. J Comput Assist Tomogr 21:110–114

Kefer JM, Coche E, Vanoverschelde J-LJ, Gerber B (2007) Diagnostic accuracy of 16-slice multidetector-row CT for detection of in-stent restenosis vs detection of stenosis. European Radiology 17:87–96

Kim RJ, Hillenbrand HB (2000) Evaluation of myocardial viability by MRI. Herz 25:417–430

Kirchgeorg MA, Prokop M (1998) Increasing spiral CT benefits with postprocessing applications. Eur J Radiol 28:39–54

Klessen C, Post F, Meyer J, Thelen M, Kreitner KF (2000) Depiction of anomalous coronary vessels and their relation to the great arteries by magnetic resonance angiography. European Radiology 10:1855–1857

Knez A, Becker A, Becker C, Leber A, Reiser M, Steinbeck G (2002) Determination of coronary calcium with multi-slice spiral computed tomography: a comparative study with electron-beam CT. Int J Cardiovasc Imaging 18:295–303

Kolipaka A, Chatzimavroudis GP, White RD, O'donnell TP, Setser RM (2005) Segmentation of non-viable myocardium in delayed enhancement magnetic resonance images. Int J Cardiovasc Imaging (formerly Cardiac Imaging) 21:303–311

Kühnel C, Hennemuth A, Boskamp T, Oeltze S, Bock S, Krass S et al. (2006) New software assistants for cardiovascular diagnosis. Köllen Druck+Verlag GmbH, Bonn, pp 491–498

Kuszyk BS, Heath DG, Ney DR, Bluemke DA, Urban BA, Chambers TP, Fishman EK (1995) CT angiography with volume rendering: imaging findings. AJR Am J Roentgenol 165:445–448

Langenhuysen RGA, Philipse PH (2001) Multiple archive storage server – white paper, September 26. Rogan Medical Systems

Lawler LP, Pannu HK, Fishman EK (2005) MDCT evaluation of the coronary arteries 2004: how we do it – data acquisition, postprocessing, display, and interpretation. AJR Am J Roentgenol 184:1402–1412

Leber AW, Knez A, White CW, Becker A, Ziegler F von, Muehling O, Becker C, Reiser M, Steinbeck G, Boekstegers P (2003) Composition of coronary atherosclerotic plaques in patients with acute myocardial infarction and stable angina pectoris determined by contrast-enhanced multislice computed tomography. Am J Cardiol 91:714–718

Leber AW, Knez A, von Ziegler F, Sirol M, Nikolaou K, Ohnesorge B, Fayad ZA, Becker CR, Reiser M, Steinbeck G, Boekstegers P (2006) Accuracy of 64-slice computed tomography to classify and quantify plaque volumes in the proximal coronary system: a comparative study using intravascular ultrasound. J Am Coll Cardiol 47:672–677

Leclerc X, Godefroy O, Pruvo JP, Leys D (1995) Computed tomographic angiography for the evaluation of carotid artery stenosis. Stroke 26:1577–1581

Ligabue G, Fiocchi F, Ferraresi S, Rossi R, Modena MG, Ratti C, Torricelli P, Romagnoli R (2007) Does 16-slice multidetector computed tomography improve stent patency and in-stent restenosis evaluation? J Cardiov Med 8:438–444

Liu Y, Hopper KD, Mauger DT, Addis KA (2000) CT angiographic measurement of the carotid artery: optimizing visualization by manipulating window and level settings and contrast material attenuation. Radiology 217:494–500

Lorensen WE, Cline HE (1987) Marching cubes: a high resolution 3D surface construction algorithm. Proceedings of the 14th annual conference on computer graphics and interactive techniques, pp 163–169

Lu B, Dai RP, Jiang SL et al. (2001) Effects of window and threshold levels on the accuracy of 3D rendering techniques in coronary artery EBCT angiography. Acad Radiol 8:754–761

Magnusson M, Lenz R, Danielsson PE (1991) Evaluation of methods for shaded surface display of CT volumes. Comput Med Imaging Graph 15:247–256

Mahnken AH, Buecker A, Wildberger JE, Ruebben A, Stanzel S, Vogt F, Gunther RW, Blindt R (2004) Coronary artery stents in multislice computed tomography: in vitro artifact evaluation. Invest Radiol 39:27–33

Maintz D, Juergens KU, Wichter T, Grude M, Heindel W, Fischbach R (2003) Imaging of coronary artery stents using multislice computed tomography; in vitro evaluation. European Radiology 13:830–835

Maintz D, Seifarth H, Raupach R, Flohr T, Rink M, Sommer T, Özgün M, Heindel W, Fischbach R (2006) 64-Slice multidetector coronary CT angiography: in vitro evaluation of 68 different stents. European Radiology 16:818–826

Marks MP, Napel S, Jordan JE, Enzmann DR (1993) Diagnosis of carotid artery disease: preliminary experience with maximum-intensity-projection spiral CT angiography. AJR Am J Roentgenol 160:1267–1271

Meinhardt G (2006) Cardiology requirements for PACS – defining future needs. Imaging Management 6:26–27

Meyers SP, Talagala SL, Totterman S, Azodo MV, Kwok E, Shapiro L, Shapiro R, Pabico RC, Applegate GR (1995) Evaluation of the renal arteries in kidney donors: value of three-dimensional phase-contrast MR angiography with maximum-intensity-projection or surface rendering. AJR Am J Roentgenol 164:117–121

Murakami T, Kashiwagi T, Nakamura H, Tsuda K, Azuma M, Tomoda K, Hori S, Kozuka T (1993) Display of MR angiograms: maximum intensity projection versus three-dimensional rendering. Eur J Radiol 17:95–100

Nagel E, Klein C, Paetsch I, Hettwer S, Schnackenburg B, Wegscheider K et al. (2003) Magnetic resonance perfusion measurements for the noninvasive detection of coronary artery disease. Circulation 108:432

Nakanishi T, Ito K, Imazu M, Yamakido M (1997) Evaluation of coronary artery stenoses using electron-beam CT and multiplanar reformation. J Comput Assist Tomogr 21:121–127

Nakanishi T, Kohata M, Miyasaka K, Fukuoka H, Ito K, Imazu M (2000) Virtual endoscopy of coronary arteries using contrast-enhanced ECG-triggered electron beam CT data sets. AJR Am J Roentgenol 174:1345–1347

Nakanishi T, Kayashima Y, Inoue R, Sumii K, Gomyo Y (2005) Pitfalls in 16-detector row CT of the coronary arteries. Radiographics 25:425–440

Namdar M, Hany TF, Koepfli P, Siegrist PT, Burger C, Wyss CA et al. (2005) Integrated PET/CT for the assessment of coronary artery disease: a feasibility study. J Nucl Med 46:930–935

Napel S, Marks MP, Rubin GD, Dake MD, McDonnell CH, Song SM, Enzmann DR, Jeffrey RB Jr (1992) CT angiography with spiral CT and maximum intensity projection. Radiology 185:607–610

Napel S, Rubin GD, Jeffrey RB Jr (1993) STS-MIP: a new reconstruction technique for CT of the chest. J Comput Assist Tomogr 17:832–838

Ney DR, Fishman EK, Magid D (1990a) Three-dimensional imaging of computed tomography: techniques and applications. Ezquerra NF 498–506. Los Alamitos, California, IEEE Computer Society Press. Proceedings of the First Conference on Visualization in Biomedical Computing

Ney DR, Fishman EK, Magid D Drebin RA (1990b) Volumetric rendering of computed tomography data: principles and techniques. IEEE Computer Graphics and Applications 9:24–32

Ochi T, Shimizu K, Yasuhara Y, Shigesawa T, Mochizuki T, Ikezoe J (1999) Curved planar reformatted CT angiography: usefulness for the evaluation of aneurysms at the carotid siphon. AJNR Am J Neuroradiol 20:1025–1030

Oeltze S, Preim B (2004) Visualization of anatomic tree structures with convolution surfaces. Proceedings Joint IEEE/EG Symposium on Visualization, pp 311–320

Oeltze S, Grothues F, Hennemuth A, Preim B (2006) Integrated visualization of morphologic and perfusion data for the analysis of coronary artery disease. Euro Vis, pp 131–138

Ohtake Y, Belyaev A, Alexa M, Turk G, Seidel HP (2003) Multi-level partition of unity implicits. ACM Transactions on Graphics (TOG) 22:463–470

Pelanek GA (1997) A DICOM cardiology exchange. In: Primer A, Kennedy TE, Nissen SE, Simon R, Thomas JD, Tilkemeier PL (eds) Digital cardiac imaging in the 21st Century. The Cardiac and Vascular Information Working Group, Bethesda, Maryland

Pollak T, Heuser H, Niederlag G, Brüggenwerth G, Kaulfuss K (2000) Evaluation of 7 PC-based diagnostic workstations. Gell G, Holzinger A, and Wiltgen M 144, 114–125. Graz, Österreichische Computer Gesellschaft. Proceedings of the 18th International EuroPACS Conference

Prokop M, Shin HO, Schanz A, Schaefer-Prokop CM (1997) Use of maximum intensity projections in CT angiography: a basic review. Radiographics 17:433–451

Rankin SC (1998) Spiral CT: vascular applications. Eur J Radiol 28:18–29

Rankin SC (1999) CT Angiography. Eur Radiol 9:297–310

Reimann AJ, Rinck D, Birinci-Aydogan A, Scheuering M, Burgstahler C, Schroeder S, Brodoefel H, Tsiflikas I, Herberts T, Flohr T, Claussen CD, Kopp AF, Heuschmid M (2007) Dual-source computed tomography: advances of improved temporal resolution in coronary plaque imaging. Investigative Radiology 42:196–203

Rensing BJ, Bongaerts AH, van Geuns RJ, van Ooijen PM, Oudkerk M, de Feyter PJ (1999a) Intravenous coronary angiography using electron beam computed tomography. Prog Cardiovasc Dis 42:139–148

Rensing BJ, Bongaerts AH, van Geuns RJ, van Ooijen PM, Oudkerk M, de Feyter PJ (1999b) In vivo assessment of three dimensional coronary anatomy using electron beam computed tomography after intravenous contrast administration. Heart 82:523–525

Ropers D, Baum U, Pohle K, Anders K, Ulzheimer S, Ohnesorge B, Schlundt C, Bautz W, Daniel W, Achenbach S (2003) Detection of coronary artery stenoses with thin-slice multi-detector row spiral computed tomography and multiplanar reconstruction. Circulation 107:664–666

Rubin GD (1994) Three-dimensional helical CT angiography. RadioGraphics 14:905–912

Rubin GD, Dake MD, Napel S, Jeffrey RB Jr, McDonnell CH, Sommer FG, Wexler L, Williams DM (1994) Spiral CT of renal artery stenosis: comparison of three-dimensional rendering techniques. Radiology 190:181–189

Rubin GD, Dake MD, Semba CP (1995) Current status of three-dimensional spiral CT scanning for imaging the vasculature. Radiol Clin North Am 22:51–70

Scheffel H, Alkadhi H, Plass A, Vachenauer R, Desbiolles L, Gaemperli O, Schepis R, Frauenfelder T, Schertler T, Husmann L, Grunenfelder J, Genoni M, Kaufmann PA, Marincek B, Leschka S (2006) Accuracy of dual-source CT coronary angiography: first experience in a high pre-test probability population without heart rate control. Eur Radiol 16:1739–1747

Schmid M, Achenbach S, Ludwig J, Baum U, Anders K, Pohle K, Daniel WG, Ropers D (2006) Visualization of coronary artery anomalies by contrast-enhanced multi-detector row spiral computed tomography. Int J Cardiol 111:430–435

Schmidt P (1999) From humble beginnings: the history of cardiac X-ray image management. Medicamundi 43:10–15

Schroeder S, Kopp AF, Baumbach A, Meisner C, Kuettner A, Georg C, Ohnesorge B, Herdeg C, Claussen CD, Karsch KR (2001) Noninvasive detection and evaluation of atherosclerotic coronary plaques with multislice computed tomography. J Am Coll Cardiol 37:1430–1435

Schroeder S, Kopp AF, Ohnesorge B, Loke-Gie H, Kuettner A, Baumbach A, Herdeg C, Claussen CD, Karsch KR (2002) Virtual coronary angioscopy using multislice computed tomography. Heart 87:205–209

Schumann C, Steffen Oeltze, Ragnar Bade, Bernhard Preim (2007) Visualisierung von Gefäßsystemen mit MPU Implicits. In: Bildverarbeitung für die Medizin, Informatik aktuell

Seifarth H, Raupach R, Schaller S, Fallenberg EM, Flohr T, Heindel W, Fischbach R, Maintz D (2005) Assessment of coronary artery stents using 16-slice MDCT angiography: evaluation of a dedicated reconstruction kernel and a noise reduction filter. Eur Radiol 15:721–726

Selle D, Preim B, Schenk A, Peitgen HO (2002) Analysis of vasculature for liver surgical planning. IEEE Transactions on Medical Imaging, pp 1344–1357

Sheth T, Dodd JD, Hoffman U, Abbara S, Finn A, Gold HK, Brady TJ, Cury RC (2007) Coronary stent assessability by 64 slice multi-detector computed tomography. Catheter Cardiovasc Interv 69:933–938

Sigwart U, Puel J, Mirkovitch V, Joffre F, Kappenberger L (1987) Intravascular stents to prevent occlusion and restenosis after transluminal angioplasty. N Engl J Med 316:701–706

Soyer P, Heath D, Bluemke DA, Choti MA, Kuhlman JE, Reichle R, Fishman EK (1996) Three-dimensional helical CT of intrahepatic venous structures: comparison of three rendering techniques. J Comput Assist Tomogr 20:122–127

Sturm B, Powell KA, Stillman AE (2003) Registration of 3D CT angiography and cardiac MR images in coronary artery disease patients. Int J Cardiovasc Imaging 6:281–293

Takahashi M, Ashtari M, Papp Z, Patel M, Goldstein J, Maguire WM, Eacobacci T, Khan A, Herman PG (1997) CT angiography of carotid bifurcation: artifacts and pitfalls in shaded-surface display. AJR Am J Roentgenol 168:813–817

Terwisscha van Scheltinga J (2001) Technical background. In: Rogalla P, Terwisscha van Scheltinga J, Hamm B (eds) Virtual endoscopy and related 3D techniques. Springer-Verlag, Berlin Heidelberg New York

Thomas JD, Nissen SE (1996) Digital storage and transmission of cardiovascular images: what are the costs, benefits and timetable for conversion? Heart 76:13–17

Traversie E, Tramarin R (2003) Intracoronary imaging with multislice spiral computed tomography. New Engl J Med 348:e5

Udupa JK (1999) Three-dimensional visualization and analysis methodologies: a current perspective. Radiographics 19:783–806

Udupa JK, Hung H-M (1990) Surface versus volume rendering: a comparative assessment. Ezquerra NF 83–91 Los Alamitos, California, IEEE Computer Society Press. Proceedings of the First Conference on Visualization in Biomedical Computing

van der Putten N, Gerritsen M, Dijk WA, den Boer A (1997) HEMA-PACS: een goedkoop PACS voor coronaire angiografie beelden. Klinische fysica 3:21–23 (in Dutch, English abstract available)

van Geuns RJ, Wielopolski PA, Rensing BJ, van Ooijen PM, Oudkerk M, de Feyter PJ (1999) Magnetic resonance imaging of the coronary arteries: anatomy of the coronary arteries and veins in three-dimensional imaging. Coron Artery Dis 10:261–267

van Ooijen PMA, Feyter PJ, Oudkerk M (1997) An introduction to three-dimensional cardiac image rendering and processing. Cardiology 4:312–319

van Ooijen PM, Oudkerk M, van Geuns RJ, Rensing BJ, de Feyter PJ (2000a) Coronary artery fly-through using electron beam computed tomography. Circulation 102:E6–10

van Ooijen PMA, Bongaerts AHH, Oudkerk M (2000b) From PACS to internet/intranet, information-systems, multimedia and telemedicine. Gell G, Holzinger A, and Wiltgen M 144, 77–83. Graz, Österreichische Computer Gesellschaft. Proceedings of the 18th International EuroPACS Conference

van Ooijen PMA, Nieman K, de Feyter PJ, Oudkerk M (2002) Non-invasive coronary angioscopy using electron beam computed tomography and multi detector computed tomography. AJC 90:998–1002

van Ooijen PMA, Ho KYAM, Dorgelo J, Oudkerk M (2003a) Coronary artery imaging with multidetector CT: visualization issues. Radiographics 23:e16

van Ooijen PMA, van Geuns RJ, Rensing B, Bongaerts AH, de Feyter PJ, Oudkerk M (2003b) Noninvasive coronary imaging using electron beam CT: surface rendering versus volume rendering. AJR Am J Roentgenol 180:223–226

van Ooijen PMA, Dorgelo J, Zijlstra F, Oudkerk M (2004) Detection, visualization and evaluation of anomalous coronary anatomy on 16-slice multidetector-row CT. European Radiology 14:2163–2171

van Ooijen PM, de Jonge G, Oudkerk M (2007) Coronary fly-through or virtual angioscopy using dual-source MDCT data. Eur Radiol 17:2852–2859

Verdonck B (1996) Blood vessel segmentation, quantification and visualization for 3D MR and spiral CT angiography. l'Ecole Nationale Superieure des Telecommunications

Watt A (1993) 3D computer graphics. Addison-Wesley, Wokingham, UK

Wiese TH, Rogalla P (2001) Virtual endoscopy of the vessels. In: P Rogalla, Terwisscha van Scheltinga J, Hamm B (eds) Virtual endoscopy and related 3D techniques. Springer-Verlag, Berlin Heidelberg New York

Zuiderveld KJ (1995) Visualization of multimodality medical volume data using object-oriented methods. Universiteit Utrecht, The Netherlands

Subject Index

A

B

C

D

E

Q

R

S

T

U

V

W

X

Z

List of Contributors

STEPHAN ACHENBACH, MD, PhD
Department of Internal Medicine II
University of Erlangen
Ulmenweg 18
91054 Erlangen
Germany
Email: stephan.achenbach@uk-erlangen.de

MARGARET ACKERMAN, MD, PhD
Division of Emergency Medicine
Department of Medicine
McMaster University
1280 Main Street West
Hamilton, Ontario
Canada
Email: mackerma@mcmaster.ca

HATEM ALKADHI, MD
PD, Institute of Diagnostic Radiology
University Hospital Zurich
Raemisstrasse 100
8091 Zurich
Switzerland
Email: hatem.alkadhi@usz.ch

CHRISTOPH R. BECKER, MD
Department of Clinical Radiology
Klinikum Grosshadern
University of Munich
Marchioninistrasse 15
81377 Munich
Germany
Email: christoph.becker@med.uni-muenchen.de

TOBIAS BOSKAMP, PhD
MeVis Research
Universitätsallee 29
28359 Bremen
Germany
Email: tboskamp@mevis.de

ANDRÉ BROEKEMA, BSc
Department of Radiology
University Medical Center Groningen
University of Groningen
Hanzeplein 1, P. O. Box 30.001
9700 RB Groningen
The Netherlands
Email: a.broekema@rad.umcg.nl

NICO BRUINING, PhD, FESC
Department of Cardiology (Thoraxcenter)
Erasmus MC
Dr. Molewaterplein 40
3015 GD Rotterdam
The Netherlands
Email: n.bruining@erasmusmc.nl

PAWEL BUSZMAN, MD, PhD
Upper Silesian Medical Center
Coronary Care Unit
Ul. Ziolowa 47,
40-635 Katowice
Poland
Email: pbuszman@katowice.onet.pl

PIM J. DE FEYTER, MD, PhD
Thoraxcenter Bd 410
University Hospital Rotterdam
P. O. Box 2040
3000 CA Rotterdam
The Netherlands
Email: p.j.defeyter@erasmusmc.nl

GONDA J. DE JONGE, MD
Department of Radiology
University Medical Center Groningen
University of Groningen
Hanzeplein 1, P.O. Box 30.001
9700 RB Groningen
The Netherlands
Email: g.de.jonge@rad.umcg.nl

Wilfred F. A. den Dunnen, MD, PhD
Department of Pathology and Laboratory Medicine
University Medical Center Groningen
University of Groningen
Hanzeplein 1, P. O. Box 30.001
9700 RB Groningen
The Netherlands
Email: w.f.a.den.dunnen@path.umcg.nl

Sebastiaan de Winter, BSc
Department of Cardiology (Thoraxcenter)
Erasmus MC
Dr. Molewaterplein 40
3015 GD Rotterdam
The Netherlands

Riksta Dikkers, MD, PhD
Department of Radiology
University Medical Center Groningen
University of Groningen
Hanzeplein 1, P. O. Box 30.001
9700 RB Groningen
The Netherlands
Email: r.dikkers@rad.umcg.nl

Robert R. Edelman, MD
Department of Radiology G507
Evanston Hospital
2650 Ridge Avenue
Evanston IL 60201
USA
Email: Redelman@enh.org

Raimund Erbel, MD
Professor, West German Heart Center Essen
Department of Cardiology
University Duisberg-Essen
Hufelandstrasse 55
45122 Essen
Germany
Email: erbel@uk-essen.de

Thomas G. Flohr, PhD
Siemens Healthcare
Computed Tomography Division
Siemensstrasse 1
91301 Forchheim
Germany
and
Institute for Diagnostic Radiology
Eberhard-Karls-University
Tübingen, Germany
Email: thomas.flohr@siemens.com

Bob Goedhart, PhD
Medis Medical Imaging Systems B.V.
Schuttersveld 9
2316 XG Leiden
P.O. Box 384
2300 AJ Leiden
The Netherlands

Marcel J. W. Greuter, PhD
Department of Radiology
University Medical Center Groningen
University of Groningen
Hanzeplein 1, P. O. Box 30.001
9700 RB Groningen
The Netherlands
Email: m.j.w.greuter@rad.umcg.nl

Jaap M. Groen, MSc, PhD
Department of Radiology
University Medical Center Groningen
University of Groningen
Hanzeplein 1, P. O. Box 30.001
9700 RB Groningen
The Netherlands
Email: j.m.groen@rad.umcg.nl

Philippe Guyon, MD
Centre Cardiologique du Nord
32–36 Avenue des Moulins Gémeaux
93200 Saint Denis
France

Sandra S. Halliburton, MD, PhD
Imaging Institute
Cardiovascular Imaging Lab
Cleveland Clinic Foundation
9500 Euclid Avenue
Cleveland, OH 44195-0001
USA
Email: HALLIBS@ccf.org

Ronald Hamers, PhD
Department of Cardiology
Department of Radiology
Erasmus MC
Dr. Molenwaterplein 40
3015 GD Rotterdam
The Netherlands
Email: r.hamers@erasmusmc.nl

Anja Hennemuth, MSc
MeVis Research
Universitätsallee 29
28359 Bremen
Germany
Email: anja.hennemuth@mevis.de

Christopher Herzog, MD, PhD
Department of Radiology
Rotkreuzklinikum Munich
Winthirstrasse 9
80639 Munich
Germany
Email: c.herzog@radiologie-muenchen.de

Udo Hoffman, MD
Department of Radiology
Massachusetts General Hospital
55 Fruit Street
Boston, MA 02114
and
Harvard School of Public Health
677 Huntington Avenue
Boston, MA 02115
USA
Email: uhoffman@partners.org

Johannes P. Janssen, MSc
Division of Image Processing (LKEB)
Department of Radiology
Leiden University Medical Center
Albinusdreef 2
2300 RC Leiden
The Netherlands
Email: j.p.janssen@lumc.nl

Willi A. Kalender, MD, PhD
Professor, Institute of Medical Physics
University of Erlangen-Nürnberg
Krankenhausstrasse 12
91054 Erlangen
Germany
Email: willi@imp.uni-erlangen.de

Matthew T. Keadey, MD
Department of Emergency Medicine
Emory University
531 Asbury Lane
Atlanta, GA 30322–1006
USA
Email: Matthew.Keadey@emoryhealthcare.org

Gerhard Koning, MSc
Division of Image Processing (LKEB)
Department of Radiology
Leiden University Medical Center
Albinusdreef 2
2300 RC Leiden
The Netherlands
Email: g.koning@lumc.nl

Wisnu Kristanto, MSc
Department of Radiology
University Medical Center Groningen
University of Groningen
Hanzeplein 1, P.O. Box 30.001
9700 RB Groningen
The Netherlands
Email: w.kristanto@rad.umcg.nl

Caroline Kuehnel, MSc
MeVis Research
Universitätsallee 29
28359 Bremen
Germany
Email: caroline.kuehnel@mevis.de

Alexandra J. Lansky, MD
Cardiovascular Research Foundation
Center for Interventional Vascular Therapy
New York-Presbyterian Hospital
Columbia University
161 Fort Washington Avenue 5th FL
New York, NY 10032
USA
Email: alansky@crf.org

Debiao Li, PhD
Professor, Department of Radiology
Northwestern University Medical School
737 North Michigan Avenue Ste 1600
Chicago, Illinois 60611
USA
Email: d-li2@northwestern.edu

Guido Ligabue, MD
Cattedra e Servizio di Radiologia
Piliclinico di Modena
Via del Pozzo 71
41100 Modena
Italy
Email: ligabue.guido@unimore.it

Jurgen Ligthart, BSc
University Hospital Rotterdam
Thoraxcenter Bd 410
P.O. Box 2040
3000 CA Rotterdam
The Netherlands

Martin J. Lipton, MD, PhD, Professor Emeritus
Department of Radiology
University of Chicago
5801 South Ellis Avenue
Chicago, IL 60637
USA
Email: mlipton@partners.org

Riccardo Marano, MD
Department of Clinical Sciences and Bioimaging
Section of Radiology
G. d'Annunzio University
"SS. Annunziata" Hospital
Via dei Vestini
I-66013 Chiety
Italy
Email: r.marano@rad.unich.it

Cynthia H. McCollough, PhD
Associate Professor of Radiologic Physics
Department of Radiology, Mayo Clinic
200 First Street SW
Rochester, MN 55905-0001
USA
Email: mccollough.cynthia@mayo.edu

Stefan Möhlenkamp, MD
West German Heart Center Essen
Department of Cardiology
University Duisberg-Essen
Hufelandstrasse 55
45122 Essen
Germany
Email: stefan.moehlenkamp@uk-essen.de

Bernd Ohnesorge, PhD
Vice president in Medical Solutions
Siemensstrasse 1
91301 Forchheim
Germany
and
Siemens Limited China, Healthcare
Siemens International Medical Park
278 Zhou Zhu Road, SIMZ, Nanhui District
Shanghai 2013118, P. R. China
Email: Bernd.Ohnesorge@siemens.com

Matthijs Oudkerk, MD, PhD
Professor of Radiology
Department of Radiology
University Medical Center Groningen
University of Groningen
Hanzeplein 1, P. O. Box 30.001
9700 RB Groningen
The Netherlands
Email: m.oudkerk@rad.umcg.nl

Gilbert L. Raff, MD
Department of Cardiology
William Beaumont Hospital
3601 W 13 Mile Road
Royal Oak, MI 48073
USA
Email: graff@beaumont.edu

Paolo Raggi, MD, PACP, FACC
Departments of Radiology
and Cardiology
Emory University
Atlanta, GA 30322
USA
Email: praggi@emory.edu

Andrei Rareş, PhD
Division of Image Processing (LKEB)
Department of Radiology
Leiden University Medical Center
Albinusdreef 2
2300 RC Leiden
The Netherlands

Gautham P. Reddy, MD
Department of Radiology
University of California
505 Paranassus Avenue
San Francisco, CA 94143-2204
USA
Email: gautham.reddy@radiology.ucsf.edu

Michael R. Rees, MD, PhD
Professor
Bangor University
Bangor
Gwynedd, LL57 2DG
United Kingdom
Email: m.rees@bangor.ac.uk

Johan H. C. Reiber, PhD
Professor of Medical Imaging
Director, Division of Image Processing (LKEB)
Department of Radiology
Leiden University Medical Center
Albinusdreef 2
2300 RC Leiden
The Netherlands
Email: J.H.C.Reiber@lumc.nl

Geoffrey D. Rubin, MD
Professor Radiology, Diagnostic Radiology
Department of Radiology
Stanford University
300 Pasteur Drive
Stanford, CA 94305
USA
Email: grubin@stanford.edu

Jos R. T. C. Roelandt, MD
Professor, Department of Cardiology (Thoraxcenter)
Erasmus MC
Dr. Molewaterplein 40
3015 GD Rotterdam
The Netherlands

Jean-Louis Sablayrolles, MD
Centre Cardiologique du Nord
32–36 Rue de Moulins Gémeaux
93200 Saint Denis
France
Email: jl.sablayrolles@ccncardio.com

Axel Schmermund, MD, FESC
Associate Professor of Internal Medicine
and Cardiology
Cardioangiologisches Centrum Bethanien
Im Prüfling 23
60389 Frankfurt/Main
Germany
Email: A.Schmermund@ccb.de

U. Joseph Schoepf, MD
Department of Radiology
Medical University of South Carolina
169 Ashley Avenue
Charleston, SC 29403–5836
USA
Email: schoepf@musc.edu

Leslee J. Shaw, PhD
Departments of Radiology and Cardiology
Emory University School of Medicine
1364 Clifton Road NE
Atlanta GA 30322
USA
Email: leslee.shaw@emory.edu

Valentin E. Sinitsyn, MD, PhD
Professor, Department of Tomography
Cardiology Research Center
Cherepkovskaya Street 15A
121 552 Moscow
Russia
Email: vsin@online.ru
vsin@orc.ru
vsin@tomography.ru
vsin@mail.ru

William Stanford, MD
Professor Emeritus
Department of Radiology
University of Iowa
200 Hawkins Drive
Iowa City, IA 52242
USA
Email: william-stanford@uiowa.edu

Arthur E. Stillman, MD, PhD, FAHA
Professor
Director of the Division of Cardiothoracic Imaging
Department of Radiology
Emory University Hospital
1365 Clifton Road NE
Atlanta GA 30322
USA
Email: aestill@emory.edu

Albert J. H. Suurmeijer, MD, PhD
Department of Pathology and
Laboratory Medicine
University Medical Center Groningen
University of Groningen
Hanzeplein 1
P.O. Box 30.001
9700 RB Groningen
The Netherlands
Email: a.j.h.suurmeijer@path.azg.nl

Giuseppe Tarulli, MD
Department of Radiology
Humber River Regional Hospital
Church street site
200 Church Street
Toronto, Ontario
Canada

Allen J. Taylor, MD
Division of Cardiology
Walter Reed Army Medical Center
6900 Georgia Avenue NW
Washington, DC 20307
USA
Email: allen.taylor@na.amedd.army.mil

Joan C. Tuinenburg, MSc
Division of Image Processing (LKEB)
Department of Radiology
Leiden University Medical Center
Albinusdreef 2
2300 RC Leiden
The Netherlands
Email: J.C.Tuinenburg@lumc.nl

Edwin J. R. van Beek, MD, PhD
Professor, Department of Radiology
University of Iowa
200 Hawkins Drive
Iowa City, IA 52242
USA
Email: edwin-vanbeek@uiowa.edu

Peter M. A. van Ooijen, PhD
Department of Radiology
University Medical Center Groningen
University of Groningen
Hanzeplein 1, P. O. Box 30.001
9700 RB Groningen
The Netherlands
Email: p.m.a.van.ooijen@rad.umcg.nl

Rozemarijn Vliegenthart Proença, MD, PhD
Department of Radiology
University Medical Center Groningen
University of Groningen
Hanzeplein 1, P. O. Box 30.001
9700 RB Groningen
The Netherlands
Email: r.vliegenthart@rad.umcg.nl

Lewis Wexler, MD
Department of Radiology
Stanford University
300 Pasteur Drive
Stanford, CA 94305
USA
Email: lwexler@stanford.edu

Charles S. White, MD
Professor of Radiology and Medicine
Chief of Thoracic Radiology
Department of Diagnostic Radiology
University of Maryland Medical Center
22 S. Greene Street
Baltimore, MD 21201
USA
Email: cwhite@umm.edu

Jacqueline C. M. Witteman, PhD
Associate Professor of Cardiovascular Epidemiology
Department of Epidemiology and Biostatistics
Erasmus MC
P.O. Box 1738
3000 DR Rotterdam
The Netherlands
Email: j.witteman@erasmusmc.nl

Felix Zijlstra, MD, PhD
Professor, Thorax Center
Department of Cardiology
University Hospital Groningen
P. O. Box 30.001
9700 RB Groningen
The Netherlands
Email: f.zijlstra@thorax.umcg.nl

Medical Radiology Diagnostic Imaging and Radiation Oncology

Titles in the series already published

Diagnostic Imaging

Innovations in Diagnostic Imaging
Edited by J. H. Anderson

Radiology of the Upper Urinary Tract
Edited by E. K. Lang

The Thymus - Diagnostic Imaging, Functions, and Pathologic Anatomy
Edited by E. Walter, E. Willich, and W. R. Webb

Interventional Neuroradiology
Edited by A. Valavanis

Radiology of the Lower Urinary Tract
Edited by E. K. Lang

Contrast-Enhanced MRI of the Breast
S. Heywang-Köbrunner and R. Beck

Spiral CT of the Chest
Edited by M. Rémy-Jardin and J. Rémy

Radiological Diagnosis of Breast Diseases
Edited by M. Friedrich and E. A. Sickles

Radiology of Trauma
Edited by M. Heller and A. Fink

Biliary Tract Radiology
Edited by P. Rossi. Co-edited by M. Brezi

Radiological Imaging of Sports Injuries
Edited by C. Masciocchi

Modern Imaging of the Alimentary Tube
Edited by A. R. Margulis

Diagnosis and Therapy of Spinal Tumors
Edited by P. R. Algra, J. Valk and J. J. Heimans

Interventional Magnetic Resonance Imaging
Edited by J. F. Debatin and G. Adam

Abdominal and Pelvic MRI
Edited by A. Heuck and M. Reiser

Orthopedic Imaging
Techniques and Applications
Edited by A. M. Davies and H. Pettersson

Radiology of the Female Pelvic Organs
Edited by E. K. Lang

Magnetic Resonance of the Heart and Great Vessels
Clinical Applications
Edited by J. Bogaert, A. J. Duerinckx, and F. E. Rademakers

Modern Head and Neck Imaging
Edited by S. K. Mukherji and J. A. Castelijns

Radiological Imaging of Endocrine Diseases
Edited by J. N. Bruneton in collaboration with B. Padovani and M.-Y. Mourou

Radiology of the Pancreas
2nd Revised Edition
Edited by A. L. Baert. Co-edited by G. Delorme and L. Van Hoe

Trends in Contrast Media
Edited by H. S. Thomsen, R. N. Muller, and R. F. Mattrey

Functional MRI
Edited by C. T. W. Moonen and P. A. Bandettini

Emergency Pediatric Radiology
Edited by H. Carty

Liver Malignancies
Diagnostic and Interventional Radiology
Edited by C. Bartolozzi and R. Lencioni

Spiral CT of the Abdomen
Edited by F. Terrier, M. Grossholz, and C. D. Becker

Medical Imaging of the Spleen
Edited by A. M. De Schepper and F. Vanhoenacker

Radiology of Peripheral Vascular Diseases
Edited by E. Zeitler

Radiology of Blunt Trauma of the Chest
P. Schnyder and M. Wintermark

Portal Hypertension
Diagnostic Imaging and Imaging-Guided Therapy
Edited by P. Rossi. Co-edited by P. Ricci and L. Broglia

Virtual Endoscopy and Related 3D Techniques
Edited by P. Rogalla, J. Terwisscha van Scheltinga and B. Hamm

Recent Advances in Diagnostic Neuroradiology
Edited by Ph. Demaerel

Transfontanellar Doppler Imaging in Neonates
A. Couture, C. Veyrac

Radiology of AIDS
A Practical Approach
Edited by J. W. A. J. Reeders and P. C. Goodman

CT of the Peritoneum
A. Rossi, G. Rossi

Magnetic Resonance Angiography
2nd Revised Edition
Edited by I. P. Arlart, G. M. Bongartz, and G. Marchal

Applications of Sonography in Head and Neck Pathology
Edited by J. N. Bruneton in collaboration with C. Raffaelli, O. Dassonville

3D Image Processing
Techniques and Clinical Applications
Edited by D. Caramella and C. Bartolozzi

Imaging of the Larynx
Edited by R. Hermans

Pediatric ENT Radiology
Edited by S. J. King and A. E. Boothroyd

Imaging of Orbital and Visual Pathway Pathology
Edited by W. S. Müller-Forell

Radiological Imaging of the Small Intestine
Edited by N. C. Gourtsoyiannis

Imaging of the Knee
Techniques and Applications
Edited by A. M. Davies and V. N. Cassar-Pullicino

Perinatal Imaging
From Ultrasound to MR Imaging
Edited by F. E. Avni

Diagnostic and Interventional Radiology in Liver Transplantation
Edited by E. Bücheler, V. Nicolas, C. E. Broelsch, X. Rogiers and G. Krupski

Imaging of the Pancreas
Cystic and Rare Tumors
Edited by C. Procacci and A. J. Megibow

Imaging of the Foot & Ankle
Techniques and Applications
Edited by A. M. Davies, R. W. Whitehouse and J. P. R. Jenkins

Radiological Imaging of the Ureter
Edited by F. Joffre, Ph. Otal and M. Soulie

Radiology of the Petrous Bone
Edited by M. Lemmerling and S. S. Kollias

Imaging of the Shoulder
Techniques and Applications
Edited by A. M. Davies and J. Hodler

Interventional Radiology in Cancer
Edited by A. Adam, R. F. Dondelinger, and P. R. Mueller

Imaging and Intervention in Abdominal Trauma
Edited by R. F. Dondelinger

Radiology of the Pharynx and the Esophagus
Edited by O. Ekberg

Radiological Imaging in Hematological Malignancies
Edited by A. Guermazi

Functional Imaging of the Chest
Edited by H.-U. Kauczor

Duplex and Color Doppler Imaging of the Venous System
Edited by G. H. Mostbeck

Multidetector-Row CT of the Thorax
Edited by U. J. Schoepf

Radiology and Imaging of the Colon
Edited by A. H. Chapman

Multidetector-Row CT Angiography
Edited by C. Catalano and R. Passariello

Focal Liver Lesions
Detection, Characterization, Ablation
Edited by R. Lencioni, D. Cioni, and C. Bartolozzi

Imaging in Treatment Planning for Sinonasal Diseases
Edited by R. Maroldi and P. Nicolai

Clinical Cardiac MRI
With Interactive CD-ROM
Edited by J. Bogaert, S. Dymarkowski, and A. M. Taylor

Dynamic Contrast-Enhanced Magnetic Resonance Imaging in Oncology
Edited by A. Jackson, D. L. Buckley, and G. J. M. Parker

Contrast Media in Ultrasonography
Basic Principles and Clinical Applications
Edited by E. Quaia

Paediatric Musculoskeletal Disease
With an Emphasis on Ultrasound
Edited by D. Wilson

MR Imaging in White Matter Diseases of the Brain and Spinal Cord
Edited by M. Filippi, N. De Stefano, V. Dousset, and J. C. McGowan

Imaging of the Hip & Bony Pelvis
Techniques and Applications
Edited by A. M. Davies, K. Johnson, and R. W. Whitehouse

Imaging of Kidney Cancer
Edited by A. Guermazi

Magnetic Resonance Imaging in Ischemic Stroke
Edited by R. von Kummer and T. Back

Diagnostic Nuclear Medicine
2nd Revised Edition
Edited by C. Schiepers

Imaging of Occupational and Environmental Disorders of the Chest
Edited by P. A. Gevenois and P. De Vuyst

Virtual Colonoscopy
A Practical Guide
Edited by P. Lefere and S. Gryspeerdt

Contrast Media
Safety Issues and ESUR Guidelines
Edited by H. S. Thomsen

Head and Neck Cancer Imaging
Edited by R. Hermans

Vascular Embolotherapy
A Comprehensive Approach
Volume 1: *General Principles, Chest, Abdomen, and Great Vessels*
Edited by J. Golzarian. Co-edited by S. Sun and M. J. Sharafuddin

Vascular Embolotherapy
A Comprehensive Approach
Volume 2: *Oncology, Trauma, Gene Therapy, Vascular Malformations, and Neck*
Edited by J. Golzarian. Co-edited by S. Sun and M. J. Sharafuddin

Vascular Interventional Radiology
Current Evidence in Endovascular Surgery
Edited by M. G. Cowling

Ultrasound of the Gastrointestinal Tract
Edited by G. Maconi and G. Bianchi Porro

Parallel Imaging in Clinical MR Applications
Edited by S. O. Schoenberg, O. Dietrich, and M. F. Reiser

MRI and CT of the Female Pelvis
Edited by B. Hamm and R. Forstner

Imaging of Orthopedic Sports Injuries
Edited by F. M. Vanhoenacker, M. Maas and J. L. Gielen

Ultrasound of the Musculoskeletal System
S. Bianchi and C. Martinoli

Clinical Functional MRI
Presurgical Functional Neuroimaging
Edited by C. Stippich

Radiation Dose from Adult and Pediatric Multidetector Computed Tomography
Edited by D. Tack and P. A. Gevenois

Spinal Imaging
Diagnostic Imaging of the Spine and Spinal Cord
Edited by J. Van Goethem, L. van den Hauwe and P. M. Parizel

Computed Tomography of the Lung
A Pattern Approach
J. A. Verschakelen and W. De Wever

Imaging in Transplantation
Edited by A. Bankier

Radiological Imaging of the Neonatal Chest
2nd Revised Edition
Edited by V. Donoghue

Radiological Imaging of the Digestive Tract in Infants and Children
Edited by A. S. Devos and J. G. Blickman

Pediatric Chest Imaging
Chest Imaging in Infants and Children
2nd Revised Edition
Edited by J. Lucaya and J. L. Strife

Color Doppler US of the Penis
Edited by M. Bertolotto

Radiology of the Stomach and Duodenum
Edited by A. H. Freeman and E. Sala

Imaging in Pediatric Skeletal Trauma
Techniques and Applications
Edited by K. J. Johnson and E. Bache

Image Processing in Radiology
Current Applications
Edited by E. Neri, D. Caramella, C. Bartolozzi

Screening and Preventive Diagnosis with Radiological Imaging
Edited by M. F. Reiser, G. van Kaick, C. Fink, S. O. Schoenberg

Percutaneous Tumor Ablation in Medical Radiology
Edited by T. J. Vogl, T. K. Helmberger, M. G. Mack, M. F. Reiser

Liver Radioembolization with ^{90}Y Microspheres
Edited by J. I. Bilbao, M. F. Reiser

Pediatric Uroradiology
2nd Revised Edition
Edited by R. Fotter

Radiology of Osteoporosis
2nd Revised Edition
Edited by S. Grampp

Gastrointestinal Tract Sonography in Fetuses and Children
A. Couture, C. Baud, J. L. Ferran, M. Saguintaah and C. Veyrac

Intracranial Vascular Malformations and Aneurysms
2nd Revised Edition
Edited by M. Forsting and I. Wanke

High-Resolution Sonography of the Peripheral Nervous System
2nd Revised Edition
Edited by S. Peer and G. Bodner

Imaging Pelvic Floor Disorders
2nd Revised Edition
Edited by J. Stoker, S. A. Taylor, and J. O. L. DeLancey

Coronary Radiology
2nd Revised Edition
Edited by M. Oudkerk and M. F. Reiser

Integrated Cardiothoracic Imaging with MDCT
Edited by M. Rémy-Jardin and J. Rémy

Multislice CT
3rd Revised Edition
Edited by M. F. Reiser, C. R. Becker, K. Nikolaou, G. Glazer

MRI of the Lung
Edited by H.-U. Kauczor

Imaging in Percutaneous Musculoskeletal Interventions
Edited by A. Gangi, S. Guth, and A. Guermazi

Springer

MEDICAL RADIOLOGY Diagnostic Imaging and Radiation Oncology

Titles in the series already published

RADIATION ONCOLOGY

Lung Cancer
Edited by C. W. Scarantino

Innovations in Radiation Oncology
Edited by H. R. Withers and L. J. Peters

Radiation Therapy of Head and Neck Cancer
Edited by G. E. Laramore

Gastrointestinal Cancer – Radiation Therapy
Edited by R. R. Dobelbower, Jr.

Radiation Exposure and Occupational Risks
Edited by E. Scherer, C. Streffer, and K.-R. Trott

Interventional Radiation
Therapy Techniques – Brachytherapy
Edited by R. Sauer

Radiopathology of Organs and Tissues
Edited by E. Scherer, C. Streffer, and K.-R. Trott

Concomitant Continuous Infusion
Chemotherapy and Radiation
Edited by M. Rotman and C. J. Rosenthal

Intraoperative Radiotherapy – Clinical Experiences and Results
Edited by F. A. Calvo, M. Santos, and L. W. Brady

Interstitial and Intracavitary Thermoradiotherapy
Edited by M. H. Seegenschmiedt and R. Sauer

Non-Disseminated Breast Cancer
Controversial Issues in Management
Edited by G. H. Fletcher and S. H. Levitt

Current Topics in Clinical Radiobiology of Tumors
Edited by H.-P. Beck-Bornholdt

Practical Approaches to Cancer Invasion and Metastases
A Compendium of Radiation Oncologists' Responses to 40 Histories
Edited by A. R. Kagan with the Assistance of R. J. Steckel

Radiation Therapy in Pediatric Oncology
Edited by J. R. Cassady

Radiation Therapy Physics
Edited by A. R. Smith

Late Sequelae in Oncology
Edited by J. Dunst, R. Sauer

Mediastinal Tumors. Update 1995
Edited by D. E. Wood, C. R. Thomas, Jr.

Thermoradiotherapy and Thermochemotherapy
Volume 1:
Biology, Physiology, and Physics
Volume 2:
Clinical Applications
Edited by M. H. Seegenschmiedt, P. Fessenden and C. C. Vernon

Carcinoma of the Prostate
Innovations in Management
Edited by Z. Petrovich, L. Baert, and L. W. Brady

Radiation Oncology of Gynecological Cancers
Edited by H. W. Vahrson

Carcinoma of the Bladder
Innovations in Management
Edited by Z. Petrovich, L. Baert, and L. W. Brady

Blood Perfusion and Microenvironment of Human Tumors
Implications for Clinical Radiooncology
Edited by M. Molls and P. Vaupel

Radiation Therapy of Benign Diseases
A Clinical Guide
2nd Revised Edition
S. E. Order and S. S. Donaldson

Carcinoma of the Kidney and Testis, and Rare Urologic Malignancies
Innovations in Management
Edited by Z. Petrovich, L. Baert, and L. W. Brady

Progress and Perspectives in the Treatment of Lung Cancer
Edited by P. Van Houtte, J. Klastersky, and P. Rocmans

Combined Modality Therapy of Central Nervous System Tumors
Edited by Z. Petrovich, L. W. Brady, M. L. Apuzzo, and M. Bamberg

Age-Related Macular Degeneration
Current Treatment Concepts
Edited by W. E. Alberti, G. Richard, and R. H. Sagerman

Radiotherapy of Intraocular and Orbital Tumors
2nd Revised Edition
Edited by R. H. Sagerman and W. E. Alberti

Modification of Radiation Response
Cytokines, Growth Factors, and Other Biolgical Targets
Edited by C. Nieder, L. Milas and K. K. Ang

Radiation Oncology for Cure and Palliation
R. G. Parker, N. A. Janjan and M. T. Selch

Clinical Target Volumes in Conformal and Intensity Modulated Radiation Therapy
A Clinical Guide to Cancer Treatment
Edited by V. Grégoire, P. Scalliet, and K. K. Ang

Advances in Radiation Oncology in Lung Cancer
Edited by B. Jeremić

New Technologies in Radiation Oncology
Edited by W. Schlegel, T. Bortfeld, and A.-L. Grosu

Multimodal Concepts for Integration of Cytotoxic Drugs and Radiation Therapy
Edited by J. M. Brown, M. P. Mehta, and C. Nieder

Technical Basis of Radiation Therapy
Practical Clinical Applications
4th Revised Edition
Edited by S. H. Levitt, J. A. Purdy, C. A. Perez, and S. Vijayakumar

CURED I • LENT
Late Effects of Cancer Treatment on Normal Tissues
Edited by P. Rubin, L. S. Constine, L. B. Marks, and P. Okunieff

Radiotherapy for Non-Malignant Disorders
Contemporary Concepts and Clinical Results
Edited by M. H. Seegenschmiedt, H.-B. Makoski, K.-R. Trott, and L. W. Brady

CURED II • LENT
Cancer Survivorship Research and Education
Late Effects on Normal Tissues
Edited by P. Rubin, L. S. Constine, L. B. Marks, and P. Okunieff

Radiation Oncology
An Evidence-Based Approach
Edited by J. J. Lu and L. W. Brady

Primary Optic Nerve Sheath Meningioma
Edited by B. Jeremić, and S. Pitz

Springer

MIX
Papier aus verantwortungsvollen Quellen
Paper from responsible sources
FSC® C105338

If you have any concerns about our products,
you can contact us on
ProductSafety@springernature.com

In case Publisher is established outside the EU,
the EU authorized representative is:
Springer Nature Customer Service Center GmbH
Europaplatz 3, 69115 Heidelberg, Germany

Printed by Libri Plureos GmbH
in Hamburg, Germany